The Massachusetts General Hospital Handbook of Pain Management

Third Edition

The Massachusetts General Hospital Handbook of Pain Management

Third Edition

Editor

Jane C. Ballantyne, MD, FRCA
Associate Professor
Department of Anesthesia
Harvard Medical School
Chief, Division of Pain Medicine
Department of Anesthesia & Critical Care
Massachusetts General Hospital
Boston, Massachusetts

Foreword by

Howard L. Fields, MD, PhD

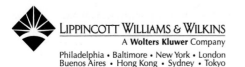

LIPPINCOTT WILLIAMS & WILKINS
A **Wolters Kluwer** Company

Philadelphia • Baltimore • New York • London
Buenos Aires • Hong Kong • Sydney • Tokyo

Acquisitions Editor: Brian Brown
Developmental Editor: Maria McAvey
Project Manager: Alicia Jackson
Senior Manufacturing Manager: Benjamin Rivera
Marketing Manager: Angela Panetta
Cover Designer: Terry Mallon
Production Services: Laserwords Private Limited
Printer: RR Donnelley-Crawfordsville

© **2006 by LIPPINCOTT WILLIAMS & WILKINS**
530 Walnut Street
Philadelphia, PA 19106 USA
LWW.com

2nd edition, © 2002 Department of Anesthesia and Critical Care
Massachusetts General Hospital, Published by Lippincott Williams &Wilkins

Printed in the United States

Library of Congress Cataloging-in-Publication Data

The Massachusetts General Hospital handbook of pain management / editor,
Jane Ballantyne ; foreword by Howard L. Fields.-- 3rd ed.
    p. ; cm.
  Includes bibliographical references and index.
  ISBN 0-7817-6224-3 (alk. paper)
  1. Pain--Treatment--Handbooks, manuals, etc. 2. Analgesia--Handbooks,
manuals, etc. I. Title: Handbook of pain management. II. Ballantyne, Jane,
1948- III. Massachusetts General Hospital.
  [DNLM: 1. Pain--therapy--Handbooks. WL 39 M414 2005]
RB127.M389 2005
616'.0472--dc22

                                                          2005017775

    To purchase additional copies of this book, call our customer service
department at (800) 639-3030 or fax orders to (301) 824-7390. International
customers should call (301) 714-2324.
    Visit Lippincott Williams & Wilkins on the Internet: at LWW.com.
Lippincott Williams & Wilkins customer service representatives are available
from 8:30 am to 6 pm, EST.

                                                10 9 8 7 6 5 4 3 2 1

Contents

I. General Considerations

II. Diagnosis of Pain

III. Therapeutic Options: Pharmacolgic Approaches

IV.   Therapeutic Options: Nonpharmacolgic Approaches

V.   Acute Pain

VI.   Chronic Pain

VII.   Pain Due to Cancer

VIII.   Special Situtations

Appendices

Contributing Authors

Salahadin Abdi, MD, PhD   *Assistant Professor, Department of Anesthesia & Critical Care, Harvard Medical School; Director, MGH Pain Center, Massachusetts General Hospital, Boston, Massachusetts*

Shihab U. Ahmed, MO, MPH   *Instructor, Department of Anesthesia & Critical Care, Harvard Medical School; Assistant, Department of Anesthesia & Critical Care, Massachusetts General Hospital, Boston, Massachusetts*

Ramin Amirnovin, MD   *Functional & Stereotactic Fellow, Department of Neurosurgery, Harvard Medical School and Massachusetts General Hospital, Boston, Massachusetts*

Lainie Andrew, PhD   *Associate Clinical Professor, Craniofacial Pain Center, Tufts University School of Dental Medicine; Consulting Psychologist, Department of Psychiatry, Massachusetts General Hospital, Boston, Massachusetts*

Martin Andrew Aquadro, MD, DMD, FACP, FACPM   *Assistant Professor, Department of Anesthesia, Harvard Medical School; Director, Cancer Pain Service; Director, Head & Neck Pain Clinic; Associate Anesthesiologist, MGH Pain Center, Massachusetts General Hospital, Boston, Massachusetts*

Joseph F. Audette, MA, MD   *Instructor, Department of Physical Medicine & Rehabilitation, Harvard Medical School; Director, Outpatient Pain Services, Department of Physical Medicine & Rehabilitation, Spaulding Rehabilitation Hospital, Boston, Massachusetts*

Allison Bailey, MD   *Instructor, Department of Physical Medicine & Rehabilitation, Harvard Medical School; Staff Physiatrist, Department of Physical Medicine & Rehabilitation, Spaulding Rehabilitation Hospital, Boston, Massachusetts*

Zahid H. Bajwa, MD   *Assistant Professor, Department of Anesthesia & Neurology, Harvard Medical School; Director, Education & Clinical Pain Research, Beth Israel Deaconess Medical Center, Boston, Massachusetts*

Jane C. Ballantyne, MD, FRCA   *Associate Professor, Department of Anesthesia, Harvard Medical School; Chief, Division of Pain Medicine, Department of Anesthesia & Critical Care, Massachusetts General Hospital, Boston, Massachusetts*

Steven A. Barna, MD   *Instructor, Department of Anesthesia, Harvard Medical School; Medical Director, MGH Pain Clinic, Department of Anesthesia & Critical Care, Massachusetts General Hospital, Boston, Massachusetts*

J. Andrew Billings, MD   *Associate Professor & Co-Director, Department of Palliative Care, Harvard Medical School; Director, Palliative Care Service, Massachusetts General Hospital, Boston, Massachusetts*

David F. Black, MD   *Assistant Professor, Department of Neurology, Mayo Clinic College of Medicine, Rochester, Minnesota*

Delbert R. Black, MS, MD   *Attending Anesthesiologist, Valley Anesthesiology Consultants, Ltd., Phoenix, Arizona*

Gary Jay Brenner, MD, PhD   *Director, Pain Medicine Fellowship Instructor, Department of Anesthesia & Critical Care, Harvard Medical School and Massachusetts General Hospital, Boston, Massachusetts*

Onassis A. Caneris, MD   *Director, Interventional Pain & Spine Treatment Center, Department of Neurology, Cincinnati, Ohio*

Lucy L. Chen, MD   *Instructor, Department of Anesthesia & Critical Care, Harvard Medical School; Assistant in Anesthesia, Department of Anesthesia & Critical Care, Massachusetts General Hospital, Boston, Massachusetts*

G. Rees Cosgrove, MD   *Associate Professor, Department of Surgery (Neurosurgery), Harvard Medical School, Boston, Massachusetts; Chairman, Neurosurgery, Lahey Clinic, Burlington, Massachusetts*

Sarah Cox, BSc, FRCP   *Honorary Senior Lecturer, Imperial College Medical School; Consultant, Department of Palliative Medicine, Chelsea & Westminster Hospital, London, United Kingdom*

Fred Michael Cutrer, MD   *Assistant Professor, Neurology, Mayo College of Medicine; Consultant, Department of Neurology, Mayo Clinic, Rochester, Minnesota*

Dennis Dey, MD, PhD   *Staff Neurologist, Department of Neurology, Western Maryland Health System, Cumberland, Maryland*

Constance M. Dahlin, APRN, BC, PCM   *Adjunct Faculty, Department of Nursing, MGH Institute of Health Professions; Nurse Practitioner, Palliative Care Service, Massachusetts General Hospital, Boston, Massachusetts*

Alexandre F. M. DaSilva, DDS, DMedSc   *Research Fellow, Martinos Center for Biomedical Imaging, Department of Radiology, Harvard Medical School and Massachusetts General Hospital, Boston, Massachusetts*

Isabelle Decosterd, MD   *Assistant Professor, Departments of Biology and Medicine, Lausanne University; Director,*

Anesthesiology Pain Research Group, Departments of Anesthesia, Cell Biology, and Morphology, Lausanne University Hospital, Lausanne, Switzerland

Thomas F. DeLaney, MD *Associate Professor, Radiation Oncology, Harvard Medical School; Medical Director, Northeast Proton Therapy Center, Radiation Oncology, Massachusetts General Hospital, Boston, Massachusetts*

Annabel D. Edwards, APRN, BC *Adult Nurse Practitioner, Department of Anesthesia & Critical Care, MGH Pain Center, Massachusetts General Hospital, Boston, Massachusetts*

Emad N. Eskandar, MD *Assistant Professor, Department of Surgery, Harvard Medical School; Assistant Visiting Neurosurgeon, Department of Neurosurgery, Massachusetts General Hospital, Boston, Massachusetts*

Jasmin M. Field, MD *Clinical Instructor, Department of Anesthesia & Critical Care, Harvard Medical School and Massachusetts General Hospital, Boston, Massachusetts*

Scott Fishman, MD *Professor, Department of Anesthesia & Pain Medicine, University of California, Davis, California; Chief, Division of Pain Medicine, UC Davis Medical Center, Ambulatory Care Center, Sacramento, California*

Jatinder Gill, MD *Instructor, Department of Anesthesia, Harvard Medical School; Assistant, Department of Anesthesia & Critical Care, Massachusetts General Hospital, Boston, Massachusetts*

Asteghik Hacobian, MD, MA *Clinical Associate, Department of Anesthesia & Critical Care, Massachusetts General Hospital, Boston, Massachusetts; Director, Interventional Spine Medicine, Barrington, New Hampshire*

Karla Hayes, MD *Instructor, Departments of Anesthesia and Psychiatry, Harvard University, Cambridge, Massachusetts; Assistant Psychiatrist, Departments of Anesthesia and Psychiatry, Massachusetts General Hospital, Boston, Massachusetts*

Eugenia-Daniela Hord, MD *Clinical Instructor, Departments of Anesthesia and Neurology, Harvard Medical School, Boston, Massachusetts*

Eija Kalso, MD, PhD *Professor, Institute of Clinical Medicine, University of Helsinki; Chief, Pain Clinic, Department of Anesthesia & Intensive Care Medicine, Helsinki University Central Hospital, Helsinki, Finland*

Lisa S. Krivickas, MD *Assistant Professor, Department of Physical Medicine & Rehabilitation, Harvard Medical School; Associate Chief, Department of Physical Medicine & Rehabilitation, Massachusetts General Hospital, Boston, Massachusetts*

Ronald J. Kulich, PhD   *Attending Psychologist, Departments of Anesthesia, Psychiatry, and Dental Medicine, Harvard Medical School and Tufts School of Dental Medicine; Attending Psychologist, Departments of Anesthesia and Psychiatry, Massachusetts General Hospital, Boston, Massachusetts*

Alyssa A. LeBel, MD   *Assistant Professor, Departments of Anesthesia and Neurology, Harvard Medical School; Associate, Departments of Anesthesia and Neurology, Pain Service, Children's Hospital, Boston, Massachusetts*

Elizabeth Loder, MD, FACP   *Assistant Professor, Department of Medicine, Harvard Medical School; Director, Headache & Pain Programs, Spaulding Rehabilitation Hospital, Boston, Massachusetts*

S. Jane Marshall, MRCP   *Specialist Registrar, Department of Palliative Medicine, St. Christopher's Hospice, London, United Kingdom*

Patricia W. McAlary, EdD, APRN-BC   *Program Director, Spaulding Pain Rehabilitation Program, Spaulding Rehabilitation Hospital, Boston, Massachusetts*

Bucknam McPeek, AB, MD   *Associate Professor, Department of Anesthesia, Harvard Medical School; Honorary Anaesthetist, Department of Anesthesia, Massachusetts General Hospital, Boston, Massachusetts*

Theresa H. Michel, DPT, DSc, CCS   *Clinical Associate Professor, Department of Physical Therapy, Graduate Programs in Physical Therapy, MGH Institute of Health Professions; Clinical Associate, Physical Therapy Services, Massachusetts General Hospital, Boston, Massachusetts*

Jeffrey A. Norton, MD   *Staff Phsycisian, Division of Pain Medicine, New England Neurological Association, North Andover, Massachusetts; Medical Director, Pain Management Services, Northeast Rehabilitation Hospital, Salem, New Hampshire*

Anne Louise Oaklander, MD   *Assistant Professor, Departments of Anesthesia and Neurology, Harvard Medical School; Assistant, Departments of Neurology and Pathology, Massachusetts General Hospital, Boston, Massachusetts*

May C. M. Pian-Smith, MD, MS   *Assistant Professor, Department of Anesthesia, Harvard Medical School; Co-Chief, Division of Obstetric Anesthesia, Department of Anesthesia & Critical Care, Massachusetts General Hospital, Boston, Massachusetts*

Andrew Tyler Putnam, MD   *Assistant Professor, Department of Medicine, Georgetown University; Attending Physician, Department of Medicine, Lombardi Cancer Center, Washington, District of Columbia*

James P. Rathmell, MD   *Professor, Department of Anesthesia, University of Vermont College of Medicine; Director, Center for Pain Medicine, Fletcher Allen Health Care, South Burlington, Vermont*

Andrew S. C. Rice, MB, BS, MD, FRCA   *Reader in Pain Research, Departments of Anaesthetics, Intensive Care, and Pain Medicine, Imperial College; Honorary Consultant in Chronic Pain Management, Pain Service, Chelsea & Westminster Hospital, London, United Kingdom*

Daniel M. Rockers, PhD   *Director, Functional Restoration Center, Sacramento Pain Clinic, Sacramento, California*

Elizabeth Ryder, RN, MSN   *Clinical Nurse Specialist, Department of Anesthesia & Critical Care, Massachusetts General Hospital, Boston, Massachusetts*

Thomas T. Simopoulos, MD, MA   *Clinical Instructor, Department of Anesthesia, Harvard Medical School; Director, Acute & Interventional Pain Services, Department of Anesthesia, Beth Israel Deaconess Medical Center, Boston, Massachusetts*

Jan Slezak, MD   *Clinical Associate, Department of Anesthesia & Critical Care, Massachusetts General Hospital, Boston, Massachusetts, Director, Interventional Spine Medicine, Barrington, New Hampshire*

Milan P. Stojanovic, MD   *Assistant Professor, Department of Anesthesia, Harvard Medical School; Director, Interventional Pain Program, Department of Anesthesia & Critical Care, Massachusetts General Hospital, Boston, Massachusetts*

Jeffrey Uppington, MB, BS, FRCA   *Professor, Department of Anesthesia & Pain Medicine, University of California, Davis, California; Vice Chairman, Department of Anesthesia & Pain Medicine, UC Davis Medical Center, Sacramento, California*

Barth L. Wilsey, MD   *Associate Clinical Professor, Department of Anesthesia & Pain Medicine, UC Davis Medical Center; Director, Anesthesiology Pain Management, Sacramento VA Medical Center, Sacramento, California*

Harriët Wittink, PhD, MS, PT   *Faculty, Departments of Physiotherapy Research and Physical Therapy, Academy of Health Sciences Utrecht, Utrecht University of Professional Education, Utrecht, The Netherlands*

Clifford J. Woolf, MD, PhD   *Richard J. Kitz Professor, Department of Anesthesia Research, Program in Neuroscience, Harvard Medical School; Director, Neural Plasticity Research Group, Massachusetts General Hospital, Boston, Massachusetts*

Foreword

After three decades of progress in mapping the neural mechanisms of pain, a revolution is underway in the clinical practice of pain management: increasing numbers of physicians are taking responsibility for the relief of their patients' pain. *The Massachusetts General Hospital Handbook of Pain Management* provides an integrated and useful overview of the knowledge base required for effective treatment of pain. The book is now in its third edition and has been updated on the basis of changes in drug availability and changes in the philosophy that guides treatment choices.

Several factors have contributed to the revolution in pain management. Perhaps the most important factor is the evolution of attitude in individuals who are no longer willing to suffer pain in silence. Pain has moved progressively from the realm of the moral to that of the medical. Scientific discoveries that explain some of the most puzzling features of pain have facilitated this change in attitude. Dramatic advances have been made in the understanding of the neural basis of pain and pain treatment. For example, several crucial transducer molecules have been discovered that convert chemical signals of tissue damage and intense thermal stimuli to coded electrochemical messages in the peripheral and central nerve cells that confer pain sensitivity; these concepts are described in Chapter 2. In addition, the central nervous system pathways that transmit the information to higher centers have been described, and, remarkably, we can now visualize the metabolic trace of neural activity produced in the brain of awake human subjects by painful stimuli. Beyond transduction and the transmission pathways, there are well-described brain circuits through which psychological factors can selectively amplify or suppress pain signals (see Chapter 1). This discovery of brain circuits has done much to explain the tremendous variability of pain severity reported by different patients with similar injuries. The public at large is familiar with the idea that endogenous opioid substances (endorphins) in the brain can produce bliss and pain relief. The objective description of pathways and mechanisms helps remove pain from the realm of the purely personal, making it less of a burden that one is expected to bear with resignation, like fear of death, and more of a sign of disease, like fever or bleeding. Clearly, the latter are matters of shared concern for both patient and physician.

This growth in our knowledge of neural mechanisms has been paralleled by increased interest on the part of physicians in actively treating pain. Although relief from pain is accepted as a major goal for physicians, many doctors traditionally assume that pain relief *per se* is a simple task for which no special training is required. In fact, although acute pain is generally managed in an adequate manner, many health care professionals continue to manage cancer pain inadequately, and chronic pain remains a major challenge. Fortunately, there has been increasing recognition among physicians that persistent pain is a serious and complex problem that often requires the skills of a variety of health care professionals for optimal assessment and treatment. Multidisciplinary pain clinics, a concept originated by the late John J. Bonica at the University of Washington, have now spread around the world, and it is unusual to find an academic medical center that does not have a pain management service. Appendix II of this handbook provides a useful list of resources.

This third edition of *The Massachusetts General Hospital Handbook of Pain Management* both reflects and supports the revolution in pain management by providing a broad introduction to the diagnostic complexities, assessment tools, and multiple treatment modalities that are now available. Master its contents and you will have gone far toward the goal of optimal care for patients with pain.

Howard L. Fields, MD, PhD

Preface

This edition of the Massachusetts General Hospital Handbook of Pain Management is dedicated to the memory of Pat Wall, who died in 2001, months after delivering the first annual Beecher Lecture at MGH. He set our imaginations free when he proposed that pain was not simply a hard-wired signal but rather an infinitely malleable system that is capable of adjusting to any number of pathologic and psychological changes. In Boston, in the 1950s and 1960s, he was working closely with Ronald P. Melzak at MIT and with Henry K. Beecher on the other side of the Charles River at MGH. Their ideas helped sow the seeds for the development of the science of pain, and we keep them in our debt as we endeavor to advance this science and apply it to the relief of suffering.

Jane C. Ballantyne

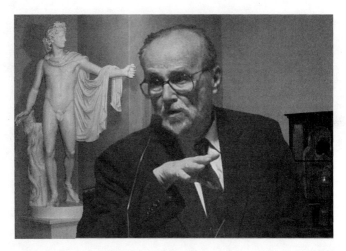

Patrick Wall after lecturing the Ether Dome at MGH in 2001. The Ether Dome is the historic birthplace of anesthesia.

Acknowledgments

We are greatly indebted to Purdue Pharma for their generous and unrestricted grant toward establishing the MGH Purdue Pharma Pain Program. Purdue's support strengthens our academic mission and is a mark of their recognition that discovery and knowledge form the foundations of good clinical care. Purdue has been committed to promoting appropriate pain management for more than two decades, working closely with MGH and a number of other organizations to increase awareness of the problem of persistent pain and its cost to individuals and to society.

We would like to express our gratitude to Tina Toland for her editorial support and authorship of the appendices.

Definitions and Abbreviations

Addiction a disorder characterized by compulsive use of a drug, resulting in physical, psychological, and/or social dysfunction to the user and in continued usage despite the dysfunction

Adjuvant analgesic a drug that has a primary indication other than pain but has an analgesic effect in some painful conditions or is capable of decreasing the side effects of analgesics; commonly administered in combination with one of the primary analgesics (e.g., opioids)

Allodynia pain associated with a stimulus, such as light touch, that does not normally provoke pain

Analgesia absence of pain; commonly used to mean pain relief

Anesthesia absence of sensation

Arthralgia pain in a joint, usually due to arthritis or arthropathy

Breakthrough pain pain that breaks through the analgesia achieved by long-acting medications

Causalgia see **CRPS II**

CNS **Central nervous system**

Central pain pain that originates from lesions of the central nervous system, usually the spinothalamocortical pathway

Central sensitization a long-term potentiation of pain signals associated with NMDA receptor activation and with the induction of specific genes; a CNS response to prolonged painful stimulation

Chronic pain pain that persists a month beyond the usual course of an acute injury or disease; this definition varies between the various treating clinicians

CNMP **Chronic Nonmalignant Pain**

CNTP **Chronic Nonterminal Pain** embraces chronic nonmalignant pain and chronic pain due to cancer (not associated with terminal illness)

Complex Regional Pain Syndrome (CRPS) a chronic neuropathic pain syndrome characterized by its association at some point with evidence of edema, changes in skin blood flow, abnormal sudomotor activity in the region of pain, allodynia, hyperalgesia or hyperpathia

COX cyclooxygenase, an enzyme in the pathway from arachidonic acid to prostaglandin, prostacyclin, and thromboxane

Coxib collective term for a new class of selective NSAIDs known as COX-2 antagonists

CRPS I [formally known as **reflex sympathetic dystropy (RSD)**]; a painful condition that is associated with a continuous burning pain and sympathetic overactivity in an extremity after trauma but without major nerve injury; this condition is not limited to the distribution of a single peripheral nerve and is apparently disproportional to the inciting event

CRPS II (formally known as **causalgia**) a condition characterized by burning pain, allodynia, and hyperpathia, often accompanied by vasomotor, sudomotor, and late trophic changes, occurring after partial injury of a nerve (or one of its major branches) in part of a limb (usually hand or foot) innervated by the damaged nerve

CSF   Cerebrospinal Fluid

DEA   Drug Enforcement Agency

Deafferentation pain   pain resulting from loss of sensory input to the CNS; the pain may arise in the periphery (e.g., peripheral nerve avulsion) or in the CNS itself (e.g., spinal cord lesions and multiple sclerosis)

Dysesthesia   an unpleasant, abnormal sensation, spontaneous or evoked, that is considered unpleasant

Drug dependence   (also known as **physical dependence**) this relates to the expression of a withdrawal syndrome upon sudden drug cessation; it occurs with the use of both addictive and nonaddictive drugs (e.g., opioids, local anesthetics, and clonidine)

Drug tolerance   this occurs when a fixed dose of a drug produces a decreasing effect so that a dose increase is required to maintain a stable effect; the effect occurs particularly with opioids

EMG   Electromyography

EDX   Electrodiagnostic Testing (also known as **EMG**)

FDA   Federal Drug Agency

Fibromyalgia   a pain syndrome that diffuses through the body and that is characterized by predictable tender areas within muscles

Hypalgesia   (same as **hypoalgesia**) an increased pain threshold (a decreased sensitivity to noxious stimulation)

Hypesthesia   an increased detection threshold (a decreased sensitivity to stimulation); the definition excludes the special senses

Hyperalgesia   a decreased pain threshold (an exaggerated painful response to a pain provoking stimulus)

Hyperesthesia   a decreased detection threshold (an increased sensitivity to stimulation); the definition excludes the special senses

Hyperpathia   increased pain either after repetitive stimulation or due to decreased pain threshold

IASP   International Association for the Study of Pain

Meralgia paresthetica   a dysesthesia in an area of lateral femoral cutaneous nerve innervation

Myofascial pain   pain stemming from muscles

Neuralgia   nerve pain along a specific anatomically distinct nerve or nerves

Neuraxis   the spinal cord and brain; the term neuraxial drug delivery is commonly used to encompass intrathecal and/or epidural delivery, although, strictly, the term should include intraventricular delivery

Neuritis   inflammation of a nerve or nerves

Neuropathy   a disturbance of function or pathologic change in individual nerves or groups of nerves; *mononeuropathy* involves a single nerve, *mononeuropathy multiplex* involves several nerves, and *polyneuropathy* involves several nerves bilaterally or symmetrically

Neuropathic pain   pain initiated or caused by a primary lesion or dysfunction in the nervous system; these pain-producing lesions may involve the peripheral and central nervous systems and may include injury from chemicals, radiation, or trauma and involvement of nerves in disease processes such as tumor infiltration and inflammation

NMDA *N*-methyl-D-aspartate a synthetic agonist of the NMDA receptor. This receptor is involved in the wind-up phenomenon, in the central sensitization, and in the development of opioid tolerance

Nocebo a negative placebo effect; for example, undesirable side effects (e.g., nausea); nocebo effects are thought to be the result of an individual's expectations of adverse effects from a treatment as well as from conditioned responses

Nociceptive pain pain arising from activation of nociceptors

Nociceptor a receptor that is preferentially sensitive to noxious stimuli or to stimuli that become noxious if prolonged; this term may also be used to refer to the entire nociceptive primary afferent

NSAID   Nonsteroidal antiinflammatory drug

Opiate an opioid drug

Opioid a substance that is active at endogenous opioid receptors; it includes opiates (drugs) and endogenous opioids (e.g., endorphins and enkephalins)

Pain an unpleasant sensory and emotional experience associated with actual or potential tissue damage or that is described in terms of damage

Pain threshold the lowest intensity of stimulus that is perceived as being painful

Pain tolerance level the greatest level of pain that a subject is able to tolerate

Paresthesia an abnormal sensation, spontaneous or evoked, that is not necessarily considered unpleasant; the term dysesthesia specifically refers to an unpleasant abnormal sensation

PCA   patient-controlled analgesia

Peripheral neuropathy any disease of the peripheral nerves; the symptoms of a neuropathy may include numbness, weakness, pain (often burning), and loss of reflexes

Phantom pain pain felt in an anatomic structure that has been surgically or traumatically removed

Physical dependence see **Drug dependence**

Placebo a drug or therapy that simulates medical treatment but has no specific action on the condition being treated

Preemptive analgesia analgesic treatment provided before and during painful stimulation that aims to attenuate the development of hypersensitive pain states

Pseudoaddiction a phenomenon of drug-seeking behavior that results from undertreatment with analgesics; the condition resolves when the dose of the drug the patient seeks is increased appropriately; it should be distinguished from true addiction, where drug-seeking behavior continues despite adequate and appropriate dosing

Psychogenic pain pain inconsistent with the likely anatomic distribution of the presumed generator or pain existing with no apparent organic pathology despite extensive evaluation

Radicular pain pain that is evoked by stimulation of nociceptive afferent fibers in spinal nerves, their roots or ganglia, or by other neuropathic mechanisms; the symptom is caused by ectopic impulse generation; it is distinct from radiculopathy, which includes a focal neurological deficit

Radiculopathy   a pathologic condition of the nerve root (or multiple nerve roots) that results in conduction blockade and produces sensory and motor changes and pain in the area of its distribution; distinct from radicular pain, but the two changes may arise together

Referred pain   pain perceived as arising in an area remote from its source; this is thought to occur because the nerve supply to both areas (i.e., the area pain is perceived and the area pain is produced) converge proximally in the CNS

Reflex sympathetic dystrophy (RSD)   see **CRPS I**

Somatic pain   pain that arises from stimulation of nerves in the skin and musculoskeletal system, including bone, ligament, joint, and muscle

TCA Tricyclic antidepressant

Tolerance   see drug tolerance

Trigeminal neurlagia   a condition that produces sharp pain in the face because of abnormal firing of the trigeminal nerve; also know as tic douloureux

Trigger point   a focal loci of pain within a muscle or connective tissue. Prolonged stimulation of these areas can generate a pattern of pain that is referred distally

VAS Visual or verbal analog scale   pain assessment tools utilizing analogs [either a measured line (visual) or a numeric scale (verbal)] to represent pain

Visceral pain   pain due to stimulation of nerves endings in viscera; these nerves characteristically respond to stretch more than to other changes (e.g., cutting, inflammation, and crushing); pain is usually referred to other areas (e.g., flank, skin, perineum, legs, and shoulders)

WHO   World Health Organization

Wind-up   sensitization of dorsal horn spinal neurons by persistent C-fiber stimulation. This neuronal sensitization progressively increases throughout the duration of C-fiber stimulation, and therefore, "wind-up," and is dependent on activation of NMDA receptors.

SELECTED READINGS

Mersky H. Classification of chronic pain. Description of chronic pain syndromes and definition of pain terms. *Pain* 1986; (Suppl. 3):S1.

Merskey N, Bogduk N. *Classification of chronic pain, IASP Task Force on Taxonomy,* 2nd ed. Seattle, WA: IASP Press, 1994: 209–214.

Portenoy RK, Kanner RM. Definition and assessment of pain. In: Portenoy RK, Kanner RM, eds. *Pain management: theory and practice.* Philadelphia: F.A. Davis, 1996:3–18.

General Considerations

Neurophysiologic Basis of Pain

Gary Jay Brenner

Severe pain is world destroying.
—*Elaine Scarry from The Body in Pain*

One of the most important functions of the nervous system is to provide information about potential and actual bodily injury. Nearly a century ago, in 1906, Sir Charles Sherrington defined **nociception** as the sensory detection of a noxious event or a potentially harmful environmental stimulus. He explicitly distinguished nociception from pain, a complex human experience that involves sensory, psychologic, and cognitive components. **Pain** is currently defined by the International Association for the Study of Pain (IASP) as "an unpleasant sensory and emotional experience associated with actual or potential tissue damage." The pain system may be grossly divided into the following components:

- **Nociceptors**, the specialized receptors in the peripheral nervous system that detect noxious stimuli, **primary nociceptive afferent fibers**, normally Aδ and C fibers, which transmit information about noxious stimuli to the **dorsal horn** of the spinal cord
- **Ascending nociceptive tracts**, for example, the spinothalamic and spinohypothalamic tract (SHT), which convey nociceptive

stimuli from the dorsal horn of the spinal cord to higher centers in the central nervous system (CNS)

- **Higher centers in the CNS** that are involved in discrimination of pain, affective components of pain, memory components of pain, and motor control related to the immediate aversive response to painful stimuli
- **Descending systems** that allow higher centers of the CNS to modify nociceptive information at multiple levels

I. NOCICEPTORS

1. Definitions

Although somewhat confusing, the term **nociceptor** is used to refer both to the free nerve terminals of primary afferent fibers that respond to painful, potentially injurious stimuli and to the entire apparatus (sensory neuron, including free terminals) capable of transducing **and** transmitting information about noxious stimuli. In this chapter, the term **nociceptor** is used to refer to the entire nociceptive primary afferent.

Free nerve terminals contain receptors capable of transducing chemical, mechanical, and thermal signals. Recently, for example, a membrane receptor that responds to noxious heat has been cloned (it has been designated TRPV1), and, interestingly, this receptor is also stimulated by capsacin, the molecule responsible for the "hot" sensation associated with hot peppers. Nociceptive terminals innervate a wide variety of tissues and are present in both somatic and visceral structures including the cornea, tooth pulp, muscles, joints, respiratory system, cardiovascular system, digestive system, urogenital system, and meninges, as well as skin.

Nociceptors may be divided according to three criteria: degree of myelination, type(s) of stimulation that evokes a response, and response characteristics. There are two basic classes of nociceptors based on their degree of myelination and conduction velocity. A-delta fibers (Aδ) are thinly myelinated and conduct at a velocity of 2 to 30 m per second. C fibers are unmyelinated and conduct at a velocity of less than 2 m per second (see Table 1). Aδ and C nociceptors can be further divided according to the stimuli they sense. These nociceptors may respond to mechanical, chemical, or thermal (heat and cold) stimuli, or a combination (polymodal). For example, C-fiber mechanoheat receptors respond to noxious mechanical stimuli and intermediate heat stimuli (41°C to 49°C), have a slow conduction velocity, and constitute most nociceptive afferent fibers. Aδ mechanoheat receptors can be divided into two subtypes. Type I receptors have a high heat threshold (>53°C) and conduct at relatively fast velocities (30 to 55 m per second). These receptors detect pain during high-intensity heat responses. Type II receptors have a lower heat threshold and conduct at slower velocity (15 m per second). Some receptors respond to both warmth and thermal pain. Some C and Aδ fibers are mechanically insensitive but respond to heat, cold, or a variety of chemicals (e.g., bradykinin, hydrogen ions, serotonin, histamine, arachidonic acid, and prostacyclin).

Table 1. Classification of fibers in peripheral nerves

Fiber Group	Innervation	Mean Diameter (μm)	Mean Conduction Velocity (m/sec)
A-α	Primary muscle spindle motor to skeletal muscle	15	100
A-β	Cutaneous touch and pressure afferent fibers	8	50
A-γ	Motor to muscle spindle	6	20
A-δ	Mechanoreceptors, **nociceptors**, thermoreceptors	<3	15
B	Sympathetic preganglionic	3	7
C	Mechanoreceptors, **nociceptors**, thermoreceptors, sympathetic postganglionic	1	1

From Bonica JJ. Anatomic and physiologic basis of nociception and pain. In: Bonica JJ, ed. *The management of pain*, 2nd ed. Philadelphia, PA: Lea & Febiger, 1990:31, with permission.

2. Primary Afferent Fibers

The neural impulses originating from the free endings of nociceptors are transmitted via primary afferent nerves to the spinal cord, or, if originating from the head and neck, the impulses are transmitted via cranial nerves to the brainstem. Most primary afferent fibers of innervating tissues below the head have cell bodies located in the **dorsal root ganglion** (DRG) of spinal nerves. Primary afferent fibers of cranial nerves V, VII, IX, and X (the sensory cranial nerves) have cell bodies in their respective sensory ganglia.

Most nociceptors are C fibers, and 80% to 90% of C fibers respond to nociceptive input. The differences in conduction velocities and response characteristics of Aδ and C fibers may explain the typical subjective experience of pain associated with a noxious stimulus: a first pain (so-called epicritic pain) that is rapid, well localized, and pricking in character (Aδ), followed by a second pain (so-called protopathic pain) that is burning and diffuse (C fiber). Visceral afferent nociceptive fibers (Aδ and C) travel with sympathetic and parasympathetic fibers; their cell bodies are also found in the DRG. Muscle is also innervated by both Aδ and C fibers, and, interestingly, muscle pain appears to be limited in quality to that of a cramp.

3. Dorsal Horn Synapses and Biochemical Mediators

Primary afferent nociceptors enter the spinal cord via Lissauer tract and synapse on neurons in the dorsal horn (see Fig. 1). Lissauer tract is a bundle of predominantly (80%) primary afferent fibers, consisting mainly of Aδ and C fibers that penetrate the spinal cord en route to the dorsal horn. After entering the spinal cord, Aδ and C fibers run up or down one or two segments before synapsing with second-order neurons in the dorsal horn. The dorsal horn synapse is an important site of further processing and integration of the incoming nociceptive information. The dorsal horn may be a point at which nociceptive information is conducted to higher centers, or a point at which nociceptive information is inhibited by descending systems. The responsiveness of dorsal horn neurons may change in response to prior noxious afferent input, particularly repetitive input (central sensitization).

Biochemical Mediators

Numerous neurotransmitters and other biochemical mediators are released in the dorsal horn. These substances are derived from three main sources:

- primary afferent fibers
- interneurons
- descending fiber systems

The neurochemistry of the dorsal horn is complicated, and there are qualitative differences between the pharmacology of acute pain and that of the facilitated pain states associated with

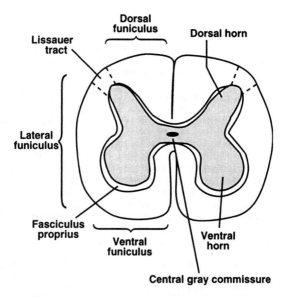

Figure 1.   Diagrammatic cross section of the spinal cord.

chronic noxious stimulation. Some of the neurochemical mediators can be categorized as excitatory or inhibitory, although many serve complex and mixed functions. For example, the endogenous opioid dynorphin may be inhibitory or excitatory depending on the state of the nervous system. The following are examples of excitatory and inhibitory substances active in the dorsal horn.

Excitatory Neuromediators

- The excitatory amino acids glutamate and aspartate
- The neuropeptides substance P (SP) and calcitonin gene–related peptide (CGRP)
- Growth factor brain-derived neurotrophic factor (BDNF)
- Bradykinin

Inhibitory Neuromediators

- Endogenous opioids such as enkephalin and β-endorphin
- γ-aminobutyric acid (GABA)
- Glycine

Cells of the dorsal horn possess specific receptors for the substances listed earlier, as well as receptors for a multitude of other neurochemicals (some probably undiscovered). Of particular note is the receptor for glutamate, the **N-methyl-D-aspartate (NMDA)** receptor, which is widely distributed in the dorsal horn. There are now extensive experimental data implicating the NMDA receptor in the generation and maintenance of facilitated pain states.

4. Peripheral Sensitization

Prolonged noxious stimulation can sensitize nociceptors. Sensitization refers to a decreased threshold as well as to an increased response to suprathreshold stimulation. It is observed following direct nerve injury and inflammation and is the result of a complex set of transcriptional and posttranslational changes in the primary nociceptive afferents. Sensitization of the entire nociceptive pathway can arise secondary to changes in the CNS (central sensitization) or the periphery (peripheral sensitization). Once sensitization is established, it is often impossible to clinically separate central from peripheral contributions to the process of sensitization. The related topics on hyperalgesia, allodynia, inflammation, and nerve injury are briefly discussed in the following text.

(i) Hyperalgesia

Tissue damage activates nociceptors; if the damage is prolonged and intense, it can generate a state in which there is a lowered threshold to painful stimuli. This state is termed **hyperalgesia**. In hyperalgesic areas, one can clinically observe an increased response to noxious stimuli. There are alterations in both the subjective and the neurophysiologic responses to stimuli. Thus, a lowered pain threshold and an increased response to painful stimuli are not only subjectively experienced by the patient, but also demonstrated by the nociceptors. **Primary hyperalgesia** is hyperalgesia at the site of injury; **secondary hyperalgesia** refers to hyperalgesia at the site surrounding the injured tissue. Secondary hyperalgesia is thought to reflect changes occurring in the CNS and would therefore be an example of central sensitization.

(ii) Allodynia

In addition to developing a lowered threshold for noxious stimuli following tissue damage (hyperalgesia), patients may also suffer a postinjury state in which normally innocuous stimuli are perceived as painful. This phenomenon is termed **allodynia**. For example, a very light touch in the area of a burn or in an area associated with postherpatic neuralgia can generate excruciating pain. Like hyperalgesia, allodynia is thought to be caused by plastic changes in both primary sensory fibers and spinal cord neurons.

(iii) Inflammation

Inflammation is the characteristic reaction to injury and results in **rubor**, **calor**, **dolor**, **tumor**, and **functio laesa** (i.e., redness, heat, pain, swelling, and loss of function). During an inflammatory response, activation of nociceptive pathways can lead to sensitization, resulting clinically in spontaneous and increased stimulation-induced pain (i.e., hyperalgesia and allodynia). Release of prostaglandins, cytokines, growth factors, and other mediators by inflammatory cells can directly stimulate nociceptors. The precise nature of this interaction between the immune system and nervous system and the manner in which this can lead to pathologic pain states, however, remains to be clarified. The critical observation is that inflammation is an important cause of both acute and chronic alteration in pain processing and sensation.

(iv) Nerve injury

Direct neural trauma can also lead to pathologic pain states characterized by **spontaneous pain** (i.e., pain occurring in the absence of any stimulus), hyperalgesia, and allodynia. Such **neuropathic pain** states can arise following injury to peripheral or central elements of the pain system. A clinical example of this pain state is complex regional pain syndrome type I (CRPS I), formerly called reflex sympathetic dystrophy (RSD), in which an apparently minor injury can lead to sensitization of pain processing in a region including but not limited to that involved in the injury.

II. ASCENDING NOCICEPTIVE PATHWAYS

1. Topographical Arrangement of the Dorsal Horn (Laminae of Rexed)

The gray matter of the spinal cord can be divided into ten laminae (I–X) (the laminae of Rexed) on the basis of the histologic organization of the numerous types of cell bodies and dendrites. The dorsal horn is composed of laminae I–VI (see Fig. 2). Most nociceptive input converges on lamina I (marginal zone), lamina II (substantia gelatinosa), and lamina V in the dorsal horn. However,

Lissauer tract

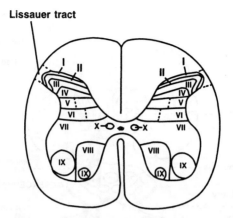

Figure 2.   Laminae of Rexed I through X of the spinal cord.

some primary visceral and somatic nociceptive afferent fibers
synapse in other laminae. Cutaneous mechanoreceptor Aδ afferent fibers synapse in laminae I, II, and V; visceral mechanoreceptor Aδ fibers synapse in laminae I and V; cutaneous nociceptor C
fibers synapse in laminae I and II; and visceral nociceptive C
fibers synapse in many laminae including I, II, IV, V, and X. The
ascending spinal pathways involved with nociceptive transmission arise mainly from laminae I, II, and V (see Fig. 3). These
pathways include the spinothalamic tract (STT), SHT, spinoreticular tract (SRT), and spinopontoamygdala tract.

2. Dorsal Horn Projection Neurons

The **second-order neurons** in the pain pathway are the
dorsal horn projection neurons (or their equivalent in cranial
pathways). These neurons have their cell bodies in the spinal
cord (or cranial nerve nuclei in the head and neck) and are
classified according to their response characteristics. High-
threshold (HT), also called nociceptive–specific (NS), cells respond exclusively to noxious stimuli; these cells receive input
only from nociceptors (i.e., Aδ and C fibers). The receptive
fields of these HT cells are small and are organized somatotopically, being most abundant in lamina I. Other cells respond to a range of stimuli from innocuous to noxious; they are
called wide dynamic range (WDR) cells and integrate information from Aβ (nonnoxious stimuli), Aδ, and C fibers. These cells
have larger receptive fields, are the most prevalent cells in the
dorsal horn, and are found in all laminae, with a high concentration in lamina V. The convergence of sensory information
onto a single dorsal horn neuron is essential for the coding of
stimulus intensity in terms of output frequency by these second-
order neurons.

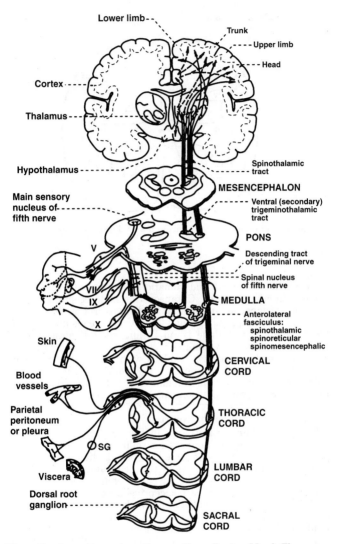

Figure 3.   Ascending pain pathways. (From Bonica JJ, ed. *The management of pain*, vol. 1. Philadelphia, PA: Lea & Febiger, 1990:29, with permission.)

3. Spinothalamic Tract

The STT (Fig. 3) is the most important of the ascending pathways for the transmission of nociceptive stimuli and is located in the anterolateral quadrant of the spinal cord. The cell bodies of STT neurons reside in the dorsal horn; most of their axons cross midline in the ventral white commissure of the spinal cord to ascend in the opposite anterolateral quadrant; however, some do remain ipsilateral. Neurons from more distal regions of the body (e.g., the sacral region) are found more laterally and neurons from more proximal regions (e.g., the cervical region) are found more medially within the STT as it ascends. STT neurons segregate into medial and lateral projections to the thalamus (see section entitled The Limbic System).

Neurons that project to the **lateral thalamus** arise from laminae I, II, and V, and from there synapse with fibers that project to the somatosensory cortex. The fibers are thought to be involved in sensory and discriminative aspects of pain.

Neurons projecting to the **medial thalamus** originate from the deeper laminae VI and IX. The neurons send collateral projections to the reticular formation of the brainstem and midbrain, to the periaqueductal gray (PAG) matter and the hypothalamus, or directly to other areas of the basal forebrain and somatosensory cortex. These neurons are thought to be involved with autonomic reflex responses, state-of-arousal, and emotional aspects of pain.

4. Spinohypothalamic Tract

Nociceptive and nonnociceptive information from neurons within the dorsal horn is conveyed to diencephalic structures, such as the hypothalamus, directly by a recently discovered pathway—the **SHT**. This pathway projects to the region of the brain (the hypothalamus) that is involved in autonomic functions such as sleep, appetite, temperature regulation, and stress response. In fact, most SHT neurons (60%) project to the contralateral medial or lateral hypothalamus and, therefore, are presumed to have a considerable role in autonomic and neuroendocrine responses to painful stimuli. Therefore, the SHT appears to form the anatomic substrate that coordinates reflex autonomic reactions to painful stimuli. Some of the connections of SHT, for example, to the suprachiasmatic nucleus that partly controls the sleep/wake pattern may account for behaviors such as difficulty in sleeping with painful conditions, particularly chronic pain. Most SHT neurons respond preferentially to mechanical nociceptive stimulation, and a smaller number respond to noxious thermal stimulation. The fibers of the SHT cross midline in the supraoptic decussation. The SRT and the spinaoponoamygdala tract are also likely involved with state-of-arousal and emotional aspects of pain.

5. Cranial Nerves

The transmission of pain in the head and neck has many of the same characteristics as the nociceptive system that has first-order synapses in the dorsal horn of the spinal cord. The face and oral cavity are richly innervated with nociceptors. The primary nociceptive afferent fibers for the head originate mainly from cranial nerve V, as well as from cranial nerves VII, IX, and X, and from the upper cervical spinal nerves. The primary afferent fibers of the cranial nerves project mainly to nuclei of the trigeminal system, whereas the upper cervical nerves project to second-order neurons in the dorsal horn of the spinal cord; from there, projections continue to the supraspinal systems.

(i) The trigeminal system (V)

The trigeminal system receives afferent input from the three divisions of the trigeminal nerve (i.e., ophthalmic, maxillary, and mandibular) that serve the entire face as well as the dura and the vessels from a large portion of the anterior two thirds of the brain. The trigeminal system has three sensory nuclei, all of which receive projections from cells that have cell bodies located within the trigeminal ganglion, a structure similar to DRG. The three nuclei are the mesencephalic, the main sensory, and the spinal trigeminal nuclei. The third nucleus is further divided into the subnucleus oralis, the subnucleus interpolaris, and the subnucleus caudalis. The subnucleus caudalis (also known as the medullary dorsal horn) extends caudally from the medulla to the level of the upper cervical segments of the spinal cord (C3-C4).

The trigeminal nuclei give rise to several ascending pathways. The axons of cell bodies in the main sensory nucleus and subnucleus oralis project either ipsilaterally, forming the dorsal trigeminothalamic tract, or contralaterally, in the ventral trigeminothalamic tract. Both tracts terminate in the thalamus. The subnucleus caudalis also contributes to the trigeminothalamic tracts and has direct projections to the thalamus, reticular formation, and hypothalamus.

(ii) The glossopharyngeal nerve (IX)

The glossopharyngeal nerve conveys impulses associated with tactile sense, thermal sense, and pain from the mucous membranes of the posterior third of the tongue, tonsil, posterior pharyngeal wall, and Eustachian tubes.

(iii) The vagus nerve (X)

The vagus nerve conveys impulses associated with tactile sense from the posterior auricular skin and external auditory meatus and those associated with visceral sensation from the pharynx, larynx, trachea, esophagus, and thoracic and abdominal viscera via the STT and the fasciculus solitarius (sensory tract of VII, IX, and X).

6. Central Sensitization

Just as prolonged noxious stimulation of nociceptors can result in altered pain states (peripheral sensitization), repetitive stimulation of second-order (and higher) neurons can also alter pain processing (**central sensitization**). Hyperalgesia and allodynia are manifestations of central and peripheral sensitization (see section entitled Peripheral Sensitization). The ability of the neural tissue to change in response to various incoming stimuli is a key function of the nervous system and is termed **neural plasticity**. Presumably, this function has some evolutionary or protective advantage, although in clinical pain practice we often see a disadvantage—the development of chronic pain. Both short-term and long-term plastic changes occur in the dorsal horn. **Wind-up** is an increase in the ratio of outgoing to incoming action potentials of a dorsal horn neuron with each successive nociceptive stimulus. It occurs in response to repetitive C-fiber stimulation and is reversed as soon as the stimulation ceases. Wind-up is an example of a short-term plastic change. Central sensitization (including wind-up) is associated with NMDA receptor activation. In the case of persistent states of sensitization, various mechanisms are likely involved including the induction of novel patterns of gene expression.

III. SUPRASPINAL SYSTEMS: INTEGRATION AND HIGHER PROCESSING

Integration of pain in higher centers is complex and poorly understood. At a basic level, the integration and processing of painful stimuli may fall into the following broad categories:

Discriminative component: This component is somatotopically specific and involves the primary (SI) and secondary (SII) sensory cortex. This level of integration allows the brain to define the location of the painful stimulus. Integration of somatic pain, as opposed to visceral pain, takes place at this level. The primary and secondary cortices receive input predominantly from the ventrobasal complex of the thalamus, which is also somatotopically organized.

Affective component: The integration of the affective component of pain is very complex and involves various limbic structures. In particular, the cingulate cortex is involved in the affective components of pain (i.e., it receives input from the parafascicular thalamic nuclei and projects to various limbic regions). The amygdala is also involved in the integration of noxious stimuli.

Memory components of pain: Recent evidence has demonstrated that painful stimuli activate the CNS regions such as the anterior insula.

Motor control and pain: The supplemental motor area is thought to be involved in the integration of the motor response to pain.

1. Thalamus

The thalamus is a complex structure that acts as the relaying center for incoming nociceptive stimuli. Two important divisions of the thalamus receive nociceptive input. First is the **lateral division**, formed by the ventrobasal complex in which NS input from NS and WDR neurons synapses. It is somatotopically organized and projects to the somatosensory cortex. Second is the **medial division**, which consists of the posterior nucleus and the centrolateral nucleus. It is thought that these nuclei project to limbic structures involved in the affective component of pain because there is no NS information conveyed by them to higher cortical regions.

The **medial and intralaminar nuclei** receive input from many ascending tracts, particularly the STT and the reticular formation. There is little evidence of somatotopic organization of these nuclei. The **ventrobasal thalamus** is organized somatotopically and can be further subdivided into (a) the **ventral posterior lateral nucleus**, which receives input mainly from the STT and from the dorsal column system and somatosensory cortex, to which it projects, and (b) the ventral **posterior medial nucleus**, which receives input from the face via the trigeminothalamic tract and projects to the somatosensory cortical regions of the face. Input to the **posterior**

thalamus comes mainly from the STT, spinocortical tract, and dorsal column nuclei. The receptive fields are large and bilateral and lack somatotopic organization. The posterior nuclei project to the somatosensory cortex and appear to have a role in the sensory experience of pain. The STT also sends projections to the **centrolateral nucleus**, an area that is involved in motor activity.

2. Hypothalamus

The hypothalamus receives innocuous and noxious stimuli from all over the body, including deep tissues such as the viscera (see section entitled Spinohypothalamic Tract). The hypothalamic neurons are not somatotopically organized and, therefore, do not provide discriminatory aspects and localization of pain. Some hypothalamic nuclei send projections to the pituitary gland via the hypophyseal stalk, brainstem, and spinal cord. The gland regulates both the autonomic nervous system and neuroendocrine response to stress, including pain.

3. The Limbic System

The limbic system consists of subcortical regions of the telencephalon, mesencephalon, and diencephalon. It receives input from the STT, the thalamus, and the reticular formation, and it projects to various parts of the cerebral cortex, particularly the frontal and temporal cortex. The limbic system is involved in the motivational and emotional aspects of pain, including mood and experience.

4. Cerebral Cortex

The somatosensory cortex and cingulate cortex are involved in pain. The somatosensory cortex is the most important area for nociception and is located posterior to the central sulcus of the brain. It receives input from the various nuclei of the thalamus, particularly the ventral posterior lateral and medial nuclei and the posterior thalamus. The somatosensory cortex is cytoarchitecturally organized and, therefore, has an important role in the discriminatory aspect and localization of pain. Afferent fibers from the somatosensory cortex travel back to the thalamus and contribute to the descending nociceptive system.

5. The Cingulate Cortex

The cingulate cortex is a component of the limbic system. The limbic system receives sensory and cortical impulses and activates visceral and somatic effectors; it contributes to the physiologic expression of behavior and emotion. The limbic system includes the subcallosal, cingulate, and parahippocampal gyri and hippocampal formation, as well as the following subcortical nuclei: amygdala, septal nuclei, hypothalamus, anterior thalamic nuclei, and nuclei in the basal ganglia. Recent work has demonstrated that the cingulate gyrus is activated in humans by painful stimuli. Cingulate cortex lesions have been used in an attempt to alleviate pain and suffering.

IV. PAIN MODULATION

Figures 4 and 5 illustrate the pathways involved in the modulation of nociceptive information. The evidence for descending controls came from two basic observations. The first observation, in the late 1960s, was that neurons in the dorsal horn of decerebrate animals are more responsive to painful stimuli with spinal cord blockade. The second observation, in the late 1980s, was that electrical stimulation of the PAG matter profoundly relieved pain in animals. So great was the analgesia produced by the stimulation that surgery could be performed on these animals without apparent pain. Furthermore, the animals behaved normally in every other way and there was no observed effect on other sensory modalities. These studies were pivotal in demonstrating an anatomic basis for the "natural equivalent" of **stimulation-induced analgesia**. Furthermore, subsequent studies demonstrated that small concentrations of morphine, when injected into regions such as the PAG matter, produced considerable analgesia. Interestingly, both **stress-induced analgesia** and **stimulation-induced analgesia** can be reversed by opioid antagonists. There are a number of brain centers that are involved in the intrinsic modulation of noxious stimuli, including the somatosensory cortex, the hypothalamus (i.e., paraventricular nucleus and lateral hypothalamus), the midbrain PAG matter, areas in the pons including the lateral tegmental area, and the raphe magnus. Electrical stimulation of these regions in humans (some cases) and in animals produces analgesia.

Fibers from these central structures descend directly or indirectly (e.g., PAG matter to raphe magnus) via the dorsolateral funiculus to the spinal cord and send projections to laminae I and V. Activation of the descending analgesic system has a direct effect on the integration and passage of nociceptive information at the level of the dorsal horn. Blockade of the dorsolateral funiculus (with cold or sectioning) increases the response of nociceptive second-order neurons following activation by painful stimuli.

1. Descending Systems

The descending system appears to have three major functionally interrelated components: the opioid, noradrenergic, and serotonergic systems.

(i) The opioid system

The opioid system is involved in descending analgesia. Opioid precursors (i.e., proopiomelanocortin, proenkephalin, and prodynorphin) and their respective peptides (beta-endorphin, met- and leu-enkephalin, and prodynorphin) are present in the amygdala, the hypothalamus, the PAG matter, the raphe magnus, and the dorsal horn. With the recent advent of opioid receptor cloning, knowledge is steadily increasing about the action sites of the various opioids (i.e., on μ, δ, and κ receptors).

(ii) The noradrenergic system

Noradrenergic neurons project from the locus caeruleus and other noradrenergic cell groups in the medulla and pons. These projections are found in the dorsolateral funiculus. Stimulation of these areas produces analgesia, as does the administration (direct or intrathecal) of an α_2-receptor agonist such as clonidine.

(iii) The serotonergic system

Many neurons in the raphe magnus are known to contain serotonin (5-hydoxytryptamine or 5-HT), and they send projections to

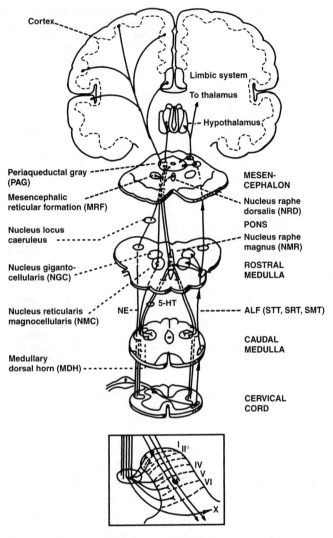

Figure 4. Descending pain pathways. 5-HT, serotonin; NE, noradrenergic input; ALF, anterolateral fasciculus; STT, spinothalamic tract; SRT, spinoreticular tract; SMT, spinomesencephalic tract. (From Bonica JJ, ed. *The management of pain*, vol. 1. Philadelphia, PA: Lea & Febiger, 1990:108, with permission.)

the spinal cord via the dorsolateral funiculus. Pharmacologic blockade, or lesioning, of the raphe magnus can reduce the effects of morphine, and administration of 5-HT to the spinal cord produces analgesia.

ASCENDING   **DESCENDING**

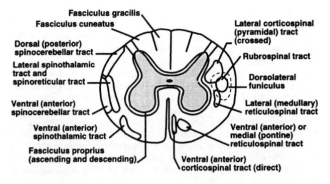

Figure 5.   Cross section of the spinal cord showing the location of the ascending pain pathways (e.g., the spinothalamic tract). The descending pain pathways are in the dorsolateral funiculus (not shown) of the spinal cord.

2. "On" and "Off" Cells: a Component of Descending Analgesia

Nociceptive cells in the dorsal horn can be activated or inhibited following stimulation of the PAG matter. Given this observation, it is reasonable to posit the existence of brain centers that provide both excitatory and inhibitory descending output. The raphe magnus, and other brain regions known to be involved in descending modulation (e.g., the PAG), appear to generate such output. Several types of neurons involved in control of nociceptive information reside in the raphe magnus; in particular, there are neurons named "on" cells and "off" cells on the basis of apparent function.

"On" cells are active before a nocifensive withdrawal reflex (e.g., tailflick). These cells are stimulated by nociceptive input; they are excited by stimulation and are inhibited by morphine. "On" cells facilitate nociceptive transmission in the dorsal horn. "Off" cells shut off before a nocifensive withdrawal reflex. These cells are inhibited by noxious stimuli; they are excited by electrical stimulation and by morphine. It has been postulated that opioids act to inhibit inhibitory interneurons (GABAergic) that act on "off" cells and, in this way, produce a net excitatory effect on these cells. These cells inhibit nociceptive transmission in the dorsal horn.

3. Projections to the Dorsal Horn

The nerve fibers that originate in nuclei that are involved in modulation of pain terminate in the dorsal horn predominately in laminae I and II and in other laminae, including IV, V, VI, and X. Therefore, there is a circuitry of projecting neurons acting directly or indirectly via interneurons on afferent fibers as well as projecting neurons such as the STT neurons.

V. CONCLUSION

The neuroanatomy and neurochemistry of the pain system are extremely complex. Unfortunately, we have only a basic understanding of the physiology of pain processing and an even more incomplete knowledge of the mechanisms through which pathology of the nervous system results in persistent hyperexcitable states. Neuroanatomic techniques have taught us a great deal about the "connectivity" of the system. New techniques have enabled the study of individual cells and specific cell populations in an attempt to elucidate roles in both ascending and descending systems. Sophisticated imaging, for example, functional magnetic resonance imaging (MRI), and positron emission tomography (PET) have allowed investigation of *in vivo* brain activity in the presence of acute and chronic pain. Therefore, fundamental neuroscientific and clinical studies hold the promise of a better understanding of the pain system in both resting and pathologic states.

SELECTED READINGS

Fields HL. *Pain: mechanisms and management*, 2nd ed. New York: McGraw-Hill, 2002.

Kruger L, ed. *Pain and touch*. San Diego, CA: Academic Press, 1996.

Scarry E. *The body in pain: the making and unmaking of the world*. Oxford, England: Oxford University Press, 1985.

Sherrington CS. *The integrative action of the nervous system*. New York: Scribner, 1906.

Simone DA. Peripheral Mechanisms of Pain Perception. In: Abram E, ed. *The atlas of anesthesia, pain management*. Philadelphia, PA: Churchill Livingston, 1998:1.1–1.11.

Waldman SD, Winnie AP, eds. Part I: anatomy and physiology of pain: clinical correlates. In: *Interventional pain management*. Philadelphia, PA: WB Saunders Company, 1996:1–72.

Wall PD, Melzack R. *Textbook of pain*. Philadelphia, PA: Churchill Livingstone, 1999.

Woolf CJ. Pain: moving from symptom control toward mechanism-specific pharmacologic management. *Ann Intern Med* 2004;140: 441–451.

Pain Mechanisms and Their Importance in Clinical Practice and Research

Isabelle Decosterd and Clifford J. Woolf

After great pain, a formal feeling comes
The Nerves sit ceremonious, like Tombs
The stiff Heart questions was it He, that bore,
And Yesterday, or Centuries before?
—*Emily Dickinson, 1830–1886*

It has become increasingly clear from animal models and from preclinical and clinical studies that multiple mechanisms operating at different sites and with different temporal profiles induce chronic pain syndromes. Identification of these mechanisms may provide the best lead to effective treatment of pain. Although primary disease factors initiate pain mechanisms, it is the molecular and structural reorganization of the pain pathways and not the disease factors that produce chronic pain. The identification of etiologic or disease/causative factors is obviously important, but it is also essential to differentiate them from pain mechanisms. Because a particular disease may activate several different distinct pain mechanisms, a disease-based classification is useful primarily for disease-modifying therapy, but less so for pain therapy. Similarly, symptoms are not equivalent to mechanisms, although they may reflect them. The same symptom may be produced by a number of different mechanisms, and a single mechanism may elicit different symptoms.

In this chapter, we propose a new way of analyzing pain on the basis of the current understanding of pain mechanisms and show its implications for assessing pain in individual patients and for evaluating new forms of diagnosis and therapy.

1. Response to Acute Painful Stimuli

Acute pain is initiated by a subset of highly specialized primary neurons, the high-threshold nociceptors, and innervating peripheral tissues (i.e., skin, muscle, bone, and viscera). The peripheral terminals of these sensory neurons are adapted so as to be activated only by intense or potentially damaging peripheral noxious stimuli. These afferents, including both unmyelinated C fibers and light-myelinated Aδ fibers, are functionally distinct from the low-threshold sensory fibers, which are normally activated only in response to nondamaging, low-intensity, innocuous stimuli (A fibers). Nociceptor transduction mechanisms involve activation of temperature ion channel transducers of the transient receptor potential (TRP) family [e.g., the heat/capsaicin vanilloid TRP type 1 (TRPV1) sensor, the heat vanilloid TRP type 2 (TRPV2) sensor, the cold/menthol sensor melastatin TRP type 8 (TRPM8), and the cold TRP ankyrin transmembrane protein 1 (TRPA1, also mentioned as ANKTM1) sensor], sodium and potassium channels sensitive to intense mechanical deformation or stretch of the membrane [e.g., mammalian degenerin channel (MDEG), K^+ channel type 1 (TREK-1)], or chemosensitive ion channels and metabotropic receptors [e.g., acid-sensing ionic channels (ASICs), TRPV1, bradykinin receptors BK1 and BK2, ATP-gated ion channel type 3 (P2X3), ATP G-protein coupled receptors type 2 (P2Y2), prostaglandin E-receptor (EP-R)] that are activated by protons, purines, amines, peptides, growth factors, prostaglandins, and cytokines released from damaged tissue or inflammatory cells. Activation of the ion channel transducers leads to inward currents in the peripheral terminal and thereby to action-potential generation, which is conducted from the periphery to the spinal cord. Invasion of the central axon terminals of primary afferents in the superficial dorsal horn by action potentials leads to an inrush of calcium and a synaptic release of the excitatory amino acid transmitter glutamate. Glutamate generates fast synaptic potentials in dorsal horn neurons via the α-amino-3 hydroxy-5 methyl-4 isoxazole proprionic acid receptor (AMPA)/kainate ionotropic receptors, and this is boosted and prolonged by the N-methyl-D-aspartate (NMDA) receptor–ion channel. These synaptic potentials encode information about the onset, intensity, quality, location, and duration of the peripheral noxious stimulus. The input is conveyed, after considerable excitatory and inhibitory processing in the dorsal horn, via projection neurons to higher centers where it is integrated in the cortex into an acute pain sensation. Such nociceptive pain (normal pain sensitivity) has an adaptive protective role, both warning of potential tissue damage and eliciting strong reflex and behavioral avoidance responses.

2. Peripheral Sensitization

The sensitivity of the peripheral terminal of nociceptors is not fixed, and its activation either by repeated peripheral stimulation or by changes in the chemical milieu of the terminal can sensitize the primary sensory neuron. This phenomenon is referred to as **peripheral sensitization**. Peripheral sensitization reflects changes both in transduction channel thresholds and kinetics and in terminal membrane excitability. These changes occur in response to the direct activation of the transduction channels, to the process of autosensitization, and to extrinsic sensitizing stimuli such as inflammatory mediators. Autosensitization of TRPV1, for instance, involves entry of calcium through the ion channel, leading to activation of protein kinase C within the cytoplasm of the peripheral terminal. Protein kinase C (PKC) in turn phosphorylates TRPV1, leading to a reduction in its threshold for activation from 43°C to 38°C. Heterosensitization is driven by sensitizing agents such as prostaglandin E_2, bradykinin, 5-HT, and nerve growth factors that activate, via their G-protein–coupled or tyrosine kinase receptors, intracellular kinases that phosphorylate and thereby augment the activity state of voltage-gated sodium channels such as Nav1.8, a sensory neuron–specific sodium channel.

3. Central Sensitization and Modulation

In addition to changes in the sensitivity of the nociceptor peripheral terminal, an augmentation of nociceptive synaptic transmission in the dorsal horn of the spinal cord occurs and contributes to increased pain sensitivity, the phenomenon of **central sensitization**.

Intense input from nociceptors to the spinal cord evokes an immediate sensation of pain that lasts for the duration of the noxious stimulus and reflects direct activation of an action-potential output in projection neurons. Such input, however, also induces an activity-dependent functional modulation of sensory processing in the dorsal horn that leads to pain hypersensitivity. This is called **central sensitization**. The increased excitability is triggered by the peripheral nociceptor input, releasing excitatory amino acid and neuropeptide neurotransmitters, which act on the spinal cord neuron postsynaptic receptors to produce synaptic currents, and to activate intracellular signal transduction cascades in these neurons. These processes include activation of several protein kinases (PKA and PKC), calcium/calmodulin-dependent protein kinase (CaMK), and the mitogen-activated protein kinases (MAPKs). Both serine/threonine and tyrosine kinases, by phosphorylating NMDA and AMPA/kainate receptors, increase membrane excitability by altering channel kinetics and by increasing insertion of receptors in the subsynaptic membrane. This boost in synaptic excitability recruits previous subthreshold inputs to the dorsal horn neurons, amplifying responses both to noxious and nonnoxious stimuli. The changes are not restricted to the activated synapse but spread to adjacent synapses and are responsible for the pain produced after peripheral injury by low-threshold afferent inputs (allodynia) as well as for the spread of pain hypersensitivity to regions beyond the site of tissue injury (secondary hyperalgesia/extraterritorial pain). Central sensitization is a major contributor to inflammatory and neuropathic pain hypersensitivity. Modulation of synaptic transmission begins immediately after intense nociceptor input as a result of ion-channel phosphorylation and the trafficking of receptors from intracellular stores to the membrane, but, in addition, a longer latent central sensitization occurs that is sustained for prolonged periods by transcriptional changes in dorsal horn neurons. After peripheral inflammation, for example, central plasticity is driven initially by input from sensitized afferents innervating the inflamed tissue and then, after several hours, is sustained by an induction of cyclooxygenase-2 (COX2) in dorsal horn neurons. This leads to a synthesis of prostaglandin E2 (PGE2) in the spinal cord, which alters presynaptic and postsynaptic excitability. The central induction of COX2 is mediated by a humoral signal originating from the peripheral inflammation, and it acts by local interleukin-1 β production in the central nervous system (CNS). After peripheral nerve injury, central sensitization is driven by the **ectopic activity** in injured fibers resulting from changes in the expression, distribution, or activity of voltage-gated ion channels. **Changes or switches in the phenotype of primary sensory neurons** contribute to these central functional changes in synaptic transmission. In addition to changes in the levels of constitutively expressed neuromodulators, novel expression also occurs so that subpopulations of dorsal root ganglion (DRG) cells that do not normally express neuromodulators, such as substance P or brain-derived neurotrophic factor (BDNF), begin to do so. For example, substance P, which is normally expressed only in nociceptors, begins to be expressed in low-threshold sensory neurons after both inflammation and nerve injury. This means that whereas central sensitization is normally evoked only by nociceptor input, after nerve injury/inflammation, input from A fibers also produces this phenomenon.

4. Disinhibition

In addition to the activity-dependent increase in membrane excitability triggered by peripheral input, a decrease in phasic and tonic inhibition can also produce changes in dorsal horn excitability. This **disinhibition** may result from a downregulation of inhibitory transmitters and from a disruption of descending inhibitory pathways. Furthermore, nerve injury, by virtue of injury discharge and ectopic activity, may lead to cell death in the superficial lamina of the dorsal horn, where inhibitory interneurons are heavily concentrated.

5. Structural Reorganization of Central Connections

After nerve injury, another anatomical change occurs, including loss of some small fiber sensory neurons and a **structural reorganization of central connections**. The reorganization involves the sprouting or growth of the central terminals of low-threshold mechanoreceptors from their normal termination site in the deep dorsal horn into lamina II, the site of termination of nociceptor C-fiber terminals. The sprouted low-threshold A fibers make synaptic contact in lamina II with neurons that normally receive nociceptor input, and this new pattern of synaptic input provides an anatomic substrate for tactile pain hypersensitivity.

6. Overview

A complex system of mechanistic changes occurs following the activation of the somatosensory pathways by both peripheral inflammatory and nerve lesions. An increase in the gain of the

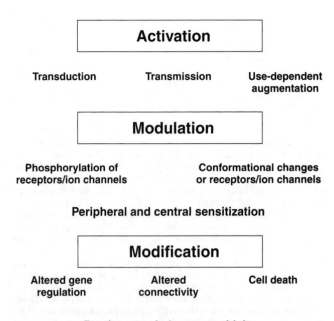

Activation

Transduction   Transmission   Use-dependent
                                                augmentation

Modulation

Phosphorylation of   Conformational changes
receptors/ion channels   or receptors/ion channels

Peripheral and central sensitization

Modification

Altered gene   Altered   Cell death
regulation   connectivity

Persistent pain hypersensitivity

Figure 1. Summary of the three forms of neural plasticity that can
produce pain hypersensitivity, highlighting the molecular and cellular
changes implicated in pain mechanisms. (From Woolf CJ, Salter MW.
Neuronal plasticity: increasing the gain in pain. *Science*
2000;288:1765–1769, with permission.)

nociceptive system, in the periphery and in the CNS, is due to
activity-dependant plasticity and manifests as a widely distributed but transient pain hypersensitivity. With time, the changes
evolve so that a number of different mechanisms that can induce
pain hypersensitivity are recruited. Three different forms (i.e.,
activation, modulation, and modification) of neural plasticity
that produce pain hypersensitivity are summarized in Figure 1.
Activation is directly linked to noxious stimuli and involves
transduction and transmission of the signal. Modulation involves
peripheral and central sensitization. Modification of the system
includes changes in gene regulation, altered connectivity, and
cell death. Persistent pain states may be associated with those
mechanisms where changes are irreversible.

II. TOWARD A NEW CONCEPTUAL APPROACH FOR THE UNDERSTANDING OF PAIN

The current clinical evaluation of pain uses an etiologic or
disease-based approach. We advocate that this approach be modified to incorporate a mechanism-based diagnosis of pain. There
is no doubt that identifying the causative disease is essential,
particularly where disease-modifying treatment is required. But

in most patients with persistent pain, the disease or pathology cannot be treated, and the injury is not reversible. In such cases, it is helpful to consider pain as the disease and to attempt to identify the mechanisms responsible for the pain rather than categorizing the patient primarily on the basis of underlying disease or the symptoms they complain of.

Given that the mechanisms operating to produce pain in normal and pathologic conditions are better understood, it is now appropriate to assess how such mechanisms fit into the overall schema of pain production and treatment. The basal pain sensitivity of an individual represents the pain experienced either spontaneously (i.e., in the absence of any identifiable stimulus) or evoked directly by, and within a short period of, a defined stimulus. In normal situations there is no spontaneous or background pain, and pain is elicited only by intense or noxious stimuli. The amplitude of the pain, beyond a clear threshold level, is determined by the intensity of the stimulus, and the localization and timing of the sensation reflect the site and duration of the stimulus. This situation constitutes a state of pain **normosensitivity**. This state is distinct from pain **hypersensitivity**, in which pain may arise spontaneously, apparently in the absence of any peripheral stimulus, or the response to noxious stimuli is exaggerated (**hyperalgesia**), may persist, radiate, or become excessively amplified (**hyperpathia**) and normally innocuous stimuli may begin to produce pain (**allodynia**). Normosensitivity is also distinct from pain **hyposensitivity**, in which pain sensitivity is reduced and suprathreshold noxious stimuli fail to elicit any pain response.

The aim of a mechanism-based approach is to first evaluate basal pain sensitivity by eliciting key aspects of the nature of the patient's symptoms. Figure 2 shows how basal pain sensitivity can be qualitatively assessed by selectively eliciting the nature of symptoms. This assessment can be accomplished using a relatively brief, semi directed interview (together with simple sensory testing to evoke symptoms) designed specifically to establish if the patient has normo-, hypo-, or hyper-basal pain sensitivity, and the extent to which the pain is spontaneous or evoked. The goal of the assessment is to characterize the clusters of symptoms, their onset and evolution, and to identify, where possible, the mechanisms responsible for the symptoms. Careful questioning, rather than the usual global assessments, will produce a new sort of clinical pain record based on the nature of the reported pain to supplement the standard history and physical. The approach may be adopted to aid treatment selection, where treatment efficacy correlates with pain mechanisms (see Section IV).

III. IMPLICATIONS FOR THERAPEUTIC APPROACHES

The conventional assessment of pain syndromes includes the causative disease, anatomical referral pattern of the pain, and a quantitative global evaluation [such as the visual analog scale (VAS)]. This approach groups patients into categories or syndromes such as neuropathic pain, headache, osteoarthritic pain, or cancer pain. Contemporary preclinical basic science has successfully elucidated the molecular mechanisms of action of current analgesics [i.e., opiates, nonsteroidal antiinflammatory drugs (NSAIDs),

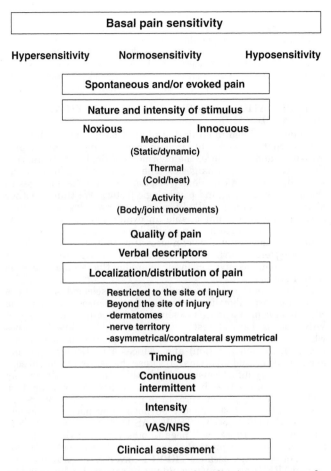

Figure 2. Canvas for an interview-based qualitative assessment of pain. (From Woolf CJ, Decosterd I. Implications for recent advances in the understanding of pain pathophysiology for the assessment of pain in patients. *Pain* 1999;6:S141–S147, with permission.)

and sodium-channel blockers] and their effect on pain mechanisms. Yet there is an extremely poor correlation between the efficacy of such analgesics and pain syndromes in clinical practice. The increasingly popular measure of the number needed to treat (NNT) is an efficacy index representing the number of patients needed to treat with a certain drug to obtain one patient with a defined degree (e.g., 50%) of pain relief. The NNT has been studied in different pain categories and is a good example of the lack of specificity and predictive value of the current pain classifications. The NNT measure of efficacy does not reveal any consistent differences across different pain conditions for different drug classes observed.

The goal of a mechanism-based assessment of pain is to provide a classification in which the categorization of patients into mechanism-based subpopulations of patients will aid the rational treatment of pain. We believe that breaking down pain into components that reflect some of the major different mechanisms may help identify how and why certain treatments work and may reveal useful correlations between pain mechanisms and treatments.

IV. IMPLICATIONS FOR EVALUATION OF EFFICACY OF NEW THERAPIES

A major problem in clinical studies of pain is the high intra- and interpatient variability in pain scoring using global outcome measures and, therefore, the enormous difficulty in evaluating the efficacy of novel analgesics. The usual explanations for the variability are the complexity of pain mechanisms, changes in the primary disease, and psychologic factors. We think another approach is therefore called for, one that provides new clinical outcome measures that enable an evaluation of whether new analgesics have an action on particular pain mechanisms. In rodent experimental models of neuropathic pain, the analgesic response differs in a manner that correlates with the different pain mechanisms involved, and we predict that similar patterns occur in patients.

If a new therapy is provided to patients selected only on the basis of a particular disease (e.g., diabetic neuropathy), and the clinical outcome measure is a simple global pain measure (e.g., a VAS score of pain at rest), it is simply not possible to assess whether or not the treatment acts on a particular mechanism (e.g., central sensitization) and reduces a particular symptom (e.g., tactile or cold allodynia). Because the degree of central sensitization may differ considerably in this cohort of patients, any treatment that acts only on central sensitization will produce highly varied responses across the population. Once drugs are available that act specifically on novel pharmacologic targets such as the DRG-specific TRPV1, ASIC, Nav1.8 receptors and ion channels, patients will need to be selected on the basis of a reasonable assessment that their pain involves one of these targets. For example, because TRPV1 is involved in encoding heat pain, a TRPV1 antagonist would not be expected to have any effect on a patient with tactile allodynia. The selection of patients based on current categories, because they are not mechanism-based, is likely to include patients with quite different mechanisms, only one of which may respond to a mechanism-specific drug treatment. In this case, patient nonresponders may produce a false-negative result by diluting out the benefit in a subgroup with the targeted mechanism.

V. CONCLUSION

In the past decade, neurobiologic research has enormously increased our knowledge of the fundamental mechanisms responsible for producing chronic pain. On the other hand, changes in clinical pain management have been slow. The challenge now is to bridge the gap between basic research and clinical practice by utilizing new inputs from basic science for the classification, assessment, diagnosis, and treatment of pain.

SELECTED READINGS

Decosterd I, Allchrone AJ, Woolf CJ. Differential analgesic sensitivity of two distinct neuropathic pain models. *Anesth Analg* 2004;99: 457–463.

Jordt SE, McKemy DD, Julius D. Lessons from peppers and peppermint: the molecular logic of thermosensation. *Curr Opin Neurobiol* 2003;13:487–492.

Siddall PJ, Cousins MJ. Persistent pain as a disease entity: implications for clinical management. *Anesth Analg* 2004;99:510–520.

Sindrup SH, Jensen TS. Efficacy of pharmacological treatments of neuropathic pain: an update and effect related to mechanism of drug action. *Pain* 1999;83:389–400.

Scholz J, Woolf CJ. Can we conquer pain? *Nat Neurosci* 2002; (Suppl. 5): 1062–1067.

Woolf CJ, Decosterd I. Implication for recent advances in the understanding of pain pathophysiology for the assessment of pain in patients. *Pain* 1999;6:S141–S147.

Woolf CJ, Salter MW. Neuronal plasticity: increasing the gain in pain. *Science* 2000;288:1765–1769.

The Placebo Effect

Eija Kalso

Placebo Domino in regione vivorum.
—*Psalm 116:9*

I. THE POWERFUL PLACEBO

Patrick D. Wall writes about the placebo response in *Textbook of Pain*. He argues that the word *placebo* alludes to Psalm 116:9: "*Placebo Domino in regione vivorum*," which is the first line of the vespers for the dead. Priests and friars harassed the people for money to sing vespers for the dead. Placebo was an expression of contempt for the unpopular and expensive prayers, as Francis Bacon writes in 1625: "Instead of giving Free Counsell sing him song of placebo." Three years later, Burton writes in *Anatomy of Melancholy*, "An empiric oftentimes, or a silly chirurgeon, doth more strange cures than a rational physician because the patient puts more confidence in him." Now, nearly four hundred years later, the placebo response is still used in medicine and the mechanisms of this phenomenon are beginning to be understood.

The first chairperson of the department of anesthesia at the Massachusetts General Hospital, Henry Beecher, published his classic study, "The Powerful Placebo," in 1955. In that communication, he surmised that patients' expectations of benefit were sufficient to achieve therapeutic benefit. He also suggested that the overall analgesic effect of morphine is composed of its drug effect plus a placebo effect. Some fifty years later, with help from modern imaging technology, research has been able to provide evidence to support Beecher's hypothesis and to suggest a neurobiologic mechanism for the phenomenon. Recent research has also shown that the placebo effect is far from nonspecific. Depending on the condition, the placebo effect can be highly targeted and somatotopically organized.

II. MECHANISMS OF PLACEBO ANALGESIA

1. Cognitive Theory

The cognitive theory states that the expectations of patients play an important role in the placebo response. A patient's expectation is one of the best predictors of outcome in pain management. In 1978, Levine et al. suggested that placebo analgesia could be at least partially mediated by endogenous opioids because the effect was inhibited by the opioid antagonist naloxone. Later, it was suggested that expectation of pain relief could trigger the release of endogenous opioids in the central nervous system (CNS).

2. Conditioning Theory

The conditioning theory states that learning through association is important in the placebo response. Further, the conditioning theory proposes that the placebo response is a conditioned response that can be elicited by stimuli that produce a reduction in symptoms through prior conditioning. It has been suggested that a classical conditioning response operates in the placebo response. Ivan Pavlov first described the classical conditioning response in dogs. He reported that dogs that were given morphine in a certain experimental chamber displayed morphinelike effects when placed again in the same chamber although morphine was not available. Repeated associations between active analgesics, pain relief, and the therapeutic environment can produce a conditioned placebo analgesic response.

3. Endogenous Opioids

As already stated, endogenous opioids may be at least partially responsible for placebo analgesia because naloxone, an opioid antagonist, has been shown in studies to reverse placebo analgesia. Amanzio and Benedetti studied the expectation-activated and the conditioning-activated systems in opioid analgesia in an elegant set of experiments. They used the human experimental model of ischemic pain and evoked placebo analgesic responses with cognitive expectation cues, with drug conditioning (morphine or ketorolac), and with cues and drug conditioning combined. Expectation cues produced placebo responses that were completely blocked by the opioid antagonist naloxone. Expectation cues together with morphine conditioning produced placebo responses that were completely antagonized by naloxone. Morphine conditioning in the absence of expectation cues elicited a naloxone-reversible placebo effect. However, the placebo effect elicited by ketorolac conditioning with expectation cues was only partially blocked by naloxone. Ketorolac conditioning alone with no expectation cues produced placebo responses that were naloxone insensitive. The authors concluded that expectation triggers the release of endogenous opioids, whereas conditioning activates specific subsystems. If conditioning is performed specifically with opioids, the conditioning part of the placebo analgesia is mediated by endogenous opioids.

The role of endogenous opioids in placebo analgesia was recently examined with positron emission tomography (PET). Healthy volunteers were exposed to noxious and nonnoxious heat stimuli in the presence of no treatment, saline, or remifentanil, a potent short-acting opioid. The volunteers rated the pain intensity while in a PET camera. They were told that a new, strong analgesic was being compared with an opioid. The results of the study showed that both opioid and placebo analgesia activated a similar neural circuit, including the rostral part of the anterior cingulate cortex, prefrontal cortex, and brainstem, areas that are involved in the modulation of pain. The study also suggested that the high interindividual variation in placebo response might be related to an individual's capacity to activate this network. Interestingly, those individuals who had a good placebo response also showed stronger activations in this network during remifentanil analgesia.

4. Dopamine

Dopamine has also been suggested to mediate expectation-related placebo effects. A study of patients with Parkinson disease using PET and $[^{11}C]$ raclopride binding showed that the placebo-induced release of endogenous dopamine correlated with symptom relief. The magnitude of response of dopamine was comparable to that of therapeutic doses of levodopa. In this study, the release of endogenous dopamine could be due to either expectation or conditioning, or both.

5. Somatotopic Organization

In 1999, Benedetti et al. further explored the role of the opioid system in target-directed expectations of analgesia. They stimulated both the feet and the hands with subcutaneous capsaicin. Specific expectation of analgesia were induced by applying a placebo cream on one of these body parts and by letting the subject expect that this was a powerful local anesthetic. The results suggested that a highly organized and somatotopic network of endogenous opioids linked expectation, attention, and body schema.

6. Therapist–Patient Interaction

The placebo response can be augmented by a good physician–patient interaction. The physician's expectations and the patient's perception of these expectations have also been shown to influence the placebo effect.

III. THE PLACEBO EFFECT AND CLINICAL RESEARCH

The control group in a clinical trial should tell us what would have happened to the patients had they had no treatment; that is, what is the natural course of the disease and/or how the new treatment compares with an established treatment, should there be one? Several important factors operate in the control group. Some of them are shown in Table 1. It was Henry Beecher who first suggested, in 1955, that the therapeutic benefit of placebo effects could not be ignored in clinical trials. He suggested adding a placebo group so that the possible placebo component of experimental or control treatments could be compared to the placebo

Table 1. Sum of effects in the control group

1. Waiting list = natural course – negativity because nothing is being done
2. Visits without treatment = natural course + doctor/nurse and patient interaction
3. Placebo treatment = natural course + interaction + expectation that there will be an effect
4. Active control = natural course + interaction + expectation + actual effect

(simulated treatment) and to no treatment, thereby improving the sensitivity of the trial. The use of placebos in clinical trials quickly became standard. The blanket inclusion of a placebo group in all trials has recently been questioned, partly on ethical grounds, and on the grounds that there is possibly no significant placebo effect, except in the case of analgesic trials. What problems would be caused by the omission of the placebo group in analgesic trials? The new analgesic could be compared with a standard analgesic such as morphine or acetaminophen. At the end of the study, the statistics would probably indicate that the treatments are equally effective. Could one argue that the new drug is equally effective as morphine? Yes, one could, but the counterargument would be that the study was unable to detect any difference. The importance of including a placebo treatment arm is to show whether the study is sensitive, that is, whether it can demonstrate a difference between two treatments, should there be one.

In an analysis of 12,000 patients in acute postoperative pain of at least moderate severity, the mean percentage of patients who achieved at least 50% pain relief with placebo was 18%. In studies of topical nonsteroidal analgesics for strains and sprains, 50% pain relief was achieved with 40% of the patients receiving placebo. This high placebo response rate may reflect the high recovery rate for this condition.

In studies on chronic pain, the fraction of placebo responders (at least 50% pain relief) has varied from 18% to 36%. The response rate with placebo is lower if the outcome is harder to achieve, for instance, free of pain at 2 hours after treatment of migraine compared with moderate to severe pain that is reduced to no pain or mild pain.

Crossover studies can be particularly challenging about the placebo response because the order of treatment can make a considerable difference. A good example is a double-blind crossover study by Moulin et al., in which oral morphine was compared with placebo for treatment of musculoskeletal pain. When morphine was given as the second treatment following a 6-week treatment with an active placebo (benztropine), the patients had no appreciable effect with morphine, whereas the analgesic effect was clear when morphine was given as the first treatment. Similarly, Laska and Sunshine reported that previous analgesic experience predicted the efficacy of placebo. They showed that the patients who had received a high-strength analgesic thought that the placebo was much more effective than did the patients who had received a lower-strength analgesic before the placebo.

IV. NOCEBO

In the placebo treatment arm, the patients often report adverse effects similar to those in the active treatment arm. Such adverse placebo effects have been termed **nocebo** effects. The cognitive and conditioning mechanisms that operate in the nocebo response are similar to those in the placebo response. It is important to take this into consideration when designing clinical trials. Patient information and focused questions about adverse effects may affect the results. It is also noteworthy that patients often experience symptoms such as feeling tired, sweating, and constipation at baseline before the study has started. To enhance true blinding, active placebos are sometimes used. An active placebo simulates the active study drug through adverse effects but has no specific action on the condition being treated.

V. THE PLACEBO EFFECT IN THE CLINIC

Recent research has shown that placebo analgesia has a neurophysiologic basis and that individuals show considerable variation in the placebo response. Therefore, it is obvious that a placebo cannot be used to test whether the patient has "real" pain on not. A placebo medication cannot be used as an alternative treatment to analgesic drugs. However, the mechanisms that have been shown to operate in placebo analgesia, particularly the therapist–patient interaction, can be used to improve the effectiveness of evidence-based therapies. The importance of the therapist–patient interaction has been recognized for a long time, but its neurobiologic basis is now better understood. If caregivers use methods that are effective, that they believe in, and if they convey this conviction to the patient, the therapy will be more effective than that provided by skeptics!

VI. CONCLUSION

The last few years have taught us much about the neurobiologic mechanisms of the placebo effect. This information is essential for the future design of clinical trials in pain management. Understanding the placebo effect has also helped us appreciate the role of the therapeutic interaction in everyday clinical management of pain.

SELECTED READINGS

Amanzio M, Benedetti F. Neuropharmacological dissection of placebo analgesia: expectation-activation opioid systems versus conditioning-activated specific subsystems. *J Neurosci* 1999;19:484–494.

Beecher HK. The powerful placebo. *JAMA* 1955;159:1602–1606.

Benedetti F, Arduino C, Amanzio M. Somatotopic activation of opioid systems by target-directed expectations of analgesia. *J Neurosci* 1999;19:3639–3648.

Benedetti F, Pollo A, Lopiano L, et al. Conscious expectation and unconscious conditioning in analgesic, motor, and hormonal placebo/nocebo responses. *J Neurosci* 2003;23:4315–4323.

Fields HL, Price DD. Toward a neurobiology of placebo analgesia. In: Harrington A, ed. *The placebo effect: an interdisciplinary exploration.* Cambridge, MA: Harvard UP, 1997:93–116.

Hrobjartsson A, Gotzsche PC. Is the placebo powerless: an analysis of clinical trials comparing placebo with no treatment. *N Engl J Med* 2001;344:1594–1602.

Kalso E, Moore RA. Five easy pieces on evidence-based medicine (2): Why randomized and (placebo) controlled? *Eur J Pain* 2000;4:321–324.

Laska E, Sunshine A. Anticipation of analgesia: a placebo effect. *Headache* 1973;13:1–11.

Levine JD, Gordon NC, Fields HL. The mechanisms of placebo analgesia. *Lancet* 1978;2:654–657.

Moulin DE, Iezzi A, Amireh R, et al. Randomised trial of oral morphine for chronic non-cancer pain. *Lancet* 1996;347:143–147.

Pavlov I. *Conditioned reflexes.* London, England: Oxford Press, 1927.

Petrovic P, Kalso E, Petersson KM, et al. Placebo and opioid analgesia–Imaging a shared neuronal network. *Science* 2002;295:1737–1740.

Turner JA, Deyo RA, Loeser JD, et al. The importance of placebo effects in pain treatment and research. *JAMA* 1994;271:1609–1614.

Wall PD. The placebo and the placebo response. In: Wall P, Melzack R, eds. *Textbook of pain.* Edinburgh: Churchill Livingstone, 1999: 1419–1430.

Diagnosis of Pain

The History and Clinical Examination

Jan Slezak and Asteghik Hacobian

To each his suff'rings; all are men,
Condemn'd alike to groan;
The tender for another's pain,
Th' unfeeling for his own.
—*Thomas Gray, 1716–1771*

The key to accurate diagnosis is a comprehensive history and detailed physical examination. Combined with a review of the patient's previous records and diagnostic studies, the findings from these steps lead to a differential diagnosis and appropriate treatment. In pain medicine, most patients have seen multiple providers, have had various diagnostic tests and unsuccessful treatments, and are finally referred to the pain clinic as a last resort. With advances in research and better education of primary care providers, this trend is beginning to change, and more patients are being referred to pain management specialists at an earlier stage, with better outcomes as a result.

I. PATIENT INTERVIEW

1. Pain History

(i) Development and Timing

The pain history should reveal the pain location, time of onset, intensity, character, associated symptoms, and factors aggravating and relieving the pain.

It is important to know when and how the pain started. The pain onset should be described and recorded (e.g., sudden, gradual, or rapid). If the pain started gradually, identifying an exact time of onset may be difficult. In the case of a clear inciting event, the date and circumstances of the pain onset may help determine its cause. The condition of the patient at the onset of pain should be noted if possible. In cases of injuries from motor vehicle crashes or work-related injuries, the state of the patient before and at the time of the injury should be clearly understood and documented.

The time of onset of the pain can be important. If the pain event is of short duration, as in acute pain, the treatment should cause has usually resolved and the treatment should focus on optimal long-term pain management.

(ii) Intensity

The various methods used to measure pain intensity are described in Chapter 6. Because the complaint of pain is purely subjective, it can only be compared to the individual's own pain over a period; it cannot be compared to another individual's report of pain. Several scales are used for reporting the so-called level of pain. The most commonly used scale is the visual analog scale (VAS) of pain intensity. Patients using this scale are instructed to place a marker on a 100-mm continuous line between "no pain" and "worst pain imaginable." The mark is measured using a standard ruler and recorded as a numeric value between 0 and 100. An alternative method of reporting the intensity of pain is by using a verbal numeric rating scale. The patient directly assigns a number between 0 (no pain) and 10 (the worst pain imaginable). The verbal numeric rating scale is frequently used in clinical practice. Another commonly used method is a verbal categoric scale, with intensity ranging from no pain through mild, moderate, and severe to the worst possible pain.

(iii) Character

The patient's description of the character of pain is quite helpful in distinguishing between the different types of pain. For example, burning or "electric shocks" often describe neuropathic pain, whereas cramping usually represents nociceptive visceral pain (e.g., spasm, stenosis, or obstruction). Pain described as throbbing or pounding suggests vascular involvement.

(iv) Evolution

The pattern of pain spread from the onset should also be noted. Some types of pain change location or spread farther out from the original area of insult or injury. The direction of the spread also provides important clues to the etiology and, ultimately, the diagnosis and treatment of the condition. An example of this is the complex regional pain syndrome (CRPS), which can start in a limited area such as a distal extremity and then spread proximally and, in some instances, even to the contralateral side.

(v) Associated Symptoms

The examiner should ask about the presence of associated symptoms, including numbness, weakness, bowel and/or bladder dysfunction, edema, cold sensation, and/or loss of use of the extremity because of pain.

(vi) Aggravating and Relieving Factors

Aggravating factors should be elicited because they sometimes explain the pathophysiologic mechanisms of pain. Various stimuli can exacerbate pain. Exacerbating mechanical factors such as different positions or activities such as sitting, standing, walking, bending, and lifting may help differentiate one cause of pain from another. Biochemical changes (e.g., glucose and electrolyte levels and hormonal imbalance), psychological factors (e.g., depression, stress, and other emotional problems), and environmental triggers (e.g., dietary influences and weather changes, including barometric pressure changes) may surface as important diagnostic clues. Relieving factors are also important. Certain positions will alleviate pain better than others (e.g., in most cases of neurogenic claudication, sitting is a relieving factor, whereas standing or walking worsens the pain). Pharmacologic therapies and "nerve blocks" help the clinician determine the diagnosis and select the appropriate treatment.

(vii) Previous Treatment
The patient should be asked about previous treatment attempts. Knowing the degree of pain relief, the duration of treatment, and the dosages and adverse reactions of medications helps avoid repeating procedures or using pharmacologic management that has not helped in the past. The list should include all treatment modalities, including physical therapy, occupational therapy, chiropractic manipulation, acupuncture, psychological interventions, and visits to other pain clinics.

2. Medical History

(i) Review of Systems
A review of systems is an integral part of comprehensive evaluation for chronic and acute pain. Some systems could be directly or indirectly related to the patient's presenting symptoms, whereas others are important in the management or treatment of the painful condition. Examples are the patient with a history of bleeding problems, who may not be a suitable candidate for certain injection therapies; or someone with impaired renal or hepatic function who may need adjustments in their medication dosage.

(ii) Past Medical History
Past medical problems, including conditions that have resolved, should be reviewed. Previous trauma and any past or present psychological or behavioral issues should be recorded.

(iii) Past Surgical History
A list of operations and complications should be made, preferably in chronologic order. Because some painful chronic conditions are sequelae of surgical procedures, this information is important for diagnosis and management.

3. Drug History

(i) Current Medications
The practitioner must prescribe and intervene on the basis of medications the patient is currently taking because complications, interactions, and side effects need to be taken into account. A list should be made of medications, including pain medications. The list should include nonprescription and alternative medications (e.g., acetaminophen, aspirin, ibuprofen, and vitamins).

(ii) Allergies
Allergies, both to medications and nonmedications (e.g., latex, food, and environmental factors), should be noted. The nature of

a specific allergic reaction with each medication or agent should be clearly explored and documented.

4. Social History

(i) General Social History

Understanding the patient's social structure, support systems, and motivation is essential in analyzing psychosocial factors. Whether a patient is married, has children, and works makes a difference. Level of education, job satisfaction, and general attitude toward life are important. Smoking and a history of drug or alcohol abuse are important in evaluating and designing treatment strategies. Lifestyle questions about how much time is taken for vacation or is spent in front of a television, favorite recreations and hobbies, exercise, and sleep give the practitioner a more comprehensive overview of the patient.

(ii) Family History

A complete family history, including health status of the patient's parents, siblings, and offspring, offers important clues for understanding a patient's biologic and genetic profile. The existence of unusual diseases should be noted. A history of chronic pain, substance abuse, and disability in family members (including the spouse) should be ascertained. Even clues that have no direct genetic or biologic basis may help by revealing coping mechanisms and codependent behavior.

(iii) Occupational History

The highest level of education completed by the patient and the degrees obtained should be identified. The specifics of the present job and previous employment should be noted. The amount of time spent in each job, reasons for leaving, any previous history of litigation, job satisfaction, and whether the patient works full-time or part-time are important in establishing the occupational framework. Whether the patient has undergone disability evaluation, functional capacity assessment, or vocational rehabilitation is also relevant.

II. PATIENT EXAMINATION

The clinical examination is a fundamental and valuable diagnostic tool. Over the past few decades, advances in medicine and technology and a better understanding of the pathophysiology of pain have dramatically improved the evaluation process. The lack of exact diagnosis in most patients presenting to the pain clinic underscores the need for detail-oriented examinations.

Improper coding and inadequate documentation to support charges billed to Medicare for evaluation and management services incur various sanctions. Complying with regulations using appropriate documentation will not only result in higher reimbursement but also provide protection against fraud and abuse. The level of evaluation and management services that can be coded depends on the complexity of examination, which in turn reflects the nature of the presenting problem and the clinical judgment of the provider. Types of examinations include either general multisystem (ten organ systems—musculoskeletal, nervous, cardiovascular, respiratory, ear/nose/mouth/throat, eyes, genitourinary, hematologic/lymphatic/immune, psychiatric, and integumentary) or single-organ-system examinations. In pain medicine, the most commonly examined systems are the musculoskeletal and nervous systems.

If interventional pain management is part of a diagnostic or therapeutic plan, the evaluation should reveal whether the patient has risk factors for the procedure being considered. Coagulopathy, untreated infection, and preexisting neurologic dysfunction should be documented before placement of the needle or the catheter, or before implantation of a device. Extra caution is needed when administering medications such as (a) local anesthetics to a patient with seizure disorder, (b) neuraxial anesthetics to a patient who may tolerate vasodilatation poorly, or (c) administration of glucocorticoids to patients with diabetes. Preanesthetic evaluation should assess the patient's ability to tolerate sedation or anesthesia if indicated for a procedure.

The following sections outline a physical examination that incorporates the musculoskeletal and neurologic assessments relevant to pain practice. The examination starts with the evaluation of single systems and commonly proceeds from head to toe.

1. General Examination

(i) Constitutional Factors

Height, weight, and vital signs (i.e., blood pressure, heart rate, respiratory rate, body temperature, and pain level) should be measured and recorded. Appearance, development, deformities, nutrition, and grooming are noted. The room should be scanned for the presence of assistive devices brought by the patient. Patients who smoke or drink heavily may carry an odor. Observing a patient who is unaware of being watched may detect discrepancies that were not seen during the evaluation.

(ii) Pain Behavior

Note facial expression, color, and grimacing. Speech patterns suggest emotional factors as well as intoxication with alcohol, and with prescription or nonprescription drugs. Some patients attempt to convince the practitioner that they are suffering a great deal of pain by augmenting their verbal presentation with grunting, moaning, twitching, grabbing the painful area, exaggerating the antalgic gait or posture, or tightening muscle groups. This, unfortunately, makes the objective examination more difficult.

(iii) Skin

Evaluate for color, temperature, rash, and soft tissue edema. Trophic changes of skin, nails, and hair are frequently seen in advanced stages of complex regional pain syndrome. In patients with diabetes, vascular disease, and peripheral neuropathy, search for defects that might be a chronic source of bacteremia requiring treatment before hardware implantation (i.e., spinal cord stimulator or an infusion pump device).

2. Systems Examination

(i) Cardiovascular System

A systolic murmur with propagation suggests aortic stenosis, and the patient may not tolerate the hypovolemia and tachycardia that accompany rapid vasodilatation (e.g., after administration of neuraxial local anesthetics and sympathetic or celiac plexus blockade). The patient with irregular rhythm may have atrial fibrillation and may be treated with anticoagulants. The pulsation of arteries (diabetes, complex regional pain syndrome, and thoracic outlet syndrome), venous filling, presence of varicosities and capillary return must be checked. Vascular claudication must be distinguished from neurogenic claudication in patients referred with a diagnosis of lumbar spinal stenosis. Growth in utilization of interventional cardiology procedures, such as coronary artery stenting, has increased the population of younger patients on new antiplatelet agents.

(ii) Lungs

Examination of lungs may reveal abnormal breath sounds such as crackles, which may be a sign of congestive heart failure and low cardiac reserve. Rhonchi and wheezes are signs of chronic obstructive pulmonary disease. Caution in performing blocks around chest cavity is advised because there is an increased risk of causing pneumothorax.

(iii) Musculoskeletal System

The musculoskeletal system examination includes inspection of gait and posture. Deformities and deviation from symmetry are observed. After taking the history, the examiner usually has an idea about the body part from which the symptoms originate. If this is not the case, a brief survey of structures in the relevant region might be necessary. Positive tests warrant further and more rigorous evaluation of the affected segment. Palpation of soft tissues, bony structures, and stationary or moving joints may reveal temperature differences, presence of edema, fluid collections, gaps, crepitus, clicks, and tenderness. Functional comparison of left and right side, checking for normal curvature of the spine, and provocation of usual symptoms with maneuvers can help identify the mechanisms and location of the pathologic process. Examination of the range of motion may demonstrate hyper or hypomobility of the joint. Testing active movement will determine range, muscle strength, and willingness of the patient to cooperate. Passive movements, on the other hand, when performed properly, test for pain, range, and end-feel. Most difficulties arise when examining patients who are in constant pain, because these patients tend to respond to most maneuvers positively, therefore making the specificity of tests low.

Specific Tests

- **Straight Leg Raising (SLR, Lasègue):** SLR tests the mobility of dura and dural sleeves from L4 to S2. The sensitivity of this test to diagnose lumbar disc herniation ranges between 0.6 and 0.97, with a specificity of 0.1 to 0.6. Tension on the sciatic nerve begins at 15 to 30 degrees elevation in supine position. This puts traction on the nerve roots L4 to S2 and on the dura. End of range is normally restricted by hamstring muscle tension at 60 to 120 degrees. More than 60 degrees of elevation causes movement in the sacroiliac joint and, therefore, may be painful in sacroiliac joint disorders.

- **Basic sacroiliac tests** causing pain in the buttock: Sacroiliac tests are performed to determine when pain occurs in the buttock.

  (a) Pushing the ilia outward and downward in supine position, with the examiner's arms crossed. If gluteal pain results, the test is repeated with the patient's forearm placed under lumbar spine to stabilize the lumbar joints.

  (b) Forcibly compressing ilia to the midline with the patient lying on the painless side stretches posterior sacroiliac ligaments.

  (c) Exert forward pressure on the center of the sacrum in a prone position.

  (d) Patrick or FABER test (pain due to ligamentous strain)— Flexion, Abduction, and External Rotation of femur in the hip joint while holding down the anterior superior iliac spine on the contralateral side provides stretching of the anterior sacroiliac ligament.

  (e) Force lateral rotation in the hip joint with the knee held in 90-degree flexion in a supine position.

- **Spinal flexibility:** Spinal flexion, extension, lateral bending, and rotation may be limited and/or painful in zygoapophyseal joint, discogenic, muscular, and ligamentous pain.

- **Adson test:** Adson test has been advocated for diagnosis of thoracic outlet syndrome. The examiner evaluates the change of radial artery pulsation in a standing patient with arms resting at the side. Ipsilateral head rotation during inspiration may cause vascular compression by the anterior scalene muscle. During *modified Adson test,* the patient's head is rotated to the contralateral side. Pulse change suggests compression by the middle scalene muscle. Both tests are considered unreliable by some because the findings may be found positive in approximately 50% of the healthy population.

- **Tinel test:** Tinel test involves percussion of the carpal tunnel. If positive, it gives rise to distal paresthesiae. It can be performed at other locations (e.g., cubital or tarsal tunnel), where it might be suggestive of nerve entrapment. **Phalen test** is positive for carpal tunnel syndrome when a passive flexion in the wrist for 1 minute followed by sudden extension results in sensation of paresthesiae.

(iv) Neurologic Examination

Table 1 summarizes localization of cervical and lumbar radicular nerves.

The **motor system** evaluation starts with observation of **muscle** bulk, tone, and presence of spasm. Muscle strength is tested in upper and lower extremities. Weakness might be caused by un-willingness of the patient to cooperate, fear of pain provocation, poor effort, reflex neural inhibition in the painful limb, or an or-ganic lesion. Further information is obtained by examination of **deep tendon reflexes**, clonus, and pathologic reflexes such as the Babinski. Evaluation of **coordination** and fine motor skills may reveal associated dysfunction.

The integrity of **cranial nerve function** is tested by the ex-amination of visual fields, pupils and eye movement, facial sen-sation, facial symmetry and strength, hearing (e.g., use tuning fork, whisper voice, or finger rub), spontaneous and reflex palate movement, and tongue protrusion.

Sensation is tested to light touch (Aβ fibers), pinprick (Aδ fibers), and hot and cold stimuli (Aδ and C fibers). Tactile sensa-tion can be evaluated quantitatively with von Frey filaments. We have found the sharp end of a broken sterile wooden cotton-tipped swab to be a convenient and safe tool for testing sensation to pinprick. The following are often observed in neuropathic pain conditions:

- **Hyperesthesia**—increased sensitivity to stimulation, ex-cluding the special senses
- **Dysesthesia**—an unpleasant abnormal sensation, either spontaneous or evoked
- **Allodynia**—pain caused by stimulus that normally does not provoke pain
- **Hyperalgesia**—an increased response to a stimulus that is normally painful
- **Hyperpathia**—a painful syndrome characterized by an ab-normally painful reaction to stimulus (especially a repetitive one), and an increased threshold
- **Summation**—a repetitive pinprick stimulus applied in in-tervals of more than 3 seconds, with a gradually increasing sensation of pain with each subsequent stimulus

(v) Mental Status Examination

The mental status examination is a part of the neuropsychiatric assessment. Examine the level of consciousness, orientation, speech, mood, affect, attitude, and thought content. The **Mini-Mental Status Exam** (MMSE) of Folstein is a useful guide for documenting a level of mental function. Five areas of mental status are tested: orientation, registration, attention and calculation, recall, and lan-guage. Each correct answer is given 1 point. A maximum score on the Folstein is 30. A score of less than 23 is abnormal and suggests cognitive impairment.

III. INCONSISTENCIES IN THE HISTORY AND PHYSICAL EXAMINATION

Inconsistencies in the history and physical examination, vague description of symptoms, and evidence of intense suffering, together with inappropriate pain behavior may suggest symptom exaggera-tion, malingering for compensation and other gains, or psychogenic pain. The frequently cited **Waddell** nonorganic signs may raise sus-picion in patients with lower back pain. It may be warranted to pro-ceed with the SF-36 Health Survey or other instruments designed to

Table 1. Cervical and lumbar radicular localization

	Spinal Nerve					
	C5	C6	C7	L4	L5	S1
Disc Level	C4/5	C5/6	C6/7	L3/4 (L4/5)	L4/5 (L5/1)	L5/1
Sensory changes	Lateral upper arm	Lateral forearm and first, second, and half of third digits	Third digit	Medial leg and medial foot	Dorsal foot	Lateral foot
Deep tendon reflex	Biceps	Brachioradialis	Triceps	Patellar	None	Achilles
Muscle tested	Deltoid and biceps	Wrist extensors	Triceps, wrist, and finger extensors	Foot inversion	Dorsiflexion of toes and foot	Plantar flexion and eversion

identify underlying problems or issues. The Waddell nonorganic signs are grouped into five categories:

(a) Tenderness
- Widespread superficial sensitivity to light touch over lumbar spine
- Bone tenderness over a large lumbar area

(b) Simulation
- Axial loading, during which light pressure is applied to the skull in the upright position
- Simulated rotation of lumbar spine with the shoulders and pelvis remaining in the same plane

(c) Distraction
- Greater than 40 degrees' difference in sitting versus supine SLR

(d) Regional disturbance
- Motor—generalized giving way or cogwheeling resistance in manual muscle testing of lower extremities
- Sensory—nondermatomal loss of sensation to pinprick in lower extremities

(e) Overreaction
- Disproportionate pain response to testing (e.g., pain behavior with assisted movement using cane or walker, rigid or slow movement, rubbing or grasping the affected area for more than 3 seconds, grimacing, and sighing with shoulders rising and falling).

IV. CONCLUSION

The history and physical examinations are the foundations for pain evaluation and treatment and are essential elements of good pain management. They need to be tailored to the individual patient, the complexity of the pain problem, and the medical condition of the patient. This chapter outlines a standard history and physical examination that can be applied to most patients presenting in the pain clinic.

SELECTED READINGS

Benzon H. *Essentials of pain medicine and regional anesthesia.* Philadelphia, PA: Churchill Livingstone, 1999.

Kanner R. *Pain management secrets.* Philadelphia, PA: Hanley & Belfus, 1997.

Ombregt L. *A system of orthopaedic medicine.* London, England: WB Saunders, 1997.

Raj P. *Pain medicine: a comprehensive review.* St. Louis, MO: Mosby-Year Book, 1996.

Tollison D. *Handbook of pain management.* Philadelphia, PA: JB Lippincott, 1994.

5

Diagnostic Imaging and Pain Management

Onassis A. Caneris

I have a little shadow that goes in and out with me,
And what can be the use of him is more than I can see.
He is very, very like me from the heels up to the head;
And I see him jump before me when I jump into my bed.
—*Robert Louis Stevenson, 1850–1894*

In recent years, there have been advances in understanding the pathophysiology and mechanisms of pain; concomitantly, there have been advances in diagnostic imaging. Diagnostic imaging is an essential tool for the pain physician, who uses it to understand, diagnose, and treat pain. Although plain x-rays remain the mainstay of diagnostic imaging, advanced modalities including computerized tomography (CT), magnetic resonance imaging (MRI), and nuclear medicine studies have proved to be valuable diagnostic tools for patients with pain. There has been an increasing interest in understanding the dynamic nature of pain processes; functional imaging modalities, including positron emission tomography (PET) scanning and functional magnetic resonance imaging (fMRI), have added to our knowledge in this area. Over the past decade, the use of new technologies has resulted in a 50% increase in health care costs. It becomes increasingly important for the pain physician to have a clear understanding of imaging studies and to optimize the use of diagnostic imaging. A radiologist or imaging specialist can help pain physicians select the most cost-effective test and identify causative pathology.

I. IMAGING TECHNIQUES AND STUDIES

1. Plain Films

Plain x-rays (static x-rays) generate two-dimensional (2D) images that primarily display skeletal tissue, and, in addition, soft tissue anatomy is either seen or inferred. Contemporary x-ray technology generally produces high-quality images with minimal radiation exposure. X-rays produced as electrons from a cathode are accelerated by electric current toward an anode target. The x-ray beam is differentially absorbed as it passes through a section of the patient and then goes on to expose the film. Radiopaque contrast materials given orally, locally, intravenously, and intrathecally may be used to aid the study. Most contrast materials used with plain x-rays are iodine based. Plain x-rays remain the first-line examination for many conditions.

2. Fluoroscopy

The principles of fluoroscopy are the same as those of plain x-rays. The primary difference is that the transmitted radiation is viewed on a fluorescent screen rather than on a static film and that the patient can be imaged in real time in fluoroscopy. The image is generally amplified by an image intensifier. Fluoroscopy can be used both in diagnostic studies and in assisting therapeutic treatment.

3. Computerized Tomography

The prototype CT scanner was developed in the 1960s. First-generation scanners took days to collect data and then hours to reconstruct the images. In the early 1970s, CT scanning for imaging the brain became available. Today's fourth-generation scanners have considerably improved on quality, and the imaging time is considerably shortened. In CT imaging, the x-ray tube produces a beam of energy that passes through a single section of the patient. This beam is then detected by a circular array of detectors on the opposite side. Both the detector and the x-ray source rotate around an axis of the patient and produce exposures at small intervals of rotation. Subsequently, computer reconstruction results in a display of the targeted area. The resolution can be as low as 0.5 mm. Intravenous contrast can be used to enhance the imaging of vascular structures and normal tissues.

CT scanning offers the advantage of three-dimensional (3D) images, but they are generally in standard cross-sectional or axial planes. Quantitative CT scanning is particularly useful in measuring bone density for the assessment of osteoporosis. 3D CT scan also allows postreconstruction images to be rotated at various angles. CT scan displays soft tissues fairly well and is used for soft tissue imaging if MRI (which provides superior soft tissue contrast) is not available or if the patient cannot tolerate MRI because of claustrophobia or because it is a more lengthy process.

4. Magnetic Resonance Imaging

As early as the 1940s and 1950s, nuclear magnetic resonance (NMR) was used to image chemical compounds by exposing them to strong magnetic fields. By the mid-1980s, clinical NMR had become common, and the name was changed to MRI because of public anxiety engendered by the word *nuclear*.

A major difference between MRI scanning and CT scan as well as x-rays is that MRI uses no ionizing radiation. In MRI, signals are obtained by subjecting the tissues to strong magnetic fields, which influence hydrogen ions in the tissues to align in a certain direction. Tiny radio frequency signals are emitted as the hydrogen ions "relax" when the magnetic field is removed. The image represents the intensities of the electromagnetic signals emitted from the hydrogen nuclei in the patient. A tissue such as fat, which is rich in hydrogen ions, gives a bright signal, whereas bone gives a void or essentially no signal. Abnormal tissue generally has more free water and displays different magnetic resonance (MR) characteristics.

The MR signal is a complex function of the concentration of deflected normal hydrogen ions, buildup and relaxation times of the magnetic field (T1 and T2, respectively), flow or motion within the sample, and the MR sequence protocol. Three types of MR sequences are used: spin echo, gradient echo, and inversion recovery. MRI is easily able to provide multiplanar images. Its advantage over CT scan is its superior contrast of soft tissues, especially neural tissues. The addition of gadolinium as a contrast material aids in defining tumors and inflammatory processes.

5. Myelography

Injection of radiocontrast material into the intrathecal space, followed by imaging using conventional x-ray techniques or CT scanning, provides diagnostic information about potential structural abnormalities affecting the spinal nerves. When noninvasive imaging with either MRI or CT scanning does not provide adequate information, myelography, which was once the gold standard for assessing the spine, remains an option for diagnosing structural spine disease. It is also useful for imaging patients who have had spinal instrumentation, which tends to produce extensive artifact on CT imaging.

Postmyelogram CT imaging is sometimes useful for detecting subtle spinal nerve impingement caused by far-posterior lateral intervertebral disc herniation that has been missed by MRI. Its disadvantages are that it is invasive and, unlike MRI, it uses ionizing radiation.

6. Bone Scans and Nuclear Medicine

The field of nuclear medicine followed the discovery of radioactivity in 1896. There are three types of radioactive emissions: positive particles (α particles), negative particles (β particles), and high-penetration radiation (γ radiation). The scintillation events are detected by a scintillation camera and are mapped in 2D space. Nuclear medicine uses the tracer principle, which essentially tags certain physiologic substances in the body and measures its distribution and flow or its presence in a target system. A radiopharmaceutical agent is injected into the patient and the radioactive decay is detected by a detection device (e.g., a γ counter).

Bone scans are commonly used to evaluate complaints of skeletal pain. Radiopharmaceuticals labeled with technetium 99 m localize areas of increased bone turnover and blood flow that represent increased rates of osteoblastic activity. Bone scans are more sensitive than x-rays in detecting skeletal pathology. One third of patients with pain and known malignant disease with normal x-rays have metastatic lesions on bone scans. The specificity of bone scans is not high, which can sometimes be a problem.

7. Discography

Discography involves injecting the nucleus pulposus of an intervertebral disc with contrast material under fluoroscopic guidance. This process can provide objective structural and anatomic information about the intervertebral disc. In addition, it can provide subjective information on whether a specific disc is the source of a patient's axial lumbar pain. This information is helpful in recommending specific treatment modalities.

8. Positron Emission Tomography

In PET, positron emissions are detected with a circular array of detectors. The number of decays is displayed to produce an image of specific metabolic processes. PET is an excellent tool for quantification of various metabolic and physiologic changes and processes, making it a functional imaging device. PET scanning is being increasingly used to unravel pain processes, and the literature on PET scanning and functional neuroimaging of pain is growing.

9. Functional Magnetic Resonance Imaging

In the early 1990s, a number of centers reported that MRI could be used for functional imaging of the human brain. Functional imaging, including fMRI, has helped identify mechanisms that are critical targets for more effective and specific treatments for neuropathic pain. The technique utilizes the principle that functional activation of brain regions are reflected by increases in the blood oxygen level dependent (BOLD) signal in fMRI. This modality has been used to examine the contribution of thalamic and cortical areas to the human pain experience. The cortical areas identified include the primary and secondary somatosensory cortex (S1 and S2), the anterior insula, and the anterior cingulate cortex. Abnormal pain evoked by innocuous stimuli (allodynia) has been associated with the amplification of the thalamic, insular, and SII responses.

II. HEADACHE

Headache is a frequent presentation in both the primary care physician's office and the pain clinic. The pain physician must be familiar with the indications for imaging in the assessment of patients with headache. Most patients who complain of headache and whose neurologic examinations reveal normal findings show normal findings from a CT imaging study. Careful history and neurologic examination are crucial before deciding whether to order a diagnostic test.

1. Primary Headache

In patients who present with a history characteristic of primary headache without additional neurologic symptoms and with normal findings from neurologic examinations, it is exceedingly rare to find imaging abnormalities, as confirmed by clinical studies.

2. Secondary Headache

Subarachnoid hemorrhage should be considered in patients without chronic headache but with an initial presentation of the "worst headache of my life." Emergent noncontrast CT scanning is the evaluation of choice because it is sensitive to the presence of acute blood. When there is new headache plus fever, lumbar puncture may be indicated. Before proceeding to lumbar puncture, a noncontrast CT scan is needed to exclude space-occupying lesion—a contraindication to lumbar puncture. Noncontrast CT scanning is also indicated in acute trauma because it best identifies acute hemorrhage and lesions of the bone.

Contrast CT scanning is indicated when there is clinical suspicion of vascular lesions, neoplastic lesions, or inflammatory conditions.

Plain x-rays are less helpful in evaluating chronic headache. In this setting, MRI scanning is preferred because it has a high degree of sensitivity for intracranial pathology. Diagnostic criteria and imaging for secondary headache are discussed in Chapter 28.

(i) Neoplasia

Forty percent of patients with newly diagnosed brain tumors present with a chief complaint of headache. Increased intracranial pressure due to obstructed cerebrospinal fluid (CSF) flow can produce headaches. Larger parenchymal tumors may not produce headaches. In patients with headache and focal or lateralizing neurologic symptoms, MRI with contrast is the study of choice.

(ii) Carotid Artery Dissection

Symptoms of carotid artery dissection include new-onset unilateral headache with associated anterior cervical pain. Fluctuating hemispheric neurologic deficits and Horner syndrome may be present. Carotid dissections are most common in association with trauma; fibromuscular dysplasia may also predispose to carotid dissection. The most common location for dissection is several centimeters above the carotid bifurcation.

Arterial angiography is usually most effective in making the diagnosis, but MRI and magnetic resonance angiography (MRA) may also be helpful, particularly in follow-up examinations. MRI scanning demonstrates high signal intensity, which usually represents a clot or low arterial flow.

(iii) Cerebrovenous and Sinus Occlusive Disease

The most common presenting symptom of venous or sinus occlusive disease is headache; more than 75% of these patients generally complain of headache. Occlusive disease frequently results in increased intracranial pressure. Cerebral ischemia may also result. Cavernous sinus thrombosis produces severe retroorbital or periorbital pain with proptosis and ophthalmoparesis. Traditional contrast angiography is usually the imaging study of choice, but traditional angiography is being replaced by MRA and MRI.

(iv) Hydrocephalus

Both CT scan and MRI are appropriate for evaluating hydrocephalus. Aqueductal stenosis is apparent as dilatation of the third and lateral ventricles, with a normal-appearing fourth ventricle. MRI is the imaging study of choice.

Imaging studies tend to be normal in pseudotumor cerebri. Diagnosis is made by examination of the CSF with careful manometry and by identification of increased intracranial pressure.

(v) Low-Pressure Headache

Postural headaches can be caused by diminished intracranial pressure. These headaches are most commonly seen after lumbar puncture but can also be seen after trauma or can occur "spontaneously." CT scan and MRI findings tend to be normal. Isotope cysternography may demonstrate the site of dural leakage of CSF.

(vi) Chiari Malformation

Patients with Chiari malformations frequently present with headache as a primary symptom. Additional neurologic complaints are often associated with Chiari malformations. MRI is the imaging modality of choice. Three types have been identified. In type 1, the cerebellar tonsils are displaced caudally into the cervical spinal canal. In type 2, there is additional caudal displacement of the lower cerebellum and the brainstem; anatomic abnormalities are seen in the fourth ventricle, and there is associated meningomyelocele. In type 3, either encephalocele or spina bifida is also present.

III. CRANIOFACIAL PAIN SYNDROMES

1. Trigeminal Neuralgia

Severe unilateral paroxysmal lancinating pain in the distribution of the trigeminal nerve is characteristic of trigeminal neuralgia. Trigeminal neuralgia is idiopathic. The imaging studies generally show no abnormalities. In patients with trigeminal neuropathy and trigeminal neuropathic pain in which atypical features exist, it is important to evaluate for other diagnostic possibilities. MRI is the imaging modality of choice. Occasionally, vascular malformations, aneurysms, and tumors cause trigeminal neuropathy. Multiple sclerosis is sometimes associated with neuropathic facial pain, in which case lesions of increased T2-weighted signal intensity on MRI may be seen in the trigeminal brainstem dorsal root entry zones.

2. Glossopharyngeal Neuralgia

The characteristic pain of glossopharyngeal neuralgia is similar to that of trigeminal neuralgia but is located unilaterally in the posterior tongue throughout the tonsillar area and sometimes in the auricular area. It is also most frequently idiopathic. In isolated glossopharyngeal neuralgia, the imaging studies rarely show abnormalities. In patients with evidence of associated pathology, particularly at the brainstem, MRI with contrast medium is the imaging study of choice.

IV. CENTRAL PAIN SYNDROMES

Central neuropathic pain can result after an injury to the primary somatosensory nervous system. Constant burning neuropathic pain is typically seen. Infarction, trauma, and radiation are frequent causes.

1. Thalamic Pain Syndromes

Injury to the thalamus, specifically to the ventral posterolateral nucleus, typically results in constant burning pain in the contralateral hemicorpus, including the face, arm, trunk, and leg. This pain most frequently results from thalamic infarction but can also result from hemorrhage, trauma, or space-occupying lesions including tumor, infection, and abscess. Imaging reveals signal abnormalities in the thalamus contralateral to the site of pain. A "pseudothalamic pain syndrome" can result after injury to the thalamocortical white-matter tract. Clinical presentation is similar, but MRI reveals abnormalities in the thalamocortical radiations. In exceptional cases, the MR image is normal and pathology can only be delineated using functional imaging studies.

2. Spinal Cord Injury

Injury to the spinal cord at any level can result in a central pain syndrome. Damage to the spinothalamic tract frequently results in central neuropathic pain. Considerable central neuropathic pain accompanies spinal cord injury in 25% of patients. Causes include trauma, space-occupying lesions including neoplasms, demyelinating processes including multiple sclerosis, and syringomyelia. MRI is the imaging modality of choice. In multiple sclerosis, lesions of increased T2-weighted signal intensity are seen in the white-matter tracts of the spinal cord. In syringomyelia, MRI reveals a central cavity that shows high signal intensity on T2-weighted images and diminished signal on T1-weighted images.

V. VERTEBRAL AXIS PAIN

Low back pain is a common presentation in both primary care and pain clinics. Pathologic processes affecting the lumbar spine include disc degeneration, degrees of intervertebral disc herniation, facet joint osteoarthosis, vertebral fracture, vertebral dislocation, spondylolisthesis, and osteoporosis. Degenerative causes of low back pain may be difficult to distinguish from other common causes such as spasm or inflammation of muscle or soft tissue. Less common causes include intradural and extradural neoplasms, infections, and congenital abnormalities of the spine.

The history and physical examination are the basis of the evaluation, but imaging studies may be needed to make a definitive diagnosis.

The primary rationale for radiographic imaging of low back pain is to exclude or define serious pathology. Most low back pain originates from soft tissues, and imaging studies are not helpful. In older patients, imaging studies frequently reveal abnormalities that may or may not be responsible for the pain. Plain x-rays can help diagnose spondylolysis (pars interarticularis defects, usually at L5 or sometimes L4), ankylosing spondylitis, fractures, and, occasionally, degenerative disc disease. When neurologic signs or symptoms are present, including those of sciatica, MRI is the imaging modality of choice. MRI without contrast material can detect herniation of lumbar discs with compression of nerve roots causing radicular symptoms.

In patients with a previous history of lumbar surgery, it is imperative to also obtain a contrast–enhanced study, which helps differentiate recurrence of disc herniation from epidural scar tissue; the latter is detected by T1-weighted signal enhancement after administration of contrast. In patients with a clinical complaint of lumbar claudication and suspected spinal stenosis, both CT scan and MRI are appropriate. CT scan offers the advantage of superior imaging of bony hypertrophic changes of the lumbar spine.

1. Plain X-Ray Evaluation of Low Back Pain

Plain x-ray provides an assessment of the configuration and alignment of the lumbar vertebral spine with a high degree of accuracy. There have been a number of natural history and comparative studies evaluating the usefulness of plain x-rays in evaluating low back pain. In a large retrospective study reviewing 1,000 lumbar spine radiographs of patients with low back pain, more than one half of the radiographs were normal. In another study of 780 patients, only 2.4% had unique diagnostic findings on plain radiographs.

Most episodes of low back pain resolve within 6 weeks. Evidence-based guidelines recommend that radiographs are not indicated for a first presentation of low back pain (see Chapter 27). General recommendations for radiographs in patients with low back pain are as follows:

- For a first episode of low back pain for fewer than 6 weeks, with improvement with or without active treatment, no radiographs are indicated unless an atypical clinical finding or special psychological or social circumstances exist. Atypical history includes age of more than 65 years, history suggesting a high risk for osteoporosis, symptoms of persistent sensory deficit, pain-worsening despite treatment, intense pain at rest, fever, chills, unexplained weight loss, and recurrent back pain with no radiographs within the last 2 years. Atypical physical findings include considerable motor deficit and unexplained deformity.
- For recurrent low back pain, radiographs are not indicated if a previous radiographic study had been done within 2 years.

In general, anteroposterior and lateral views are the only views needed initially. In patients with chronic pain or additional history and physical findings suggesting stenosis or instability, flexion and extension films may be helpful.

2. MRI and Low Back Pain

MRI has high sensitivity for detecting pathology of the lumbar spine. A poor correlation exists between the severity of pain symptoms and the extent of morphologic changes seen on MRI studies: a statistically significant percentage of healthy individuals without lumbar pain have degenerative changes on MRI (as many as 50% to 60%) and even disc herniation (as many as 20%). Careful attention must be paid to correlating clinical symptoms with radiographic findings; otherwise, imaging findings may be used inappropriately to justify unneeded intervention or treatment.

Age-related morphologic changes occur in the lumbar spine throughout life. There is a decrease in concentration of water and glycosaminoglycans in the intervertebral disc, and there is an increase in concentration of collagen. On the MRI, these changes show up as a loss of signal intensity on T2-weighted images, a reduction in the height of vertebral bodies, a reduction in the height of the intervertebral discs, and a reduction in the caliber of the spinal canal. The onset of degenerative processes of the lumbosacral spine seems to be consistently marked by tears of the annulus fibrosis, and by MRI and histologic changes of the vertebral bone marrow adjacent to the intervertebral spaces. Facet degeneration rarely occurs in the absence of disc degeneration, and it seems likely that facet osteoarthropathy results from the added stress of increased loading after disc space narrowing has occurred. Multiple studies have found an association between degenerated disc and facet osteoarthritis using imaging criteria.

In patients with radicular symptoms, the clinical evaluation can usually predict the spinal nerve involved. The actual spinal pathology, however, cannot be predicted with clinical evaluation alone, and MRI examination can be of assistance. A spinal nerve can be compressed by a disc either at the traversing segment by central disc herniation or at the exiting segment by a lateral disc herniation. In these circumstances, imaging is beneficial for defining the site of pathology. Symptomatic patients may have neuroimaging abnormalities at more than one spinal level.

3. Pain after Lumbar Surgery

In patients who have had previous back surgery and now complain of recurrent radicular pain, the differential diagnosis includes the following:

- Incorrect original diagnosis or concomitant disease
- Spinal nerve or dorsal root ganglion pathology, including axonal injury or persistent neurapraxic injury
- Retained or recurrent intervertebral disc fragment
- Epidural fibrosis
- Central sensitization
- Complex regional pain syndrome

Fibrosis is a natural consequence of surgical procedures. Numerous reports suggest that fibrosis and adhesions cause compression or tethering of the spinal nerves and their roots, which in turn causes recurrent radicular pain and physical impairment. The literature repeatedly suggests that fibrosis is the major cause of recurrent symptoms when no alternative bone or disc pathology can be found. It has also been suggested that fibrosis may be causal in as many as 25% of patients with failed back surgery syndrome.

Recurrent radicular pain is radicular pain occurring 6 months or later after primary surgery after a successful initial result (e.g., at 1 month postoperatively). A considerable association between the size of the peridural scar and the incidence of pain has been demonstrated. MRI with and without contrast helps differentiate recurrent or retained disc fragment from epidural scarring. The criteria used to identify epidural fibrosis by MRI include the following:

- Epidural scar is isointense or hypointense relative to the intervertebral disc on T1-weighted images on an MRI scan.
- Peridural scar tends to form in a curvilinear pattern surrounding the dural tube, with homogenous intensity.
- Traction of the dural tube toward the side of the soft tissue is more characteristic of scar.
- Scar tissue is seen to consistently enhance immediately after the injection of contrast material, regardless of its location.

The criteria used to identify recurrent herniated disc by MRI include the following:

- Recurrent herniated disc material is isointense to the intervertebral disc on T1-weighted images. There tends to be a more variable appearance on T2-weighted images.
- Recurrent herniations tend to have a polypoid configuration with a smooth outer margin.
- Recurrent disc material does not enhance within the first 10 to 20 minutes after administration of contrast material.

4. Arachnoiditis

Arachnoiditis, which is distinct from epidural scar formation, involves inflammatory and scar tissue within the dura surrounding the spinal nerves. The MRI characteristics of arachnoiditis show three different possible patterns. The first is centrally clumped spinal nerve roots in the thecal sac seen on T1-weighted images, the second is peripheral adhesions of roots to the thecal sac, and the third is an increased soft tissue signal within the thecal sac below the conus. Arachnoiditis typically presents as polyradicular lower extremity pain.

5. Metastatic Disease of the Spine

Severe back pain is a common presentation of metastatic disease of the lumbar spine. The most common tumors that metastasize to bone and therefore to the lumbar spine are lung, prostate, and breast. Multiple myeloma and breast cancer typically are osteolytic, whereas prostate cancer tends to cause osteosclerotic changes. Bone scans are sensitive for detecting metastatic involvement of the lumbar spine. The correlation between the severity of bone scan and the intensity of pain is generally poor.

When spinal cord compression resulting from epidural metastatic disease is suspected, MRI is the imaging modality of choice and contrast enhancement is recommended. Back pain is a common presentation of spinal cord compression. When considerable reduction of vertebral body height is seen, concomitant epidural involvement is common. Disruption of the pedicle on imaging suggests metastatic disease and, when seen on a plain radiograph, warrants thorough investigation.

6. Infectious Processes of the Vertebral Spine

Plain x-rays can be used to assess osteomyelitis. Characteristic changes include loss of end-plate definition, associated soft tissue swelling, destruction of vertebral bodies, and loss of intervertebral disc height. MRI detects involvement of the disc space. Occasionally, the MRI is negative and radionucleotide imaging studies can help establish the diagnosis. The characteristics of osteomyelitis on MRI include decreased signal intensity, a loss of delineation and demarcation of the vertebral end plate on T1-weighted images, and increased signal intensity in the intervertebral disc on T2-weighted images.

VI. CONCLUSION

Imaging studies are indispensable tools for the pain physician, who must use them not only as appropriate diagnostic tools but also in a cost-effective manner. Consultation with the department of radiology may be helpful when a diagnosis is uncertain.

SELECTED READINGS

Atlas SW, ed. *Magnetic resonance imaging of the brain and spine.* New York: Raven Press, 1996.

Modic MT, Masaryk TJ, Ross JS, eds. *Magnetic resonance imaging of the spine.* Chicago, IL: Year Book Medical, 1989.

Osborn AG. *Diagnostic neuroradiology.* St Louis, MO: Mosby, 1994.

Assessment of Pain

Alyssa A. LeBel

When you can measure what you are speaking about, and express it in numbers, you know something about it; but when you cannot measure it, when you cannot express it in numbers, your knowledge of it is of a meager and unsatisfactory kind; it may be the beginning of knowledge, but you have scarcely, in your thoughts, advanced to the stage of science.
—*William Thompson Lord Kelvin, 1824–1907*

Pain is a complex multidimensional symptom determined not only by tissue injury and nociception but also by previous pain experience, personal beliefs, affect, motivation, environment, and, at times, pending litigation. **There is no objective measurement of pain**. Self-report is the most valid measure of the individual experience of pain. The pain history is key to the assessment of pain and includes the patient's description of pain intensity, quality, location, timing, and duration, as well as ameliorating and exacerbating conditions. Frequently, pain cannot be seen, defined, or felt by the physician, and the physician must assess the pain from a combination of factors. The most important of these factors is the patient's report of the pain, but other factors such as personality and culture, psychological status, the existence of secondary gain, and the possibility of drug-seeking behavior should also be considered. Reports of pain may not correlate with the degree of disability or findings on physical examination. However, it is important to remember that to the patients and their families, distress, suffering, and pain behaviors are often not distinguished from the pain itself.

Diagnosis and measurement of acute pain require frequent and consistent assessment as part of daily clinical care to ensure rapid titration of therapy and preemptive interventions. Chronic pain is often more diagnostically challenging than acute pain, but no less compelling. Application of a structured history and comprehensive physical examination will define treatable problems and identify complicating factors. Somatic, visceral, neuropathic, or combined pain problems suggest specific diagnoses and interventions. An understanding of pain pathophysiology guides rational and appropriate treatment.

I. PAIN HISTORY

The general medical history may contribute considerably and is always included as part of the pain assessment. This is described in Chapter 4. The specific pain history includes three main issues—intensity, location, and pathophysiology. The following questions help define these issues:

- What is the time course of the pain?
- Where is the pain?
- What is the intensity of the pain?
- What factors relieve or exacerbate the pain?
- What are the possible generators of the pain?

1. Pain Assessment Tools

As previously stated, pain cannot be objectively measured. The intensity of pain is one of the most difficult and perhaps frustrating characteristics of pain to pinpoint. Several tests and scales are available. Some of the more commonly used tools are the following:

(i) Unidimensional Self-report Scales

In practice, self-report scales serve as very simple, useful, and valid methods for assessing and monitoring patients' pain.

VERBAL DESCRIPTOR SCALES. The patient is asked to describe his or her pain by choosing from a list of adjectives that reflect gradations of pain intensity. The five-word scale consists of **mild, discomforting, distressing, horrible,** and **excruciating**. Disadvantages of this scale include limited selection of descriptors and the fact that patients tend to select moderate descriptors rather than the extremes.

VERBAL NUMERIC RATING SCALES. These are the most simple and frequently used scales. On a numeric scale (most commonly 0 to 10, with 0 being "no pain" and 10 "the worst pain imaginable"), the patient picks a number to describe the pain. Advantages of numeric scales are their simplicity, reproducibility, easy comprehensibility, and sensitivity to small changes in pain. Children as young as 5 years old, who are able to count and have some concept of numbers (e.g., "8 is larger than 4"), can use this scale.

VISUAL ANALOG SCALES. Visual analog scales (VAS) are similar to the verbal numeric rating scales, except that the patient marks on a measured line, one end of which is labeled "no pain" and the other end "worst pain imaginable," where the pain falls. Visual scales are more valid for research purposes, but are used less clinically because they are more time-consuming to conduct than verbal scales and require motor control.

FACES PAIN RATING SCALE. Evaluating pain in children can be very difficult because of the child's inability to describe pain or to understand pain assessment forms. This scale depicts six sketches

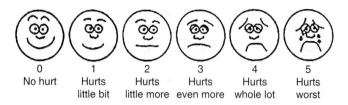

Figure 1. Wong–Baker FACES Pain Rating Scale. Explain to the person undergoing the rating that each face depicts a person who feels happy because he has no pain (hurt) or who feels sad because he has some or a lot of pain. Face 0 is very happy because he does not hurt at all. Face 1 hurts just a little bit. Face 2 hurts a little more. Face 3 hurts even more. Face 4 hurts a whole lot. Face 5 hurts as much as you can imagine, although you do not have to be crying to feel this bad.

of facial features, each with a numeric value, 0 to 5, ranging from a happy, smiling face to a sad, teary face (see Fig. 1). To extrapolate this scale to the VAS, the value chosen is multiplied by two. This scale may also be beneficial for mentally impaired patients. Average children as young as 3 years can reliably use this scale.

(ii) Multiple Dimension Instruments

These instruments provide more complex information about the patient's pain. They are especially useful for assessment of chronic pain. Because they are time consuming, they are most frequently used in outpatient and research settings.

MCGILL PAIN QUESTIONNAIRE. McGill pain questionnaire (MPQ) is the most frequently used multidimensional test. Descriptive words from three major dimensions of pain (i.e., sensory, affective, and evaluative) are further subdivided into 20 subclasses, each containing words of varying degrees. Three scores are obtained, one for each dimension, and a total score is calculated. Studies have shown the MPQ to be a reliable instrument in clinical research.

BRIEF PAIN INVENTORY. In brief pain inventory (BPI), patients are asked to rate the severity of their pain at its "worst," "least," or "average," within the past 24 hours and at the time the rating is done. The inventory also requires the patients to represent the location of their pain on a schematic diagram of the body. The BPI correlates with the scores of activity, sleep, and social interactions. It is cross-cultural and a useful method for clinical studies (see Fig. 2).

MASSACHUSETTS GENERAL HOSPITAL PAIN CENTER PAIN ASSESSMENT FORM. Massachusetts General Hospital (MGH) Pain Center pain assessment form (see Fig. 3) combines many of the foregoing assessment instruments and is given to all patients on initial consultations at the MGH Pain Center. It elicits information about pain intensity, its location (body diagram), quality of pain, therapies tried, and past and present medications. It takes 10 to 15 minutes to complete and is an extremely valuable instrument. Its disadvantages are that it is time-consuming to complete and is not applicable if there are language constraints.

(iii) Pain Diaries

A diary of a patient's pain is useful in evaluating the relation between pain and daily activity. Pain can be described using the numeric rating scale, during activities such as walking, standing, sitting, and routine chores. The evaluation can be done on an hourly basis. Use of medication and alcohol, and emotional responses of the patient and family may also be recorded. Pain diaries may reflect a patient's pain more accurately than a retrospective description that may significantly over- or underestimate pain.

2. Pain Location

The location and distribution of pain are extremely important characteristics that help in understanding the pathophysiology of the pain complaint. Body diagrams, found in some of the assessment instruments, can prove very useful. Although the clinician can view the patient's perception of the topographic area of pain, the patient may show psychological distress either by poorly localizing the pain or by magnifying the pain to other areas of the body.

Is the pain localized or referred? Localized pain is pain confined to its site of origin, without radiation or migration. Referred pain usually arises from visceral or deep structures and radiates to other areas of the body. A classic example of referred pain is shoulder pain from phrenic nerve irritation (causes include liver metastases from pancreatic cancer) (see Table 1).

Is pain superficial/peripheral or visceral? Superficial pain, arising from tissues rich in nociceptors, such as skin, teeth, and mucous membranes, is easily localized and limited to the affected part of the body. Visceral pain arises from internal organs, which contain relatively few nociceptors. Visceral afferent information may converge with superficial afferent input at the spinal level, referring the perception of visceral pain to a distant dermatome. Visceral pain is diffuse and often poorly localized. In addition, it often has associated autonomic components such as diaphoresis, capillary vasodilation, hypertension, or tachycardia.

3. Pain Etiology

By taking a complete history and by answering the two questions described in preceding text (Is pain superficial/peripheral or visceral? Is the pain localized or referred?), the clinician can begin to formulate the etiology of the pain complaint. By doing so, the rest of the history, as well as the physical examination, can be tailored to systematically explore the aspects of pain, such as symptoms and physical signs, common to the particular type of pain in question.

Types of Pain

The various types of pain tend to present differently (e.g., nociceptive pain is associated with tissue injury due to trauma, surgery, inflammation or tumor; neuropathic pain is invariably associated with sensory change; and radicular pain is often associated with radiculopathy). History and physical examination help identify these differences. Because the different types of pain tend to respond to different treatments, the identification of

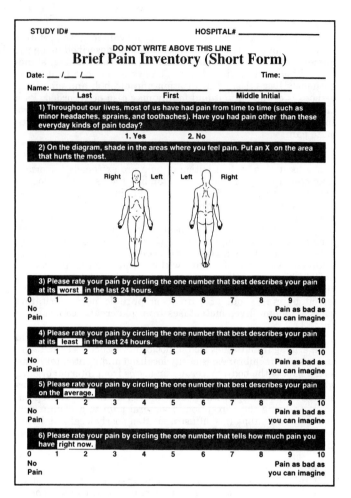

Figure 2.   Brief pain inventory (see text). (Adapted from Zempsky WT, Schecter NL. What's new in the management of pain in children. *Ped Clin North Am* 1989;36:823–836, with permission.)

the pain type during pain assessment is important. Pain can be categorized as follows:

- **Nociceptive**—pain arising from activation of nociceptors; nociceptors are found in all tissues except the central nervous system (CNS); the pain is clinically proportional to the degree of activation of afferent pain fibers and can be acute or chronic (e.g., somatic pain, cancer pain, and postoperative pain).

7) What treatments or medications are you receiving for your pain?

8) In the last 24 hours, how much relief have pain treatments or medications provided? Please circle the one percentage that most shows how much relief you have received.

| 0% | 10% | 20% | 30% | 40% | 50% | 60% | 70% | 80% | 90% | 100% |
| No Relief | | | | | | | | | | Complete Relief |

9) Circle the one number that describes how, during the past 24 hours, pain has interfered with your:

A. General activity

| 0 | 1 | 2 | 3 | 4 | 5 | 6 | 7 | 8 | 9 | 10 |
| Does not interfere | | | | | | | | | Completely Interferes | |

B. Mood

| 0 | 1 | 2 | 3 | 4 | 5 | 6 | 7 | 8 | 9 | 10 |
| Does not interfere | | | | | | | | | Completely Interferes | |

C. Walking ability

| 0 | 1 | 2 | 3 | 4 | 5 | 6 | 7 | 8 | 9 | 10 |
| Does not interfere | | | | | | | | | Completely Interferes | |

D. Normal work (includes both work outside the home and housework)

| 0 | 1 | 2 | 3 | 4 | 5 | 6 | 7 | 8 | 9 | 10 |
| Does not interfere | | | | | | | | | Completely Interferes | |

E. Relations with other people

| 0 | 1 | 2 | 3 | 4 | 5 | 6 | 7 | 8 | 9 | 10 |
| Does not interfere | | | | | | | | | Completely Interferes | |

F. Sleep

| 0 | 1 | 2 | 3 | 4 | 5 | 6 | 7 | 8 | 9 | 10 |
| Does not interfere | | | | | | | | | Completely Interferes | |

G. Enjoyment of life

| 0 | 1 | 2 | 3 | 4 | 5 | 6 | 7 | 8 | 9 | 10 |
| Does not interfere | | | | | | | | | Completely Interferes | |

Pain Research Group • Department of Neurology • University of Wisconsin-Madison

Figure 2. *Continued.*

- **Neuropathic**—pain caused by nerve injury or disease, or by involvement of nerves in other disease processes such as tumor or inflammation; the pain may occur in the periphery or in the CNS
- **Sympathetically mediated**—pain that is characterized at some point with evidence of edema, changes in skin blood flow, abnormal sudomotor activity in the region of pain, allodynia, hyperalgesia, or hyperpathia

M.G.H. PAIN CENTER
PAIN ASSESSMENT FORM

Information About the Pain

1. What is the problem you would like us to help you with?

2. Please mark the event or events that led to your present pain: (If you experience more than one kind of pain, please write in separate sets of answers for each type of pain you have.)

____ Accident ____ Cancer

____ Other injury ____ ____ No obvious cause

____ Following an operation ____ Other disease ____

____ Other ____

3. For how long have you had this pain?

4. How often does the pain occur?
____ Continuously (nonstop)

____ Several times a day

____ Once or twice a day

____ Several times a week

____ Less than 3 or 4 times per month

5. How has the *intensity* of the pain changed throughout the time you have had it?

____ Increased ____ Decreased ____ Stayed the same

6. The following five words represent pain of increasing intensity:

1	2	3
Mild	Discomforting	Distressing

4	5
Horrible	Excruciating

To answer each question below, write the *number* of the most appropriate word in the space beside the question.

a. Which word describes your pain at its worst? ____
b. Which word describes your pain at its least? ____
c. Which word describes your pain right now? ____
d. Which word describes how your pain is most of the time? ____

7. Location of the Pain (please shadow in the affected areas).

8. Quality of the Pain

Below is list of words that are often used to describe pain. After each descriptive word, indicate with a checkmark whether this word describes a particular quality of your pain and, if it does, the intensity of that quality.

	None (not at all)	Mild	Moderate	Severe
Throbbing	0)	1)	2)	3)
Shooting	0)	1)	2)	3)
Stabbing	0)	1)	2)	3)
Sharp	0)	1)	2)	3)
Cramping	0)	1)	2)	3)
Gnawing	0)	1)	2)	3)
Hot-Burning	0)	1)	2)	3)
Aching	0)	1)	2)	3)
Heavy	0)	1)	2)	3)
Tender	0)	1)	2)	3)
Splitting	0)	1)	2)	3)
Tiring/Exhausting	0)	1)	2)	3)
Sickening	0)	1)	2)	3)
Fearful	0)	1)	2)	3)
Punishing/Cruel	0)	1)	2)	3)

9. Which of the following have an effect on your pain? Please indicate whether it makes the pain *better, worse,* or has *no effect.*

____ Heat ____ Cold
____ Sitting ____ Standing
____ Walking ____ Fatigue
____ Coughing ____ Anxiety/emotions
____ Vibration ____ Massage/rubbing
____ Climate ____ Alcoholic beverages
____ Noise
____ Lying down
____ Particular position or movement explain: ____
____ Caffeinated drinks (coffee, tea, colas)

10. How does the pain affect your activity in these different areas:
Work-school–
Household chores–
Social interactions–
Leisure–
Sexual activity–

11. What is your current employment status?

12. Do you have pending a settlement about disability, workers' compensation, or a legal matter?

____ yes ____ no

If yes, briefly explain: ____

13. What treatments have you tried for your pain?
____ Surgery ____ TENS unit
____ Nerve block ____ Exercise program
____ Brace ____ Trigger point injection
____ Physical therapy ____ Acupuncture
____ Relaxation training ____ Chiropractic therapy
____ Biofeedback ____ Psychotherapy/counseling
____ Hypnosis
Other ____ ____ Massage

14. What specialists have you seen for your pain (e.g., orthopedic surgeon, neurologist, neurosurgeon, psychiatrist)?

15. Pain Medications and Other Treatments

A. What are the medications you are currently taking for pain?

	Drug	Dose	Frequency
1.			
2.			
3.			
4.			

B. What other medications have you taken in the past for pain?

	Drug	Effect on Pain
1.		
2.		
3.		
4.		

Figure 3.　The Massachusetts General Hospital (MGH) Pain Center's pain assessment form.

C. Are you allergic to any medications (including local anesthetics)?

        Drug   *Type of Reaction*

D. What other medications are you currently taking?

16. Name, address, and phone number of your primary care physician:

17. Name, address, and phone number of the physician who referred you to us:

Figure 3. *Continued.*

- **Deafferentation**—chronic pain resulting from loss of afferent input to the CNS; pain may arise in the periphery (e.g., peripheral nerve avulsion) or in the CNS (e.g., spinal cord lesions and multiple sclerosis)
- **Neuralgia**—lancinating pain associated with nerve damage or irritation along the distribution of a single nerve (e.g., trigeminal nerve) or multiple nerves
- **Radicular**—pain that is evoked by stimulation of nociceptive afferent fibers in spinal nerves, their roots or ganglia, or by other neuropathic mechanisms; the symptom is caused by ectopic impulse generation; this pain is distinct from radiculopathy, but the two often arise together
- **Central**—pain arising from a lesion in the CNS usually involving the spinothalamic cortical pathways (e.g., thalamic infarct); pain is usually constant, with a burning, electrical quality and is exacerbated by activity or changes in the weather; hyperesthesia and hyperpathia and/or allodynia are invariably present; pain is highly resistant to treatment
- **Psychogenic**—pain inconsistent with the likely anatomic distribution of the presumed pain generator, or pain existing with no apparent organic pathology despite extensive evaluation
- **Referred**—pain often originates from a visceral organ (Table 1); it may be felt in body regions remote from the site of pathology; the mechanism of pain may be the spinal convergence of visceral and somatic afferent fibers on spinothalamic neurons; common manifestations are cutaneous and deep hyperalgesia, autonomic hyperactivity, tenderness, and muscular contractions.

II. PHYSICAL EXAMINATION

A complete examination is required, including a general physical examination followed by a specific pain evaluation and neurologic, musculoskeletal, and mental status assessments. It is

Table 1.   Examples of referred pain

Origin of Pain	Region of Pain Referral
Head (dura mater or vessels)	
Anterior cranial fossa	Ipsilateral forehead
Middle cranial fossa	Ipsilateral supraorbital region, temples
Posterior cranial fossa	Ipsilateral ear, postauricular region, occiput
Pharynx	Ipsilateral ear
Chest	
Esophagus	Substernal region
Heart	Left arm, epigastric
Abdomen	
Visceral pain	Segmental muscle spasms
Cholecystitis	Upper abdominal muscles
Appendicitis	Lower abdominal muscles
Renal colic	L2-L3 segments
Subphrenic region	Shoulder pain
Liver	Right phrenic region
Kidney	Lower thorax and back
Ureter	
Upper (renal pelvis)	Groin, testis, or ovary
Terminal	Scrotum/labia
Pelvis	
Prostate	Lower back
Uterus	Lower back
Ovary	Anterior thigh
Lower extremity	
Peroneal entrapment at fibula	Dorsum of foot
Other	
Unilateral cordotomy	Pain applied to analgesic side produces pain in symmetrical contralateral body part

From Brass LM, Stys K. *Handbook of neurological lists.* New York: Churchill-Livingstone, 1991, with permission.

important not to limit the examination to the painful location and surrounding tissues and structures.

1. General Physical Examination

This physical consists of the usual head-to-toe examination, as described in Chapter 4. Important points to note are

- Appearance—obese, emaciated, histrionic, flat affect;
- Posture—splinting, scoliosis, kyphosis;
- Gait—antalgic, hemiparetic, using assistive devices;
- Expression—grimacing, tense, diaphoretic, anxious;
- Vital signs—sympathetic overactivity (e.g., tachycardia, hypertension), temperature asymmetries.

It is also important to watch how a patient dresses and moves. Favoring an extremity or protecting a part of the body is not advisable unless the relevant movements are elicited despite these drawbacks. Some elements of the comprehensive examination may be missed if a clinician is fearful of invading the patient's privacy.

2. Specific Pain Evaluation

Following general examination, the clinician evaluates the painful areas(s) of the body. The history will often direct the search for physical findings. Inspection of the skin may reveal changes in color, flushing, edema, hair loss, presence or absence of sweat, atrophy, or muscle spasm. Inspection of nails may show dystrophic changes. Nerve root injury may be manifest as goose flesh (cutis anserina) in the affected dermatome. Palpation allows mapping of the painful area and detection of any change in pain intensity within the area during the examination and helps define the pain type and trigger points. Patient responses, both verbal and nonverbal, should be noted, as well as the appropriateness of the responses and their correlation with affect. Factors that reproduce, worsen, or decrease the pain are sought.

While conducting the physical examination, it is important to identify any changes in sensory modalities and pain processing that may have occurred. These changes may be manifest as anesthesia, hypesthesia, hyperesthesia, analgesia, hypoalgesia, allodynia, hyperalgesia, or hyperpathia. Please refer to *Definitions and Abbreviations* for definitions of these terms.

3. Neurologic Examination

Subtle physical findings are often found only during the neurologic examination. It is essential to conduct a comprehensive neurologic examination when first assessing a patient with pain to identify associated, and possibly treatable, neurologic disease. The examination can be performed in 5 to 10 minutes. Later in the course of treatment, the neurologic examination can be more focused and briefer.

Mental function is assessed by evaluating the patient's orientation to person, place, and time; short-term and long-term memory; choice of words used to describe symptoms and to answer questions; and educational background.

The **cranial nerves** should be examined, especially in patients complaining of head, neck, and shoulder pain symptoms. Table 2 lists the function of each cranial nerve.

A simple assessment of **spinal nerve function** should also be carried out. Spinal nerve sensation is determined by the use of cotton or tissue paper for light touch, and pinprick for sharp pain and proprioception. Potentially painful peripheral neuropathies are listed in Table 3. Spinal nerve motor function is determined by deep tendon reflexes, the presence or absence of the Babinski reflex, and tests of muscle strength. Table 4 lists sensory and motor manifestations of common root syndromes.

Coordination is assessed by testing balance, rapid hand movement, finger-to-nose motion, toe-to-heel motion, gait, and Romberg test. Cerebellar dysfunction can often be detected during these maneuvers. Table 5 lists pain disturbances due to various disease processes that can affect gait.

Table 2.   Neurologic examination of cranial nerves

Cranial Nerves	Function
I—Olfactory nerve	Smell
II—Optic	Vision
III—Oculomotor	
Parasympathetic	Sphincter muscle of iris, ciliary muscle
Motor	Superior, inferior, and medial rectus muscles; inferior oblique and levator palpebrae superioris muscle
IV—Trochlear	Superior oblique
V—Trigeminal	
Motor	Muscles of mastication
Sensory	Face, mucosa of nose, mouth, dura, and cornea
VI—Abducens	Lateral rectus muscle
VII—Facial	
Motor	Muscles of expression
Parasympathetic	Lacrimal gland, salivary glands, and mucous membranes of mouth
Sensory	Sensation to parts of external ear, auditory canal, and tympanic membrane
	Taste to anterior two thirds of tongue
VIII—Vestibulocochlear	Equilibrium and hearing
IX—Glossopharyngeal	
Parasympathetic	Parotid gland
Motor	Stylopharyngeal muscle
Sensory	Sensation to posterior one third of tongue, pharynx, middle ear, and dura
X—Vagus	
Parasympathetic	Viscera of thorax and abdomen
Motor	Muscles of pharynx and larynx
Sensory somatic	Dura and auditory canal
Sensory visceral	Viscera of thorax and abdomen
XI—Accessory	
Motor	Muscles of larynx, sternocleidomastoid, and trapezius
XII—Hypoglossal	Intrinsic muscles of tongue, genioglossus, hypoglossus, and styloglossus

Sensory examination in the patient with neuropathic pain extends beyond routine discrimination of sharp and dull sensations and requires testing for mechanical and thermal allodynia, summation and after-sensation, hyperalgesia, and hyperpathia.

Sensory Testing

- Dynamic allodynia: lightly rub fingertip, foam, or cotton swab across skin.
- Static allodynia: slowly apply perpendicular pressure to blunt device (cotton swab).

Table 3. Painful sensory neuropathies

Endocrinologic
Diabetes mellitus
Hypothyroidism

Metabolic
Uremia
Thiamine deficiency
Acute intermittent porphyria

Toxic
Vincristine
Acrylamide
Heavy metals
Organic solvents

Infectious/inflammatory
HIV-related painful neuropathies
Herpes zoster—acute and chronic postherpetic neuralgia
Guillain–Barré syndrome
Chronic inflammatory polyneuropathy

Immunologic
Polyarteritis nodosa
Cryoglobulinemia
Systemic lupus erythematosus

Physical
Brachial plexopathies
Compressive

Neoplastic
Multiple myeloma
Cancer (including nonmetastatic effects and carcinomatosis)

Genetic
Fabry disease
Tangier disease
Familial dysautonomias (Riley–Day syndrome, inherited sensory
    neuropathy III)
Amyloidosis

- Thermal allodynia: Warm/cold test tube or tuning fork.
- Hyperalgesia: single pinprick; multiple pinpricks for summation/ aftersensations.

Pain of psychogenic origin will usually result in a neurologic examination that does not correlate with findings typical of organic pathology. Abnormal pain distributions, such as glove or stocking patterns, and exact hemianesthesia are common in patients with psychogenic pain.

4. Musculoskeletal System Examination

Abnormalities of the musculoskeletal system are often evident on inspection of the patient's posture and muscular symmetry. Muscle atrophy usually indicates disuse. Flaccidity indicates extreme weakness, usually from paralysis, and abnormal movements indicate neurologic damage or impaired proprioception.

Table 4.   **Pain-induced disturbances of gait**

Diagnosis	Symptoms
Intermittent claudication	Pain on walking a specific distance, arterial insufficiency
	Pain appears sooner with increasing intensity of work
	Pain disappears after rest
	Pain localized to calf
Cauda equina (neurogenic claudication, spinal stenosis)	Pain on walking after varying distances
	Patient usually older
	Pain usually bilateral
	Radicular in character
	Pain localized to saddle area, upper thigh, and calf
	Pain in back on sneezing
	Pain does not usually disappear on cessation of walking
	Pain improves when leaning forward
Hip disease	Pain worsens with first few steps
Inguinal region	Pain increases on prolonged standing
	Usually after appendectomy, hernia repair
Meralgia paresthetica	Pain in the lateral aspect of the thigh
Long bones	Localized pain
	Evidence of tumor/osteoporosis, Paget disease, pathologic fracture
	After surgical procedure—anterior compartment syndrome
Feet	
Foot deformities	Pain after walking or standing
Calcaneal spur	Pain in the plantar aspect of foot (prevents walking)
Achilles tendinitis	
Tarsal tunnel syndrome	

From Mumenthaler M. *Neurologic differential diagnosis.* New York: Thieme-Stratton, 1925:118–119, with permission.

Limited range of motion of a major joint can indicate pain, disc disease, or arthritis. Palpation of muscles will help in evaluating range of motion and in determining whether trigger points are present. Coordination and strength are also tested.

5. Assessment of Psychological Factors

Complete assessment of pain includes analysis of the psychological aspects of pain and the effects of pain on behavior and emotional stability. Such assessment is challenging because many patients are unaware of or are reluctant to present psychological issues. It is also more socially acceptable to seek medical

Table 5. Common painful root syndromes

Root	Sensory Loss	Motor Changes	
		Weakness	Decreased Deep Tendon Reflexes
Upper extremity			
C5	Lateral aspect of upper arm	Deltoid and biceps	None/biceps
C6	Thumb and index finger	Biceps and brachioradialis	Brachioradialis and biceps
C7	Middle finger	Triceps and pronator teres	Triceps
Lower extremity			
L4	Medial calf	Quadriceps	Knee
L5	Medial half of foot and lateral calf	Peroneal, anterior and posterior tibial and toe extension	Internal hamstring
S1	Lower posterior calf and lateral foot	Plantar flexion	Ankle

than psychiatric care. Initially, the use of a descriptive pain questionnaire such as the MPQ may provide some evidence of a patient's affective responses to pain. For example, words such as "aching" and "tingling" refer to sensory aspects of pain, whereas words such as "agonizing" and "dreadful" suggest negative feelings and do not aid in characterizing the pain sensation. For a better description of psychological evaluation in pain management, see Chapter 15.

A patient's personality greatly influences his or her response to pain and choice of the coping strategy. Some patients may benefit from the use of strategies of control such as distraction and relaxation. Patients who have an underlying anxiety disorder may be more likely to seek high doses of analgesics. Therefore, inquiry regarding a patient's history of coping with stress is often useful.

As part of the pain history, the clinician should include questions about some of the common symptoms in patients with chronic pain: depressed mood, sleep disturbance, preoccupation with somatic symptoms, reduced activity, reduced libido, and fatigue. Standardized questionnaires, such as the Minnesota Multiphasic Personality Inventory (MMPI), may expand the assessment. On this inventory patients with chronic pain characteristically score very high on the depression, hysteria, and hypochondriasis scales. However, the MMPI may reflect functional limitation secondary to pain, as well as psychological abnormality associated with chronic pain, limiting its interpretation for some patients suspected of having psychogenic pain.

A number of psychological processes and syndromes predispose patients to chronic pain. Predisposing disorders include major depression, somatization disorder, conversion disorder, hypochondriasis, and psychogenic pain disorder. The diagnosis of somatization disorder is quite specific, although many patients with chronic pain may "somatize" (focus on somatic complaints). Somatization disorder as such requires a history of physical symptoms of several years' duration, beginning before the age of 30 years and including complaints of at least 14 specific symptoms for women and 12 for men. These symptoms are not adequately explained by physical disorder, injury, or toxic reaction.

Psychogenic pain may occur in susceptible individuals. In some patients, pain may ameliorate more unpleasant feelings, such as depression, guilt, or anxiety, and distract the patient from environmental stress factors. Historic features that suggest a psychogenic component to chronic pain include the following:

- Multiple locations of pain at different times
- Pain problems dating since adolescence
- Pain without obvious somatic cause (especially in the facial or perineal area)
- Multiple, elective surgical procedures
- Substance abuse (patient and/or significant other)
- Social or work failure

Psychogenic pain is clearly distinct from malingering. Malingerers have an obvious, identifiable environmental goal in producing symptoms, such as evading law enforcement, avoiding work, or obtaining financial compensation. Patients with

THE CLINICAL JOURNAL OF PAIN

Subscription Reply Card

THE CLINICAL JOURNAL OF PAIN

SAVE 10%

The **Clinical Journal of Pain** explores all aspects of pain and its effective treatment, bringing you the insights of leading anesthesiologists, surgeons, internists, neurologists, orthopedists, psychiatrists and psychologists, clinical pharmacologists, and rehabilitation medicine specialists. Each bimonthly issue presents timely and thought-provoking articles on clinical dilemmas in pain management; valuable diagnostic procedures; promising new pharmacological, surgical, and other therapeutic modalities; psychosocial dimensions of pain; and ethical issues of concern to all medical professionals. The journal also publishes Special Topic issues on subjects of particular relevance to the practice of pain medicine.

☑ **YES**, please begin my subscription to *Clinical Journal of Pain* at the rate checked below.

9 issues per year • ISSN: 0749-8047 • www.clinicalpain.com

Editor-in-Chief:
Dennis C. Turk, PhD

	In the U.S.	Outside the U.S.
Individual	❏ $~~282.00~~ $255.00	❏ $~~282.00~~ $255.00
Institutional	❏ $~~498.00~~ $449.00	❏ $~~498.00~~ $449.00
In-training	❏ $~~123.00~~ $112.00	❏ $~~123.00~~ $112.00

Add $8.00 for air freight delivery outside the U.S., Canada, and Mexico.

Subscribe up to 3 years at the DISCOUNTED current rate! ❏ 3 years ❏ 2 years ❏ 1 year

Please indicate method of payment:

❏ Check payable to Lippincott Williams & Wilkins

❏ VISA ❏ MasterCard ❏ AMEX ❏ Discover ❏ Diners Club

Card #_____Exp. Date_____

Signature_____

Name_____

Address_____

City/State/Prov._____

Country_____Zip/Postal Code_____

Phone_____

E-mail_____

Your e-mail address will be used if we need to contact you regarding your order.
You will also receive product updates and special offers from LWW.com.

Individual subscription rates include print and access to the online version. Institutional rates are for print only; online subscriptions are available via Ovid. Prices in U.S. funds and subject to change. Prices include a handling charge. Please indicate sales tax when applicable. In Canada, add 7% GST. Institutional rates apply to libraries, hospitals, corporations, and partnerships of three or more individuals. Subscription will begin with the currently available issue unless you request otherwise.

Four Easy Ways to Order!

❶ VISIT www.LWW.com available on

❷ FAX 1-301-223-2400

❸ CALL 1-800-638-3030 or 1-301-223-2300 (outside the U.S. and Canada)

❹ MAIL this card

LIPPINCOTT
WILLIAMS & WILKINS
P.O. Box 1600
Hagerstown, MD 21741-1600
USA

S5ANS053   I5S053ZZ

psychogenic pain make illness and hospitalization their primary goals. Being a patient is their primary way of life. Such patients are unable to stop symptom production when it is no longer obviously beneficial.

The physical examination in patients with psychological factors exacerbating pain may be perplexing. Some findings may not correspond to known anatomic or physiologic information. Examples of such findings include the following:

- manual testing inconsistent with patient observation during sitting, turning, and dressing
- grasping with three fingers
- antagonist muscle contraction on attempted movement
- decreased tremor during mental arithmetic exercises
- a positive Romberg sign with one eye closed
- vibration sense absent on one side of midline (e.g., right side of skull or sternum)
- inconsistency of timed vibration when affected side is tested first
- patterned miscount of touches
- difficulty touching the good limb with the bad
- a slight difference in sensation on one side of the body.

Useful neurologic signs are deep tendon reflexes, motor tone and bulk, and the plantar response. Observation is crucial. Pain drawings at multiple time intervals are also useful in evaluating on a patient with chronic pain of unclear etiology.

III. DIAGNOSTIC STUDIES

The diagnosis and understanding of a patient's pain complaint can usually be obtained after a thorough history and physical examination. Diagnostic and physiologic studies are used to support a clinician's suspicion, as well as to assist in the diagnosis. Some of the more common studies used for pain assessment are described in following text.

Conventional radiography is used to diagnose bony abnormalities such as pathologic fractures seen in bony metastases; spine pathology, including spondylolisthesis, stenosis, and osteophyte formation; and in bone tumors. Some soft-tissue tumors and bowel abnormalities can also be seen. X-rays of the painful area have usually been obtained by the referring physician.

A **computerized tomography** scan is most often used to define bony abnormalities, and **magnetic resonance imaging** best shows soft-tissue pathology. Spinal stenosis, disk herniation or bulge, nerve root compression, and tumors in all tissues can be diagnosed, as well as some causes of central pain, such as CNS infarcts or plaques of demyelination.

Diagnostic blocks may differentiate somatic pain from visceral pain and confirm the anatomic location of peripheral nerve pain. These blocks may help localize painful pathology or contribute to the diagnosis of complex regional pain syndrome (CRPS). They are also necessary precedents to neurolytic blocks for malignant pain or radiofrequency lesions. The various diagnostic blocks are described in detail in Chapter 12.

Drug challenges are used to predict drug treatment utility and help in the assessment of pain etiology. For example, brief intravenous infusions of opioids, lidocaine, and phentolamine are used to predict opioid sensitivity in nonmalignant chronic pain and sensitivity to sodium channel blockade in neuropathic pain, and to assess the potential reversibility of the sympathetic component of pain in CRPS. The value of this type of testing in predicting treatment efficacy is debatable. In most reports, chronic treatment has been limited to responders, which precludes validation of the infusion as a predictive test.

Various **neurophysiologic tests** are used to help in the diagnosis of pain syndromes and related neurologic disease. These tests are described in Chapter 7. The neurophysiologic tests most commonly used in pain clinics come under the general category of Quantitative Sensory Testing (QST), and these tests specifically evaluate patients' responses to carefully quantified physical stimuli.

Thermography is a noninvasive way of displaying the body's thermal patterns. A normal thermal pattern is relatively symmetric. Tissue pathology is associated with chemical and metabolic changes that may cause abnormal thermal patterns by altering vascularity, such as in CRPS. The patterns of color difference seen are not specific for underlying central or peripheral pathology.

Myelography is the injection of radiopaque dye into the subarachnoid space to visualize spinal cord/column abnormalities radiographically, such as disk herniation, nerve root impingement, arachnoiditis, and spinal stenosis. Major disadvantages of this procedure are postdural-puncture headache and meningeal irritation.

Bone scanning is the use of a radioactive compound to detect a number of bone lesions, including neoplastic, infectious, arthritic, traumatic, Paget disease, and the osteodystrophy of reflex sympathetic dystrophy. The radioactive compound accumulates in areas of increased bone growth or turnover. It is a very sensitive test for subtle bone abnormalities that may not appear on conventional radiographs.

The removal of small punch **skin biopsies** (immunolabeled to show the cutaneous sensory nerve endings) has provided a new tool with which to directly visualize the cutaneous endings of pain neurons. Although currently available at only a few centers, this technique is replacing sural nerve biopsy for the diagnosis of sensory neuropathies. The technique appears to be helpful for diagnosing focal painful nerve injuries. Research has shown that various painful neuropathic conditions are associated with loss of nociceptive innervation in the painful region of the skin. Skin biopsies are only minimally invasive, can be repeated, and can be performed in areas other than those innervated by the sural nerve.

Functional brain imaging, such as positron emission tomography and functional magnetic resonance imaging (fMRI), is an investigative tool, at present, with provocative findings about the cortical and subcortical processing of pain information. The fMRI shows pain to be remarkably distributed at the cortical level.

IV. CONCLUSION

The assessment of pain can be challenging and intensive but is an essential component of pain management and allows the pain physician to devise optimal treatment of some of the most complex pain issues of patients. It is important to treat the patient as a complete person and not just the painful location. Believing the patient and establishing rapport with the patient are of the utmost importance. A systematic approach, grounded in knowledge of anatomy and physiology, will assist the clinician in determining the pathophysiology of the patient's pain complaint. With this essential knowledge, therapy can be formulated, promptly initiated, and easily reassessed.

SUGGESTED READINGS

Beecher HK. *Measurement of subjective responses.* New York: Oxford University Press, 1959.

Bovie J, Hansson P, Lindblom U, eds. *Touch, temperature and pain in health and disease: mechanisms and assessments*, Vol. 3. Seattle, WA: IASP Press, 1994.

Carlsson AM. Assessment of chronic pain I: aspects of the reliability and validity of the visual analogue scale. *Pain* 1983;16:87–101.

Galer BS, Dworkin RH. *A clinical guide to neuropathic pain.* Minneapolis, MN: McGraw-Hill, 2000.

Gracely RH. Evaluation of multidimensional pain scales. *Pain* 1992; 48:297–300.

Katz J. Psychophysical correlates of phantom limb experience. *J Neurol Neurosurg Psychiatry* 1992;55:811–821.

Lowe NK, Walder SM, McCallum RC. Confirming the theoretic structure of the McGill pain questionnaire in acute clinical pain. *Pain* 1991;46:53–60.

McGrath PA. *Pain in children: nature, assessment and treatment.* New York: Guildford Press, 1990.

Melzack R, Katz J. Pain measurement in persons in pain. In: Wall PD, Melzack R, eds. *Textbook of pain*, 4th ed. New York: Churchill Livingstone, 1999.

Melzack R. The McGill questionnaire: major properties and scoring methods. *Pain* 1975;1:277–299.

Price DD, Bush FM, Long S, et al. A comparison of pain measurement characteristics of mechanical visual analogue and simple numerical rating scales. *Pain* 1994;56:217–226.

7

Neurophysiologic Testing in Pain Management

Annabel D. Edwards and Lisa S. Krivickas

As to pain, I am almost ready to say the physician who has not felt it is imperfectly educated.
—*R. Weir Mitchell*

I. INTRODUCTION

When physiologists learned that nerve transmission is based on electrical principles, they began to devise ways to measure neuronal activity. Pain signals are communicated through the peripheral and central nervous systems and are interpreted supraspinally. The understanding that small and large sensory fibers play different roles in various pain states has led to differential nerve fiber testing. Parts of the nervous system that are not normally involved in pain messaging, such as the sympathetic and parasympathetic systems, can become involved in certain disease states, after injury, and/or following sensitization. Neuronal activity in various afferent systems can overlap and connect or change functionally (both anatomically and at a cellular and molecular level), creating a particularly complex challenge for the diagnosis and treatment of some pain problems. Evaluation of such a potentially confusing network of neurons can be a challenge.

Neurophysiologic testing is broad in scope and has developed over a long time. Although electrodiagnostic studies were said to have been performed by Swammerdam in the 1600s, it was not until the mid-1900s that the testing progressed to the point of clinical usefulness. Electrodiagnostic studies can assess the function of large-diameter sensory and motor nerve fibers, localize focal peripheral nerve lesions, and evaluate overall peripheral nerve function. Autonomic nervous system (ANS) testing helps elucidate the role of sympathetic and parasympathetic nerves in the processing and modulation of pain states, although there is no clearly defined pattern of ANS response that is recognized as demonstrating the presence of "chronic pain." Quantitative sensory testing (QST) techniques [warm sensation (WS) and cool sensation (CS), hot pain (HP) and cold pain (CP), electrical stimulation, etc.], although not as objective as electrodiagnostic testing, can help evaluate the function of small-diameter nerve fibers (nociceptive fibers) in the entire sensory pathway, and cannot be used to localize nerve lesions. Used in combination, these neurophysiologic tests can provide information about the neuronal mechanism(s) involved in pain.

Neurophysiologic testing is useful because it

- helps detect underlying pathology;
- helps define pain mechanisms;
- helps anatomically localize pain instigators;
- helps focus treatments on mechanisms;
- helps predict if patients will respond to particular treatments by clarifying mechanisms;
- used sequentially, helps monitor disease progress and response to treatment;
- may have medico-legal applications;
- advances pain research by providing quantitative and reproducible measurements of pain and its various mechanisms.

In clinical practice, neurophysiologic testing is useful when a diagnosis is elusive or when a pain problem has been refractory to treatment. Neurophysiologic testing can be time-consuming and is not appropriate for all patients. Patients should be tested only if their condition is likely to be better managed because of the results. Figure 1 summarizes the utility of various tests for different parts of the nervous system.

II. ELECTRODIAGNOSTIC TESTING

Electrodiagnostic testing is used to diagnose peripheral nervous system disorders. These include radiculopathies, plexopathies, mononeuropathies, and generalized peripheral neuropathies. Occasionally, myopathic disorders such as myotonic dystrophy type II present with pain as a chief complaint. A more focused treatment plan can be devised by localizing the source of a patient's pain to a specific location in the peripheral nervous system. A normal electrodiagnostic evaluation can also help narrow the differential diagnosis when the pain is of unclear etiology. Electrodiagnostic studies are normal in patients with only central nervous system pathology and in those with only small fiber neuropathy or sources of pain.

Routine electrodiagnostic evaluations [often referred to as EMG (electromyogram)] comprise nerve conduction studies (NCSs) and needle electrode examination (NEE). An electrodiagnostic study must include both components to provide a complete assessment of peripheral nervous system function. The results can assist in determining the severity of a lesion and the prognosis for recovery.

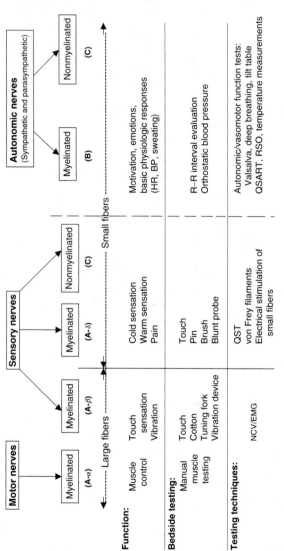

Figure 1. The peripheral nerve fibers. NCV, nerve conduction velocity; EMG, electromyography; QST, quantitative sensory testing; QSART, quantitative sudomotor axon reflex testing; RSO, resting sweat output.

1. Nerve Conduction Studies

NCSs are performed by electrically stimulating a nerve and then by recording a response from either the nerve itself or a muscle it innervates. The two basic types of NCS are motor and sensory. An additional category of study is called the "late response," which includes detection of a characteristic wave (F wave) or a reflex (H reflex). The parameters assessed in NCSs are the amplitude of the response, the latency (time between nerve stimulation and response generation), and the nerve conduction velocity (NCV). These parameters are compared with established sets of normal values. The amplitude reflects the number of intact axons, and the distal latency and conduction velocity reflect the integrity of the myelin sheath. Therefore, amplitude is reduced in axonal nerve lesions, and conduction velocity is reduced in demyelinating lesions.

Motor NCSs are performed by stimulating a motor nerve and by recording a compound motor action potential (CMAP) from the belly of a muscle innervated by that nerve. For example, the median motor study is performed by stimulating the median nerve at the wrist and by recording a CMAP from the abductor pollicis brevis (APB) muscle, as pictured in Figure 2. The nerve is then stimulated at a more proximal site so that a conduction velocity may be calculated between the two sites of stimulation.

Sensory NCSs are performed by stimulating sensory nerves and by recording sensory nerve action potentials (SNAPs). For example, the median sensory study is performed by stimulating the median nerve at the wrist and by recording a SNAP from the digital nerves of the second finger. SNAPs are much smaller in amplitude than CMAPs because they are nerve-generated potentials rather than muscle-generated potentials.

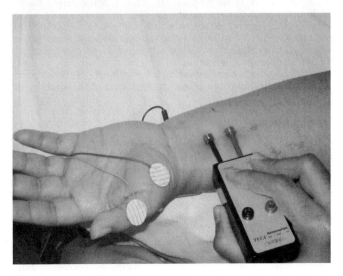

Figure 2.   The median motor study being performed by stimulating the median nerve at the wrist.

When assessing the results of NCSs, amplitude measurements are as important, if not more important, than NCV because most nerve lesions are primarily axonal rather than demyelinating. Amplitudes correspond to clinical symptoms such as pain, weakness, and sensory loss, whereas demyelination itself does not cause any symptoms.

2. Needle Electrode Examination

The NEE involves inserting a needle electrode into the muscle belly to look for evidence of denervation or of a myopathic disorder. The electrical activity of the muscle at rest and the electrical activity generated by voluntary activation of the muscle are assessed. When the muscle is relaxed, the electromyographer looks at insertional activity (the response of the muscle to small movements of the electrode) and for spontaneous activity that can include fasciculations, positive sharp waves, fibrillation potentials, complex repetitive discharges, and myotonic discharges. When the muscle is activated, the size and shape of voluntary motor units and their firing pattern are assessed. When a muscle is denervated, the motor units are reduced in number but fire excessively fast; this is called "reduced recruitment." In myopathic disorders, a large number of motor units fire at a normal rate despite minimal force production; this is called "early recruitment." In chronic neuropathic disorders, motor units become excessively large. In myopathic disorders, the motor units are smaller than normal.

3. Findings in Nerve Injury

The EMG findings following nerve injury depend on the severity of the injury and its chronicity. With an axonal nerve injury or neuropathy, sensory and motor amplitudes will be reduced on NCS, and the NCV may be slightly slow. When a mixed nerve, such as the median nerve, is involved, sensory fibers are usually involved to a greater extent than motor fibers. In demyelinating neuropathies, NCV will be considerably slowed and distal latencies and F wave latencies will be prolonged. Needle examination will show decreased recruitment, with rapidly firing motor units in both axonal and demyelinating neuropathies. In axonal nerve lesions, fibrillation potentials and other forms of abnormal spontaneous activity are present. In chronic axonal neuropathies, reinnervation produces motor unit remodeling so that the remaining motor units are increased in size.

4. Timing

Under normal circumstances, the EMG study should not be performed sooner than 3 weeks postinjury because it often takes this long for fibrillation potentials to develop in denervated muscle. In addition, the process of wallerian degeneration must occur before NCS amplitudes reach their nadir. Following an acute axonotmetic or neurotmetic lesion, CMAP amplitudes recorded distal to the lesion begin to decline at 3 days and reach their nadir at 7 days; SNAP amplitudes begin to drop at 6 days and reach their nadir at 11 days. If an EMG study is performed too soon following a nerve injury, a severe axon loss lesion may be incorrectly diagnosed as a less severe axonal or demyelinating lesion.

III. QUANTITATIVE SENSORY TESTING

QST has a major application in pain management practice and perhaps an even bigger role in pain research. It specifically tests high-threshold pain and temperature-sensing mechanisms, provides information on the function of the entire afferent pain pathway (from receptor to brain), is noninvasive, and is relatively simple to perform. These are considered psychophysical tests because they lack the objectivity seen in electrodiagnostic and ANS studies. In cases where NCS and EMG may be normal, however, QST results can demonstrate hypoesthesia or hyperalgesia. When using QST methods to look for small fiber neuropathy, diagnostic sensitivity has been reported as ranging from 67% to 100%. There is no single listing of tests that fit into the category of QST, but common tests measure responses to thermal (warm, cool, hot, and cold), mechanical (light touch and pinprick), vibratory, and electrical stimuli. They primarily explore the function of the primary nociceptive afferents, the Aδ and C fibers, and Aβ fibers. Each fiber type responds to specific kinds of stimuli allowing for tests to be chosen to elucidate their functioning. For example, Aδ fibers are activated by cold perception and by HP and CP stimuli, C fibers by warm perception and by HP and CP stimuli, and the Aβ fibers by vibration.

Measured stimuli (most commonly thermal) are used to invoke pain responses. In abnormal pain states such as allodynia and hyperalgesia, there are alterations in the pain threshold (see Chapter 1). Common findings and their association with various pain processes are listed in Table 1.

Table 1.   Pain processes and their association with test findings

Pain Processes	Test Findings
Painful neuropathies (including CRPS II)	Thermal hypesthesia, hyperesthesia, hypoalgesia or hyperalgesia
Peripheral sensitization and inflammation	Heat hyperalgesia
CRPS I	Cold or heat hyperalgesia without hypesthesia or hyperesthesia
Central sensitization	Tactile allodynia, mechanical hyperalgesia
Postherpetic neuralgia	Thermal hypoesthesia and hyperalgesia (anesthesia dolorosa)
Sympathetically mediated pain (CRPS I and II)	Changes in sudomotor reflexes (QSART), sweat output (RSO), and vasomotor function

CRPS, complex regional pain syndrome; QSART, quantitative sudomotor axon reflex testing; RSO, resting sweat output.
For definition of terms, see *Definitions and Abbreviations*.

QST relies on subjective responses to calibrated sensory stimuli. The responses are, therefore, susceptible to confounding factors that can lead to inaccuracy. These include the following:

- Unwillingness or inability to pay attention and to respond accurately
- Distractions and discomfort during testing
- Inability to understand directions and use equipment properly
- Medical problems (known and unknown)
- Use of medications

Other potential confounding factors include faulty equipment, failure to adhere to standard protocols, and the lack of normative data for particular testing sites or techniques. There is considerable variation between centers in the testing methods that are used. A continuing important challenge for pain clinicians and researchers is to reach a consensus on testing methodology so that results are broadly applicable across patient populations. Some of the equipment used for QST is expensive and requires careful maintenance, a quiet testing space, and a person willing to spend the time to become proficient in its use.

As is usual for most neurologic examinations, testing should be done on the pain site and on contralateral and remote sites for comparison.

1. Thermal Stimuli

Pain and temperature sensitivities are closely related because they are both transmitted to higher brain centers by small, high-threshold fibers (C and Aδ) via the lateral spinothalamic tracts. To test thermal thresholds, specific devices have been built that can activate temperature changes on a small-surface thermode that is placed flat against the skin. A computer regulates the thermal changes such that the rate and extent of change are controlled within specific limits. The device is very safe when used in the traditional clinical testing modes. In research, the usual clinical restrictions can be bypassed, allowing for more varied patterns and degrees of thermal exposure. Clinical testing variables that need to be controlled include the size of the thermode used, the site chosen for testing, and the pattern of stimuli delivered. There are suggested testing sites based on the pain area and normative data for result comparisons. For example, to test the S1 dermatome, the thermode is placed on the dorsum of the foot proximal to the fourth and fifth toes, spaced equally between them. Basic protocols have been described to help standardize testing and should be used by all centers doing such clinical testing. The thresholds measured with this device are identified as WS, CS, HP, and CP. One is usually able to detect a temperature change from baseline (WS and CS) within 1°C to 2°C up or down. HP is typically felt at approximately 45°C. CP threshold is quite variable but can occur starting at approximately 10°C or less.

2. Vibration Stimuli

The vibration test measures the sensitivity of the larger Aβ fibers. The head of the vibration device must make a solid, even, and balanced contact on the testing site. The amount of pressure applied at the site must be as reliably controlled as possible because extra pressure can alter nerve function readings. Vibration devices usually have a range of at least 0 to 130 μ, and they must be able to deliver vibration stimuli at a rate of 0.1 to 4 μ per second. Again, site selection is critical and the literature identifies recommended sites. For example, to test the S1 dermatome, the device is placed on the plantar surface of the foot between the fourth and fifth toes on the metatarsal head.

3. Mechanical Stimuli

One of the most common ways to quantify sensitivity to mechanical stimuli is through the use of von Frey hairs (or similar filaments). The testing units are commonly made of nylon filaments of graduated diameter that, when pressed down on the skin hard enough to cause them to bend, exert a reproducible and reliable calibrated force. The filaments usually come in sets that span a range of force from 4.5 mg to 447 g. Some practitioners present the values of the force in terms of either tension (g per cm) or pressure (g per cm^2). Testing through the whole range of the filaments is time-consuming. In most clinical situations, a few representative filaments are selected for screening purposes to detect early stages of, for example, diabetic peripheral neuropathy. Changes in pain thresholds and areas of primary and secondary hyperalgesia can be detected.

Mechanical stimuli can be used to test for **summation**, which can be detected in neuropathic pain states (e.g., spinal cord injury and post-herpetic–neuralgia), and nociceptive pain states (e.g., fibromyalgia and temporomandibular disorders). The rhythmic application of a pinprick to the same site on the skin over a period of at least eight repetitions, each being delivered within 2 to 3 seconds of the previous one, will cause a considerable escalation of discomfort in a person with hyperalgesia. The amount of force used needs to be just enough to cause a slight pricking sensation. Testing can also be done with blunt stimuli, as from an **algometer**, which looks similar to a drill press.

Testing for tactile allodynia can be accomplished using several modalities, including a cotton-tipped applicator, camel's hair brush, or a finger.

4. Electrical Stimuli

Sensory nerve perception thresholds can be measured using a simple-to-operate electrical device. The machines generate stimuli of 5 Hz, 250 Hz, and 2,000 Hz. The 5-Hz stimulus is purported to activate the C fibers, 250 Hz the Aβ fibers, and the 2,000 Hz the Aδ fibers. The machines can generate a current ranging from approximately 0.1 to 9.99 mA. Research results indicate that these studies can help isolate nerve root pathology. There is still some debate about the accuracy of the claim that the specific levels of stimuli, as described, actually activate the specified nerve fiber types. In general, low CPT (current perception threshold) measures are associated with inflammation or neuritis and reflect a hyperesthetic state. Abnormally elevated CPT measures reflect a hypoesthetic state, such as found in neuropathy, and indicate a loss of nerve function.

IV. AUTONOMIC TESTING

Small fiber sensory neuropathy causing severe neuropathic pain is often accompanied by ANS dysfunction. Causes include diabetes, monoclonal gammopathies, amyloidosis, acquired immune deficiency syndrome (AIDS), nutritional deficiency, Tangier disease, Fabry disease, and the hereditary sensory and autonomic neuropathies (HSANs). Routine EMG testing can be normal in patients with a purely small fiber neuropathy because motor and sensory NCSs assess conduction along large-diameter myelinated nerve fibers only. Therefore, in patients with symptoms suggesting neuropathic pain who have normal NCSs, autonomic testing can be useful in attempting to diagnose small-fiber neuropathy. This testing should also be considered in patients with other symptoms suggesting dysautonomia, such as syncope, orthostatic hypotension, gastrointestinal or urologic disturbances, and sweating disorders. Autonomic tests can be divided into two categories: those that assess sudomotor and those that assess cardiovagal and adrenergic function. Testing of sudomotor function is most valuable in patients with suspected small-fiber neuropathy because these patients are most likely to have abnormalities in vasomotor function and sweating. Abnormalities in cardiovagal and adrenergic function are less common.

1. Sudomotor Function

Assessment of sudomotor function in the distal extremity can provide objective evidence of a small-fiber neuropathy. The term sudomotor refers to the sympathetic pathways involved in sweat production. Three tests are available to assess sudomotor function. The simplest, but least reliable, test is the **sympathetic skin response**. This test can be performed using standard EMG equipment. Because of the large intersubject variability and the habituation of the response with repeated stimuli, only the absence of a response indicates abnormality. The **quantitative sudomotor axon reflex test** (QSART) is relatively a new test with high sensitivity and reliability. A special sweat capsule is attached to the skin, and acetylcholine is iontophoresed through the skin to produce a sweat response. The sweat is then collected in the capsule and quantified. A third, older method of assessing sudomotor function is the **thermoregulatory sweat test** (TST). The TST is sensitive and reliable but quite messy and must be performed in a special heat tent or sweat chamber. A powder that changes color when exposed to sweat is applied to the skin over the entire body, allowing areas of anhidrosis to be mapped.

2. Cardiovagal and Adrenergic Function

Three commonly used tests of cardiovagal and adrenergic function are the heart rate response to deep breathing, the heart rate and blood pressure responses to the Valsalva maneuver, and head-upright tilt. The heart rate response to deep breathing is determined by parasympathetic function only, whereas the response to Valsalva maneuver and head-upright tilt are mediated by a combination of sympathetic and parasympathetic function.

V. CONCLUSION

This chapter describes some of the neurophysiologic tests used in pain management and research. Some of these tests (chiefly those used to aid in the diagnosis of disease) need to be conducted by experienced personnel and are usually available only in the hospital setting. The most useful tests in the pain clinic are those that are incorporated in QST. QST is essentially noninvasive and causes little discomfort, which makes it widely applicable. Although the tests are time-consuming, which restricts their clinical use, it is sometimes helpful to use the tests to document treatment effects and, in some cases, to optimize treatment.

SELECTED READINGS

Chong PST, Cros DP. Technology literature review: quantitative sensory testing. *Muscle Nerve* 2004;29:734–747.

Cobb, M. Exorcizing the animal spirits: Jan Swammerdam on nerve function. *Nat Rev Neurosci* 2002;3:395–400.

Cruccu G, Anand P, Attal N, et al. EFNS guidelines on neuropathic pain assessment. *Eur J Neurol* 2004;11:153–162.

Jaradeh SS, Prieto TE. Evaluation of the autonomic nervous system. *Phys Med Rehabil Clin N Am* 2003;14(2):287–305.

Lefaucheur JP, Creange A. Neurophysiological testing correlates with clinical examination according to fibre type involvement and severity in sensory neuropathy. *J Neurol Neurosurg Psychiatry* 2004;75: 417–422.

Verdugo R, Ochoa JL. Quantitative somatosensory thermotest. A key method for functional evaluation of small caliber afferent channels. *Brain* 1992;115(Pt. 3):893–913.

Zaslansky R, Yarnitsky D. Clinical applications of quantitative sensory testing (QST). *J Neurol Sci* 1998;153:215–238.

Therapeutic Options: Pharmacologic Approaches

8

Nonsteroidal Antiinflammatory Drugs

Jane C. Ballantyne and Steven A. Barna

Take an aspirin and call me in the morning.
—*Twentieth-century physician*

The nonsteroidal antiinflammatory drugs (NSAIDs), including aspirin, are the most widely used analgesics in the United States and worldwide. Although they are considered weak analgesics, NSAIDs are used for the treatment of headaches, menstrual cramps, arthritis, and a wide range of minor aches and pains. NSAIDs have also become popular for use in the surgical population, especially since the advent of injectable preparations. Because of their predominantly peripheral site of action, they are useful in combination with opioids and other centrally acting analgesics for severe pain, both acute and chronic. This chapter reviews the use of NSAIDs for acute and chronic pain—indications, efficacy, side effects, and contraindications.

I. PHARMACOLOGY

The NSAIDs are a heterogeneous group of compounds consisting of one or more aromatic rings connected to an acidic functional group (see Fig. 1). The chemical families of the commonly used NSAIDs are outlined in Table 1. The NSAIDs are weak organic acids (pKa 3 to 5.5), act mainly in the periphery, bind extensively to plasma albumin (95% to 99% bound), do not readily cross the blood–brain barrier, are extensively metabolized by the liver, and have low renal clearance (<10%). Acetaminophen is not strictly an antiinflammatory drug but is included in this group of drugs because it shares many of the properties of the NSAIDs. In contrast to the true NSAIDs, acetaminophen is nonacidic, is a phenol derivative, and readily crosses the blood–brain barrier. It acts mainly in the central nervous system, where prostaglandin inhibition produces analgesia and antipyresis. Its peripheral and antiinflammatory effects are weak.

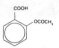

Aspirin

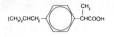

Indomethacin

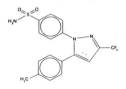

Celecoxib

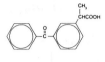

Ketoprofen

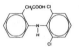

Diclofenac

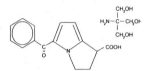

Ketorolac tromethamine

Diflunisal

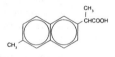

Naproxen

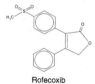

Rofecoxib

Paracetamol

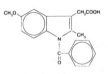

Ibuprofen

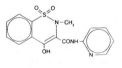

Piroxicam

Figure 1.   Chemical structures of commonly used nonsteroidal anti-inflammatory drugs.

**Table 1.   Classification of commonly
used antipyretic analgesics**

I. **Carboxylic acid and enolic acid groups (pKa 3–5.5)**
   A. **Carboxylic acid containing**
      salicylates
      *aspirin, diflunisal, salicylic acid, salsalate, sodium salicylate,
         choline magnesium trisalicylate*
      2-propionic acid derivatives
      *naproxen, ibuprofen, ketoprofen, flurbiprofen, fenoprofen,
         carprofen, nabumetone[a]*
      indoleacetic acid derivatives
      indomethacin, suldinac
      phenylacetic acid derivatives
      diclofenac, alclofenac, fenclofenac
      pyrroleacetic acid derivatives
      ketorolac, tolmetin
      N-phenylanthranilic acid derivatives
      mefenamic acid
   B. **Enolic acid containing**
      enolic acid pyrazolone derivatives
      phenylbutazone, aminopyrine, antipyrine, piroxicam
II. **Benzenesulfonic acid derivatives**
      celecoxib, rofecoxib, valecoxib
III. **Phenol group (pKa 9–10)**
      para-amino-phenol derivatives
      paracetamol/acetaminophen, phenacetin

[a]A nonacidic prodrug metabolized to a structural analog of naproxen and
thought to be associated with less GI toxicity than the acidic NSAIDs.

NSAIDs are powerful inhibitors of prostaglandin synthesis
through their effect on cyclooxygenase (COX) (see Fig. 2).
Prostaglandins have many effects, and the therapeutic and toxic
effects of NSAIDs can be accounted for by the ability of these
drugs to inhibit prostaglandin and thromboxane synthesis (see
Table 2). Prostaglandins themselves are not thought to be important pain mediators, but they do cause hyperalgesia by sensitizing
peripheral nociceptors to the effects of various mediators of pain
and inflammation such as somatostatin, bradykinin, and histamine. Therefore, NSAIDs primarily treat hyperalgesia or secondary pain, particularly the pain resulting from inflammation.

Two isoforms of COX have been recognized: an inducible
isoenzyme (COX-2) and the constitutive enzyme (COX-1). COX-1
is expressed in most tissues under physiologic conditions, whereas COX-2 is induced by mediators of inflammation under pathologic conditions (see Fig. 3). COX-1 has a protective effect in the
stomach because it is the source of prostaglandins E_2 and I_2,
which are cytoprotective in the gastrointestinal epithelium.
COX-2 is the source of the same prostaglandins in the mediation
of inflammation.

A new subclass of NSAIDs has recently been released for clinical use—the selective COX-2 inhibitors, known also as *coxibs*.
These drugs were developed in the hope of being able to reduce

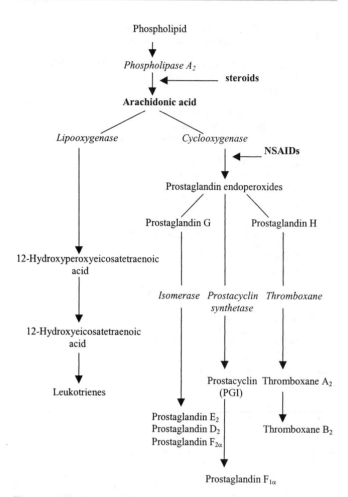

Figure 2.   A schematic diagram showing the metabolism of phospholipid and arachidonic acid. Nonsteroidal antiinflammatory drugs (NSAIDs) inhibit cyclooxygenase and thereby suppress the synthesis of prostaglandin E, prostacyclin, and thromboxane and alter the balance between these eicosanoids and the leukotrienes.

NSAID side effects, particularly the damaging gastrointestinal (GI) effects. The first drugs (celecoxib and rofecoxib) became available in the United States in 1999; valdecoxib followed more recently. Early clinical trials and clinical experience confirmed the analgesic efficacy and favorable side-effect profile of these drugs with regard to their effects on the gastric mucosa and on platelets, although some of the early trial results have now been brought into question. Coxibs do not seem to have any advantage in terms of renal effects, and serious concerns have arisen over a

Table 2. Prostaglandin and thromboxane actions

Fever vascular smooth muscle relaxation (predominant action) (PGI_1 and PGE) and contraction (PGI_1 and TXA)

Increased capillary permeability (LTB)

Uterine smooth muscle contraction (PGE and PGI_2)

Bronchial smooth muscle relaxation (PGE) and contraction (PGI_2 TXA, LTC, LTD)

Increased GI contraction and motility (PGI_1 and PGI)

Protection of GI tract by inhibiting gastric acid secretion and enhancing gastric mucous secretion (PGI_1 and PGI)

Regulation of renal blood flow and sodium/potassium exchange (PGI_1 and PGI)

Marked potentiation of the effects of other mediators of inflammation and pain (serotonin, bradykinin, and histamine) (PGI_1 and PGI)

Sensitization of nociceptors (PGI_1 and PGI)

Inhibition of platelet aggregation (PGI)

Increased platelet aggregation (TXA)

Constriction of vascular smooth muscle (TXA)

PGI, prostacyclin; PGE, prostaglanin E; PGF, prostaglanin F; TXA, thromboxane A; LTB, leukotriene B; LTC, leukotriene C; LTD, leukotriene D.

possible increase in the risk of myocardial infarction and thrombotic stroke when coxibs are taken continuously for long periods. In 2004, the manufacturers of rofecoxib withdrew the drug from the market because new trials substantiated the fears of adverse cardiovascular effects. Similar concerns arose in connection with the other coxibs, and in 2005 valdecoxib was also withdrawn. The coxibs will be used with greater caution now that their cardiovascular (and other) risks are better understood.

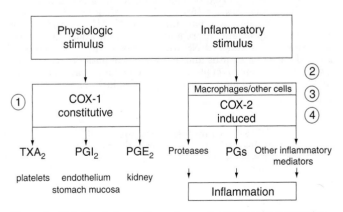

Figure 3. Relation between the pathways leading to the generation of prostaglandins, thromboxanes, and other eicosanoids by COX-1 or COX-2.

Table 3.   Principal adverse effects of long-term NSAID therapy

- Dyspepsia, peptic ulcer disease
- Diarrhea, gastrointestinal hemorrhage
- Renal dysfunction and failure—acute papillary necrosis, chronic interstitial nephritis, decreased renal blood flow, decreased glomerular filtration rate, salt and water retention
- Inhibition of platelet aggregation; increased bleeding time
- Altered liver function tests, jaundice
- Drug interactions
- Impaired cartilage repair in osteoarthritis

II. ADVERSE EFFECTS AND CONTRAINDICATIONS

Unfortunately, the NSAIDs are not free of bothersome, and sometimes even dangerous, adverse effects (see Table 3). Many patients cannot tolerate these drugs because of their GI effects. Surveys suggest that more than 100,000 patients are hospitalized and 16,500 die each year in the United States secondary to NSAID-associated GI events, the elderly being particularly affected.

1. Gastrointestinal Effects

Prostaglandins inhibit acid secretion by blocking the activation of parietal cells by histamine. At the same time, prostaglandins are cytoprotective because they stimulate mucus production from the upper GI tract. By inhibiting prostaglandins, NSAIDs cause gastroduodenal mucosal lesions and ulcers. Gastritis, resulting in abdominal pain, nausea and vomiting, and, sometimes, diarrhea, is an extremely common side effect of NSAIDs that occurs particularly in persons with a propensity to peptic ulceration and that occasionally results in catastrophic GI bleeding and death. Upper GI studies demonstrate a 15% to 30% prevalence of ulcers in the stomach or duodenum of patients taking NSAIDs regularly (see Table 4). Symptomatic ulcers and ulcer complications associated with the use of standard NSAIDs may occur in 1% of patients treated for 3 to 6 months and in 2% to 4% of patients treated for 1 year. Eighty percent of patients with GI toxicity have no preceding symptoms and most have few or no risk factors.

Table 4.   Cumulative prevalence of endoscopically visualized ulcers after 12 weeks of therapy with various NSAIDs (%)

Celecoxib 200 mg bid	8.5%
Rofecoxib 25 mg/d	4.7%
Naproxen 500 mg bid	40.7%
Ibuprofen 800 mg tid	28.5%

It is accepted practice to withhold NSAIDs from patients with known peptic ulcer disease. The risk of GI toxicity can be scored using the ARAMIS (Arthritis, Rheumatism, and Aging Medical Information System) scoring system (see Table 5). This system provides a guide for assessing patients' suitability for NSAID treatment or for concomitant prophylactic treatment. Prostaglandin analogs such as misoprostol; parietal cell inhibitors (acid inhibitors) such as omeprazole; and histamine antagonists such as ranitidine and cimetidine can provide useful prophylaxis against NSAID-induced GI symptoms. The coxibs, which appear to be associated with less GI toxicity than standard NSAIDs, are a good choice for patients with a history of GI symptoms or sensitivity to NSAIDs. However, they are expensive, require a prescription, and are now associated with significant safety concerns. The combination of a standard NSAID with GI prophylaxis is thought to be equally effective in terms of efficacy and freedom from GI toxicity, and should certainly be maintained as an option.

2. Decreased Hemostasis

The decreased hemostasis associated with NSAIDs is largely due to platelet dysfunction. Cyclooxygenase inhibition also inhibits the endogenous procoagulant thromboxane. Platelets are especially susceptible to cyclooxygenase inhibition because they have little or no capacity for protein biosynthesis and therefore cannot regenerate the enzyme. The literature confirms that bleeding time is consistently prolonged in patients receiving long-term treatment with standard NSAIDs, but the consensus is that such prolongation is not excessive and that values remain below the upper limits of normal. COX-2 is not present in platelets, and it appears that the coxibs are not associated with platelet dysfunction.

3. Surgical Bleeding

The degree of risk of perioperative bleeding in patients treated with standard NSAIDs is not clear. Some studies show increased blood loss in patients treated with standard NSAIDs, whereas

Table 5. The ARAMIS model for estimating the risk of gastric ulceration while taking nonselective NSAIDs

Step 1	Start at a score of 0
Step 2	Add 0.3 for every 5 y of patient age over 50 y
Step 3	Add 1.2 if the patient is receiving a corticosteroid
Step 4	Add 1.4 if the patient has reported a previous NSAID-related GI side effect
Step 5	Add 0.5 if the patient has substantial disability

A score >1.5 is considered a high risk and a contraindication for the use of nonselective NSAIDs at MGH.

The ARAMIS rating system is an evidence-based scale, which assesses risk in patient populations. It has been validated prospectively. The scale is for chronic use over a 12-month period.

others fail to show this effect. The coxibs are not likely to affect platelets, and most trials show no difference between COX-2 inhibitors and placebo in postoperative blood loss. Increased bleeding in standard NSAID-treated patients undergoing major abdominal surgery, hysterectomy, and tonsillectomy has been reported. Notably, several reports of perioperative bleeding associated with the use of the potent injectable NSAID ketorolac appeared in the literature shortly after the drug was launched. Most commonly, this was GI bleeding, but hematoma formation and hemarthrosis after knee surgery also were reported. It is likely that the reported high incidence of GI hemorrhage associated with ketorolac was a function of the excessively high doses used before the manufacturers recommended a lower dose. However, this will be difficult to determine because physicians now use extreme caution and avoid using potent NSAIDs perioperatively, or they use conservative doses.

4. Renal Dysfunction and Failure

Prostaglandins in the kidney contribute to the maintenance of renal blood flow and glomerular filtration, to the modulation of renin release and tubular ion transport, and to the excretion of water. In normal, sodium-repleted, well-hydrated individuals, the role of prostaglandins in the kidney is less important than in patients with abnormal renal function, hypovolemia, or abnormal serum electrolytes, in whom local synthesis of vasodilating prostaglandins is important in maintaining renal homeostasis. In these patients, NSAID administration may decrease the glomerular filtration rate and result in the release of renin from the juxtaglomerular cells, leading to further reduction in renal blood flow and a disturbance of renal function. The most common clinical picture is of a small and rapidly reversible fall in the glomerular filtration rate, which occasionally progresses to acute renal failure. Sodium and water retention, hyperkalemia, hypertension, papillary necrosis, and the nephrotic syndrome are other possible consequences of the renal disturbance.

Although NSAID-induced renal dysfunction is extremely rare in healthy patients, it is a significant risk for patients with renal compromise, and this risk increases with prolonged and excessive NSAID use. The older patients; patients with chronic renal dysfunction, congestive heart failure, ascites, or hypovolemia; and patients treated with nephrotoxic drugs such as the aminoglycosides and vancomycin, are at particular risk. Early human studies suggest that the coxibs have similar renal effects to those of standard NSAIDs. Therefore, this new class of drugs does not appear to spare the kidneys.

5. Cardiovascular Effects

An increase in thrombotic events associated with long-term, continuous coxib use was observed during prerelease trials, years before the recent withdrawal of rofecoxib and valdecoxib. However, it was felt that the benefits of reduced GI bleeding outweighed the cardiovascular risk. This was despite the fact that one large trial of rofecoxib (the Vioxx Gastrointestinal Outcomes Research or VIGOR trial) found a fivefold increase in myocardial infarction, which, it was proposed, was due to either chance or the lack of protective effect from the control drug naproxen. (Epidemiologic studies of the possible cardioprotective effect of naproxen are inconclusive, and, in fact, a recent release of data from a large, long-term coxib study using naproxen as a control suggests that cardiovascular risk may apply equally to continuous long-term naproxen use.) Two other large trials—the Celecoxib Long-term Arthritis Safety Study (CLASS) and the Therapeutic Arthritis Research and Gastrointestinal Event Trial (TARGET)—included patients who were taking aspirin in addition to the study drug. A difference in GI events was shown only in patients not taking aspirin. Although the studies were not powered sufficiently to show a difference in cardiovascular events, in the CLASS and TARGET trials, there was a tendency toward more cardiovascular morbidity in patients taking the coxib without aspirin. It appears, then, that the deleterious cardiovascular effects of the coxibs may occur when there is no protection from aspirin, yet the gastroprotective effect is lost when aspirin is added.

The exact mechanism of effect of adverse cardiovascular events associated with coxib use has not been fully elucidated. It has recently been proposed that COX-2 might be hemodynamically induced by laminar shear stress, offering protection through prostaglandin I_2 inhibition of the products of atherosclerotic plaque rupture. Prolonged use of coxibs would remove this protective effect.

There is a great deal of uncertainty about the cardiovascular safety of the coxibs, and this uncertainty may now spread to the standard NSAIDs. Presently, it would seem that in view of the long experience and apparent safety of standard NSAIDs used as recommended by the manufacturers (up to 10 days), and the fact that the use of standard NSAIDs in the recent coxib trials differed in that it was continuous and prolonged, there is no reason to believe that it is unsafe to continue to use the standard NSAIDs as directed by the manufacturers. The safety of coxibs, on the other hand, is likely to come under continued scrutiny.

6. Drug Interactions

NSAIDs are highly bound to albumin in plasma, and adverse drug interactions could potentially occur because of this high degree of binding. However, NSAIDs do not seem to alter the effects of the oral hypoglycemic drugs or warfarin. Warfarin doses may need to be altered because of the platelet effects of NSAIDs, and concomitant use may be contraindicated. Reduced doses of NSAIDs are recommended in patients with severe hypoalbuminea. NSAIDs may also reduce the diuretic and natriuretic effects of furosemide as well as the antihypertensive effects of the thiazide diuretics, α-adrenergic antagonists, and angiotensin-converting enzyme inhibitors, probably because of inhibition of renal or vascular prostaglandin synthesis.

7. Others

Other adverse effects are less common. The incidence of immune-related hypersensitivity is low, the most serious effect being dose-dependent, potentially fatal hepatic necrosis. Borderline increases of one of more liver tests occur in up to 15% of individuals taking

NSAIDs. In 1% of individuals, the levels of ALT (alanine aminotransferase) or AST (aspartate aminotransferase) may increase by three times. Asthma can occur in susceptive individuals, not because of hypersensitivity but rather because of blockade of the cyclooxygenase pathway leading to exaggerated leukotriene effects. Some patients display intolerance to NSAIDs in the form of vasomotor rhinitis, angioneurotic edema, generalized urticaria, asthma, laryngeal edema, hypotension, and even shock. Despite the resemblance to anaphylaxis, these reactions do not appear to be immunologically based. Celecoxib and valdecoxib have cross-sensitivity with sulfa drugs and can cause an allergic reaction in persons who are allergic to sulfa drugs.

NSAIDs are known to impede cartilage repair, which has become a problem for some patients with osteoarthritis taking NSAIDs for long periods of time (i.e., years). Those individuals taking indomethacin for more than 1 to 2 years have been shown to have increased radiologic joint deterioration compared to placebo. NSAIDs adversely affect osteogenesis in animals. Although impaired bone remodeling and delayed fracture healing have not been firmly established in humans, many surgeons prefer to avoid the use of NSAIDs in patients who have undergone bone fusion, particularly in the spine. No human studies to date document that the coxibs have these negative effects. A study in rabbits showed no such negative effect. Standard NSAIDs may also be associated with an increased rate of miscarriage if used near the time of conception. However, they are unlikely to be harmful to nursing infants.

By way of summary, contraindications are listed in Table 6.

III. USE IN SPECIFIC POPULATIONS

The NSAIDs are commonly prescribed by physicians for acute and chronic pain, particularly for pain due to surgery and trauma, and pain due to joint disease. Commonly used NSAIDs and their doses are presented in Appendix VIII.

1. Perioperative Patients

(i) Domestic Use—Cautions

Patients should be advised to stop taking NSAIDs before surgery, chiefly because of their platelet effects and their propensity

Table 6. Contraindications to NSAID use

History of peptic ulcer disease or intolerance to NSAIDs

Bleeding, bleeding diatheses, or anticoagulant therapy

Renal failure, renal dysfunction, or risk factors for renal dysfunction (i.e., hypovolemia, sodium depletion, congestive heart failure, hepatic cirrhosis, concurrent use of nephrotoxic drugs including aminoglycocides)

Old age, particularly in the presence of any of the preceding[a]

Prophylactic use in major surgery (i.e., preoperative or intraoperative use, particularly if there is a potential for bleeding)

[a]The elderly (>60 years) appear to be especially vulnerable to the effects of prostaglandin inhibition by NSAIDs.

to increase surgical bleeding. Aspirin, the platelet effects of which are not reversible, should be stopped for up to 10 days before elective surgery. Other NSAIDs have rapidly reversible platelet effects, and 24 hours' cessation is probably sufficient, although 2 to 3 days' cessation is usually advised. Acetaminophen, which has only mild peripheral effects and does not affect platelets, can be substituted. Spinal and epidural instrumentation and catheter placement appear to be safe, even if aspirin and other NSAIDs are not discontinued. Because the coxibs do not have platelet effects, it is not considered necessary to stop them before surgery

(ii) Postoperative and Acute Pain

NSAIDs are extremely useful and often underutilized for acute and postoperative pain. Broadly, there are two indications in this population: (a) as a sole analgesic for mild pain, and (b) as an adjunct to other analgesics in severe pain.

(A) MILD PAIN. The efficacy of NSAIDs for mild acute pain is well established by countless randomized controlled trials. However, until recently, their widespread applicability in postoperative pain was limited because of the lack of availability of parenteral formulations and the limitations this placed on the use of NSAIDs in patients who cannot take oral medications. Prompted by the availability of rectal and parenteral preparations, the value of NSAID treatment in postoperative patients has now been realized, and both enteral and parenteral preparations are being used preoperatively, intraoperatively, and postoperatively, providing useful postoperative analgesia. The use of NSAIDs allows for complete avoidance, or minimal use, of opioids during and after minor surgery, thus avoiding the opioid-induced side effects (nausea and somnolence) that commonly delay recovery and discharge. NSAID side effects are rare in the relatively healthy day-surgery population, and with short-term use. NSAIDs (unless contraindicated) are arguably the treatment of choice for pain after minor surgery and late in the postoperative course after major surgery. Acetaminophen is a popular choice, particularly in infants because it does not cause GI irritation.

(B) ADJUNCT USE AND OPIOID SPARING. For more severe acute pain, NSAIDs alone may be ineffective, but in conjunction with other modes of pain treatment, they have an important role. Opioids will probably always hold a place in the management of acute somatic pain because they are highly effective and are the only analgesics that have no ceiling effect. However, their side effects, particularly respiratory depression, severely limit their use. There are many ways to reduce opioid requirement, including the use of local nerve blocks, epidural and intrathecal anesthesia and analgesia, and nonopioid analgesics, including NSAIDs. In fact, a multimodal approach, using a combination of appropriate pain treatments, would seem the best approach in terms of achieving synergy between different modes of treatment and reducing the side effects of each.

Multiple controlled trials confirm the opioid-sparing effects of NSAID usage in postoperative pain. Whether this reduction in opioid consumption can be translated into a significant difference in the incidence of opioid-associated side effects, or with improved

Table 7.   Adverse effects of NSAIDs in surgical patients

Gastrointestinal hemorrhage *(occasionally catastrophic)*

Renal dysfunction or failure

Decreased hemostasis and hematoma formation

Asthma in susceptible individuals *(due to blockade of the cyclooxy-genase pathway, leading to exaggerated effects of the metabolites of the lipooxygenase pathway—that is, leukotrienes)*

Anaphylaxis *(risk of immune-related anaphylactoid reactions is small, although some individuals suffer anaphylaxislike symptoms that are unrelated to an immune process)*

Decreased healing of gastrointestinal anastomoses *(proposed)*

Delayed fracture healing *(not established in humans, but demonstrated in animals)*

overall outcome, is less clear. Obviously, there are groups of patients in whom opioid treatment and opioid side effects are particularly undesirable, including the very young, those with preexisting ventilatory compromise, and those with a strong history of opioid-induced side effects.

(C) ADVERSE EFFECTS.   The adverse effects of NSAIDs in surgical patients are summarized in Table 7.

(D) TIMING OF ADMINISTRATION.   There is no consensus regarding timing of NSAID doses in patients undergoing surgery, even though speed of onset influences the usefulness of the drugs. In studies that specifically examine the issue of timing of doses and effects, the benefit of NSAIDs was not seen until 4 hours or more after the parenteral administration of an NSAID (ketorolac or other), and effectiveness continued to improve even after administration. Is it advisable, then, to start NSAID treatment preoperatively? Pretreatment was superior in terms of efficacy where this was assessed in dental patients. However, in a large meta-analysis of the general surgical population, no measurable difference was found between the same dose given preoperatively versus postoperatively. Moreover, as already discussed, NSAID pretreatment may be ill-advised before major surgery because of the risks of hypovolemia, hypotension, bleeding, and renal compromise. The question of when to treat is a complex one that needs to be addressed by research into the clinical benefit versus cost benefit of pretreatment with NSAIDs. Currently, it is probably better to offer preoperative oral NSAIDs to patients undergoing minor surgery and to reserve injectable NSAIDs for the end of surgery or for postoperative use.

(E) KETOROLAC.   Ketorolac was introduced in the United States in 1990 and was the first NSAID with US Food and Drug Administration approval for parenteral use in postoperative patients. Ketorolac differs from other NSAIDs in two respects: it is both injectable and highly efficacious, with efficacy close to that of morphine. For these reasons, it has been widely adopted for use in acute and postoperative pain. Unfortunately, ketorolac's potency extends to its side effects, and there are many reported cases of problems associated with its use, possibly caused by inappropriately high doses or by the failure to recognize its con-traindications. The most common and serious side effects have been gastrointestinal bleeding, other bleeding problems, and reversible renal dysfunction. Ketorolac has been found to be as effective as morphine and other opioids for surgery ranging in severity from simple outpatient procedures to major operations. At the same time, investigators have demonstrated the efficacy of other NSAIDs, traditionally considered weak analgesics, to be equal to that of ketorolac for mild pain.

2. Patients with Chronic Noncancer Pain

By far, the commonest indication for NSAIDs is joint pain. Other indications for NSAID use in patients with chronic non-cancer pain are myalgias, headache, and mild to moderate pain of any etiology.

(i) Joint Pain

The NSAIDs are the first-line pharmacologic treatment of inflammatory joint diseases, including osteoarthritis, rheumatoid arthritis, anklyosing spondylitis, and scleroderma. They are used to treat both pain and inflammation in these diseases. So effective are they in improving quality of life for these patients that the significant risk of GI toxicity has been accepted despite the occurrence of many deaths each year from catastrophic GI bleeding in this population. The coxibs offer hope of greater safety for those patients with arthritides who obtain significant pain relief from NSAIDs. Despite concerns over the coxibs' cardiovascular safety, until there is a better alternative, these drugs can be considered a useful option for many patients, such as the elderly, whose risk of catastrophic GI bleeding outweighs their cardiovascular risk. In fact, if the drug companies had not chosen to introduce the coxibs as "blockbuster" therapies, but instead focused on these more limited indications, there would probably have been no need to withdraw from the market.

(ii) Other Indications

NSAIDs are useful therapy for myalgias and other muscle pains that may occur in conjunction with joint pain, particularly back pain. Perhaps the commonest indication for NSAIDs in noncancer patients in the pain clinic is headache. Acetaminophen and NSAIDs are a useful first-line treatment for both migraine and tension headaches. Even if NSAID therapy alone is not sufficient for headaches, their combination with other treatments, such as vasoconstrictors (caffeine, ergotamine, sumatriptan), is often useful. In addition to the previously mentioned indications, NSAIDs can be tried as a first-line treatment of any mild to moderate pain. The choice of NSAID for whatever indication is largely a matter of trial and error. The older, cheaper NSAIDs (e.g., aspirin, indomethacin, and phenylbutazone) are often poorly tolerated because of their GI effects. They also need frequent dosing. Aspirin is the oldest and cheapest of the NSAIDs and maintains its place as a useful analgesic despite its side-effect profile. Several formulations (e.g., buffered and enteric coated) that are less toxic to the GI tract are available. Ibuprofen is the most popular of the newer NSAIDs, is less toxic than the older drugs, but still needs 4-to-6-hourly dosing to maintain therapeutic levels. Naproxen and diflusinal are widely used for chronic pain because they are long acting and only twice-daily dosing is required. Nabumetone (a nonacidic prodrug metabolized to a structural analog of naproxen) is minimally toxic to the GI tract and has been the treatment of choice when GI side effects are a problem. The coxibs could also be used when GI side effects are a problem, not forgetting that GI prophylaxis together with standard NSAIDs can be used as well (see section entitled Gastrointestinal Effects). Despite these logical considerations, it is often necessary to try out different NSAIDs before finding the best drug for an individual patient.

3. Patients with Cancer

In patients with cancer pain, acetaminophen and NSAIDs are used as a first-line therapy for mild to moderate pain, in combination with opioids for more severe pain, and specifically for bone and inflammatory pain in advanced cancer.

(i) The World Health Organization Guidelines

In 1986, the World Health Organization (WHO) released a set of guidelines under the title "Cancer Pain Relief." The central component of this guideline is the "three-step analgesic ladder" (see Chapter 32, Fig. 1). The three-step ladder became the guiding principle for cancer pain treatment in many parts of the world, recommending initial treatment with nonopioid analgesics, alone or with adjuvant (anticonvulsants, antidepressants, etc.); advancing to mild opioids, alone or in combination with nonopioid analgesics and adjutants; then to potent opioids, alone or in combination. Although new drugs and techniques have in some measure altered the way we might wish to treat cancer pain, the basic principles in the WHO guideline are still a sound basis for cancer pain treatment. One question that arises is whether, since the advent of more potent NSAIDs, the step two in the ladder (the use of opioid with or without nonopioid analgesic with or without adjuvant) should be abandoned in favor of simply continuing step one (the use of nonopioid analgesics with or without adjuvant) for mild to moderate pain. However, there is still a safety issue, and at present, opioid/nonopioid combinations maintain their place for mild to moderate cancer pain because these combinations have synergy and the ability to reduce the side effects of each drug. The advent of more potent, safer NSAIDs may well change the way we treat moderately severe or even severe cancer pain.

(ii) The Role of NSAIDs in Advanced Cancer

In advanced cancer, NSAIDs are particularly useful for bone pain (due to distention of the periosteum by metastases), for soft tissue pain (due to compression or distention of tissues), and for visceral pain (due to irritation of the pleura or peritoneum). Of particular concern in these patients are the platelet effects of NSAIDs and the risk of inducing bleeding. Many of these patients suffer general debilitation, with resultant effects on protein synthesis, including the synthesis of clotting factors. They commonly have thrombocytopenia or pancytopenia due to the underlying malignancy or prior therapy. The coxibs may be substituted for standard NSAIDs in patients at risk because they appear not to affect platelet function.

IV. CONCLUSION

NSAIDs are useful analgesics with a predominantly peripheral action that can provide sole treatment of mild pain or complement the central effects of opioids and neuraxial analgesics for more severe pain. Were it not for their side effects, which are occasionally catastrophic, NSAIDs would be more widely used. Several developments in NSAID pharmacology are leading toward the formulation of more efficacious and safer drugs. The coxib story, which is still unfolding, has been a setback, but the search continues for safer alternatives to standard NSAIDs and the hope of improving acute and chronic pain management using NSAIDs.

SELECTED READINGS

FitzGerald GA. Coxibs and cardiovascular disease. *N Engl J Med* 2004;351:1709–1711.

Gajraj N. Cyclooxygenase-2 inhibitors. *Anesth Analg* 2003;96: 1720–1738.

Gilron I, Milne B, Hong M. Cyclooxygenase-2 inhibitors in postoperative pain management: current evidence and future directions. *Anesthesiology* 2003;99:1198–1208.

Kenny GNC. Potential renal, hematological and allergic adverse effects associated with nonsteroidal anti-inflammatory drugs. *Drugs* 1992;44(Suppl. 5):31–37.

Laneuville O, Breuer DK, Dewitt DL, et al. Differential inhibition of human prostaglandin endoperoxide H synthases-1 and -2 by nonsteroidal anti-inflammatory drugs. *J Pharmacol Exp Ther* 1994; 271:927–934.

McMurray R, Hardy K. COX-2 inhibitors: today and tomorrow. *Am J Med Sci* 2002;323:181–189.

Topol EJ. Failing the public health–rofecoxib, Merck, and the FDA. *N Engl J Med* 2004;351:1707–1709.

Vane JR, Botting RM. Mechanism of action of aspirin-like drugs. *Semin Arthritis Rheum* 1997;26(6 Suppl. 1):2–10.

Weir M, Sperling R, Reicin A, et al. Selective COX-2 inhibition and cardiovascular effects: a review of the rofecoxib development program. *Am Heart J* 2003;146:591–604.

Wright J. The double-edged sword of COX-2 selective NSAIDs. *Can Med Assoc J* 2002;167:1131–1136.

Opioids

Jeffrey Uppington

Among the remedies which it has pleased Almighty God to give to man to relieve his sufferings, none is so universal and so efficacious as opium.
—*Thomas Sydenham, 1624–1689*

Opioids are the core pharmacologic treatment of pain. They are the mainstay for treatment of both acute pain and cancer pain, and although controversy still exists over their use in chronic nonterminal pain (CNTP), they are increasingly used for this indication also. Opioids are the only pain medications that have no ceiling effect and are therefore the only systemic treatment that can be used to treat severe accelerating pain. Any health care provider treating pain should understand the effects and proper usage of these important drugs.

I. TERMINOLOGY

Opiates are drugs derived from opium, which is obtained from the juice of the poppy **Papaver somniferum**. These drugs include morphine, codeine, and various semisynthetic congeners derived from morphine and codeine, and other components of opium such as thebaine. The term **opioid** applies to substances with morphine-like activity, including agonists and antagonists, as well as naturally occurring and synthetic opioid peptides. **Endorphin** is a generic term applying to the endogenous opioid peptides. There are three families of endogenous opioids—the endorphins, the enkephalins, and the dynorphins. The word **narcotic** was derived from the Greek word for stupor. Originally, **narcotic** referred to any drug that induced sleep, but it later became associated with the strong opiate analgesics. The term is no longer useful pharmacologically because it is being increasingly used in the legal and regulatory context to refer to a wide variety of abused substances.

II. ENDOGENOUS OPIOIDS

Each of the three families of opioid neuropeptides (i.e., endorphins, enkephalins, and dynorphins) is derived from a distinct precursor polypeptide and has a distinct anatomic distribution. Like peptide hormones, endogenous opioids have biologically inactive precursors that generate active agents only after enzymatic cleavage. The precursor for β-endorphin, proopiomelanocortin, also contains peptide sequences for adrenocorticotropin (ACTH) and melanocyte-stimulating hormone (MSH), illustrating the close relation between the endogenous opioids and hormone systems.

III. CLASSIFICATION OF OPIOIDS

Opioids can be classified as naturally occurring, semisynthetic, and synthetic (see Table 1). Morphine, codeine, papaverine, and thebaine are naturally occurring. The semisynthetic drugs are derived from morphine, codeine, and thebaine. The synthetic drugs structurally resemble morphine but do not occur in nature. They are produced by gradually reducing the number of

Table 1.   Classification of opioids

Naturally occurring
  Morphine
  Papaverine
  Codeine
  Thebaine

Semisynthetic
  Heroin
  Hydromorphone
  Hydrocodone
  Buprenorphine
  Oxycodone

Synthetic
  Morphinan series (e.g., levophanol and butorphanol)
  Diphenylpropylamine series (e.g., methadone)
  Benzomorphinan series (e.g., pentazocine)
  Phenylpiperidine series (e.g., meperidine, fentanyl, sufentanil, and alfentanil)

rings from the five-ring structure of morphine, through the four-ring "morphinans," the three-ring "benzomorphinans" to the two-ring "phenylpiperidines" (see Fig. 1). There are alternative classifications of opioids. The drugs may be grouped according to the specific receptors they act on (see subsequent text). Another useful distinction is whether they are agonists, antagonists, or some combination of the two (see Table 2).

IV. OPIOID RECEPTORS

Opioids act via specific receptors on cell membranes. Specific opioid receptors have been proposed through a mixture of clinical and laboratory observation. The structure of opioid receptors is currently understood at cellular, molecular, and genetic levels. It is now clear that there are three well-defined "classical" opioid receptors (i.e., μ, δ, and κ). Recently, DNA encoding for an "orphan" receptor has been identified. The "orphan" receptor has a high degree of similarity to the "classical" opioid receptors and has been named **opioid receptorlike** (ORL). There is also pharmacologic evidence for subtypes of each known receptor, and for

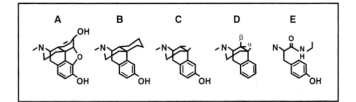

Figure 1.   Structure of morphinelike opioids. A: Morphine. B: Morphinan. C: Benzomorphan. D: Phenylpiperidine. E: Tyramine moiety of endogenous opioids. Note the progressive removal of ring structures from five-ring morphine to two-ring phenylpiperidine. (From Carr DB. Opioids. *Int Anesthesiol Clin* 1988;26:273, with permission.)

Table 2. Alternative classification of opioids

Class	Definition	Example
Agonist	A drug that, when bound to the receptor, stimulates the receptor to the maximum level; by definition, the intrinsic activity of a full agonist is unity	Morphine
Antagonist	A drug that, when bound to the receptor, fails completely to produce any stimulation of that receptor; by definition, the intrinsic activity of a pure antagonist is zero	Naloxone
Partial agonist	A drug that, when bound to the receptor, stimulates the receptor to a level below the maximum level; by definition, the intrinsic activity of a partial agonist lies between zero and unity	Buprenorphine (partial μ agonist)
Mixed agonist-antagonist	A drug that acts simultaneously on different subtypes, with the potential for agonist action on one or more subtypes and antagonist action on one or more subtypes	Nalbuphine (partial μ agonist, κ agonist, δ antagonist)

From Wall PD, Melzack R, eds. *Textbook of pain*, 3rd ed. New York: Churchill-Livingston, 1994, with permission.

other, less well-characterized opioid receptors, including ε and γ. The σ receptor is no longer considered to be an opioid receptor.

1. μ Receptors

It seems likely that morphine and morphinelike drugs produce analgesia primarily through interaction with μ-receptors. These receptors are present in large quantities in the periaqueductal gray matter (brain) and the substantia gelatinosa (spinal cord). Activation of μ receptors results in analgesia, euphoria, respiratory depression, nausea and vomiting, decreased gastrointestinal (GI) motility, tolerance, and dependence. β-endorphin has a high affinity for μ receptors, as do the enkephalins. Dynorphin also binds to the μ-receptor but not as avidly as it does to the κ receptor.

The proposed classification into μ_1 and μ_2, which provided a rationale for the hope that selective μ_1 agonists could provide analgesia without respiratory depression, did not survive the scrutiny of several laboratories.

2. κ Receptors

Activation of these receptors also causes analgesia, but less respiratory depression than μ-receptor activation. κ receptor activation produces dysphoria and hallucinations rather than euphoria. Several κ receptor subtypes have been proposed as a result of binding studies, but their actions have not been fully elucidated. Dynorphin A is the endogenous ligand for the κ receptor.

3. δ Receptors

Using selective agonists and antagonists, studies have established δ-receptor analgesia both spinally and supraspinally, although the spinal system analgesia appears more robust. δ_1- and δ_2-receptors have been proposed, based on differential sensitivity to several antagonists. The enkephalins are the endogenous ligands for the δ-receptors.

4. Opioid Receptor–like Receptors

Although the ORL receptor is accepted as a member of the opioid receptor "family" because of its structural similarity to the "classical" opioid receptors, there is no pharmacologic similarity. The receptor was called an **"orphan"** receptor because ligands of the "classical" receptors did not have the same high affinity for the "orphan" receptors. A confusion of effects of known high-affinity ligands has been reported, including antinociception, pronociception/hyperalgesia, allodynia, and no effect.

5. Cloned Receptors

The μ, δ, κ, and ORL receptors are the only opioid receptors whose genes have been identified and have been cloned, despite an intensive search for genes corresponding to opioid receptor subtypes and the less well-characterized receptors. The cloned opioid receptors have characteristics of typical G-protein–coupled receptors. There are seven hydrophobic regions that span the cell membrane, with three extracellular and three intracellular loops. There is an intracellular carboxy-terminal tail and an extracellular amino-terminal tail. The amino acid sequences of the different opioid receptors are approximately 65% identical to each other. The regions of highest similarity are the sequences predicted to lie in the seven transmembrane spanning regions and intracellular loops. The extracellular regions that differ in amino acid sequence may contain the unique ligand-binding domains for each receptor (see Fig. 2).

6. Receptor Mechanisms

Opioid receptors are coupled to G-proteins and are therefore able to affect protein phosphorylation via second messenger systems, thereby altering ion channel conductance. Opioids act both presynaptically and postsynaptically. Presynaptically, they inhibit the release of neurotransmitters, including substance P and glutamate. Postsynaptically, they can inhibit neurons by opening potassium channels that hyperpolarize the cell. There is evidence that opioids produce both short- and long-term effects on neural function. Opioids may play a distinct role during early embryonic development. Administration of opioids considerably reduces the facilitation of nociceptive processing (e.g., "windup"). Opioids (including endogenous opioids) can also affect opioid gene regulation with possible short-term and long-term effects, and local as well as distal effects.

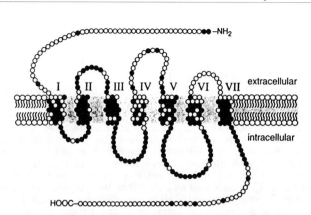

Figure 2.   Amino acid sequence identity among the three cloned opioid receptors. Comparison of the amino acid sequences of the cloned mouse δ and κ receptors and the rat p receptor reveals that approximately 65% of the residues are either identical or similar. Amino acid residues that are identical or similar among the receptors are in *black*, and those that are not similar are in *open circles*. Note that the intracellular loops and transmembrane-spanning regions I, II, III, V, and VII are very similar in amino acid sequence. In contrast, the amino and carboxy termini are very different, as are extracellular loops two and three and trans-membrane-spanning region IV. (From Goodman LS, Limbird LE, Milinoff PB, et al., eds. *Goodman and Gilman's the pharmacological basis of therapeutics*, 9th ed. New York: McGraw-Hill, 1996, with permission.)

7. Alternative Opioid Mechanisms

Not all nociceptive mechanisms are mediated by opiate receptors. It is known that *N*-methyl-D-aspartate (NMDA)-sensitive glutamate receptors are involved in nociceptive transmission in the spinal dorsal horn. Norepinephrine, serotonin, and sodium channels are also involved, and it is possible that a central nitric oxide–cyclic guanosine monophosphate signaling pathway may help mediate nociception. It appears that some opioid actions are not mediated by opioid receptors, and this is a potentially important observation in terms of understanding pain and analgesic mechanisms. Therefore, methadone, meperidine, and tramadol inhibit serotonin and norepinephrine reuptake. Methadone, meperidine, and other opioids are antagonists of the NMDA amino acid excitatory pathway. Meperidine blocks sodium channels and has local anesthetic properties.

V. OPIOID EFFECTS

1. Central Nervous System

(i) Analgesia, Mood, and Consciousness

Opioids selectively relieve pain without affecting other sensory modalities. Pain can be described as a specific sensation (i.e., burning, shooting, throbbing) or in terms of suffering (i.e., excruciating and miserable). Opioids alter the sensation of pain as well as the affective response. Patients often say that their pain is still present but that they feel more comfortable. Occasionally, patients experience euphoria or dysphoria, more so when these drugs are used for recreational purposes. Useful analgesia occurs without loss of consciousness, although high doses of opioids do produce unconsciousness, and drowsiness is a common side effect.

(ii) Respiratory Depression

Opioids of the morphine type depress respiration by acting directly on the respiratory centers in the brain stem. Equianalgesic doses of morphinelike opioids produce the same degree of respiratory depression as morphine itself. Partial agonists and agonist-antagonist opioids are less likely to cause severe respiratory depression, as are the selective κ-agonists. Therapeutic doses of morphine depress all phases of respiration, respiratory rate, and minute volume. At the same time, the responsiveness to carbon dioxide (CO_2) is decreased and, therefore, the CO_2 response curve is shifted upward and to the right. The degree of respiratory depression is dependent on opioid dose and patient status, and apnea is a true risk. Pain and stimulation counteract respiratory depression, while sedative drugs, such as the benzodiazopines, potentiate it. Natural sleep also reduces CO_2 responsiveness and is additive to the opioid effect. Unexpected respiratory depression may occur in relation to variations in serum concentration, concomitant drug use, and varying degrees of pain and stimulation. Naloxone effectively reverses the respiratory depression.

(iii) Nausea and Vomiting

Nausea and vomiting from opioids is due to the direct stimulation of the chemoreceptor trigger zone (CRTZ). The CRTZ is situated in the area postrema in the floor of the 4th medulla. There is also an associated increase in vestibular sensitivity so that opioid-induced nausea tends to be exacerbated by movement. Treatment includes opioid dosage reduction, antidopaminergics (e.g., droperidol, compazine, metoclopramide), anticholinergics (e.g., scopolamine), or serotonin antagonists (e.g., ondansetron).

(iv) Cough

Opioids depress the cough center in the medulla. There is no relation between cough suppression and respiratory depression, and effective antitussive agents are available that do not depress respiration in clinical doses, such as dextromethorphan. The antitussive receptors are less sensitive to naloxone than receptors involved in analgesia.

(v) Miosis

μ and κ-agonists constrict the pupil by exciting the Edinger-Westphal nucleus (parasympathetic) of the oculomotor nerve. Tolerance to the miotic effects occurs with long-term opioid use, but addicts, with high circulating blood concentrations of opioids, will have small pupils. The pupillary effects of opioids are altered by concomitant use of drugs, including general anesthetics. Morphine reduces intraocular pressure.

(vi) Convulsions

In animals, high doses of morphine and related opioids cause convulsions. The drugs stimulate hippocampal pyramidal cells, probably by inhibiting release of γ-aminobutyric acid (GABA) at the synaptic level. Selective δ-agonists may do the same. In humans, convulsions are rarely seen because seizure-producing doses are extremely high and not given. However, meperidine is particularly prone to produce seizure activity through its metabolite normeperidine, the accumulation of which is most likely to occur in patients with renal dysfunction and in the elderly. Meperidine-induced seizures are relatively common, and for that reason the use of meperidine is discouraged, particularly in susceptible patients, and for chronic pain. Naloxone can be used to treat seizures but is more effective in treating convulsions caused by morphine and related drugs than meperidine.

(vii) Hypothalamic Effects

Opioids can cause decrease in body temperature. The chief mechanism is alteration of the equilibrium point of the hypothalamic heat-regulating mechanism, although opioid-induced vasodilation may worsen the effect. Although shivering is not observed consistently after opioid anesthesia, it does occur frequently after inhalation anesthesia. Small doses of opioid (particularly meperidine) can attenuate or abolish this shivering through a mechanism that is poorly understood.

2. Neuroendocrine Effects

Opioids have a number of neuroendocrine effects. High-dose opioid therapy reduces release of stress hormone (i.e., glucocorticoids and catecholamines). It is not at all clear to what extent and under which conditions this is a desirable effect. Evidence is emerging that high-dose opioids may also suppress immune response, which clearly is not a desirable effect. Opioids suppress hypothalamic releasing factors, thereby suppressing the release of lutenizing hormone (LH), follicle-stimulating hormone (FSH), ACTH and β-endorphin. Cortisol and testosterone levels are thereby reduced. In women, the menstrual cycle may be disrupted, and testosterone levels may be reduced in men. Some opioids also reduce growth hormone production. During chronic opioid administration, tolerance to these effects develops. Therefore, when heroin addicts are maintained on methadone, the disrupted menstrual cycles and plasma concentrations of LH of women and the depressed testosterone levels of men return to normal.

3. Gastrointestinal System

(i) Stomach

Gastric motility is decreased, prolonging gastric emptying and increasing the risk of esophageal reflux. The passage of gastric contents through the duodenum is usually delayed. μ agonists usually decrease gastric acid secretion, but stimulation can occur. Indirect effects, such as increased secretion of pancreatic somatostatin, predominate.

(ii) Small Intestine

Biliary, pancreatic, and intestinal secretion are diminished, and the digestion of food is delayed. The duodenum is affected more than the ileum; water is absorbed more completely and the viscosity of bowel contents increases.

(iii) Large Intestine

Peristaltic propulsive waves are decreased or abolished in the colon. Bowel tone increases. Water is absorbed, which desiccates the feces and slows their passage. In postoperative patients, prolonged ileus is a problem; in patients on long-term opioids, constipation is common and these patients should take stimulant laxatives.

(iv) Biliary Tract

The sphincter of Oddi constricts, and bile duct pressure may increase. Despite this, little clinical effect is seen. Naloxone reverses the effects, as does glucagon. Atropine and nitroglycerine only partially reverse the effect. Morphine and morphine-like drugs are thought by some to have a less pronounced effect than meperidine and its derivatives, but the validity of this finding is in doubt.

4. Cardiovascular System

Opioids have a number of actions on the cardiovascular system. Histamine release and peripheral vasodilation accompany the use of morphine and of some other opioids. High doses of any opioid will reduce sympathetic output, and thus allow a greater preponderance of parasympathetic effects. The pulse rate may be slowed by stimulation of the vagal center, especially with high doses. There is little direct effect on the myocardium, but the peripheral effects may reduce myocardial oxygen consumption, left ventricular end diastolic pressure, and cardiac work. High doses, low blood volume, and the combination of other drugs such as phenothiazines accentuate the hypotensive effects.

5. Tolerance, Dependence, and Addiction

These phenomena are discussed in detail in Chapters 30 and 35. However, it is important to understand these phenomena when prescribing opioids, so a brief overview is included here. Although tolerance and physical dependence are likely, or almost inevitable, consequence of chronic opioid use, addiction is a behavioral problem that arises only in certain individuals. Tolerance is marked by the need for increasing doses to achieve the same analgesic effect and is a form of tachyphylaxis. Tolerance to side effects, other than bowel effects, also occurs. Changing from one opioid to another is often effective in reducing tolerance because of incomplete cross-tolerance between opioids (see Chapter 30). Physical dependence arises when continuous exposure to a drug is necessary to avoid withdrawal symptoms. Slow weaning of opiate drugs usually prevents withdrawal syndrome. Addiction implies socially destructive drug-seeking behavior and arises in certain individuals with a predisposition to addiction. Addiction rarely occurs in patients treated with opioids for acute pain or cancer pain, but the risk of addiction should always be considered when prescribing opioids for chronic nonmalignant pain (CNMP) (see Chapter 35). In the treatment of acute and cancer pain it is often necessary to reassure patients that the risk of their developing addiction is extremely low, and that tolerance and physical dependence are distinct from addiction.

6. Others

(i) Chest Wall Rigidity

Rapid infusion of a large bolus injection of potent opioids can induce increased muscle tone, mainly of the chest wall and abdomen. The opioids most associated with this phenomenon are fentanyl, sufentanil, and alfentanil. The mechanism of the muscle rigidity is not clear, but it is resolved with muscle relaxants or opioid antagonists.

(ii) Ureter and Bladder

The ureteral tone and amplitude of contraction may increase with therapeutic doses of opioids. The urinary voiding reflex is inhibited, external sphincter tone and bladder volume increases and urinary retention may result. Tolerance to these effects usually occurs over time.

(iii) Skin

Therapeutic doses of morphine can produce dilation of the cutaneous blood vessels. Histamine release is the likely cause. Histamine release also probably accounts for the local urticaria sometimes seen after injection. Pruritis may occur, particularly after neuraxial administration of opioids. Naloxone does not abolish the histamine effects, but it does reverse itching. Antihistamines are also effective for opioid-induced itching, even if the presumed mechanism of effect is central (as in neuraxial administration).

VI. PRECAUTIONS

1. Hepatic and Renal Diseases

In these disease processes, because of decreased metabolism and elimination of opioids, some concerns arise:

- Active metabolites of morphine and codeine, especially morphine-6-glucuronide, may accumulate
- Meperidine administration can lead to accumulation of normeperidine, causing central nervous system (CNS) excitation with tremors or seizures
- Repeated doses of propoxyphene may cause naloxone-insensitive cardiac toxicity secondary to its metabolite norpropoxyphene.

2. Respiratory Disease

One should proceed with caution when using opioids whenever respiratory reserve is diminished (e.g., emphysema, kyphoscoliosis, extreme obesity). Opioids that release histamine may precipitate bronchospasm, especially in asthmatics. Depression of the cough reflex may be deleterious in patients with copious secretions (e.g., pneumonia, bronchiectasis, postthoracotomy).

3. Head Injury

An increase in P_{CO_2} from respiratory depression can lead to elevated intracerebral pressure. Miosis, vomiting, and mental clouding, which are important clinical signs for the evaluation of head injury, may be obscured.

4. Allergic Reactions

True allergies to opioid medications are rare but do occur. More commonly, patients believe they are allergic because they have suffered a side effect, but have not had a true allergic reaction. Wheals at the injection site are from histamine release.

5. Drug Interactions

Opioid effects may be potentiated by concomitant drug use, and these effects are not unusual. In particular, the sedative and respiratory depressant effects of opioids may be exaggerated by concomitant administration of drugs with sedative properties (e.g., antihistamines, anxiolytics, antiemetics). On the other hand, the opioid sedative and respiratory depressant effects may be offset by stimulants (e.g., amphetamines, analeptics). One specific dangerous interaction is that between meperidine and the monoamine oxidase inhibitors (MAOIs). This results in a potentially fatal excitatory reaction with delirium, hyperpyrexia, and convulsions and is caused by central serotonergic overactivity secondary to blockage of neuronal uptake of serotonin by meperidine. Methadone is also associated with a number of potentially dangerous drug interactions. Methadone interactions (e.g., with desipramine, antivirals, antibiotics) arise because of methadone's ability to induce hepatic cytochrome enzymes, and the ability of other drugs to affect methadone clearance via induction and inhibition of hepatic enzyme systems.

VII. ROUTES OF ADMINISTRATION

Opioids may be administered by a number of routes, although the oral route is the route of choice in most situations. Some relatively new routes are described.

1. Oral

There is usually a significant first pass effect, so that the oral dose of opioids needs to be higher than the parenteral dose (commonly 3:1). For example, the bioavailability of oral morphine is only approximately 25%. The duration of oral opioids is prolonged by their slow absorption through the GI tract. Sustained-release forms are available that further prolong the action. The oral route is simple because of its accessibility, and relative safety is because of slow drug absorption. Opioids are also relatively easy to titrate using this route.

2. Parenteral

Intravenous (IV), intramuscular, and subcutaneous administration are the clinical parenteral routes of administration. Patient-controlled analgesia (PCA) may be used in all forms, although the IV route is most common. PCA via the subcutaneous route is chosen for home care.

3. Transdermal

Passive diffusion of certain drugs through the skin is possible. The drug is delivered via patches that contain a drug reservoir and a controlling membrane. Fentanyl has been used in this way for several years, and patches are available that deliver doses from 25 to 100 μg per hour. After initial placement of the patch, maximum blood levels may take 12 hours to be reached, after which analgesia persists for up to 72 hours (less in some patients). Patches are changed every 2 to 3 days. The liver is bypassed, blood levels are fairly constant, and the system is convenient and comfortable. The great disadvantage of the transdermal route is that rapid titration (either up or down) is impossible. However, for patients with stable pain, especially patients who cannot take oral medications, the patches are useful. This is also a useful way to give fentanyl, which is a highly specific μ-receptor agonist, thought to be particularly effective in neuropathic pain.

4. Neuraxial

The epidural, intrathecal, and intraventricular routes of administration allow for smaller doses, prolonged duration of action, and minimal systemic side effects. The aim of this form of administration is to produce a specific spinal effect called **selective spinal analgesia**. Delayed respiratory depression may occur with larger doses, particularly with morphine, which is extremely nonlipophilic and therefore subject to rostral flow in the watery cerebrospinal fluid (CSF) where this drug tends to accumulate. This occurs when drug reaches the respiratory center in the brain stem. The more lipophilic opioids tend to diffuse across lipid bilayers more readily and generally do not travel rostrally (see Chapter 21). Neuraxial opioids are used commonly to treat postoperative pain and less commonly to treat cancer pain.

5. Rectal

Morphine may be given rectally and suppositories are available. Plasma morphine concentration after oral and rectal route administration suggests that the oral to rectal potency ratio for morphine is 1:1. Thus oral and rectal doses are the same. Slow-release morphine tablets have been given rectally when patients are no longer able to swallow tablets.

6. Transmucosal

The more lipophilic opioids are readily absorbed through buccal, nasal, or gingival mucosa. First pass effects in the liver are avoided and rapid onset of action is possible. Buprenorphine, butorphanol, fentanyl (fentanyl lollipop), and sufentanil have all been given via this route.

VIII. PRINCIPLES OF OPIOID THERAPY

1. "Mild" Versus "Strong"

There is really no such thing as a "mild" opioid because all opioids can be titrated to achieve equianalgesic effects and there is no ceiling effect to any opioid. However, certain opioids have traditionally been considered "mild" either because dosing is limited by side effects (e.g., codeine's constipating effect), or more often, because they have been offered by the pharmaceutical companies in combined preparations where the secondary drug (e.g., acetaminophen or aspirin) limits dosing (e.g., Percocet, Percodan, Vicodin, and Tylenol no. 3). These combination therapies are useful for short-term management of mild to moderate pain such as acute pain after surgery or trauma, but less useful in long-term pain management because of their dose limitations. In fact, we are moving away from the World Health Organization (WHO) concept of using these drugs as second-level therapy in the treatment of cancer pain (see Chapter 32) because of their lack of titratability. Most authorities now encourage the earlier adoption of small doses of "strong" opioids (i.e., choice of any opioid) in preference to combination therapies for the treatment of chronic and cancer pain. Obviously, adjuncts can be given at the same time, but giving these as a separate preparation allows the opioid to be titrated to need.

2. The Titration Principle

For many reasons, not least of which is to avoid side effects, particularly respiratory depression, the best principle for giving opioids is to start low (standard starting doses for opioids for acute pain are presented in Chapter 21, Table 2 and for chronic pain in Appendix VII, Table 2) and titrate up (or down) in increments until optimal (maximal analgesia with acceptable side effects). The exact choice of starting dose and the size and timing of incremental increases will obviously depend on the patient's likely opioid sensitivity, which will depend in turn on the patient's medical condition and whether or not tolerance has developed.

The only exception to this principle is when PCA or IV infusions are used to treat acute severe pain when it is safer to give a monitored bolus to achieve comfort than to maintain comfort using standard or near-standard PCA or infusion doses. This approach is safer than rapidly increasing PCA or infusion doses in an effort to achieve pain relief in patients who are not only opioid naïve, but also have probably been given multiple centrally acting depressant drugs in the course of their treatment. Once these patients become comfortable and can sleep, overdose may occur if a high-dose infusion or frequent large bolus dosing is allowed to continue.

3. Choice of Opioid

Combination "mild" opioids such as Percocet, Vicodin, and Tylenol no. 3 are acceptable choices for mild to moderate short-term pain, especially considering physicians' familiarity with their use. Meperidine (Demerol) is often avoided, especially for long-term use, because of the possibility of normeperidine toxicity and because the drug's euphoric effects make it a drug that is often favored by addicts. Likewise, propoxyphene (Darvon, Darvocet) is avoided because of the possibility of norpropoxyphene toxicity (see section entitled Precautions) and because its analgesic effect at standard doses is weak. Long-term morphine use should be avoided in patients with renal dysfunction, including the older patients (>80 years), because of the likelihood of morphine-6-glucuronide accumulation. Partial agonists (e.g., buprenorphine) and mixed agonist/antagonists (e.g., pentazocine, nalorphine) are sometimes chosen because of their low potential for abuse and respiratory depression. However, pure agonists are preferred, particularly in chronic pain patients, because of their superior efficacy and easier titratability. Also difficulties arise in switching opioids when mixed agonists/antagonists are used and the effects of one drug (e.g., analgesia) are reversed by another. Otherwise, any opioid is suitable, and preference will often be dictated by physician familiarity and by patient choice. It is worth asking patients if they have received opioids in the past and have a preference because efficacy and side effects are often patient dependent and idiosyncratic.

4. Short-acting Versus Long-acting

Several choices of long-acting opioids are now available [morphine sulfate (MS Contin), oxycodone (OxyContin), fentanyl transdermal system (Duragesic), methadone] making the use of long-acting opioids highly feasible. In the treatment of prolonged pain (cancer and noncancer) it is usually preferable to base therapy on a long-acting preparation and to use short-acting drugs for "breakthrough" pain. Breakthrough pain is pain that breaks through the analgesia achieved by a long-acting medication and does so because of activity, anxiety, time of day, and so on. Long-acting (slow-release) opioid therapy is associated with less euphoria and dysphoria (therefore has less addictive potential), and is preferred for the treatment of CNTP. The use of short-acting (immediate-release) opioids in CNTP is minimized to reduce possible euphoric effects and to avoid overreliance on medication when other means of controlling pain, such as distraction or relaxation, would be preferable. Long-acting preparations may also be useful in the treatment of resolving acute pain when analgesic needs are predictable and the patient would prefer twice daily to more frequent dosing. However, such therapy should be strictly time limited, and if treatment becomes chronic, opioid therapy should only be provided under all the usual constrains of appropriately monitored chronic opioid treatment (see Chapter 30).

5. Prescribing Opioids

In the hospital setting, prescribing opioids is relatively easy, and regulatory restrictions apply particularly to the pharmacy and to those actually administering the drugs (nurses and anesthesiologists). Hospital personnel are generally comfortable with using opioids within regulatory guidelines and restrictions. Prescribing opioids for home use is much more difficult. Each state has its own regulations, and the prescribing physician must be familiar with these. The Drug Enforcement Administration (DEA) (Federal) guidelines for the prescription of controlled substances are presented in Appendix VI; U.S. Food and Drug Administration (FDA) drug schedules are presented in Appendix VII. The Massachusetts General Hospital (MGH) has a set of guidelines for prescribing opioids for CNMP, which are presented in Appendix V.

6. Controlling Side Effects

Respiratory depression is rightly the most feared of the opioid side effects. Hypoxia, apnea, and even death can occur with opioid use. However, this is much more likely to occur when opioids are used for acute rather than chronic pain. Obeying the principles of acute pain management (see Chapter 21) and the opioid titration principle (mentioned earlier) will avoid respiratory depression in most cases. Nausea and vomiting are also far less likely to be troublesome when opioids are used for chronic rather than acute pain. When they do occur, they can be treated by reducing opioid dose, switching opioid, or giving an antiemetic. Constipation is a common complication of chronic opioid treatment, to that extent that preventive treatment should always be offered in conjunction with chronic opioid therapy. This should be with stimulant laxatives [e.g., senna (Senokot), lactulose], not with bulk-forming laxatives, which do not solve the problem of slow transit time and may actually worsen the situation. Other side effects are uncommon and should be treated by dose reduction or symptomatically if necessary.

Opioid rotation—the sequential use of different opioids—has been used to manage tolerance and side effects. A number of different drugs may have to be tried before the most effective with the least side effects is found. The effectiveness of opioid rotation is based on the interindividual variation as well as incomplete cross-tolerance between opioids. Because of cross-tolerance, a lower than equipotent dose (e.g., half, or in the case of methadone, one fourth) is used in rotations (see Chapter 33).

7. Treating Overdose

Adverse reactions from excessive ingestions of opioids may result from clinical overdose, accumulation, or accidental overdose in addicts or in suicide attempts. Death is nearly always attributable to respiratory failure, but if this is being treated with ventilation, very high doses of opioid are safely tolerated. Blood pressure may fall progressively; the patient becomes flaccid and unrousable. Noncardiogenic pulmonary edema is possible and frank convulsions may occur with very large doses. The pinpoint pupils occur, unless hypoxia intervenes, and then pupils may dilate. Treatment is supportive, with ventilation and careful fluid management. Naloxone may be given to reverse the respiratory depression, but large doses given quickly can precipitate withdrawal or rebound increases in sympathetic nervous system activity. The safest approach is to dilute the standard 0.4 mg naloxone with 10 mL of fluid, and titrate carefully to effect. It should be remembered that naloxone has a short duration (a shorter half-life than most of the agonists) and renarcotization can occur. Repeat doses of naloxone or an infusion may be needed.

IX. INDIVIDUAL PREPARATIONS

The structures of some commonly used opioid agonists, partial agonists, and antagonists are shown in Figure 3. Choice of opioid should be determined as mentioned in preceding text (see section entitled Choice of Opioid). Opioid conversion doses are shown in Appendix VIII, Table 2.

1. Morphine

Morphine remains the standard with which all other opioids are compared. It is widely used and recommended as a standard by the WHO because of its wide availability and low cost. One third of morphine is bound to plasma protein and the unbound fraction is ionized at physiologic pH; thus the drug is very hydrophilic. Because of this, although it is distributed widely, it has limited ability to penetrate tissues. It is for this reason that morphine given epidurally or intraspinally can spread rostrally in CSF and cause delayed respiratory depression.

Morphine is metabolized by the liver. The major metabolites are morphine-3-glucuronide and morphine-6-glucuronide. Although morphine-3-glucuronide is inactive, morphine-6-glucuronide is more potent than morphine itself and has a longer half-life. The glucuronides are excreted by the kidneys and patients with renal dysfunction can accumulate morphine-6-glucuronide and develop prolonged opioid effects, including respiratory depression. On the other hand, patients in liver failure tolerate morphine up to the point of hepatic precoma because glucuronidation is rarely impaired. IV injection of morphine results in rapid peak plasma levels, but peak effector site (brain and spinal cord receptors) concentrations occur 15 to 30 minutes later, so there is a relatively

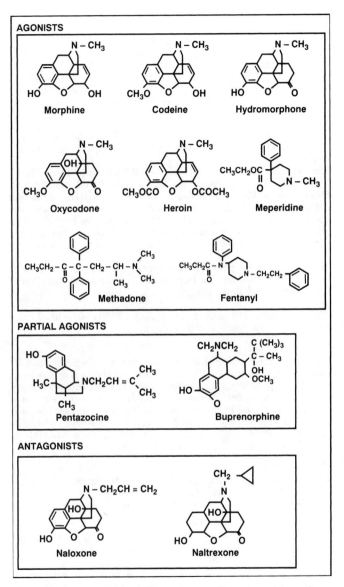

Figure 3. Structures of opioid agonists, partial antagonists, and antagonists.

slow onset of peak CNS effects. Plasma half-life after an IV bolus is 2 to 3 hours. The initial dose given intramuscularly (IM) or subcutaneously (SQ) is highly variable, although 10 mg for a 70-kg healthy patient is reasonable. The high first pass effect means that the oral dose is approximately three times that of the parenteral dose or more. Preservative free morphine (Duramorph) given in small doses epidurally (1 to 4 mg) or intrathecally (0.1 to 0.4 mg) can produce profound analgesia of long duration (up to 12 to 24 hours). These are conservative doses given at MGH for patients who are in unmonitored beds. Higher doses (up to 10 mg epidurally or 1 mg intrathecally) can be given to monitored patients in intensive care units (ICUs) or step-down units.

Preparations

Morphine sulfate: injections 1, 5, 8, 10, 15, and 30 mg per mL; oral tablets 8, 10, 15, and 30 mg; rectal suppository 5, 10, 20, and 30 mg.

Morphine sulfate controlled release (MS Contin): tablets 15, 30, 60, and 100 mg. **(Oramorph SR):** tablets 30, 60, and 100 mg.

Morphine sulfate immediate release [(MDIR), Roxanol, Rescudose, MS/L]: oral solution 2 and 4 mg per mL; oral concentrate 20 mg per mL; and tablets and capsules 15 and 30 mg.

Morphine sulfate preservative-free solution (Duramorph and Astramorph) for IV, epidural, or intrathecal use: 0.5 and 1.0 mg per mL.

Morphine sulfate preservative free (Infumorph) for continuous microinfusions for implantable epidural or intrathecal pumps: 10 and 25 mg per mL.

Formulations containing morphine for the treatment of diarrhea include paregoric and laudanum.

2. Codeine

Codeine is less potent than morphine but it has a high oral–parenteral potency ratio. Codeine is largely metabolized by the liver, and the by-products are excreted by the kidneys. Approximately 10% of codeine is demethylated to morphine. Its analgesic action is probably related to this conversion. It has a considerable antitussive action, probably involving receptors that bind codeine itself. The plasma half-life is 2 to 4 hours. Codeine is available in combination with acetaminophen or aspirin.

Preparations

Codeine phosphate: injections 15, 30, and 60 mg per mL; tablets 15, 30, and 60 mg; oral solution 3 mg per mL.

Codeine sulfate: tablets 15, 30, and 60 mg.

3. Hydrocodone

This is a semisynthetic codeine derivative with analgesic and antitussive properties, used most commonly in combination with acetaminophen in Vicodin.

Hydrocodone bitartrate (Vicodin): tablets 7.5 mg with acetaminophen 750 mg.

4. Heroin

Heroin, or diacetylmorphine, is a typical prodrug. It has no direct action itself on the opioid receptor but is rapidly metabolized to 6-monoacetylmorphine and subsequently to morphine. It is not available for clinical use in the United States but is available in Canada and the UK. Although many have touted heroin to have certain advantages over morphine, all present evidence suggests that this is not so. It does come in a preservative-free powder and has a high solubility, so high concentrations can be made, but other drugs such as hydromorphone can be substituted as a potent soluble agent.

5. Hydromorphone

This semisynthetic derivative of morphine is ten times more potent than its parent compound. After parenteral injection, levels rise rapidly but there is a slower onset of CNS effects. Plasma half-life is 2 to 3 hours after an IV dose. IM injection delays peak plasma levels and CNS effects. Oral dosing takes 45 minutes or so for peak effects. Typical doses are 2 to 6 mg orally and 1.5 mg parenterally every 3 to 4 hours.

Preparations

Hydromorphone hydrochloride (Dilaudid): injections 1, 2, and 4 mg per mL; tablets 1, 2, 3, 4, and 8 mg; suppository 3 mg; cough syrup 1 mg in 5 mL; oral liquid 1 mg per mL.

Hydromorphone hydrochloride (Dilaudid HP): highly concentrated for opioid-tolerant patients: 10 mg per mL.

6. Oxycodone

This is a synthetic thebaine derivative with a similar profile and potency to morphine. It has typically been used in combination with nonopioids (Percocet, Percodan), but more recently has been formulated as a long-acting preparation (OxyContin), which has popularized its use in cancer pain and other pain states. Immediate-release oxycodone has also become more popular, partly because it makes sense to prescribe it for breakthrough pain in patients taking OxyContin and partly because it is now perceived as a "strong," titratable opioid rather than as a "weak," nontitratable opioid (in combination therapies). OxyContin and oxycodone are a useful substitute for MS Contin and immediate-release morphine, particularly in the elderly who are sensitive to morphine-induced sedation and mental status change and to morphine-6-glucuronide accumulation. Unfortunately, OxyContin recently became fashionable as a drug of abuse, which currently places constraints on the legitimate use of this clinically useful drug.

Preparations

Oxycodone hydrochloride immediate release: (OxyIR) capsule 5mg; **(OxyFAST)** concentrated oral liquid 20 mg per mL.

Oxycodone hydrochloride controlled release (OxyContin): tablets 10, 20, 40, and 80 mg.

Oxycodone hydrochloride (Percocet): tablets 5 mg with 325 mg acetaminophen;

(Tylox): capsule 5 mg with 500 mg acetaminophen.

Oxycodone hydrochloride (Roxicet): oral solution 5 mg with 325 mg acetaminophen per 5 mL.

Oxycodone hydrochloride (Percodan): tablet 5 mg with 325 mg aspirin.

Oxycodone hydrochloride (Roxicodone): tablet 5 mg; oral solution 5 mg in 5 mL; concentrated oral solution (Intensol) 20 mg per mL.

7. Meperidine

Meperidine is 70% protein bound, which is more highly protein bound than morphine. Parenteral and oral doses are similar. The analgesic effects of meperidine are detectable approximately 15 minutes after an oral dose, reach their peak effect in 1 to 2 hours, and then gradually subside over several hours. Onset after parenteral administration of the same dose is within 10 minutes and peaks in 1 hour. Clinical duration of effective analgesia is between 2 to 4 hours. The usual initial dose is between 50 to 100 mg. The drug has vagolytic activities and is the only opioid that may produce tachycardia. Meperidine is metabolized eventually to normeperidine. This metabolite has a half-life of 15 to 20 hours and is eliminated by both the kidney and the liver. Decreased renal or hepatic function can cause normeperidine to accumulate. The half-life is extended in the older patients. Therefore, in some individuals, the metabolite can build up. Normeperidine is toxic, and large doses can cause tremors, muscle twitches, dilated pupil, hyperactive reflexes, and convulsions. If meperidine is combined with monoamine oxidase (MAO) inhibitors, a number of reactions may be seen, including severe respiratory depression or excitation, delusions, hyperpyrexia, and convulsions. Meperidine has weak local anesthetic activities. This drug is generally avoided except for short-term use because of the risk of normeperidine toxicity and because it has a high abuse potential.

Preparations

Meperidine hydrochloride (Demerol): injections 25, 50, 75, and 100 mg per mL; tablets 50 and 100 mg; syrup 50 mg in 5 mL; **(Mepergan):** injection 25 mg per mL with 25 mg promethazine. Cogeners of meperidine are **diphenoxylate hydrochloride (Lomotil)** and **loperamide hydrochloride (Imodium)**, which are used to treat diarrhea.

8. Levorphanol

This drug is a morpinium, and is the only example of this series that is commercially available. It has a long duration of action and pharmacologic effects that resemble morphine, except it may be associated with less nausea and vomiting. The average dose is 2 mg (SQ or orally) and this would be expected to last 6 to 8 hours. The oral–parenteral potency ratio is comparable to oxycodone and codeine. Levorphanol may be crushed so that it can be administered via a nasogastric tube. It is occasionally useful in cancer patients who feel nauseated by morphine and who benefit from the longer lasting effect, although it has largely been superceded by oxycodone and OxyContin.

Preparations

Levorphanol tartrate (Levo-Dromoran): injection 2 mg per mL; tablet 2 mg.

9. Methadone

This is the only opioid with prolonged activity not achieved by controlled-release formulation. It is a synthetic opioid with effects similar to those of morphine. There can be a high variability in steady state plasma levels in different individuals due to the pharmacokinetic and pharmacodynamic profile of the drug, in addition to the varying extent of liver metabolism, possibly resulting in unexpected respiratory depression. Unlike morphine, which undergoes glucuronidation, methadone undergoes N-demethylation by the liver cytochrome P-450 enzymes, the activity of which can vary widely in different people. Multiple drug interactions have been identified, so that caution should be used in patients with complex medical conditions who are receiving multiple medications, especially antivirals and antibiotics. Methadone has biphasic elimination, with a long β-elimination phase that ranges from 30 to 60 hours. Therefore, sedation and respiratory depression can outlast the analgesic action because the analgesic action equates to the α-elimination phase, which typically is usually 6 to 8 hours. This biphasic pattern helps explain why methadone is needed every 4 to 8 hours for analgesia but only once a day for opioid maintenance therapy. Cardiac toxicity, with QTc interval prolongation, can occur with high doses of methadone.

In addition to its μ and δ agonist effect, it is an NMDA inhibitor and also an inhibitor of serotonin and norepinephrine reuptake. It has been said that these properties should make methadone an ideal agent for neuropathic pain. This concept has not been fully explored with clinical trials, so it remains for the moment theoretical only. These other effects of methadone are thought to confer real benefit in terms of reducing tolerance, a property that can be useful in opioid rotations (see Chapter 32). Withdrawal symptoms are said to be less severe than those associated with morphine, and because of this and its long duration of action, methadone is used for detoxification or maintenance treatment of opioid addicts. An analog of methadone—levo-alpha-acetyl-methadol (LAAM)— is also used for the treatment of opioid dependence.

For pain relief, oral doses may vary from 2.5 to 15 mg, parenteral doses from 2.5 to 10 mg and, for addict maintenance, 40 to 100 mg daily. After an oral dose, analgesia occurs in 30 to 60 minutes. After a parenteral dose, analgesia occurs in 10 to 20 minutes, with peak effects in 1 to 2 hours. As already described, the drug is eliminated slowly, which makes it liable to accumulate. Rapid titration (up and down) is not possible, so this drug is best reserved for patients with stable pain. Although methadone is cheap and can be very effective, many physicians are uncomfortable prescribing it for outpatients because of its uncertain pharmacokinetics and safety profile.

Preparation

Methadone hydrochloride (Dolophine): injection 10 mg per mL; tablets 5 and 10 mg (40-mg specialized dose for opioid addiction); oral solution 1, 2, and 10 mg per mL.

10. Fentanyl

This is a phenylpiperidine that is 50 to 80 times as potent as morphine. It can be used as an analgesic (2 to 10 μg per kg) or anesthetic (20 to 100 μg per kg). Onset after parenteral administration is very rapid. Maximum analgesia and respiratory depression may not peak until 20 to 30 minutes after IM injection or several minutes after IV usage. Fentanyl may be given also intrathecally, epidurally, via mucous membranes, or through the skin. Transdermal fentanyl is extremely useful as a treatment of chronic pain, especially cancer pain, when the oral route cannot be used. Several fentanyl derivatives (i.e., sufentanil, alfentanil, and remifentanil) are used in anesthetic practice but not in pain practice.

Preparations

Fentanyl citrate (Sublimaze): injection 50 μg per mL.
Fentanyl transdermal system (Duragesic): patches 25, 50, 75, and 100 μg per hour.

11. Buprenorphine

This is a highly lipophilic, semisynthetic opioid with partial activity at the μ-receptor and very little activity at the κ and σ receptors. It has a high affinity but low intrinsic activity at the μ receptor. It has qualitatively similar effects to morphine in terms of analgesia, CNS, and cardiovascular system effects. However, because it is a partial agonist, it has a pharmacologic ceiling. Buprenorphine 0.4 mg is the equivalent of 10 mg of morphine IM, but buprenorphine has the longer duration of action. The dose for analgesia is 0.3 mg IM or IV every 6 hours. After IM administration, initial effects are seen at 15 minutes with a peak at 1 hour. IV administration results in shorter onset and peak times. Sublingual doses as low as 0.4 mg produce effective pain relief.

The FDA has recently approved the use of sublingual buprenorphine, either alone or in combination with naloxone, for the treatment of opioid dependence. It is the first drug available in the USA that can be used in an office-based treatment of addiction. It can be given for withdrawal from heroin or methadone, or used as maintenance for treatment of addicts.

Preparations

Buprenorphine hydrochloride (Buprenex): injection 0.3 mg per mL.
Buprenorphine hydrochloride (Subutex): sublingual tablet 2 mg and 8 mg.
Buprenorphine hydrochloride and naloxone (Suboxone): Buprenorphine 2 mg and naloxone 0.5 mg; buprenorphine 8 mg and naloxone 2 mg.

12. Nalbuphine

Nalbupine is an agonist-antagonist with its chief agonist effects at the κ site. Nalbuphine has a ceiling effect on analgesia and respiratory depression, and doses more than approximately 30 mg have no further effect. Dysphoria due to σ activation may occur. Sedative effects are similar to those of morphine. Sweating and headache may occur. The usual dose in the adult is 10 mg every 3 to 6 hours parenterally, when the onset of effect is 5 to 10 minutes and the duration of action 3 to 6 hours.

Preparations

Nalbuphine hydrochloride (Nubain): injections 10 and 20 mg per mL.

13. Tramadol

Tramadol is a synthetic centrally acting analgesic with an unusual mode of action. It has weak opioid activity at μ-, δ-, and κ receptors, with a 20-fold preference for the μ-receptor. It also has nonopioid analgesic activity via norepinephrine and serotonin reuptake inhibition. Tramadol is available in the United States only as an oral preparation. It has a low potential for addiction and respiratory depression. Its main use is in mild to moderate pain, but it can be used to treat severe pain (usually together with other nonopioid analgesics) in patients who cannot tolerate standard opioids. It is usually given as 25 to 100 mg every 4 to 6 hours orally, but the maximum daily dose should not exceed 400 mg. Dosing is limited by side effects, especially dizziness and vertigo.

Preparations
Tramadol hydrochloride (Ultram): scored tablet 50 mg.

14. Remifentanil
Remifentanil is a synthetic opioid and μ agonist, which, although chemically related to the fentanyl congeners, is unique in that it has a number of ester linkages. Because of these ester linkages, it is hydrolyzed by blood and tissue nonspecific esterases. There is a minor N-dealkylating metabolic pathway. The metabolism of the drug is not affected by pseudocholinesterase deficiency. Therefore, it is the first ultra–short-acting opiate. Because of this short action, it does not yet have a place in the treatment of chronic pain, but it is of relevance to acute pain management in the sense that any patient whose intraoperative analgesia was provided by remifentanil can be anticipated to require postoperative analgesia much sooner than with other analgesics to avoid severe pain after surgery.

Preparations
Remifentanil (Ultiva): injections 1, 2, and 5 mg per mL

15. Naloxone
Naloxone is an opioid antagonist with greatest affinity for the μ-receptor, but acting at all opioid receptors. Small doses given intravenously or IM will either prevent or promptly reverse the effects of μ-receptor agonists. In addition to reversing analgesia, patients with respiratory depression will show an increase in respiratory rate within 1 to 2 minutes. Sedative effects are also reversed and blood pressure, if low, returns to normal. The duration of action is 1 to 4 hours and the plasma half-life is approximately 1 hour. Abrupt reversal of narcotic depression with large doses of naloxone may result in nausea and vomiting, tachycardia, sweating, hypertension, tremulousness, seizures, and cardiac arrest. These effects are at least partially attributable to a sudden surge of sympathetic activity as is seen in opioid withdrawal states. Other side effects that have been reported include hypotension, ventricular tachycardia and fibrillation, and pulmonary edema. To avoid these serious and potentially dangerous side effects, it is advisable to reverse the effects of opioids slowly with repeated small doses of naloxone, titrating dose to effect. This can easily be accomplished by diluting one 0.4 mg ampule in 10 mL (0.04 mg per mL) and injecting 1 to 2 mL (0.04 to 0.08 mg) every 1 to 2 minutes. In this way it is sometimes possible to reverse respiratory depression while retaining analgesia.

Naloxone is readily absorbed from the GI tract, but the drug is almost completely metabolized by the liver before it reaches the circulation. Parenteral administration is thus needed for systemic effects. The drug may be used orally to treat constipation utilizing its localized effect on opioid receptors in the gut. Generally, dosages range from 0.8 to 4.0 mg (2 to 10 ampules) every 4 hours, four times, or until a bowel movement has occurred.

Preparations

Naloxone hydrochloride (Narcan): injections 0.02, 0.4, and 1.0 mg per mL.

X. CONCLUSION

Opioids are the most effective analgesics known, not surprisingly because we now know that endogenous opioids are responsible for natural analgesic states, and that opiate drugs produce analgesia by binding to endogenous opioid receptors. Unfortunately, there are several barriers to their use, not least of which is the risk of respiratory depression—a potentially lethal side effect of opioids. Another important barrier is the social stigma attached to opioids because of their use as recreational drugs. Careful education of health care providers, patients, and patients' relatives is often needed to allow them to understand the therapeutic value of opioids and the difference between therapeutic and recreational use. The opioids are not benign drugs and should be used with knowledge of their complex actions and adverse effects. At the same time, they are essential tools in pain management and in medicine in general, so an understanding of opioid effects is important.

SELECTED READINGS

Borsook D. Opioids and neurological effects. *Curr Opin Anaesthesiol* 1994;7:352–357.

Carr D, Lipkowski A. Mechanisms of opioid analgesic actions. In: Rogers M, Tinker JH, Covino BG, et al., eds. *Principles and practice of anesthesiology*. St. Louis, MO: Mosby-Year Book, 1993.

Cowan A. Mechanisms of opioid activity. *Curr Opin Anaesthesiol* 1992;5:529–534.

Fields HL. *Pain.* New York: McGraw-Hill, 1987:251–279.

Lambert DG. Opioid receptors. *Curr Opin Anaesthesiol* 1995;8:317–322.

Malan Jr TP. Opioid pharmacology in anesthesia pain management. *ASA Refresher Lectures* 2000:422.

Reisine T, Pasternak G. Opioid analgesics and antagonists. In: Hardman JG, Gilman A, et al., eds. *Goodman and Gilman's the pharmacological basis of therapeutics*, 9th ed. New York: McGraw-Hill, 1996.

Twycross RG. Opioids. In: Wall PD, Melzack R, eds. *Textbook of pain*, 3rd ed. Edinburgh: Churchill-Livingstone, 1999.

Adjuvant Treatments

Karla Hayes

My heart aches, and a drowsy numbness pains
My senses, as though of hemlock I had drunk,
Or emptied some dull opiate to the drains
One minute past, and Lethe-wards had sunk.
—*John Keats, "Ode to a Nightingale," 1795–1821*

The opioids and the antiinflammatory agents are the primary analgesics used in pain management. These drugs have the unique property of providing immediate (within minutes to hours) pain relief. The opioids are the only drugs indicated for the treatment of moderate to severe pain. The antiinflammatory drugs are useful for the treatment of osteoarthritis and rheumatoid arthritis, as well as for various mild to moderate acute and chronic pain conditions, and as adjuncts in the case of severe pain. The remaining categories of analgesic drugs, called **adjuvant analgesics**, have primary indications [U.S. Food and Drug Administration (FDA) approved] for nonpain diagnoses, their analgesic effects being secondary. These nonpain diagnoses include epilepsy, depression, and cardiac arrhythmia. Characteristically, the adjuvant drugs do not provide immediate pain relief; rather, their effects are noticeable only after days or weeks of therapy (see Table 1).

There are many categories of drugs in the adjuvant class, including the tricyclic antidepressants, the selective serotonin reuptake inhibitors, the sodium channel blockers, the GABAergics, the benzodiazepines, and the α-adrenergics. This chapter focuses on the use of anticonvulsants, local anesthetics, corticosteroids, and antispasmodics in the treatment of chronic pain (including cancer pain). The psychotropic medications are described in Chapter 11, and analgesics for headache are described in Chapter 28. A brief review of all the adjuvant analgesics is presented in Appendix VIII.

Adjuvant	Indicated Diagnoses
Topiramate	Diabetic neuropathy, spinal cord injury, headache
Pregabalin	Diabetic neuropathy, PHN, fibromyalgia
Oxcarbazepine	Trigeminal neuralgia
Mexiletine	Peripheral neuropathy
Carbamazepine	Trigeminal neuralgia
Gabapentin	Diabetic neuropathy, postherpetic neuralgia, migraine headache, phantom limb pain
Valproic acid	Trigeminal neuralgia, migraine headache
Lamogitrine	Trigeminal neuralgia, peripheral neuropathy, spinal cord injury, central pain
Tizanidine	Trigeminal neuralgia, chronic daily headache
Lidocaine Ointment	Postherpetic neuralgia
Lidocaine Patch	Postherpetic neuralgia
Capsaicin	Postherpetic neuralgia
Prednisolone	Rheumatoid arthritis

RCTs, randomized controlled trials.

I. GENERAL CONSIDERATIONS

The decision to begin a particular analgesic medication for any individual patient involves many issues. The potential benefit of the drug must be weighed against its side effects. The patient should be made aware of the state of evidence concerning the drug's analgesic efficacy and should have realistic expectations. A check of the patient's medical background is needed to identify areas of susceptibility, and the patient's current medications must be reviewed for drug interactions. Appropriate patient selection is important. Patient and physician should be aware that the side effects of adjunctive agents may be noticed within days of initiating treatment, whereas the analgesic effect may not be apparent for 1 to 2 weeks.

Another consideration is the drug's mechanism of action, which can direct treatment strategies if the cause of the pain is known. Over the past several years, the treatment algorithm for chronic pain has seen a shift toward a mechanism-based approach. This concept is underscored in the following statement:

"As we approach the new millennium, it is clear that we are on the brink of a major change in clinical pain management. We are poised to move from a treatment paradigm that has been almost entirely empirical to one that will be derived from an understanding of the actual mechanisms involved in the pathogenesis of pain. . . . The implications of this are immense and will necessitate major changes . . . to a mechanism-based classification. . . . The aim in the future will be to identify in individual patients what mechanisms are responsible for their pain and to target treatment specifically at those mechanisms." (Clifford Woolf, 1999)

This approach will make it possible to match a medication (with a known mechanism of action) to a pain syndrome in which this physiologic mechanism has been disrupted. In addition, this approach will allow pairing of medications with different mechanisms of action to provide synergistic effects. Finally, we will be able to use agents with the same mechanism of action in place of drugs that are effective but are not tolerated because of side effects.

II. ANTICONVULSANTS

Anticonvulsant drugs have been used in the management of pain since the 1960s, soon after they were introduced for the treatment of epilepsy. This group of medications is also known as antiepileptic drugs, and we refer to them in their commonly abbreviated form (AEDs). For years, it was thought that the primary indication for these drugs was specific neuropathic pain disorders such as trigeminal neuralgia (TN) or other syndromes that had predominately lancinating or burning pain. The newer anticonvulsants that have been introduced in recent years have been used with some success for a variety of indications. Eight anticonvulsants currently are useful in neuropathic pain states: carbamazepine, oxcarbazepine, topiramate, levetiracetam, pregabalin, zonisamide, gabapentin, and lamotrigine.

Although the mechanism of action of each AED is different, the mechanisms underlying their anticonvulsant effects likely contribute to their analgesic effects because the pathophysiology of epilepsy and neuropathic pain may be similar. AEDs have many potential side effects, and their individual side effect profiles differ. Gabapentin has a uniquely favorable side effect profile and also a lack of drug–drug interactions. It is widely used in the treatment of pain, largely because of its good safety record. It also seems effective in a wide range of pain conditions, both neuropathic and nonneuropathic.

1. Indications

The following are indications for AEDs in patients with chronic pain:

- Neuralgias–trigeminal, glossopharyngeal, and postherpetic
- Neuralgia secondary to peripheral nervous and central nervous system (CNS) infiltration by cancer
- Central pain states (e.g., thalamic pain syndrome and poststroke pain)
- Postsympathectomy pain
- Posttraumatic neuralgia
- Porphyria, Fabry disease, and others
- Painful diabetic neuropathy
- Paroxysmal pain in multiple sclerosis
- Migraine headaches
- Phantom limb pain and postamputation stump pain
- Peripheral neuropathy secondary to a variety of disease states [e.g., alcoholism, amyloidosis, diabetes mellitus, HIV/AIDS (human immunodeficiency virus/acquired immunodeficiency syndrome), malabsorption, porphyria, toxic exposure, sarcoidosis, and drug induced]

2. Clinical Guidelines

(i) Dosing Regimes

A 4- to 6-week trial is the minimum required to adequately assess the analgesic efficacy of a new drug. The patient is given instructions about dosing and a titration schedule. In general, the phrase "start low and go slow" is adhered to when a new anticonvulsant analgesic is started. This allows the body to adjust to the new drug and decreases the likelihood of major side effects. Doses are generally increased until therapeutic effects or limiting adverse effects are observed. A review of previous analgesic drug trials is valuable, with special attention being paid to pain relief and side effects. Serum levels do not appear to correlate well with pain response. Both physician and patient must understand that this process may take months to years (several medication trials). The medications should not be discontinued abruptly, but should be tapered slowly to avoid withdrawal symptoms.

(ii) Choice of Drug

On the basis of their proven efficacy, carbamazepine and gabapentin have been approved by the U.S. FDA for the management of pain. Because of its favorable side effect profile, gabapentin is often used as a first-line agent. The unfavorable side effect profile of carbamazepine and the need for monitoring of hematologic function are major drawbacks that have influenced physicians to utilize other drugs, especially oxcarbazepine, its keto-analog. Because the various anticonvulsants have different mechanisms of action, the lack of response to one drug cannot probably predict the response to another drug.

3. Drug Characteristics

(i) Carbamazepine

MECHANISM OF ACTION.   Carbamazepine is chemically and pharmacologically related to the tricyclic antidepressants. It inhibits norepinephrine uptake and prevents repeated discharges in neurons. Carbamazepine likely blocks sodium channels. This observation is consistent with its ability to relieve lancinating pain in neuralgia states.

PHARMACOLOGY.   Carbamazepine is absorbed slowly and unpredictably after oral intake. Peak concentrations are seen in 2 to 8 hours. It is moderately protein bound and has active metabolites. Metabolism is hepatic, and excretion is urinary. It has a serum half-life of 10 to 20 hours, averaging 14 hours.

RECOMMENDED DOSAGE.   Start at 200 mg per day and increase by 200 mg every 1 to 3 days to a maximum of 1,500 mg per day. If side effects are encountered, the dosage should be decreased to the previous level for several days and then gradually increased. Therapeutic dosages usually range from 800 to 1,200 mg per day. Carbamazepine is a gastric irritant and therefore should be taken with food.

ADVERSE EFFECTS.   Sedation, nausea, diplopia, and vertigo occur most frequently with carbamazepine. Hematologic abnormalities such as aplastic anemia, agranulocytosis, pancytopenia, and thrombocytopenia can occur. Other side effects include jaundice (hepatocellular and cholestatic), oliguria, hypertension, and acute left ventricular heart failure.

Baseline and periodic complete blood counts (CBCs), and liver function studies should be performed. Blood counts are obtained at baseline, then every 2 weeks for a month, monthly for 3 months, twice over the following year, and then yearly. If a patient exhibits low white cell or platelet counts, the patient should be monitored closely. The drug should be discontinued if considerable bone marrow depression develops. Liver function studies should be obtained for patients with a history of liver dysfunction. Carbemazepine should be discontinued immediately in cases of aggravated liver dysfunction or acute liver disease.

CLINICAL APPLICATIONS.   The analgesic effects of carbamazepine for TN were first reported in 1962. Analgesic efficacy has been most frequently documented in TN and in painful diabetic neuropathy. Efficacy in postherpetic neuralgia, tabetic pain, and central pain is less well documented.

(ii) Oxcarbazepine

MECHANISM OF ACTION.   Oxcarbazepine (OXC) is a 10-keto analog of carbamazepine. It reduces the number of spikes elicited by a train of high-frequency stimuli (similar to carbamazepine), probably by suppressing the generation of high-frequency firing and by prolonging the refractory period. It also likely binds to sodium channels in their inactive state, as well as increases potassium conductance and modulates high-voltage-activated calcium channels.

PHARMACOLOGY.   Following oral administration, OXC is completely absorbed and extensively metabolized to its pharmacologically active 10-monohydroxy metabolite (MHD). The half-life of the parent drug (OXC) is 2 hours, whereas the half-life of MHD is approximately 9 hours. Steady-state plasma concentrations are reached within 2 to 3 days. Food has no effect on the rate and extent of absorption.

RECOMMENDED DOSAGE.   For pain management, OXC is typically titrated more slowly than when used for epilepsy. It should be initiated at 150 mg bid and increased by 150 to 300 mg per day at weekly intervals. The recommended daily dosage for seizure control is 1,200 mg. Typical maintenance dosages for pain management are 600 to 1,200 mg per day.

ADVERSE EFFECTS.   The most commonly observed adverse events in association with OXC are dizziness, somnolence, diplopia, fatigue, ataxia, nausea, and abnormal vision. Hyponatremia can occur, so sodium levels should be monitored.

CLINICAL APPLICATIONS.   Surprisingly, there have been very few studies examining OXC and pain. Nevertheless, because of its favorable side effect profile, it is now the drug of choice for TN in the United States. It is widely used with success for a variety of neuropathic pain syndromes.

(iii) Topiramate

MECHANISM OF ACTION.   Topiramate has several mechanisms of action, which may be relevant in treating neuropathic pain. It has been shown to block voltage-gated sodium channels, inhibit high-voltage-activated L-type calcium channels, potentiate GABAergic inhibition by facilitating the action of GABA-A receptors, and block excitatory glutamate activity via the AMPA and kainate receptors.

PHARMACOLOGY.   Absorption of topiramate is rapid, with peak plasma concentrations occurring at approximately 2 hours. The relative bioavailability of topiramate from the tablet form is approximately 80% compared to the solution. The bioavailability is not affected by food. The half-life is 21 hours, with steady state reached in 4 days in patients with normal renal function. Topiramate is not extensively metabolized, and approximately 70% is eliminated unchanged in the urine. There is evidence of renal tubular reabsorption.

RECOMMENDED DOSAGE.   Start at 25 mg per day and then increase by 25 to 50 mg per week until clinical efficacy is achieved. Typical maintenance dosage is 400 to 600 mg per day, usually divided bid.

ADVERSE EFFECTS.   Side effects include the development of kidney stones (1.5%) due to carbonic anhydrase inhibition, somnolence, dizziness, ataxia, paresthesias, nervousness, abnormal vision, weight loss, and cognitive difficulties including difficulty with memory and concentration. In clinical trials, subjects lost an average of 1.7% to 7.2% of body weight depending on dosage. Weight loss peaked after 15 to 18 months of therapy, with partial return to pretreatment weight thereafter.

CLINICAL APPLICATIONS.   Topiramate is indicated for the prophylactic treatment of migraine headaches in adults. Controlled trials have also shown the drug to be effective in neuropathic pain resulting from spinal cord injuries as well as diabetic neuropathy.

(iv) Gabapentin

MECHANISM OF ACTION.   The mechanism of analgesic effect for this drug is not known. Although this drug's structure resembles that of the neurotransmitter γ-amino butyric acid (GABA), it does not interact with GABA receptors, inhibit GABA degradation, or convert into GABA. It is believed that gabapentin increases the total concentration of GABA in the brain, but the mechanism of this effect is unknown. In addition, this drug binds to a calcium channel subunit that may play a role in analgesia.

PHARMACOLOGY.   Gabapentin is not appreciably metabolized in humans. Its bioavailability is inversely proportional to dose, especially at low doses (e.g., 100 to 400 mg). At the recommended dosing schedule (300 to 600 mg tid), the differences in bioavailability are not significant (average approximately 60%). Food has no effect on the rate or extent of absorption. Gabapentin circulates largely unbound (<3% bound to plasma proteins). It is eliminated from the systemic circulation by renal excretion as unchanged drug. Elimination half-life is 5 to 7 hours and is unaltered by dose or following multiple doses. Plasma clearance is directly proportional to creatinine clearance.

RECOMMENDED DOSAGE.   Start with a 300-mg capsule at bedtime for 1 to 2 days. If the bedtime dose is tolerated, then tid dosing may be started. The dosage should be increased by 300-mg increments every 3 to 5 days until either pain relief or intolerable side effects are experienced. If maximal tid dosing (1,200 mg tid) does not provide relief, qid dosing is a reasonable next step. In fact, some experts suggest that qid dosing provides superior efficacy. Absorption of individual doses is dependent on gastrointestinal (GI) enzymes and absorption decreases abruptly at doses greater than 900 mg (excess gabapentin is eliminated in the stool). Dosing adjustments are required in subjects with renal impairment (noted in Table 2). Change in dosing is not required in hepatic insufficiency. When discontinuing the drug, it is recommended to taper gradually over at least 7 days.

ADVERSE EFFECTS. Somnolence, dizziness, ataxia, fatigue, inability to concentrate, GI disturbance, and nystagmus are the most commonly observed adverse events with gabapentin treatment. Pedal edema is listed in one study as occurring in only 1.7% of subjects, although practitioners report that it is often responsible for drug termination.

CLINICAL APPLICATIONS.   Because of its relatively benign side effect profile and lack of drug interactions, gabapentin is widely used for pain management, often as a first-line therapy. It has been available in the United States for the treatment of epilepsy since 1993, and in May 2002 the drug was approved for the treatment of postherpetic neuralgia (PHN). Other indications with proven efficacy are diabetic neuropathy, multiple sclerosis, and phantom limb pain.

(v) Lamotrigine

MECHANISM OF ACTION.   Lamotrigine is a phenyltriazine derivative that blocks voltage-dependent sodium channels and inhibits

Table 2.   Neurontin dosage based on renal function

Renal Function Creatinine Clearance (mL/min)	Total Daily Dose (mg/d)	Dosing Regimen (mg)				
≥60	900–3600	300 tid	400 tid	600 tid	800 tid	1200 tid
>30–59	400–1400	200 bid	300 bid	400 bid	500 bid	700 bid
>15–29	200–700	200 qd	300 qd	400 qd	500 qd	700 qd
<15[a]	100–300	100 qd	125 qd	150 qd	200 qd	300 qd
		Post-Hemodialysis Supplemental Dose (mg) [b]				
Hemodialysis —		125 [b]	150 [b]	200 [b]	250 [b]	350 [b]

[a]For patients with creatinine clearance <15mL/min, reduce daily dose in proportion to creatinine clearance (e.g., patients with a creatinine clearance of 7.5 mL/min should receive one-half the daily dose that patients with a creatinine clearance of 15 mL/min receive).

[b]Patients on hemodialysis should receive maintenance doses based on estimates of creatinine clearance as indicated in the upper portion of the table and a supplemental post-hemodialysis dose administered after each 4 hours of hemodialysis as indicated in the lower portion of the table.

The use of Neurontin in patients <12 years of age with compromised renal function has not been studied.

From Lori Murray, ed. *The Physicians' desk reference*. Montvale, NJ: Thomson, 2004:2563, with permission.

glutamate release from presynaptic neurons. It is also thought to modulate calcium and potassium currents. By inhibiting the pathologic release of glutamate, lamotrigine has the potential to be antinociceptive and to prevent the mechanisms responsible for the establishment of chronic pain.

PHARMACOLOGY.   Lamotrigine is rapidly and completely absorbed after oral administration, with negligible first-pass metabolism. The bioavailability is 98% and is not affected by food. Peak plasma concentrations occur from 1.4 to 5 hours after drug administration with a single-dose half-life of 24 hours. Lamotrigine is metabolized by the liver through glucuronic acid conjugation and, unlike gabapentin, there are significant drug–drug interactions with other anticonvulsants. Concurrent use of carbamazepine and lamotrigine increases carbamazepine levels and can produce toxicity. Used with valproic acid, the half-life of lamotrigine more than doubles, whereas the concentration of valproic acid decreases. The induction of hepatic glucuronidation from concurrent use of phenytoin or phenobarbital decreases the half-life of lamotrigine.

RECOMMENDED DOSAGE.   Starting dosages depend on other drugs being used concurrently, but standard recommendations suggest starting low, with a gradual dosage escalation to minimize side effects such as rash. The usual approach is to begin at 25 mg bid and then to increase by 25 mg per week until reaching 100 mg bid. After stabilization on this regimen for 7 days, the dosage may be further increased by 50 mg per week until the usual maintenance dosage of 300 to 400 mg per day, divided bid, is reached. Discontinuation should also be gradual, tapering the dosage over a minimum of 2 weeks.

ADVERSE EFFECTS.   Lamotrigine is generally well tolerated. Dizziness, nausea, headache, ataxia, diplopia, blurred vision, and somnolence are the most common side effects. The incidence of rash is approximately 9% to 10%, whereas the potential for developing a serious, life-threatening rash, including Stevens–Johnson syndrome, is estimated at 1% in pediatric patients (age less than 16 years) and 0.3% in adults. Patients must be instructed to watch for any skin changes and to discontinue the medication and contact their physician if a rash occurs.

CLINICAL APPLICATIONS.   Lamotrigine has been studied in both animals and humans with abundant evidence of effectiveness in pain control. At least ten randomized controlled trials (RCTs) have been published, seven showing efficacy and three not showing efficacy. Additionally, numerous published noncontrolled trials and case reports have examined the efficacy of lamotrigine on various types of pain and shown efficacy in complex regional pain syndromes (CRPS), TN, spinal cord injury, multiple sclerosis, and central poststroke pain.

(vi) Levetiracetam

MECHANISM OF ACTION.   Levetiracetam is a piracetam analog that reduces high-voltage N-type calcium currents, opposes the inhibition of GABA and glycine-gated currents, and affects potassium channel conductance.

PHARMACOLOGY.   Levetiracetam has almost complete bioavailability and is rapidly absorbed after oral administration. Its bioavailability is not affected by food. Peak plasma levels occur within 1 hour in healthy subjects and a steady state is established within 2 days of administration. The half-life is 7 to 8 hours in healthy volunteers and 10 to 11 hours in the older patients. Levetiracetam is predominately (95%) excreted in the urine. Most of the drug is excreted unchanged, with approximately 25% hydrolyzed to LO57, an acidic metabolite. Neither the drug nor its metabolite interacts with the P-450 isoenzymes or other common hepatic microsomal enzyme systems.

RECOMMENDED DOSAGE. Dosages of levetiracetam have ranged from 500 to 4,000 mg per day in reports. No recommendations exist for pain management. To treat seizures, the drug is initiated at 500 mg bid, with titration to the maximum recommended daily dosage of 3,000 mg by increments of 500 mg per week.

ADVERSE EFFECTS. The most common adverse events reports are somnolence, asthenia, and dizziness. Psychiatric abnormalities such as depression, nervousness, and emotional lability have been reported in a small number of patients, but these effects seem to be occurring in patients with epilepsy and not in patients taking the medication for other indications.

CLINICAL APPLICATIONS. Few studies have been done on levetiracetam and pain. Case reports and open-label trials have found it efficacious for migraine prophylaxis, postherpetic neuralgia, and generalized neuropathic pain. Animal models have shown the drug to be antihyperalgesic in neuropathic pain.

(vii) Pregabalin

MECHANISM OF ACTION. Pregabalin is a GABA analog, discovered during the search for other 3-substituted GABA compounds. It is the S-enantiomer of racemic 3-isobutyl GABA. The exact mechanism of action is presently unknown; however, it has been shown to displace radiolabeled gabapentin from its binding site. Both gabapentin and pregabalin increase neuronal GABA concentrations. Pregabalin produces a concentration-dependent increase in glutamic acid decarboxyase activity.

PHARMACOLOGY. Its pharmacologic profile is similar to that of gabapentin, with increased potency in experimental models of pain and seizure disorders. Pregabalin has an oral bioavailability of approximately 90% in healthy subjects. The half-life is approximately 5.8 hours and is not affected by food. The drug is not significantly metabolized, with 99% of it appearing in the urine unchanged.

DOSING. Dosing ranges from 150 to 600 mg per day, divided as bid or tid.

ADVERSE EFFECTS. Pregabalin is generally well tolerated. The most common adverse effects are CNS related and include dizziness, somnolence, and headache.

CLINICAL APPLICATIONS. Pregabalin was recently approved for the treatment of neuropathic pain associated with peripheral diabetic neuropathy and postherpetic neuralgia. Approval for fibromyalgia and generalized anxiety disorder may also be sought.

(viii) Zonisamide

MECHANISM OF ACTION. Zonisamide is a sulfonamide derivative structurally unrelated to other current or investigational AEDs. It has a broad spectrum of action, including blocking voltage-sensitive sodium channels, blocking voltage-dependent T-type calcium channels, facilitating serotoninergic and dopaminergic neurotransmission, blocking potassium-evoked glutamate response, and increasing GABA release from the hippocampus.

PHARMACOLOGY.   Zonisamide is rapidly absorbed and has an oral bioavailability of approximately 100%. Maximal plasma levels are reached within 2 to 6 hours after oral administration. Food delays the time to maximum concentration by 2 hours but does not affect the bioavailability. The mean half-life is 60 hours, so it takes approximately 2 weeks to reach steady state. Zonisamide is excreted primarily in the urine as parent drug and as the glucuronide of a metabolite. The plasma protein binding and concentration of zonisamide is not altered by other AEDs; however, enzyme-inducing AEDs, such as phenobarbital, phenytoin, and carbamazepine, can shorten the half-life of zonisamide by 50%.

DOSING.   Zonisamide is initially dosed at 100 mg per day. In patients who tend to be sensitive to medication side effects, the drug can be dosed at 100 mg on alternate days for the first week. After 2 weeks, the dosage may be increased to 200 mg per day for at least 2 weeks. It can be increased further to 300 mg per day and then to 400 mg per day, with the dosage being stable for at least 2 weeks to achieve steady state at each level. The usual maintenance dosage is 200 to 400 mg per day. Dosages of more than 400 mg have not been shown to be more efficacious but may result in increased weight loss.

ADVERSE EFFECTS.   The most common side effects are somnolence, ataxia, anorexia, difficulty in concentrating, agitation, and headache. The drug should not be prescribed to patients who are allergic to sulfonamides. Serious reactions such as Stevens–Johnson syndrome have occurred. Pediatric patients are at increased risk of developing oligohidrosis and hyperthermia.

CLINICAL APPLICATIONS.   There are few published studies examining zonisamide as an analgesic, but several have been conducted and have shown efficacy for treating various types of neuropathic pain and migraine headaches.

III. LOCAL ANESTHETICS

The use of local anesthetics as nerve-blocking agents—subcutaneous, along the nerve roots, or at the spinal cord—is well known. However, the use of systemic local anesthetics as adjuvant analgesics is not as common. Intravenous lidocaine has been found to be useful in the treatment of some neuropathic pain conditions, including continuous and lancinating dysesthesias. Some of the conditions include neuropathic pain due to herpes zoster, phantom limb pain, diabetic neuropathy, and various other pain complaints resulting from neuropathies.

The mechanism of pain relief appears to be the stabilization of nerve membranes. This occurs as a result of the blockade of sodium channels, which prevents the influx of sodium. The rapid influx of sodium is responsible for the initiation and propagation of depolorization in nerve fibers, which may in turn be perceived as pain.

A trial of intravenous lidocaine is often used to assess (in a timely manner) the efficacy of sodium channel blockade in a particular patient. Prior to the trial, a baseline electrocardiogram (ECG) and liver function tests should be performed. Intravenous lidocaine infusion has been found useful to predict successful relief from pain with subsequent use of mexiletine, an oral sodium channel blocker. The lidocaine infusion procedure involves administering 1 to 2 mg per kg of lidocaine (100 mg for most adults) intravenously over 10 to 15 minutes while the patient is adequately monitored. Verbal analog scores are obtained before, during, and after the test. Patients may experience tinnitus, perioral numbness, a metallic taste in the mouth, and dizziness during the trial. A 50% or greater reduction in pain warrants a trial of mexiletine or an antiepileptic with sodium channel blocking features such as oxcarbazepine or zonisamide.

Mexiletine (Mexitil) has a favorable side effect profile and is the most commonly used oral local anesthetic. Mexiletine is started at 150 mg at bedtime for approximately a week. If tolerated, the dosage is increased to 150 mg tid. If pain relief is inadequate, the dosage can be slowly escalated (every 5 to 7 days) to the maximum of 1,200 mg per day. This can result in remarkable pain relief in some patients. Possible adverse effects include arrhythmias, syncope, hypotension, ataxia, tremors, nervousness, upper GI distress, dizziness, hepatotoxicity, skin rash, visual changes, and fever/chills.

IV. CORTICOSTEROIDS

Coricosteroids are useful as adjuvant analgesics, either alone or in combination with opioids. The exact mechanism of action is not clear. A peripheral effect is apparently due to the reduction of inflammation, and a central effect may occur through altered neurotransmitter levels. In addition, corticosteroids are believed to reduce neuronal excitability by affecting cell membranes directly.

Steroids are used primarily in the management of pain due to rheumatic disease and cancer. They may reduce pain due to metastatic bone tumors, spinal cord compression, plexopathies, lymphedema, hepatomegaly, and some types of primary tumors. High dosages of steroids can be tried for 1 week. If a positive response is not observed, therapy should be terminated. If a therapeutic response is observed, therapy should be continued but should be tapered to the lowest dose that maintains the response. Prednisone (100 mg per day), methylprednisolone (100 mg per day), or prednisolone (7.5 mg per day) can be tried for 1 week and then tapered.

Steroid tapers (e.g., medrol dosepacks) are often useful in nonmalignant pain of acute onset (e.g., back pain) or for an exacerbation of a chronic pain state. The standard tapering of oral methylprednisolone is from 24 mg to 0 mg over a period of 7 days.

The numerous adverse effects of steroids are well known, ranging from osteoporosis and infections to gastric ulcerations, Cushing disease, and psychiatric symptoms. These are not first-line medications, and explicit risk–benefit analysis should precede their administration. As a general principle, steroids should not be used in combination with the nonsteriodal antiinflammatory drugs (NSAIDs).

V. ANTISPASMODICS

The two antispasmodic agents routinely used to treat chronic pain are baclofen (Lioresal) and cyclobenzaprine (Flexeril). Tizanidine (Zanaflex), an adjuvant analgesic often used in the treatment of sympathetically maintained pain, has a mechanism of action similar to that of clonidine.

1. Baclofen (Lioresal)

Baclofen is an antispasmodic drug that is often used in the treatment of spasticity associated with multiple sclerosis and spinal cord lesions. However, it is believed to possess some analgesic properties, which may augment opioid-induced analgesia. This apparently occurs through its GABA-B agonist actions. Lioresal appears to be useful in the treatment of painful spasticity, TN, and other forms of neuropathic pain, particularly lancinating pain. It should be avoided in patients with seizure disorders and impaired renal function.

Baclofen is usually started at 5 mg PO tid. Each dose can be increased by 5 mg every 3 days, to a maximum of 80 mg per day. It may also be administered intrathecally, and pump systems are sometimes implanted for continuous infusion therapy in selected patients. Common side effects include drowsiness, fatigue, vertigo, orthostatic hypotension, headaches, hypotonia, psychiatric disturbances, insomnia, slurred speech, ataxia, rash, urinary frequency, and GI distress. These can be avoided through slow titration and by avoidance of abrupt discontinuation.

2. Cyclobenzaprine (Flexeril)

Cyclobenzaprine relieves muscle spasm of local origin without interfering with muscle function. It is ineffective for muscle spasm due to CNS disease. It is indicated as an adjunct to rest and physical therapy for relief of muscle spasm associated with acute, painful musculoskeletal conditions. Relief of muscle spasm results in relief from pain, tenderness, movement limitation, and activity restriction. Cyclobenzatprine is closely related to the tricyclic antidepressants, and its side effect profile closely resembles that of the tricyclics. Common side effects are drowsiness, dry mouth, and dizziness. Tachycardia, hypertension, syncope, and GI upset have also been reported. Cyclobenzaprine should not be used with an MAOI (monoamine oxidase inhibitor). Other contraindications are similar to those of the tricyclics and include cardiac arrhythmias, hyperthyroidism, and urinary obstruction. The usual dosage is 10 mg tid, with a range of 20 to 40 mg per day in divided doses.

3. Tizanidine (Zanaflex)

Tizanidine is an α_2-agonist that decreases sympathetic transmission at the level of the dorsal horn. Its antispasmodic action is attributed to reduced facilitation of the spinal motor neurons. Following oral administration, it is completely absorbed. Its half-life is approximately 2.5 hours, and its duration of action is short (3 to 5 hours). It is indicated for sympathetically maintained pain, as well as for pain described as "lancinating, electrical, or burning." Adverse effects most commonly seen with use of Tizanidine include dry mouth, sedation, asthenia (i.e., weakness, fatigue, and/or tiredness), and dizziness. Dosage is started at 2 mg qhs and is gradually titrated to as high as 8 mg q6h to q8h as tolerated.

4. Others

Methocarbamol (Robaxin) and metaxalone (Skelaxin) are two other centrally acting skeletal muscle relaxants that are effective in treating musculoskeletal pain and muscle spasms. Both should be used with caution in patients who have severe renal or hepatic impairment. Methocarbamol is contraindicated in epilepsy. It is dosed 750 mg q4h or 1,500 mg tid. It is also available in parental form. Metaxalone is dosed 800 mg q6h to q8h. Results of the liver function tests should be monitored when this medication is used long-term.

VI. CLONIDINE

Clonidine stimulates α-adrenoreceptors in the brainstem, thereby decreasing sympathetic outflow from the CNS, with a resultant decrease in peripheral resistance, heart rate, and blood pressure. Its unique mechanism of action explains why it is the only transdermal/oral agent that employs the mechanistic treatment approach for sympathetically maintained pain. The transdermal patch (Catapres TTS) is the preferred mode of administration because it produces more consistent blood levels. Dosing of the patch starts with one TTS-1 and can increase to a maximum of two TTS-3 patches applied every 7 days. The patch should be applied every 7 days to a hairless area of the intact skin of the upper arm or chest. Subsequent patches should be applied to a different site to prevent skin irritation. Most common adverse events include dry mouth, drowsiness, fatigue, headache, lethargy, and sedation. Dizziness is not uncommon, especially in those with low baseline blood pressures.

VII. TOPICAL AGENTS

Disorders that are responsive to topical therapy include CRPS and peripheral polyneuropathy. PHN is a chronic pain syndrome that is ideally suited to treatment with topical agents for several reasons. Most patients with PHN have clearly demarcated areas of affected skin, with modest amounts of a topical preparation providing relief from pain, accompanied by few side effects. Three categories of topical agents have received the most attention: capsaicin preparations, local anesthetics, and NSAID preparations. All three categories have been demonstrated in controlled trials to be effective analgesics in subjects with PHN, but the most popular of these is the lidocaine transdermal patch (Lidoderm). Although developed for PHN, the lidocaine patch is used for a wide variety of pain conditions, including peripheral neuropathy and myofascial pain with good results. Up to three patches per day may be used. The patches are intended to be applied for 12 hours at a time, allowing the skin to then breathe for 12 hours before applying new patches.

Although controlled studies have not verified the effectiveness of such topical compounds, many drugs are being mixed into creams and ointments (e.g., ketoprofen 100 mg per mL + bupivicaine 50 mg per mL + ketamine 50 mg per mL) by pharmacies for the treatment of superficial pain. Combining agents with different mechanisms of action may increase the benefit. Use of these agents requires caution: too frequent use over too large an area can result in toxicity.

VIII. CONCLUSION

The adjuvant analgesics include a great number of drugs with various mechanisms of action. As the name implies, they were originally used as "add-on" therapy, in combination with an opioid or an antiinflammatory agent. Presently, they are often the first choice for analgesic therapy. Although studies show little progress in matching the mechanism of action of the drug to pain pathophysiology, there is anecdotal evidence of some success. For instance, although neuropathic pain appears to be resistant to pharmacologic treatment in general, certain drugs (e.g., sodium channel blockers) do seem to be effective. Randomized controlled trials provide us with the best evidence available to determine treatment strategy. Our treatment approach aims to be based on scientific evidence; yet each patient and disease is unique, therefore, our treatment must be adjusted to each individual clinical situation. This is just one of the challenges we face when treating patients with chronic pain.

SELECTED READINGS

Benedetti C, Butler SH. Systemic analgesics. In: Bonica JJ, ed. *The management of pain*, Vol 2. Philadelphia, PA: Lea & Febinger, 1990; 1640–1675.

Galer BS, Harle J, Rowbotham MC. Response to intravenous lidocaine infusion predicts subsequent responses to oral mexilitine: a prospective study. *J Pain Symptom Manage* 1996;12(3):161–167.

Max MB. Is mechanism-based pain treatment attainable? Clinical trial issues. *J Pain* 2000;(3 Suppl. 1):2–9.

McQuay H, Carroll D, Jadad AR, et al. Anticonvulsant drugs for management of pain: a systematic review. *Br Med J* 1995;311(7012): 1047–1052.

Munglani R, Hill RG. Other drugs including sympathetic blockers. In: Wall PD, Melzack R, eds. *Textbook of pain*, 4th ed. New York: Churchill-Livingstone, 1999;1233–1250.

Woolf CJ, Decosterd I. Implications of recent advances in the understanding of pain pathophysiology for the assessment of pain in patients. *Pain* 1999;82:1–7.

Psychopharmacology for the Pain Specialist

Daniel M. Rockers and Karla Hayes

It was a most repugnant undertaking to have to treat a group of complaints which, as all authors are agreed, are typified by instability, irregularity, fantasy, unpredictability—complaints which are governed by no law or rule, and whose diverse manifestations are connected to no serious theoretical formulation.
—Paul Briquet in "Traité clinique et thérapeutique de l'hystérie"

Knowledge of psychopharmacology is important for a pain practitioner because of the substantial overlap of psychiatric diagnoses with chronic pain conditions as well as the common psychopharmacologic medication groups used as analgesics. Many of these agents have multiple mechanisms of action, accounting for their dual effects. In this chapter, psychotropic medications and their role in pain treatment are reviewed. Because of the high comorbidity of depression and pain, antidepressants—the largest category—are covered first. Next, medications that directly affect cognitive functioning—antipsychotics or neuroleptics—are reviewed. Mood stabilizers, used to treat bipolar disorder and derivative conditions, are next, followed by anxiolytics and psychostimulants.

I. ANTIDEPRESSANTS

In many chronic pain cases, a patient either will be prescribed an antidepressant or will already be taking one. Antidepressants often serve a dual role: treating a mood disorder and independently addressing pain symptoms.

The earliest forms of currently used antidepressants were tricyclic antidepressants (TCAs) and monoamine oxidase inhibitors (MAOIs), each with inhibitory actions on norepinephrine (NE) and serotonin (5HT) reuptake. These antidepressants were the drugs of choice for treating depression until the 1980s, when the selective

serotonin reuptake inhibitors (SSRIs) were found to possess substantial antidepressant efficacy. SSRIs have revolutionized treatment of depression by offering efficacy with greatly reduced side
effect profiles. Over the past decade, numerous atypical antidepressants have been developed, including norepinephrine and dopamine
reuptake inhibitors (NDRIs), serotonin–norepinephrine reuptake
inhibitors (SNRIs), and serotonin-2 antagonist/reuptake inhibitors
(SARIs). These newer agents are currently undergoing clinical trials
to assess relative efficacy compared with standard TCAs and SSRIs.
When first reported as having analgesic activity, antidepressants
were thought to work by relieving the depression component of pain.
Although it is well known that relieving depression by any method
is likely to decrease pain, some antidepressants appear to have
analgesic properties of their own. A third mechanism to consider is
the potentiation or enhancement of opioid analgesia by modulating
serotonergic, noradrenergic, and cholinergic effects.

1. Cyclic Antidepressants

(i) Indications

TCAs are approved by the U.S. Food and Drug Administration
(FDA) for the treatment of major depressive disorders and secondary depression in other disorders. In treating chronic pain, they
are considered to have independent analgesic effects. Reasonable
goals for using TCAs as analgesics include decreasing pain intensity from unbearable to bearable. Some mild side effects may be
unavoidable in exchange for analgesia.

(ii) Mechanisms

All TCAs inhibit both serotonergic and noradrenergic reuptake to varying degrees. The tertiary amines have a broader
spectrum of activity than the secondary amines. The time course
of TCA analgesia varies between 1 and 120 days, suggesting that
initial early analgesia is maximized over time. Duration of TCA
analgesia also persists over time with maintenance of therapy.

(iii) Adverse Effects

Unfortunately, the TCAs interact with multiple neurotransmitter systems and, as a result, have a wide side effect profile,
including anticholinergic (constipation and dry mouth) and
cardiovascular (hypotension and tachycardia) effects. Other effects include sedation, weight gain, and sexual dysfunction.
Amitriptyline and the other tertiary amines have more side effects than nortriptyline and the other secondary amines.
Caution is advised when prescribing this class of medications
to the older patients (because of potential orthostasis leading to
falls), patients with closed-angle glaucoma, those with heart
block, arrhythmia, or recent myocardial infarction (TCAs are
antiarrhythmic, decrease contractility, and increase conduction
delays), or patients with suicidal ideation (TCAs can be fatal if
overdosed). TCA overdose is a leading cause of drug-related
overdose and death. Three to five times the therapeutic dose
of TCAs is potentially lethal; this low therapeutic index (ratio
of toxic to therapeutic dose) must make prescribers vigilant.

The low therapeutic index of TCAs is probably a large part of the reason that SSRIs are often chosen as first-line antidepressants over TCAs.

Combining TCAs with opioids can lead to decreased intestinal motility, already a problem for many patients taking opioids. Additive anticholinergic and opioid effects on the bowels can lead to treatment-resistant constipation or ileus.

(iv) Dosages and Monitoring

As a general principle, dosing should start at the low end of the dosage range and should be titrated upward in 10- to 25-mg weekly increments until a therapeutic level is reached. This dosing will minimize side effects, and patients will be less likely to reject the therapy because of side effects (see Table 1 for dosages).

2. Monoamine Oxidase Inhibitors

MAOIs (see Table 2) are rarely used anymore because of their potentially serious side effects. They are still prescribed by some psychiatrists to treat patients who have not responded to the other classes of antidepressants. Physicians who do not have training in psychiatry are advised to avoid this class of medications. Phenelzine has been shown to have adjuvant analgesic properties in patients with chronic fatigue syndrome, atypical facial pain, and migraines.

3. Selective Serotonin Reuptake Inhibitors

(i) Indications

Since the introduction of fluoxetine (Prozac) in 1987, several other SSRIs have been introduced and have revolutionized first-line therapy for depression (see Table 3). Although SSRIs initially were introduced for use in major depressive disorder, the US FDA has approved other indications for these agents, including anxiety disorders, bulimia nervosa, and obsessive compulsive disorder. In addition, SSRIs are often used by clinicians for a variety of other conditions including premenstrual syndrome, chronic fatigue syndrome, intermittent explosive disorder, and chronic pain management.

(ii) Mechanisms

The immediate effect of the SSRIs on the central nervous system (CNS) is blockade of the presynaptic serotonin reuptake pump. There have not been many studies examining the efficacy of SSRIs as analgesics. Of 20 studies examining the effect of SSRIs on pain, 12 found that SSRIs provided clinically important pain relief. When SSRIs were compared to TCAs, the latter were shown superior as analgesics in four out of six trials.

(iii) Adverse Reactions

Although SSRIs have fewer side effects than the older antidepressants, they may still cause some undesirable symptoms. Possible CNS effects include headaches, stimulation or sedation, fine tremor, and akathisia. Gastrointestinal effects include nausea, vomiting, anorexia, bloating, and diarrhea. The limited sedation associated with these agents makes them ideal for patients

Table 1. Tricyclic antidepressants

Medication	Proprietary Name	Dosage Range (mg/dl)	Anticholinergic Activity	Central Action	Hypotension	Sedation
Tertiary amines						
Imipramine	*Tofranil*	10–300	Moderate	N/S	Moderate	Moderate
Amitriptyline[a]	*Elavil*	10–300	Strong	S(N)	Strong	Strong
Clomipramine	*Anafranil*	25–300	Moderate	S(N)	Strong	Mild
Doxepin	*Sinequan*	10–300	Moderate	S	Strong	Mild
Secondary amines						
Desipramine[a]	*Norpramin*	10–300	Minimal	N	Mild	Minimal
Nortriptyline[a]	*Pamelor*	10–200	Mild	N/S	Moderate	Mild
Protriptyline	*Vivactil*	10–60	Moderate	N	Minimal	Mild
Amoxapine	*Asendin*	50–400	Minimal	N	Mild	Minimal

S, serotonergic; N, norepinephrinergic; (N), weakly norepinephrinergic quantitative sensory testing.
[a]Commonly used for neuropathic pain.

Table 2. **Monoamine oxidase inhibitors**

Medication	Proprietary Name	Dosage Range (mg/d)
Isocarboxazid	*Marplan*	30–50
Phenelzine	*Nardil*	45–90
Tranylcypromine	*Parnate*	20–60

with pain on sedating analgesics. Other serotonergic drugs should be avoided or used with caution given the possibility of causing serotonergic syndrome. Approximately 10% to 15% of patients taking an SSRI will experience sexual side effects of decreased libido, impotence, ejaculatory disturbances, and anorgasmia.

(iv) Dosages and Monitoring

No initial laboratory workup is required. Dosage titration is usually based on clinical response and side effects. Note that beneficial effects are usually not seen before 2 to 3 weeks. When discontinuing SSRIs, taper dosages slowly to avoid withdrawal symptoms.

4. Atypical Antidepressants

Other classes of antidepressants have been developed to target specific neurotransmitter interactions at the synaptic level (see Table 4). These classes of antidepressants maximize therapeutic benefits while minimizing side effects. NDRIs such as bupropion (Wellbutrin), SNRIs such as venlafaxine (Effexor) and duloxetine (Cymbalta), norepinephrine antagonist/serotonin antagonist (NASAs) such as mirtazapine (Remeron), and SARIs, represented by trazodone (Desyrel), are included in these classes (see Table 4 for dosages).

Bupropion (Wellbutrin), an NDRI, is metabolized to hydroxy-bupropion, a powerful inhibitor of both noradrenergic and dopaminergic pumps. This agent differs from most other antidepressants in that it has psychostimulant properties. There have been no controlled clinical trials of its efficacy in the treatment of chronic pain; however, its stimulating properties offer advantages in treating depression in patients on sedating drugs such as opioids.

Table 3. **Selective serotonin reuptake inhibitors**

Medication	Proprietary Name	Dosage Range (mg/d)
Fluoxetine	*Prozac*	10–80
Fluvoxamine	*Luvox*	50–300
Paroxetine	*Paxil*	10–50
Sertraline	*Zoloft*	50–200
Citalopram	*Celexa*	20–60
Escitalopram	*Lexapro*	10–40

Table 4.   Atypical antidepressants

Medication	Propietary Name	Dosage Range (mg/d)
Trazodone	*Desyrel*	50–200 (qhs)
Bupropion	*Wellbutrin*	150–400
Mirtazapine	*Remeron*	15–45
Venlafaxine	*Effexor*	150–450
Duloxetine	*Cymbalta*	30–60

Bupropion comes in a short-acting form, which is taken three times a day; sustained release, which is normally taken twice a day; and a new, extended-release, once-daily form. The typical maintenance dosage is 300 mg per day. Seizures occur in approximately 0.4% of patients at dosages of less than 450 mg per day, and in 4% of patients when dosages range from 450 to 600 mg per day. Therefore, dosages exceeding 450 mg per day should be avoided. Bupropion should also be avoided in patients with a seizure or eating disorder or in patients taking medications that may lower the seizure threshold. The most common adverse effects are headache, insomnia, upper respiratory complaints, nausea, restlessness, agitation, and irritability. Patients have survived overdoses as high as 4,200 mg.

Venlafaxine is an SNRI with some anecdotal evidence of efficacy in the treatment of chronic pain. Potential analgesia is suggested by its profile of dual inhibition of serotonin and norepinephrine reuptake that is similar to proven analgesic antidepressants such as imipramine, amitriptyline, and desipramine. Venlafaxine differs from these agents in its lack of anticholinergic, antiadrenergic, and antihistiminergic side effects, a difference that has unknown bearing on analgesia.

Venlafaxine is available in extended-release form, which is prescribed more widely than the older, short-acting version. The dosing usually starts at 37.5 to 75 mg and is slowly titrated to 225 to 450 mg per day, given once daily if using the XR form. Side effects include nausea, headache, somnolence, dry mouth, dizziness, nervousness, constipation, anxiety, anorexia, blurred vision, and sexual dysfunction. No reports of fatal overdose have been reported. Venlafaxine should not be used in conjunction with MAOIs, and it may affect hepatic metabolism of other medications.

Duloxetine is an SNRI and the latest antidepressant. It is the only antidepressant that is being marketed for patients who suffer from both depression and pain. There have been several randomized clinical trials that have shown that duloxetine is effective in treating both depression and pain in depressed patients. Dosing is recommended at 60 mg per day.

Trazodone is an SARI by virtue of blocking serotonin-2 receptors as well as serotonin reuptake. This agent was first marketed as an antidepressant, but it is used primarily for insomnia now, because of its sedating effect. Its usefulness in the treatment of chronic pain is undetermined but, given the incidence of insomnia in pain patients, Trazodone may offer at least an adjuvant role. Serzone, another SARI, was recently taken off the market owing to concerns about liver toxicity.

Dosages should begin as low as 25 mg given at bedtime, but can be increased to as high as 200 to 400 mg. Side effects include sedation, orthostatic hypotension, dizziness, headache, nausea, dry mouth, and gastrointestinal upset. There are no anticholinergic effects of SARIs. Rare cases of cardiac arrhythmias have been reported. An infrequent but serious side effect is priapism (occurring in 1/1,000 to 1/10,000 men), and patients should be warned of this before starting treatment. There have been no reported cases of death following overdose with SARIs taken alone. SARIs should not be used in conjunction with MAOIs. Also, the use of SARIs with astemizole or terfenadine may decrease hepatic P450 metabolism of these compounds, resulting in cardiac arrhythmias. Finally, SARIs may increase serum levels of triazolam (Halcion) and alprazolam (Xanax).

II. ANTIPSYCHOTICS

Indications

Antipsychotics are used to treat schizophrenia as well as psychotic symptoms associated with mood disorders and delirium. They also are commonly used to treat anxiety, insomnia, and agitation associated with dementia and personality disorders.

Antipsychotics are also known as neuroleptics because of the often-irreversible side effects seen with the older, typical agents. This class of medications has been used for more than 30 years as a part of analgesic regimens despite conflicting data. Phenothiazines such as chlorpromazine and prochlorperazine have been used for the treatment of migraine and nonmigraine headaches. Haloperidol and methotrimeprazine have been used for various malignant and nonmalignant pain conditions. Haloperidol, the most widely used typical antipsychotic, shows isomorphic similarity to meperidine and morphine. It is the only antipsychotic available in intravenous form. Thus, it is used quite frequently in the inpatient setting. Clinical studies and many case reports suggest that neuroleptics, including fluphenazine and haloperidol, might be useful in neuropathic pain, or when overwhelming suffering or distress accompanies pain. Neuroleptics are the drugs of choice for treating delirium, which is a common complication seen in cancer pain and in postoperative patients. Anxiety, cognitive impairment, insomnia, and agitation are symptoms of delirium, which can make treatment more complicated. Anxiety and cognitive impairment can interfere with obtaining an accurate pain assessment from the patient and can limit the safe escalation of opioid dosing. Neuroleptics may play a role as adjuvant analgesics in this group of patients. Although the data on this group of medications is limited, it is thought that the anxiolytic or sedating effects do not explain the analgesic effects that have been observed. The atypical neuroleptics, especially quetiapine and olanzapine, are being used to treat insomnia in patients who do not necessarily carry a primary psychiatric diagnosis.

1. Typical Neuroleptics

(i) Mechanisms

Typical neuroleptics (see Table 5) function as antipsychotics because of their dopaminergic antagonism, particularly at

Table 5.   Typical neuroleptics

Medication	Proprietary Name
Phenothiazine	
Aliphatic	
Chlorpromazine	*Thorazine*
Piperidine	
Mesoridazine	*Senentil*
Thioridazine	*Mellaril*
Piperazine	
Fluphenazine	*Prolixin*
Perphenazine	*Trilafon*
Trifluoperazine	*Stelazine*
Thioxanthenes	
Thiothixene	*Navane*
Butyrophenone	
Haloperidol	*Haldol*
Diphenylbutylpiperidines	
Pimozide	*Orap*
Dibenzoxazepine	
Loxapine	*Daxolin, Loxitane*
Dihydroindolone	
Molindone	*Moban*

postsynaptic D2 receptors, probably in pathways from the midbrain to the limbic system—temporal and frontal lobes. Typical neuroleptics also may affect cholinergic, α_1-adrenergic, and histaminic systems. These actions are responsible for many of the numerous and serious side effects of typical neuroleptics.

(ii) Adverse Reactions

Antipsychotics carry a risk of extrapyramidal symptoms, including acute dystonia, akathisia, pseudoparkinsonism, and tardive dyskinesia; those antipsychotics with the least anticholinergic effects have the greatest risk. Neuroleptics also have effects on numerous hormonal systems. Prolactin levels may be elevated by neuroleptics, with possible effects including amenorrhea, galactorrhea, and false-positive pregnancy tests in women and gynecomastia and galactorrhea in men. Neuroleptics may cause hypothalamic dysfunction [leading to syndrome of inappropriate antidiuretic hormone (SIADH) and temperature regulation difficulties] or may disrupt serum glucose levels. Neuroleptic malignant syndrome is a particularly serious, albeit rare, potential adverse event.

Anticholinergic activity may cause dry membranes, blurred vision, constipation, urinary retention, and confusion or delirium. Histaminic effects include sedation, cognitive impairment, and weight gain. A combination of dopaminergic, anticholinergic, and α_1 adrenergic effects may cause sexual dysfunction. In addition, neuroleptics may lower the seizure threshold. This effect is seen most in lower-potency agents such as chlorpromazine and least in high-potency agents such as haloperidol. Cardiovascular effects include hypotension, tachycardia, dizziness, fainting, nonspecific electrocardiogram (ECG) changes,

Table 6. Atypical neuroleptics

Medication	Proprietary Name	Dosage Range
Risperidone	*Risperdal*	1–6 mg/d
Clozapine	*Clozaril*	300–900 mg/d
Olanzapine	*Zyprexa*	5–30 mg/d
Ouetiapine	*Seroquel*	100–600 mg/d
Aripiprazole	*Abilify*	10–30 mg/d
Ziprasidone	*Geodon*	20–80 mg bid

and, rarely, arrhythmias including "torsades de pointes," and sudden cardiac death.

2. Atypical Neuroleptics

(i) Mechanisms

Atypical neuroleptics include the agents risperidone (Risperdal), clozapine (Clozaril), quetiapine (Seroquel), aripiprazole (Abilify), ziprasidone (Geodon), and olanzapine (Zyprexa) (Table 6). These agents are D2 antagonists, but to a lesser degree than typical neuroleptics. Additionally, they appear to block serotonin-2 receptors and to variable degrees the D4 receptor. Atypical neuroleptics may be more efficacious than typical neuroleptics, particularly with negative psychotic symptoms. However, no controlled studies of the use of atypical neuroleptics in the treatment of chronic pain have been conducted. Olanzapine was shown to decrease pain in a prospective trial of eight patients with cancer with anxiety and mild cognitive impairment. One advantage of atypical neuroleptics over typical neuroleptics is the lower incidence of extrapyramidal side effects.

(ii) Adverse Effects

Clozapine is considered a second-line therapy for patients because of the possibility of fatal agranulocytosis in about 1% of patients exposed to the drug. Olanzapine is similar in structure and mechanism to clozapine but does not carry the risk of leukopenia. Olanzapine has a low drug interaction potential and a reduced incidence of extrapyramidal side effects. Side effects of the atypicals vary depending on the particular agent but, in general, practitioners should monitor for sedation, weight gain, dizziness, and insulin resistance. Quetiapine is thought to carry the least risk of extrapyramidal symptoms.

(iii) Dosages and Monitoring

No routine laboratory tests are necessary for prescribing the antipsychotic agents. Be aware of the emergence of extrapyramidal side effects—and warn patients about potential tardive dyskinesia.

III. MOOD STABILIZERS

(i) Indications

Mood stabilizers are used to treat bipolar disorder, which involves alternating periods and degrees of mania and depression. Lithium is the classic agent for treating bipolar disorder. In recent years, anticonvulsants such as valproic acid, carbamazepine, and lamotrigine have taken a prominent role alongside lithium in the treatment of bipolar disorder. The overlap of this group of drugs with those used to treat neuropathic pain is striking, but the meaning has not yet been clarified.

Although bipolar disorder is not overly common in the patient with chronic pain, it does occur and can be worsened by medications that are often used to treat pain, such as antidepressants and opioids. Analgesic agents that may provoke mania include antidepressants as well as steroids. However, several agents that are specifically effective against neuropathic pain also are helpful in treating bipolar disorder (e.g., carbamazepine and gabapentin) and are thus obvious choices for the treatment of comorbid bipolar disorder and chronic pain.

(ii) Lithium

Lithium has been used extensively for treatment of migraine and cluster headaches. However, there is no evidence of efficacy in the treatment of any other type of chronic pain. Lithium remains one of the most commonly used agents for treating bipolar disorder; however, the narrow therapeutic index and negative side effects profile has led to a decrease in its use over the past five years, especially as newer medications have proven efficacious.

(iii) Anticonvulsants

Anticonvulsants are the most commonly used type of medications for neuropathic pain. They are discussed in more detail in Chapter 10. This same group of drugs is being used more widely in treating psychiatric disorders, including impulse-control disorders and behavioral disturbances associated with dementia and personality disorders.

(iv) Mechanisms

The mechanisms of action of this diverse group are understandably varied, but all are thought to act as membrane stabilizers. Phenytoin and carbamazepine slow the rate of recovery of voltage-activated Na^+ channels from inactivity. Clonazepam stimulates GABAergic pathways. Valproic acid is believed to increase GABA concentrations in the brain, whereas gabapentin's action is unknown—although it functions as a GABA analog, it does not act at GABA receptors. The action of lithium's therapeutic effects is unknown but is postulated to be endocrine, neurotransmissive, circadian, or cellular. Lithium is not a sedative, depressant, or euphoriant. Possible side effects include blood dyscrasias (although they are less common than with carbamazepine) and hepatitis.

IV. ANXIOLYTICS

Anxiety disorders may occur in a large percentage of patients with chronic pain. These disorders include panic disorder, generalized anxiety disorder, obsessive compulsive disorder, and posttraumatic stress disorder. These disorders often present with somatic symptoms including chest pain, gastrointestinal disturbances, and neurologic symptoms (i.e., headache, dizziness, syncope, and paresthesias). Treatment of chronic pain that is comorbid with an anxiety disorder should include anxiolysis as part of the analgesic strategy.

1. Benzodiazepines

Benzodiazepines are the most popular medication for anxiety and, in fact, are the most widely prescribed medication of any type. Clonazepam is considered both a psychotropic agent (anxiolytic) and a neurologic agent (anticonvulsant). This advantage suggests its possible usefulness in the pain clinic pharmacologic armamentarium.

(i) Indications

Benzodiazepines are approved for treatment of anxiety disorders, alcohol withdrawal seizures, and insomnia. They also have been used to treat akathisia, agitation (including mania), depression, catatonia, and muscle spasm.

(ii) Mechanisms

Benzodiazepines depress the CNS at the levels of the limbic system, brain stem reticular activating formation, and cortex by binding to and facilitating the action of GABA. Although not primary analgesics, benzodiazepines often have a role in the analgesic regimen.

(iii) Adverse Reactions

The most common side effects of benzodiazepines are sedation and respiratory depression. Rapid withdrawal from benzodiazepines can result in rebound insomnia, anxiety, delirium, or withdrawal. Severe withdrawal reactions include seizures, psychosis, and death. Dosages should be discontinued by gradual taper.

(iv) Dosages and Monitoring

As with any medication for which tolerance develops, dose ranges tend to be open-ended. In overdose, benzodiazepines are rarely fatal if taken alone, although they may cause respiratory depression. If taken with alcohol or barbiturates, however, benzodiazepines can be fatal, with symptoms including hypotension, depressed respiration, and coma. The choice of a specific benzodiazepine is often based on onset of action and half-life. In general, short-acting agents are used to treat insomnia and acute anxiety, whereas long-acting agents are used to treat chronic conditions. See Table 7 for half-lives.

2. Buspirone (Buspar)

Although not known to be efficacious for the treatment of pain, buspirone can be an effective anxiolytic. Buspirone acts as a 5-HT1A agonist. Buspirone may potentiate the antidepressant and antiobsessional effects of SSRIs and is also being studied for use in posttraumatic stress disorder. No laboratory studies are required before initiating treatment with buspirone. Patients may take 5 to 30 mg per day in divided doses, starting at 5 mg tid and increasing to as high as 10 mg tid. It requires 1 to 4 weeks for anxiolytic effects to appear. Buspirone has relatively few side effects; less than 10% of patients taking buspirone experience headache, dizziness, lightheadedness, fatigue, parasthesias, and gastrointestinal disturbance. Buspirone has a low potential for abuse or addiction and it does not impair psychomotor or cognitive functions. There have been no reports of withdrawal symptoms

Table 7.   Benzodiazepines onset and half-life

Medication	Proprietary Name	Onset	Half-life (hr)
Alprazolam	*Xanax*	Intermediate	6–20
Chlordiazepoxide	*Librium*	Intermediate	30–100
Clonazepam	*Klonopin*	Intermediate	18–50
Clorazepate	*Tranxene*	Rapid	30–100
Diazepam	*Valium*	Rapid	30–100
Eestazolam	*Prosom*	Intermediate	10–24
Flurazepam	*Dalmane*	Rapid-intermediate	50–160
Lorazepam	*Ativan*	Intermediate	10–20
Midazolam	*Versed*	Intermediate	2–3
Oxazepam	*Serax*	Intermediate-slow	8–12
Quazepam	*Doral*	Rapid-intermediate	50–160
Temazepam	*Restoril*	Intermediate	8–20
Triazolam	*Halcion*	Intermediate	1.5–5

or death from overdose. However, buspirone should be used with caution in patients taking MAOIs because this combination may result in elevated blood pressure. Also, buspirone inhibits the metabolism of benzodiazepines and haloperidol.

V. PSYCHOSTIMULANTS

(i) Indications

Although approved indications for psychostimulants include attention deficit disorder, Parkinson disease, and narcolepsy, they are also used for treatment-resistant depression, to augment antidepressants, and in the treatment of sedation or fatigue in terminal illness. Psychostimulants are the only immediate-acting "antidepressants." Although they have been used as so-called diet pills, psychostimulants can improve appetite in cancer treatment. Additionally, psychostimulants are used to counter iatrogenic sedation, most commonly caused by opioid analgesics. Common psychostimulants include dextroamphetamine, methylphenidate, and magnesium pemoline. Modafinil (Provigil) will be included in this category, although it is technically not a psychostimulant. It is a Schedule IV medication rather than Schedule II like the other medications in this group. Modafinil is approved by the U.S. FDA for excessive daytime sleepiness associated with narcolepsy, sleep apnea, or shift-work sleep disorder. It has been shown to be effective in improving opioid-induced sedation in patients treated for nonmalignant pain and in lessening fatigue associated with multiple sclerosis, fibromyalgia, and depression.

(ii) Mechanisms

At normal dosages, amphetamines stimulate the release of norepinephrine. As the dosage increases, amphetamines cause the release of dopamine, which accounts for the behavioral changes and the reinforcing properties. At excessive dosages, amphetamines cause the release of serotonin, which may be associated with the amphetamine psychosis. Methylphenidate blocks the reuptake of dopamine. Magnesium pemoline exhibits effects similar to amphetamines and methylphenidate. The stimulant effects appear to be mediated through dopaminergic mechanisms; however, there are also weak sympathomimetic effects. The exact mechanism of action of modafinil is unclear, but, unlike stimulants, which promote wakefulness by widespread CNS stimulation, modafinil works in selective hypothalamic areas.

(iii) Adverse Reactions

The risk factors include hypertension, tachyarrythmias, and anxiety. Liver disease is a contraindication (pemoline is not used as a first-line treatment because of reports of late-onset hepatotoxicity), as is functional psychosis, anxiety, and anorexia. The incidence of tic in patients with Tourette syndrome is 20% to 50%. Other adverse effects commonly seen include anorexia, irritation, sadness, and clingy behavior. Modafinil can cause headaches, nausea, and nervousness.

(iv) Dosages and Monitoring

Psychostimulants should be used cautiously in patients with existing drug or alcohol abuse problems. The medication should be started at a low dosage and then be increased gradually over several days. Because of the short half-life, methylphenidate must be dosed bid. Patients should not stop taking the drug abruptly. Methylphenidate is available in extended-release forms (see Table 8 for dosages).

Table 8. Psychostimulants, dosage, and cautions

Generic Name	Proprietary Name	Dosage	Cautions
Dextroamphetamine	Dexedrine, Dextrostat	5–60 mg/d	Abuse potential
Methylphenidate	Ritalin	10–30 mg/d	Same abuse potential as amphetamines Tourette syndrome is a contraindication
Magnesium pemoline	Cylert	37.5–112.5 mg/d; dose dependent on age	Long half-life (9–14 hr) means once-a-day dosing is possible Not used as first-line because of association with hepatotoxicity
Modafinil	Provigil	200 mg/d	Less abuse potential

VI. CONCLUSION

Psychopharmacologic agents can play an important role in the management of chronic pain and associated symptoms. These agents can reduce opioid requirements, address aspects of pain that opioids do not usually treat, and improve symptoms that may be side effects of opioid therapy. Without adequate familiarity of psychopharmacologic agents, the pain specialist risks limiting her or his analgesic repertoire: he or she may overlook potentially beneficial possibilities as well as potential adverse complications of polypharmacy. The ongoing revolution in development of psychoactive drugs surely will impact pain management, and these drugs are likely to gain increased prominence in the arsenal against pain.

SELECTED READINGS

Bezchlibnyk-Butler KZ, Jefferies JJ, Martin BA. *Clinical handbook of psychotropic drugs*, 4th ed. Seattle, WA: Hogrefe and Huber Publishers, 1994.

Breitbart W. Psychotropic adjuvant analgesics for pain in cancer and aids. *Psychooncology* 1998;7:333–345.

Bloom FE, Kupfer DJ, eds. *Psychopharmacology: the fourth generation of progress*. New York: Raven Press, 1995.

Ciraulo DA, Shader RI, Greenblatt DJ, et al., eds. *Drug interactions in psychiatry*, 2nd ed. Philadelphia, PA: Williams & Wilkins, 1995.

Guze B, Richeimer S, Szuba M. *The psychiatric drug handbook*. Boston, MA: Mosby–Year Book, 1995.

Hyman SE, Arana GW, Rosenbaum JF. *Handbook of psychiatric drug therapy*, 3rd ed. Boston, MA: Little, Brown and Company, 1995.

Kaplan HI, Sadock BJ, eds. *Comprehensive textbook of psychiatry*, 6th ed. Philadelphia, PA: Williams & Wilkins, 1995.

Magni G. The use of antidepressants in the treatment of chronic pain. A review of the current evidence. *Drugs* 1991;42(5):730–748.

Sindrup SH, Brosen K, Gram LF. Antidepressants in pain treatment: antidepressant or analgesic effect? *Clin Neuropharmacol* 1992;15(Suppl. 1 Pt. A):636A–637A.

Stahl SM. *Essential psychopharmacology. Neuroscientific basis and clinical applications*. Cambridge, MA: Cambridge University Press, 1996.

Zitman FG, Linssen AC, Edelbroek PM, et al. Clinical effectiveness of antidepressants and antipsychotics in chronic benign pain. *Clin Neuropharmacol* 1992;15(Suppl. 1 Pt. A):377A–378A.

Therapeutic Options: Nonpharmacologic Approaches

Diagnostic and Therapeutic Procedures in Pain Management

Milan P. Stojanovic

Take care not to get off soundings.
—*James C. White*

This chapter outlines the major diagnostic and therapeutic procedures performed at the Massachusetts General Hospital (MGH) Pain Center. Rather than attempting to cover the multitude of advances in the field of Interventional Pain Medicine over the years, this chapter serves only as an introduction to the most common procedures. For a more detailed description of procedures, readers should refer to more detailed texts.

I. GENERAL PRINCIPLES

1. Preprocedure Management

Patients are requested to consume only light meals on the day of a procedure and to take only clear liquids for 4 hours before the procedure. Baseline vital signs (including pain scale) are obtained on arrival in the clinic. If indicated, an 18- or 20-gauge intravenous (IV) catheter with a heplock is placed. An IV is placed routinely in patients undergoing procedures that are associated with a risk of sympathectomy and hypotension (e.g., lumbar sympathetic nerve block, celiac plexus block, etc.). The medical condition of the patient also could dictate that an IV should be placed (e.g., extreme anxiety, history of vasovagal syncope, and substantial cardiovascular disease). In general, premedication is avoided so that the baseline pain is not altered and so that patient cooperation is maintained. The patient is positioned appropriately, and monitors are placed as needed. Decisions about the level of monitoring needed are made on a patient-to-patient basis using similar criteria to those for IV placement. The usual monitors used are noninvasive blood pressure gauge, electrocardiograph (ECG), and pulse oximeter. Baseline verbal analog scores (VAS) and range-of-motion estimates are obtained before starting the procedure.

2. Choice of Injectate

(i) Local Anesthetic

For most of the diagnostic nerve/plexus blocks, a 1:1 mixture of equal parts 1% lidocaine and 0.25% bupivacaine are used. Lidocaine provides rapid onset of effect, while bupivacaine provides a useful prolongation of the effect so that patients can make observations that may have diagnostic value. Also, because of its prolonged action, bupivacaine may have a better effect on interrupting the "wind-up" phenomena in patients with chronic neuropathic pain. Although epinephrine can be used for somatic blocks, it should be avoided in patients with sympathetically maintained pain (SMP) because it may exacerbate their pain condition. In patients with history of anxiety, the epinephrine may cause a panic attack and is best avoided.

(ii) Steroids

The steroids currently used are depot preparations of methylprednisolone (Depo-Medrol) and triamcinolone (Aristocort), which may be irritating, and Kenalog, which is less irritating but allergenic. The doses generally range between 40 to 80 mg for epidural injection and 10 to 40 mg for peripheral nerve blocks. The steroids can be mixed with local anesthetics; however, we use small total volumes for all of our procedures performed under fluoroscopy. Studies have shown that if adequately placed under fluoroscopic guidance, even the small volumes can reach the site of pathology.

(iii) Contrast Media

Only nonionic contrast media should be used when performing epidural blocks (e.g., Isovue 300, Bracco DXS, Princeton, NJ). Standard contrast media can cause neurotoxicity and should be avoided. In case the standard contrast media is accidentally injected intrathecally, it should be irrigated with large amounts of normal saline. There is no clear consensus whether nonionic contrast should be used in patients allergic to the IV contrast solutions. If there is perceived risk of allergic reaction but the need for contrast agent is still present, the gadolinium can be used instead.

(iv) Neurolytic Agents

It is important to point out that neurolytic agents may exacerbate pain in neuropathic pain states. Therefore, their use should be mostly limited to patients with pain from cancer. Alcohol (50% to 95%) and phenol (6% to 10%) are the two agents commonly used for neurolysis. Alcohol has been extensively used as a neurolytic agent because it is effective and is easy to inject. It is the neurolytic agent of choice for injecting into the trigeminal ganglion, celiac plexus, and lumbar sympathetic chain. Occasionally, neuritis with intense burning pain is seen after alcohol neurolysis. Local anesthetics are injected prior to the neurolytic to localize the target nerve/plexus and to minimize the incidence of neuritis. The analgesic effect of phenol is almost equal to that of alcohol; however, it has the advantage of not producing neuritis. It is extremely viscous and difficult to inject (needs a larger bore needle and slow injection). Neither agent is isobaric in cerebrospinal fluid (CSF) (alcohol is hypobaric and phenol is hyperbaric); therefore, patients need to be positioned appropriately according to the baricity of the agent chosen. Neurolytic blockers have a delayed effect (up to 1 week), which generally lasts for up to 1 year.

3. Fluoroscopy Use

Recent studies strongly suggest the use of fluoroscopy for most procedures in interventional pain medicine. The fluoroscopy can improve accuracy of medication delivery, positively affect the outcomes, decrease complication rates, and improve validity of diagnostic blocks.

The radiation exposure to patients from fluoroscopy during common procedures is trivial, and not thought to be harmful. Caution is advised if fluoroscopy time exceeds 30 minutes. For the operator, most of the exposure arises from scatter, but it is very low. However, the use of a lead apron, thyroid shield, and dosimeter is recommended for the operator.

The accurate placement of needles can be challenging in obese patients and in certain complex procedures. A 25-gauge 3.5-inch or 22-gauge 6-inch spinal needle should be bent at a 20-degree angle 0.5 inch from its distal shaft to facilitate the placement. The "tunneled" or "coaxial" view can significantly help guide the needles to appropriate target points.

The negative aspiration of needles for blood return to rule out intravascular placement is a test with a high rate of false-negative results (up to 50%). Therefore, the placement of the needles should be verified with nonionic contrast injection.

4. Diagnostic Versus Therapeutic Procedures

Although therapeutic blocks are performed to potentially relieve pain for a prolonged period, diagnostic blocks are utilized

- to identify the source of pain (e.g., facet joint and disc);
- to evaluate the role of the sympathetic versus somatosensory nerves in maintaining pain;
- as a predictor of outcome for further treatment [radiofrequency denervation, intradiscal electrothermal therapy (IDET), spinal cord stimulation, and surgical treatments];
- as a predictor of drug class efficacy (e.g., IV testing of opioids and local anesthetics).

Before a diagnostic block is performed, the clinician must be sure that the patient has sustained reproducible pain and must document the activity or stimuli that evoke the pain. These factors can then be reassessed after the block and compared to the preblock state.

When performing diagnostic procedures, one should minimize patient sedation and procedure-related pain because both factors may interfere with the interpretation of effect and may lead to false-negative and false-positive results.

The use of placebo agents (e.g., saline versus local anesthetics) for diagnostic procedures is unethical and is strongly discouraged. This practice is likely to be helpful only in identifying placebo responders, not in identifying those with "real" versus psychogenic pain. Furthermore, the practice may damage the patient–physician relationship and may reduce the placebo effect of future treatments (see Chapter 3).

5. Complications

Many complications are common to all pain clinic procedures, and these are listed here.

The most common complication in the pain center setting is vasovagal syncope. Serious consequences can arise if procedures are performed in the sitting or standing position; therefore, it is advisable to perform procedures with patients lying down.

(i) General

- Syncope, including vasovagal syncope
- Infection, including cutaneous infection
- Bleeding
- Inadvertent intravascular injection
- Inadvertent puncture of viscera
- Seizure
- Nerve penetration and injury

(ii) Specific to Spine Procedures

- Inadvertent dural puncture
- Inadvertent intrathecal injection
- High spinal blockade
- Postdural puncture headache
- Epidural hematoma

- Epidural abscess; cutaneous infection; meningitis
- Spinal cord injury and paralysis

6. Postblock Management

Once the procedure is over, patients recover in the recovery room. The recovery time varies, depending on the procedure performed. Once the patients meet standard recovery room discharge criteria, they are discharged with an escort.

II. MOST COMMON PROCEDURES FOR LOW BACK PAIN

1. Epidural Steroid Injection

The presumed effect of steroid is to reduce the neuropathic pain, inflammation, swelling, and scarring. This pathology is a consequence of rupture of annulus fibrosus, causing radiculitis either by mechanical pressure from disc protrusion or by chemical irritation of the nerve root by leaking material from nucleus pulpous (phospholipase A2) resulting in radiculopathy-neuropathic pain. It has been shown that in neuropathic pain states the steroids can decrease the conduction in injured nerves. It also has been observed that steroids reduce the bulk of a scar by diminishing its hyaline portion, while leaving the fibrous skeleton intact.

The results of outcome studies for epidural steroid injection (ESI) are mixed. It is important to stress that many studies with negative outcomes did not use fluoroscopy and contrast media to verify the needle placement during the ESI. Recent, placebo-controlled studies using fluoroscopy strongly support the effectiveness of ESI, particularly the transforaminal approach. Although ESI is potentially indicated for axial (low back pain with no radiation to the leg), its role in treating that condition has not been extensively studied.

The use of fluoroscopy and contrast media is firmly supported in the case of ESI. In up to 30% of lumbar ESIs and 50% cervical ESIs, inadequate medication delivery is achieved without fluoroscopy. It is also important to place medication on the side of pathology because unilateral contrast spread is seen in 50% of the cases. There is significantly increased risk/benefit ratio if cervical ESI is performed without fluoroscopic guidance.

It seems that the transforaminal approach offers several advantages over interlaminar (see Fig. 1). This is particularly important in patients postlaminectomy. Several separate levels can be blocked at the same time.

Recent reports have revealed serious complications with the cervical transforaminal approach; this approach should be used only in carefully selected cases.

According to a recent national survey, the average number of ESIs per patient per year is five to seven. At the MGH Pain Center, we limit the number of ESIs per patient per year to four to six. Alternatively, a smaller dose of steroids per injection can be used and the total number of ESIs increased.

INDICATIONS
- Radiculopathy due to mechanical or chemical nerve root irritation
- Spinal stenosis
- Certain cases of axial low back pain (discogenic pain)

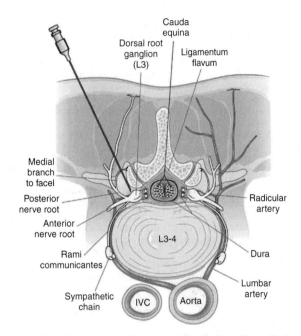

Figure 1.   Transforaminal epidural steroid injection. (From Rathmell JP. *Atlas of imaging in regional anesthesia and pain medicine.* **Philadelphia, PA: Lippincott Williams & Wilkins, 2005, with permission.)**

SPECIAL COMPLICATIONS. Intrathecal steroid injection, with potential complications such as anterior spinal artery syndrome, arachnoiditis, meningitis, urinary retention, conus medullaris syndrome, as well as a lack of effect.

BLOCK TREATMENT PROTOCOL. There is no need to repeat ESI "series of three injections" if the first procedure fails to produce any effect. If the first procedure was effective but the pain has fully or partially returned, the procedure can be repeated after 4 to 6 weeks.

PATIENT POSITION. Prone, feet over end of table, with a bunched-up pillow under abdomen (between iliac crests and costal margin) to reverse lumbar lordosis and for patient comfort is the recommended position. For the cervical approach, the pillow is placed under the chest (see subsequent text). Small support should be provided under the head if requested. Arms should be relaxed over the sides of table.

(i) Lumbar and Cervical Interlaminar Approach

TECHNIQUE
- Achieve true anteroposterior (AP) fluoroscopic view (spinous process is midline to the pedicles).
- Prepare skin with betadine and drape widely.

- Mark the skin with Kelly clamp at the interlaminar foramen so that the clamp is ipsilateral to the site of pathology but not more lateral than the lateral margin of the spinous process.
- Infiltrate the skin with 1% lidocaine (and small amount of sodium bicarbonate) using 25-gauge needle at the mark site (no need for the skin wheal).
- Insert a 22-gauge Tuohy needle in a "tunneled" view and advance it until it sits in ligamentum flavum.
- Obtain lateral fluoroscopic view and advance the needle until its tip is 3 mm posterior to the epidural space.
- Check the AP fluoroscopic view so that the needle is not more lateral than the lateral margin of the spinous process.
- Place a drop of normal saline into the hub of the needle.
- Attach the loss-of-resistance syringe to the needle. Holding the syringe with one hand and the needle with the other, press firmly on plunger, maintain positive pressure constantly while rapidly oscillating the plunger. Advance the needle slowly and steadily until sudden loss of resistance is achieved and the saline disappears from the hub of the needle (allow only minimal air to escape). Save the images of lateral fluoroscopic view for later comparison.
- Inject 0.2 to 0.5 mL of nonionic contrast media and confirm its epidural spread using lateral fluoroscopic view (see Figs. 2, 3).
- In AP fluoroscopic view, confirm adequate contrast media spread toward the site of pathology (see Fig. 4).
- Inject 2 mL of triamcinolone (40 mg per mL) with 0.5 mL of 1:1 mix of 0.25% bupivacaine and 1% lidocaine (only 40 to 80 mg triamcinolone in cervical area).
- Replace stylette in needle (to avoid tracking steroid through skin) and withdraw the needle.
- Slowly raise the patient to a sitting position; do not leave him or her unattended until he or she is safely seated in a wheelchair because the legs may be weak and may buckle.

(ii) Lumbar Transforaminal Approach

- Obtain oblique fluoroscopic view.
- The target point is just caudal to the 6 o'clock point on the projection of the pedicle above desired level entry point.
- Prepare and drape the skin in the usual manner and anesthetize the skin at the entry point.
- Enter the skin in a "tunneled" view with a 3.5-inch needle bent at a 20-degree angle that is 0.5 inch from its distal shaft and advance the needle slowly.
- The target point is a "safe triangle" with corresponding sides: (a) base = inferior border of the pedicle; (b) medial side = exiting spinal nerve; (c) lateral side = lateral border of the vertebral body.
- The final position of the needle in AP view should be just below the midpoint of the pedicle, the position being just below the ceiling of the intervertebral foramen in lateral view.

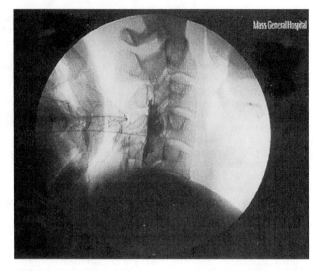

Figure 2.   Lateral fluoroscopic image of cervical epidural steroid injection with contrast media spread.

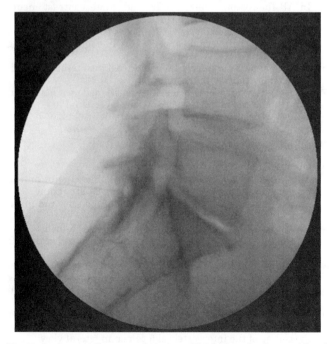

Figure 3.   Lateral fluoroscopic image of L5-S1 *interlaminar* epidural steroid injections (ESI) with contrast media spread.

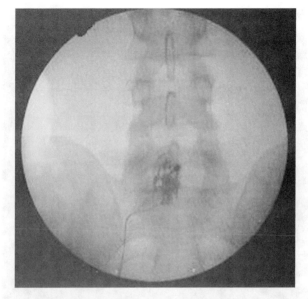

Figure 4. Anteroposterior fluoroscopic image of L5-S1 *interlaminar* epidural steroid injections (ESIs). Note the unilateral contrast spread.

- Inject 0.2 to 0.5 mL of nonionic contrast media and confirm its epidural spread using AP and lateral fluoroscopic view after negative aspiration (see Fig. 5).
- Inject slowly 1 to 2 mL of triamcinolone (40 mg per mL) with 0.5 mL of 1:1 mix of 0.25% bupivacaine and 1% lidocaine.
- Keep in mind that the artery of Adamkiewicz enters the spinal canal in proximity to the nerve root from T7 to L4 spinal levels. Injection of particulate matter into artery may lead to spinal cord infarction.
- Replace stylette in needle (to avoid tracking steroid through skin) and withdraw the needle. Slowly raise the patient to a sitting position. Do not leave the patient unattended until he or she is safely seated in a wheelchair.

(iii) Caudal Epidural Injection

- The caudal approach may be used in patients with previous laminectomy. However, this approach has several disadvantages: (a) it does not ensure medication spread to the site of pathology, and (b) higher volumes of injectate should be used; therefore, medication that reaches the site of pathology will be diluted. The transforaminal approach is better suited to patients postlaminectomy.
- The technique for this approach is achieved in lateral fluoroscopic view and final needle position should be checked by administration of contrast media.

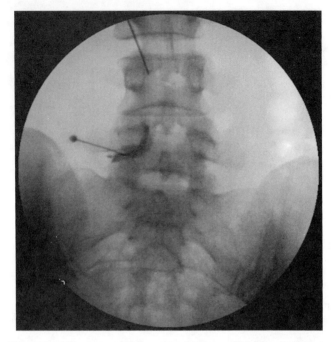

Figure 5.   Anteroposterior fluoroscopic image of L5-S1 *transforaminal* epidural steroid injections (ESIs) with contrast media spread.

(iv) Posterior S1 Foramen Approach

This approach is useful if epidural space is not otherwise accessible and especially when symptoms are confined to S1 or S2 level. Scan the sacral area briefly with the C-arm at different angles (remember that the sacrum takes off posteriorly from the lumbar spine at about 45 degrees) to see whether the posterior foramen can be made to overlie the anterior foramen. Usually only the anterior foramen is seen.

TECHNIQUE
- Position: prone using C-arm fluoroscopy for visualization.
- Using a 3.5-inch 25-gauge spinal needle, insert needle (C-arm in caudal direction) 1 inch posterior to the L5-S1 facet joint.
- The needle is advanced at 45 degrees caudally, to strike the posterior surface of the sacrum.
- The needle is then moved about until it falls through the posterior foramen.
- The posterior foramen is usually found somewhat cephalad and lateral to the superomedial border of the elliptical image of the anterior foramen.
- For epidural injections, the needle point is advanced 1 cm through the posterior foramen.
- To block the S1 root, the needle is advanced another 1 cm until a paresthesia is achieved at the anterior foramen.

- Needle position is confirmed in the lateral view with injection of the small amount of contrast media.
- Inject 1 to 2 mL of triamcinolone (40 mg per mL) slowly with 0.5 mL of 1:1 mix of 0.25% bupivacaine and 1% lidocaine.

2. Facet Joint Medial Branch Blocks

The degenerative arthropathy of facet (zygapophysial) may lead to chronic pain. The physical examination and magnetic resonance imaging (MRI) findings are nonspecific, and the best diagnostic test for facet pain is a diagnostic medial branch or intraarticular block with local anesthetics.

(i) Lumbar Facet Joint Innervation

Each lumbar facet joint is innervated by a medial branch of the posterior primary ramus of the lumbar nerve at the same level and another medial branch from one level above. For example, the L4-L5 facet joint is innervated by the medial branches of posterior primary rami of L4 and L3 nerve roots. The L5-S1 facet joint, however, is innervated by the medial branch of L4 posterior primary ramus and the dorsal ramus of the L5 nerve root.

(ii) Single-Needle Medial Branch Block

The single-needle technique seems to offer several advantages over the multiple-needle technique, including decreased procedural pain. It may even lower the rate of false positive blocks.

TECHNIQUE
- Place the patient in a prone position.
- Obtain an AP fluoroscopic image visualizing L4 and L5 transverse processes and L4-5 and L5-S1 facet joints on the affected side. The AP fluoroscopic view is the only fluoroscopic view needed for this technique.
- A 3.5-inch curved spinal needle should be inserted into the skin at the most lateral margin of the L5 transverse process. Local anesthetic for the skin should be administered through the same needle.
- The needle should be then navigated medially with the aid of its distal curve. The contact with the bone should be made at the most medial and cephalad aspect of the transverse process (at the lateral margin of the silhouette of the superior articular process—SAP) (see Fig. 6).
- A 0.3 mL of contrast (Omnipaque 240) should then be administered, making sure that the satisfactory spread without diffusion into adjacent neural structures (i.e., epidural space and intervertebral foramina) is achieved and that there is no vascular runoff. At this point, 0.3 mL of 1% to 2% lidocaine should be injected through the needle.
- After blockade of the L4 dorsal ramus medial branch, the needle should be withdrawn close to the skin without exiting it. In a manner similar to that just described, the needle should be then navigated to the L4 transverse process and the same procedure should be performed for the L3 dorsal ramus medial branch. The same procedure should be repeated for the L5 dorsal ramus, by placing the tip of the needle at the junction of the ala of the sacrum with the SAP of the sacrum.

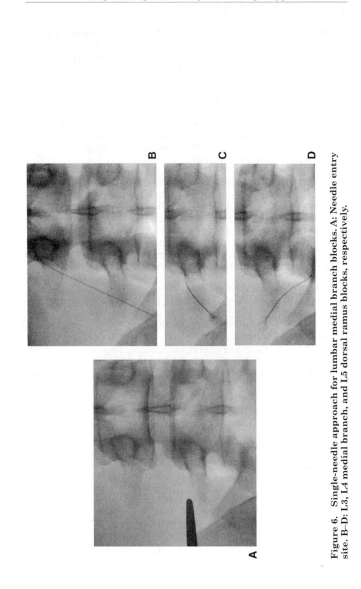

Figure 6.   Single-needle approach for lumbar medial branch blocks. A: Needle entry site. B–D: L3, L4 medial branch, and L5 dorsal ramus blocks, respectively.

(iii) Multiple-Needle Medial Branch Block

- The C arm is rotated to an oblique view until the vertical line of the facet joint is at the middle to outer one third of the endplate.
- Lidocaine (1%) is used to anesthetize the skin and the needle pathway, except the area near the target point.
- The target point of block is just caudal to the most medial portion of L2 to L5 transverse process for the L1 to L4 medial branches respectively. That is high at the "Scotty dog's eye" (see Figs. 7, 8). For the dorsal ramus of L5, the target point of the needle is at the junction of the sacral ala and the SAP. Posteroanterior (PA) view is used for the block of the L5 dorsal ramus.
- A 25-gauge, 3.5-inch spinal needle with a curved tip is used. The point of needle insertion is on the skin directly over the target point, and the tunneled view is used to advance the needle to the target point.
- Insertion is terminated once the tip of the needle strikes the bone of the target point. The final position of the needle should be confirmed in AP view. The needle tip should be at the lateral margin of the silhouette of the SAP and slightly caudal from the superior margin of the transverse process.
- Once the needle is in the correct position, 0.3 mL of contrast (Omnipaque 240) should be administered by the physician, making sure there is satisfactory spread without diffusion into adjacent neural structures (i.e., epidural space and intervertebral foramina) and that there is no vascular runoff. At this point, 0.3 mL of 1% to 2% lidocaine should be injected through the needle.

(iv) Cervical Medial Branch Block

The C2-C3 facet joint, the highest cervical facet joint, is innervated mainly by the third occipital nerve, which runs AP across the lateral surface of the C2-C3 facet joint. The medial branches of C3 and C4 dorsal rami innervate the C3-C4 facet joint. Each of these medial branches runs AP hugging the middle point of the articular pillar. The rest of the cervical facet joints have similar innervation to the C3-C4 facet joint from the medial branches at the respective levels.

SPECIAL COMPLICATIONS
- Injury and injection into carotid artery and vertebral arteries
- Seizure
- Damage to brachial plexus

TECHNIQUE. The multiple-needle technique is described but the single-needle technique also can be used in a similar fashion as for lumbar medial branch blocks.

- Patient lies in the lateral position.
- PA and lateral view of fluoroscopy is used to identify the cervical articular pillars and facet joints.
- A 25-gauge, 1.5-inch spinal needle is used.
- The target point for the block is slightly anterior to the midpoint of the C2-C3 facet joint in the lateral view and on the surface of the C2-C3 facet joint in the PA view.
- The needle end point for blocking the deeper medial branches of C3 and medial branches of C4 to C7 is at the midpoint of

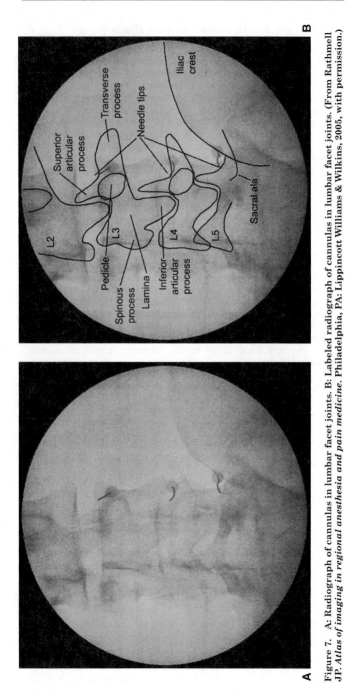

Figure 7. A: Radiograph of cannulas in lumbar facet joints. B: Labeled radiograph of cannulas in lumbar facet joints. (From Rathmell JP. *Atlas of imaging in regional anesthesia and pain medicine.* Philadelphia, PA: Lippincott Williams & Wilkins, 2005, with permission.)

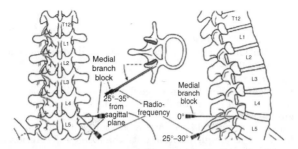

Figure 8. Landmarks for median branch block and radiofrequency lesioning for facet pain. (From Rathmell JP. *Atlas of imaging in regional anesthesia and pain medicine.* Philadelphia, PA: Lippincott Williams & Wilkins, 2005, with permission.)

the pyramid of the articular pillars in lateral view and on the lateral surface of the articular pillar in the PA view. The target point for the C7 medial branch block is high on the apex of the SAP of C7.
- Needle insertion should be carefully guided by fluoroscopy.
- Once the needle reaches the target, after negative aspiration, 0.5 mL of 1% lidocaine is injected.

3. Sacroiliac Joint Block
Although not a facet joint, sacroiliac joint block technique is similar to the facet joint injection techniques (see Fig. 9). The temptation to inject this joint is great because tenderness over the sacroiliac (SI) joint is a very common finding in patients with low back pain. In fact, this was the reason that back pain used to be treated by sacroiliac fusion, before Mixter and Barr demonstrated in the early 1930s that the herniated disc is a cause of sciatica. Because the joint is well innervated, it is no wonder that it can be the source of acute or chronic low back pain.

INDICATIONS. Because the clinical presentation is very variable (pain in the gluteal area with or without radiation to posterior

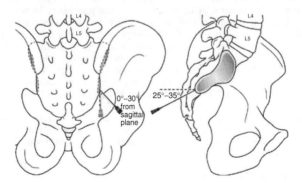

Figure 9. Sacroiliac joint block. (From Rathmell JP. *Atlas of imaging in regional anesthesia and pain medicine.* Philadelphia, PA: Lippincott Williams & Wilkins, 2005, with permission.)

thigh or knee or even down to the ankle), sacroiliac joint injection is used for the diagnosis and therapy for low back or sacral pain.

SPECIAL COMPLICATIONS

- Penetration of pelvic viscus if the needle traverses joint (remote possibility).

TECHNIQUE

- Because the joint region is easily palpable, injection in this region would seem simple. Actually it is not so, and C-arm guidance is needed.
- The patient should be in prone position, with the C-arm rotated to the oblique position until the images of anterior and posterior joints overlap.
- The insertion point is 1 inch caudally from the most caudad projection of the SI joint in the AP fluoroscopic view.
- A 25-gauge, 3.5-inch spinal needle is carried deeply into the joint. The needle tip will show its usual deviation as it does in the lumbar facet, under C-arm visualization.
- To anesthetize this joint, 2 to 3 mL of 1% lidocaine or 0.5% bupivacaine should be adequate. Steroid is an option.

III. RADIOFREQUENCY LESIONING FOR FACET PAIN

Radiofrequency lesioning (denervation) involves lesioning of small peripheral nerves with radiofrequency current. A standard technique uses high temperatures (90°C) to coagulate the peripheral nerves, whereas the new "pulse—radiofrequency" uses low (42°C to 43°C) temperatures. The technique of radiofrequency involves placement of cannulas under fluoroscopic guidance in a similar fashion as multiple-needle technique for diagnostic medial branch (Figs. 7, 8). A sensory and motor stimulation is performed once the cannulas are correctly positioned to confirm placement and to ensure that cannulas are not in close proximity to the nerve root. A small amount (0.5 mL) of local anesthetic is injected at each target site. At this point, heating at 80°C for 90 seconds is performed at each level. Pain relief usually follows an initial increase in pain for 2 to 3 days.

Many clinical studies have demonstrated pain relief and improved outcomes with radiofrequency lesioning for facet pain. The pain can recur 6 to 12 months after the procedure because of regeneration of nerves, and the procedure can be safely repeated.

Recently, a new mode of radiofrequency, a "pulse" mode, has been introduced. It uses a maximum temperature of 42°C for 120 seconds for each nerve. Although the exact mechanism of action is unclear, it seems that this treatment modality "stuns" the nerve endings, most likely by modulating the transmission in the treated nerve. The initial results of this treatment modality are encouraging, but more studies are needed.

Although radiofrequency lesioning is an excellent treatment option for lumbar and cervical facet pain, lesioning of the larger peripheral nerves can lead to worsening of pain and should be avoided.

IV. DISC PROCEDURES

Each disc consists of a central mass, the nucleus pulposus, and an outer ring, the annulus fibrosus. The annulus fibrosus is connected by Sharpey fibers into the articular surface of vertebral bodies. The inner structure of the annulus is formed of concentric lamellae of collagen fibrils. There are 10 to 12 overlapping concentric lamellae in each annulus. The lamellae are thinner and less numerous at the posterior portion of the disc. Many studies suggest that the annulus is a well-innervated structure. Degenerated discs lose nuclear hydrostatic pressure, which leads to buckling of the annular lamellae. With progressive degeneration of the disc, the annulus undergoes delamination and develops fissures. "Microfractures" of the annular collagen fibrils have been demonstrated using electron microscopy. The annular nociceptors become sensitized, with a decrease in their firing thresholds. The increased stimulation of the dorsal root ganglion by sensitized nociceptors may cause pain referred to the lower extremities. Furthermore, the damaged disc promotes the growth of nerve fibers along radial tears into the inner annulus. Degenerative disc disease (without frank protrusion) is a leading cause of back and neck pain and can afflict young as well as older patients.

1. Discography

INDICATIONS. Discography is a diagnostic procedure, best suited for diagnosis of discogenic low back pain (pain from internal disc disruption). The term discogenic pain should not be confused with disc herniation or protrusion because the pathology and treatment options differ considerably.

Provocation discography is the gold standard for the diagnosis of discogenic pain. The key diagnostic feature is reproduction of pain. Discography is performed at three to four lumbar levels, using unaffected discs as controls. Although the pattern of contrast spread is important, the concordant pain with low-pressure or low-volume disc injection is the key diagnostic finding.

SPECIAL COMPLICATIONS. The most serious complication of discography is discitis. Although rare, discitis is resistant to treatment because of limited disc blood supply. Intradiscal antibiotic administration minimizes its occurrence. Discography has been shown to be generally a safe procedure, and has not been found to produce damage to the disc.

TECHNIQUE
- The patient is placed in prone position and the lower back area is adequately prepared and draped.
- The AP fluoroscopic image is obtained first, providing good visualization of the selected disc.
- The end plates of adjacent vertebral bodies are aligned.
- The C-arm is then rotated to the oblique view, maintaining alignment of the vertebral bodies.
- The optimal end point of rotation angle is the point where the SAP image reaches the midline of the corresponding vertebral endplate.
- At this point, skin entry site is determined by the radiopaque pointer overlapping the SAP projection.
- After anesthetizing the skin with 1% lidocaine, an 18-gauge, 3.5-inch needle is inserted in a "tunneled view" toward the SAP.
- The needle tip should be advanced approximately 2 inches.
- A 22-gauge, 6-inch needle with a slightly bent tip is then inserted through the 18-gauge needle.

- Under tunneled fluoroscopic guidance, the physician steers the needle just lateral to the SAP, making sure that it is approaching the disc midline. A slightly caudally placed needle can help to avoid contact with the nerve root.
- Once the needle is entered into the disc, a "spongy" area will be encountered.
- From that point, several AP and lateral fluoroscopic views should be obtained to ensure that the needle tip is in the center of the disc.
- The L5-S1 disc level can be more difficult to approach because of the iliac crest. Maneuvering the needle bend at its distal tip around the iliac crest usually helps.
- Discography is performed once the needles are placed at all desirable levels.
- Nonionic contrast (Omnipaque 240) is appropriate for discography use, and should be mixed with 5 to 10 mg per mL of antibiotic; cefazolin is a good choice.
- Concordant pain is sought with less than 30 psi above opening pressure or with less than 1.25 mL volume of contrast administered into the disc.
- The reproduced low back pain (or pain referred to the lower extremity) under these conditions is considered to be discogenic in origin.
- The disc disruption and leakage of dye through the annular tear is usually seen with the onset of pain (see Fig. 10).
- Disc disruption alone, without reproduction of the patient's pain, is an insufficient finding for the diagnosis of discogenic pain.
- The use of postdiscography computerized tomography (CT) scan is a helpful but not absolutely necessary diagnostic tool. If used, it can be helpful in planning further treatments. The CT scan should be performed within 2 hours of discography.

2. Intradiscal Electrothermal Therapy

Intradiscal electrothermal therapy (IDET) is a new, minimally invasive approach for the treatment of discogenic low back pain. The putative mechanisms of IDET action are thermal modification of collagen fibers and destruction of sensitized nociceptors in the annular wall. Initial results with this treatment are encouraging; however, more clinical studies are needed to confirm its efficacy. IDET involves percutaneously threading a flexible catheter into the disc tissue in a fluoroscopically guided procedure. The catheter is composed of thermal resistive coil, enabling heating its distal part to the desired temperature. Considering its potential advantages over surgery, IDET could become the treatment of choice for discogenic pain, bridging the gap between conservative and surgical treatment.

INDICATIONS. Patients with discogenic pain for more than 6 months who have failed to improve from conservative treatment are considered appropriate candidates for IDET.

- Patients with severe radicular symptoms due to a herniated disc or patients with severe spinal stenosis are not good candidates.
- A severely collapsed disc (>50% of disc height), or disrupted disc might not respond well to IDET.

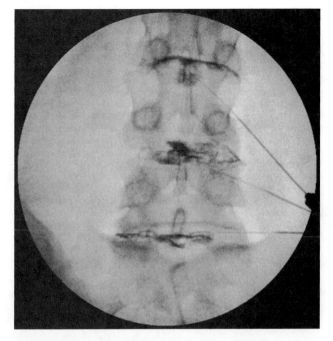

Figure 10. Anteroposterior fluoroscopic image of contrast media spread for L3, L4, and L5 discography.

- Patients older than 50 to 55 years may have an adverse effect on the disc healing process and lower success rates with treatment.
- Multilevel disc disease and history of prior spinal fusion are not contraindications for the IDET treatment.

SPECIAL COMPLICATIONS
- A possible serious complication from IDET is catheter tip shearing due to forceful manipulation.
- Inappropriate catheter handling can result in more serious complications, such as nerve damage or cauda equina injury.

TECHNIQUE
- IV sedation can be administered, but total hypnosis is avoided to maintain patient feedback.
- The technique for approaching the disc for IDET procedure is similar to discography.
- After the skin is infiltrated with local anesthetics, a 17-gauge introducer needle is inserted in the disc tissue guided by oblique fluoroscopic imaging.
- Once appropriate needle position is established by AP and lateral fluoroscopic views, the catheter is inserted through the needle. The catheter is designed to be easily navigated through the disc tissue.

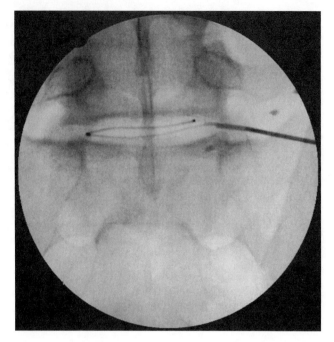

Figure 11. Anteroposterior fluoroscopic image of intradiscal electrothermal therapy (IDET) catheter placed at L5-S1 level.

- The final position of the electrode is such that the end of the catheter is placed circumferentially around the inner surface of the posterior annulus.
- The best approach to the disc is from the side opposite to the symptoms; however, some patients require ipsilateral approach if catheter navigation from the opposite side fails.
- Once the catheter is in satisfactory position, as confirmed by AP and lateral fluoroscopy (see Fig. 11), the gradual heating of the distal part of the catheter is employed utilizing a ElectroThermal Spine System generator.
- Increments in temperature are automatically achieved with a target temperature of 80°C to 90°C for 4 to 6 minutes.
- It is important to maintain maximum temperature of at least 80°C to achieve optimal results.
- A slight increase in concordant pain during heating is normal.
- Patients can be discharged home 1 hour after the procedure.

3. Percutaneous Disc Decompression

Unlike IDET, which is used for discogenic low back pain (not associated with disc protrusion), percutaneous disc decompression is used for lumbar radiculopathy caused by a minor to moderate disc protrusion. Microdiscectomy is an alternative treatment option. Percutaneous disc decompression is performed on an outpatient basis in a manner similar to IDET and can potentially replace surgery in these patients.

One of the techniques for percutaneous disc decompression, called nucleoplasty, uses "Coblation" technology, which combines ablation and coagulation of disc tissue for partial disc removal. It utilizes a radiofrequency wave to create an ionic plasma field from sodium atoms within the nucleus, which removes tissue from the treatment area via a molecular dissociation process that converts the tissue into gases that exit at the treatment site. Its "SpineWand" catheter creates small channels within the disc, thereby reducing the disc tissue mass. Nucleoplasty does not rely on heat energy to remove tissue, so thermal damage and tissue necrosis are avoided.

The alternative percutaneous disc decompression procedure, the "Dekompressor," achieves disc decompression through mechanical removal of the disc tissue with no heat involved. Technical aspects of this procedure are similar to that of lumbar discography.

Percutaneous disc decompression procedures, unlike IDET, rarely require diagnostic discography beforehand. The history, physical examination, and MRI findings are sufficient patient selection tools. Although percutaneous disc decompression is already used widely in interventional pain settings, more studies are needed to better address the patient selection criteria.

V. SYMPATHETIC NERVE BLOCKS

These techniques attempt to isolate sympathetic from somatic nerves. The following techniques are specifically for use with the C-arm fluoroscopy.

BLOCK TREATMENT PROTOCOL. Reasons for performing sympathetic blocks (SB) are (a) therapeutic to interrupt central sensitization and subsequent pain chronicity; and (b) diagnostic to identify patients with a sympathetic component of pain.

Surgical sympathectomy is no longer recommended because it is now recognized that neural destruction may worsen the pain. Spinal cord stimulation seems to produce better outcomes for sympathetically mediated pain, and recent studies support the use of SB as a predictor for spinal cord stimulation outcomes.

CONFIRMATION OF SYMPATHETIC BLOCKADE. A skin temperature change on blocked side and disappearance of psychogalvanic skin response are the most practical clinical measures in assessing adequacy of SB.

1. Stellate Ganglion Block

INDICATIONS
- Diagnosis and therapy for SMP
- Peripheral vasospastic disease, for example, Raynaud phenomenon
- Acute herpes zoster
- Acute posttraumatic or postoperative vascular insufficiency of face, neck, or upper extremities
- As an outcome predictor before spinal cord stimulator trial

SPECIAL COMPLICATIONS
- Transient nerve paralysis of the recurrent laryngeal nerve (hoarseness) or phrenic nerve (shortness of breath)
- Pneumothorax

- Hematoma
- Subarachnoid or epidural anesthesia by injection into the dural sleeve of the cervical root
- Seizures, as a result of intravascular injection of local anesthetic, including vertebral artery
- Brachial plexus blockade

PROLONGATION OF BLOCK. Intrapleural catheter treatment also can provide prolonged sympathetic blockade to the upper extremity. However, these treatments require inpatient admission.

TECHNIQUE

- Position the patient supine with the neck extended and a pillow under the shoulders. Neck extension makes the cervical spine more superficial and easier to reach, and draws the esophagus behind the trachea so it is less easily pierced by left-sided approach.
- Palpate the space between carotid pulsation and the lateral trachea, as low as possible in the neck.
- Make a skin wheal over the medial edge of carotid pulsation at this level, usually at C6 or C7 over transverse process, by C-arm fluoroscopy.
- Direct a 1.5-inch, 22- to 25-gauge spinal needle caudally and medially toward the junction of the lateral portion of bodies of C7 and T1.
- When bone is encountered, check your position (it should feel like the hard, flat top of a table), withdraw the needle 1 mm, and inject 1 mL of 300 Isovue contrast media.
- Confirm contrast spread by C-arm fluoroscopy in AP and lateral views.
- Inject in 1 mL increments total of 3 to 5 mL of 1:1 mixture of 1% lidocaine and 0.25% bupivacaine. It is not necessary to administer large amounts of local anesthetics when fluoroscopy is used (10 mL recommended in the past).
- Because of the medial placement (3 to 5 mm medial to stellate ganglion), complications of vertebral artery injection, brachial plexus block, and pneumothorax are not common. Recurrent laryngeal nerve block does occur, especially if the needle passes close to trachea.
- Horner Syndrome (i.e., ptosis, miosis, enophthalmos, often with anhidrosis and nasal congestion) is commonly produced, but does not preclude the need for testing the upper extremity sympathetic nerve block. The appearance of a Horner syndrome does not ensure an adequate block of the upper extremity.
- If only the cervical portion of the sympathetic nerves need to be blocked, then the procedure is more easily done at C6 or C5, but C-arm should be employed for accuracy.
- Patients who undergo a stellate ganglion block are asked to sip water to detect possible aspiration, prior to feeding. If hoarseness is present, oral intake should be avoided. Other potential complications should be sought before discharge.

2. Lumbar Sympathetic Blocks

Because the principal spinal segmental sympathetic supply to the lower extremities comes mainly from L1, L2, and L3, it seems logical to place a needle at L2 and to rely on volume and diffusion of local anesthetics to cover the whole outflow (see Fig. 12).

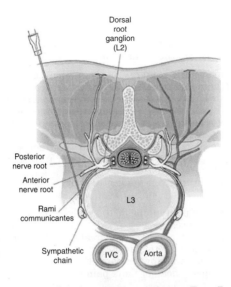

Figure 12. Lumbar sympathetic block—axial view. (From Rathmell JP.
Atlas of imaging in regional anesthesia and pain medicine.
Philadelphia, PA: Lippincott Williams & Wilkins, 2005, with permission.)

INDICATIONS
- Diagnosis and therapy for SMP of the lower extremities
- Acute peripheral vascular insufficiency
- Acute herpes zoster of the lower extremities
- As an outcome predictor before spinal cord stimulator trial

SPECIAL COMPLICATIONS
- Great vessel perforation and retroperitoneal hematoma
- Puncture of abdominal viscera, ureters, kidney, peritoneal cavity
- Inadvertent lumbar plexus injection
- Transient backache and stiffness

TECHNIQUE
- Accurate placement of the needle requires fluoroscopy.
- Position: prone, with a pillow beneath the epigastrium.
- Starting in AP fluoroscopic view, rotate obliquely the C-arm until lateral margin of the L2 transverse process overlaps with lateral margin of the vertebral body. Then rotate the C-arm in cephalad direction so that the L2 transverse process moves toward the upper end plate of L2 vertebral body.
- Mark skin projection and infiltrate the skin with lidocaine over the "waist" of the L2 vertebral body.
- A 20-guage, 12.5-cm (5-inch) curved-tip needle is inserted down to the vertebral body first in AP and then in lateral fluoroscopic view until the needle tip is 1 to 2 mm posterior to the vertebral body.
- 2 to 3 mL of Isovue 300 contrast media is administered and spread confirmed in AP, oblique, and lateral views.
- Total volume of 10 to 15 mL 0.5% lidocaine and 0.25% bupivacaine (without epinephrine) is injected.

3. Celiac Plexus Block

Because the celiac plexus is a network surrounding the celiac artery and the adjacent anterior aorta, the objective is to deposit solution anterior to the aorta. Approaches include the following:

- Bilateral posterior, antero-crural asymmetrical approach with C-arm fluoroscopy guidance described in the text that follows; right-sided needle passed between inferior vena cava and aorta toward its anterior surface, and left-sided needle passed tangential to the aorta
- Posterior retrocrural approach
- Posterior approach with transfixion of the aorta
- Anterior approach using CT scanner or ultrasound, placing needle on anterior aorta
- Transgastric approach via gastroscopy

INDICATIONS
- Treatment of pain in pancreatic cancer (and sometimes herpetic or gastric cancer)
- Pain of chronic relapsing pancreatitis, where the combination of local anesthetic and steroid is sometimes helpful
- Diagnosis and therapy for sympathetically mediated abdominal, retroperitoneal, or flank pain

SPECIAL COMPLICATIONS
- Great-vessel perforation and retroperitoneal hematoma
- Puncture of a viscus, kidneys, liver, pancreas, or peritoneal cavity
- Epidural, subarachnoid, or lumbar plexus injection, possibly with neurolytic agents
- Acute abdominal and chest discomfort, lasting about 30 minutes
- Orthostatic hypotension, as a result of profound sympathetic neural blockade, lasting for 48 hours or more, following a neurolytic injection
- Thrombosis or pressure occlusion of spinal branch of aorta, with resultant paraplegia (extremely rare)

POSTBLOCK MANAGEMENT. Regular monitoring of vital signs following a celiac plexus block for up to 4 hours with a local anesthetic block, and 24 hours or longer with a neurolytic block, may be necessary. Evaluation for the other potential complications is also necessary.

(i) Diagnostic Block

TECHNIQUE
- Place patient in prone position, with a pillow under the epigastrium.

RIGHT SIDE
- Use the same technique, as in lumbar sympathetic block, but at the L1 level (instead of L2).
- A 20-gauge, 15-cm styletted needle is passed to the upper lateral portion of body of L1, deviated laterally and caudad about 2.5 cm anteriorly to the anterior surface of L1 vertebral body.
- Aspirate carefully as you proceed.

LEFT SIDE
- An 18-gauge introducer needle is inserted to the back, 2 to 3 cm lateral to the spinous process of L1, aiming at the upper lateral margin of L1 body, using C-arm fluoroscopy visualization.
- The needle is carefully carried down to, and passed 2 to 3 cm beyond, the lateral edge of L1 vertebral body. A curved needle tip 22- to 25-gauge needle is inserted through the introducer needle. The curved tip is used to advance the needle more medially toward the celiac plexus, avoiding the aorta.
- After negative aspiration and adequate contrast media spread, 10 to 15 mL of 0.5% lidocaine or 0.25% bupivacaine (or a mixture of both) is injected on each side.

(ii) Neurolytic Block

TECHNIQUE
- Before performing a neurolytic block, a diagnostic block should be done (a day before if the scheduling condition of the patient allows) to demonstrate pain relief. If this is done just before the alcohol block, placebo effect, and duration of relief cannot be evaluated.
- Five milliliter of contrast media is injected on each side. Ideally a sausagelike pattern is produced around the aorta, but layering either anterior or posterior to aorta is satisfactory. If contrast streaks diagonally toward diaphragm, it is in the crus of the diaphragm, and alcohol injection would be ineffective. If contrast follows posteriorly toward intervertebral foramen, the needle needs to be repositioned to avoid alcohol contacting somatic nerves.
- This process of introducing the contrast is followed by 10 mL of 1% lidocaine at each side.
- After a 20-minute wait to allow the dispersal of lidocaine and contrast media (disappearance can be confirmed using fluoroscopy), 25 mL of 50% alcohol (absolute alcohol diluted with saline) is injected on each side.
- Usually, 10 mL lidocaine will protect against the irritative effect of the alcohol, but the patient may experience a brief aching in the epigastrium or back.

4. Hypogastric Plexus Block

The superior hypogastric plexus lies anterior to the L5 vertebra, innervating the organs in the pelvis and pelvic floor, including vagina, vulva, uterus, rectum, bladder, perineum, prostate.

INDICATIONS
- Pelvic cancer pain
- Nonmalignant pelvic pain

COMPLICATIONS
- Impotence
- Peripheral vascular occlusion
- Damage to the ureters

TECHNIQUE
- With patient in the prone position, the L4-L5 interspace is identified using fluoroscopy.

- A skin wheal is made with local anesthetic 5 to 7 cm from the midline at L4-L5 interspace.
- Insert 7-inch, 22-gauge, short-beveled needle through the skin wheal, aiming at the anterolateral aspect of the bottom of the L5 vertebral body.
- Guide needle in lateral fluoroscopic views just past the anterior margin of the L5 vertebral body.
- The contralateral needle is inserted in a same way under fluoroscopic guidance.
- Inject 1 to 2 mL of contrast media. In the AP view, the contrast should be just anterior to the L5-S1 intervertebral space. In the lateral view, a smooth posterior contour, corresponding to the anterior psoas fascia, indicates proper needle position.
- For diagnostic block, 5 to 10 mL of 0.25% bupivacaine is injected bilaterally after negative aspiration.
- For neurolytic block, 10 mL of 10% phenol is used unilaterally or bilaterally. A diagnostic block should be performed before the neurolytic block.

VI. EPIDURAL CATHETER PLACEMENT

We do not employ cervical epidural catheters routinely at MGH; therefore, this section of the chapter focuses on lumbar and thoracic epidural catheter techniques. Epidurally administered local anesthetics block both somatic and sympathetic nerves. However, a predominantly sympathetic block, continuous or intermittent, can be achieved using dilute local anesthetic solutions (e.g., 0.1% to 0.25% bupivacaine). Somatic blockade is achieved by increasing the local anesthetic concentration (e.g., 0.25% to 0.5% bupivacaine). For prolonged use, tunneled epidural catheters are placed.

INDICATIONS
- Pain syndromes due to peripheral vascular insufficiency, including ischemic vasospastic pain
- SMP, unilateral, or bilateral
- Acute herpes zoster and postherpetic neuralgia
- Acute thoracic or lumbar strain with radiculopathy
- Regional pain syndromes due to malignancy

SPECIAL COMPLICATIONS
- Broken epidural catheter
- Arachnoiditis

CATHETER TREATMENT MANAGEMENT. Pain relief is achieved using a continuous infusion of 0.1% bupivacaine, up to 10 mL per hour, sometimes with the addition of opioids and/or clonidine. Vital signs are closely monitored during and after the initial bolus injection or infusion. If the catheter is to be utilized for continuous block, the patient is either admitted for several days or discharged with adequate instructions. Hospital admission may be desirable for intensive in-house physical therapy. Diet and activity recommendations are based on the clinical situation.

If the catheter is to be used for cancer pain relief, 0.1% bupivacaine solution should be tried initially, but if pain relief is inadequate, 0.25% bupivacaine with or without opioids and/or clonidine may be needed. Infusions of opioid without local anesthetic are used in patients with cancer in whom local anesthetics produce undesirable effects. Vital signs are monitored as described in preceding text. Activity and diet to be followed are as tolerated. If prolonged infusions are required, the catheter is tunneled subcutaneously at the time of placement.

1. Lumbar Epidural Catheters

(i) Midline Approach

TECHNIQUE
- Patient lies in the lateral position, with maximal flexion of the back and with the knees to the abdomen.
- Obese patients should sit bent forward, with the knees to the abdomen or the legs resting on a stool. This position helps identify the midline, and may widen the posterior interspinous space.
- The spinal cord terminates at L1 or L2 in the adult; therefore, the spinous process, intervertebral space, and midline are carefully palpated below this level. An appropriate interspace is located.
- The overlying skin is prepared with antiseptic solution (such as alcohol or betadine), and a sterile, fenestrated drape is placed over the site.
- A skin wheal is made with a 0.5-inch, 25-gauge needle, using 1% lidocaine, and deeper infiltration is performed with a 1.5-inch, 22-gauge needle.
- A 17- or 18-gauge Tuohy needle is directed perpendicular or slightly cephalad in the interspinous space, bevel pointing cephalad, and advanced to the ligamentum flavum.
- The stylette is removed, and a syringe containing 3 to 4 mL of air or saline is attached to the Tuohy needle. The needle is advanced, while rapidly oscillating the plunger of the syringe, until there is a loss of resistance. Loss of resistance also may be detected with continuous pressure on the plunger, advancing until pressure is lost. We do not recommend the hanging drop method because we have noted a higher incidence of dural punctures.
- Medication or saline can be injected into the Tuohy needle to distend the epidural space. The catheter is advanced through the needle, no more than 5 cm into the epidural space.
- The Tuohy needle is removed, while maintaining the catheter in position, measuring the distance between a catheter mark and the skin, to ensure that the catheter has not been moved during the needle removal.
- The catheter is then secured to the skin with a transparent dressing, and tested for intravascular or intrathecal placement with 3 mL of 2% lidocaine with epinephrine. Aspiration is also performed for blood or CSF.
- To decrease displacement of catheter tip, it is advisable to bring the excess catheter around the flank to the epigastrium, rather than up the back and over the shoulder, as in operative cases. This is because flexing of the spine tends to pull the catheter back from the epidural space.
- The catheter is then ready for use, either with bolus or continuous infusions.

(ii) Paramedian Approach

TECHNIQUE

- A skin wheal is made 1 cm lateral, and 2 cm caudad to the interspinous space chosen.
- A 17- or 18-gauge Tuohy needle is aimed from the lateral skin wheal to the top of the target interspace, that is, the needle is aimed medially and slightly cephalad.
- The needle is advanced to the ligamentum flavum, and an air or saline-filled syringe is attached.
- After obtaining a loss of resistance, the catheter is threaded, the Tuohy needle removed and, after negative aspiration, the catheter tested and secured, as noted in previous text.

(iii) Tunneling

TECHNIQUE

- Place epidural catheter as noted in previous text.
- Anesthetize a subcutaneous tract, horizontally across one side of the back.
- Tunnel a long 14-gauge, 5.5-inch IV catheter through the tract, starting at the distal point, and emerging in the same skin nick as the epidural catheter. (Note: Do not puncture epidural catheter with IV needle.)
- Remove needle from IV catheter and thread epidural catheter through IV catheter.
- Remove IV catheter and secure epidural catheter at lateral skin exit wound, with transparent dressing.
- The epidural catheter is tested (as described earlier), and used for intermittent boluses or continuous infusion.

2. Thoracic Epidural Catheters

Procedure is performed as for lumbar epidural catheters. Choice of catheter location may vary, but technique varies only in that additional care is required in approaching the epidural space because the distances are less than those for the lumbar approach. Furthermore, the needle must be aimed in a more cephalad direction to traverse the sloping thoracic interspinous space. Management and complications are similar to those of the lumbar epidural catheters.

VII. PERIPHERAL NERVE BLOCKS

1. Trigeminal Nerve Blocks

Trigeminal nerve blocks are commonly used for the treatment of trigeminal neuralgia. At MGH, this procedure is performed by neurosurgeons. Under monitored sedation, the patient is placed in supine position with the neck extended. At a point 2.5 cm lateral to the corner of the mouth, the skin is prepared and draped in a standard sterile fashion. After anesthetizing the skin with 1% lidocaine, a 20-gauge, 13-cm Hinck needle is advanced through the anesthetized skin, in the direction of the fixed pupil in a cephalad trajectory into the foramen ovale. At this point there is often a free flow of CSF when the stylette is removed. After radiographic confirmation of needle position, 0.1 mL aliquots of a preservative-free local anesthetic (i.e., 1% lidocaine or 0.5% bupivacaine) or a neurolytic agent is injected. The patient is left in supine position if alcohol is to be injected. If phenol is chosen for the injection, the patient is moved into a sitting position with the chin on the chest so that the solution gravitates around the maxillary and mandibular divisions of the nerve and therefore spares the ophthalmic division. A similar approach can be utilized to place radiofrequency and cryotherapy probes.

2. Occipital Nerve Block

Occipital neuralgia results from stretching or entrapment of the occipital nerve. The nerve may become trapped in the fascia overlying the posterior surface of C2 or in occipital ligamentous attachments.

INDICATIONS
- Occipital neuralgia as in either tension headaches or following injury, for example, auto accidents with whiplash, falls, or work injuries

TECHNIQUE
- Position the patient in lateral decubitus position on the table and forehead in hands.
- Palpate posterior occipital protuberance and move 1.5 to 2 cm laterally and feel for occipital artery pulsation, and groove.
- Inject 2 to 3 mL 0.5% bupivacaine with 10 to 20 mg triamcinolone down to the bone and fan out. Occipital nerve analgesia should occur very rapidly.
- Inject some of the solution more caudally, for occipital muscle attachment pain and spasm, which often responds to steroid injections.

3. Suprascapular Nerve Block

INDICATIONS
- Shoulder pain secondary to rotator cuff lesions, osteoarthritis of the shoulder, or adhesive capsulitis ("frozen shoulder")
- Shoulder arthroscopy and other orthopedic manipulations of the shoulder

SPECIAL COMPLICATIONS
- Pneumothorax
- Muscle atrophy

TECHNIQUE
- Place the patient in a sitting position.
- Insert a 22-gauge, 1.5-inch needle 1 to 2 cm superior to the midpoint of the spine of the scapula and advance toward the suprascapular notch until a paresthesia is elicited.
- Inject 5 to 10 mL of local anesthetics with or without steroids.
- Position of the hand ipsilateral to the block on the contralateral shoulder can move the scapula away from the posterior chest wall and reduce the risk of pneumothorax.

4. Intercostal Nerve Blocks

INDICATIONS
- Rib fractures—acute, traumatic, and pathologic
- Chest wall metastases, or tumor

- Postthoracotomy pain or pain due to percutaneous drainage tubes
- Diagnostic or therapeutic blocks for abdominal pain versus abdominal wall pain

SPECIAL COMPLICATION
- Pneumothorax

TECHNIQUE
- Place the patient in a semilateral position, with sites to be injected made prominent by pillow under the opposite chest wall.
- Insert a posterior axillary line 5 to 7 cm lateral to vertebral spinous processes [One cannot reach the posterior division without injecting by the paravertebral approach: hazard of pneumothorax (see section entitled Selective nerve root blocks)].
- Make a skin wheal and inject with 25-gauge, 0.5-inch (or longer if necessary) needle: enter vertically to the skin, "walk" needle just below rib and 2 mm forward. Inject 3 mL of 0.5% bupivacaine with epinephrine at each rib. (Note: Anesthetic is absorbed rapidly into the systemic circulation because of the vascularity of the injection site.)
- For a neurolytic intercostal block, first block nerve proximally with 0.5% bupivacaine, then inject 2 to 3 mL 100% alcohol, lateral to anesthetized site (alcohol injection is initially very painful).

5. Lateral Femoral Cutaneous Nerve Block

Lateral femoral cutaneous nerve pain is believed to be associated with obesity or pregnancy or with the wearing of a tight belt. It is thought to be due to entrapment of the lateral femoral cutaneous nerve because it passes through the inguinal ligament. Neurolytic blocks are not recommended; however, surgical dissection may be considered.

INDICATION
- Meralgia paresthetica: burning pain, numbness, and tingling in the anterolateral aspect of the thigh

TECHNIQUE
- Place patient in the supine position.
- Palpate anterior superior iliac spine, and insert 1.5-inch, 25-gauge needle, 2 cm medial and 2 cm caudal to it.
- Proceed through fascia (feel a "pop"), and inject 10 mL 0.5% bupivacaine with 30 mg triamcinolone fanwise, from medial surface of iliac spine medially to beneath insertion point.

EVALUATION OF BLOCK. Analgesia of upper two thirds of anterolateral thigh should be produced.

6. Ilioinguinal Nerve Block

INDICATIONS
- Postherniorrhaphy pain (usually due to trauma to genitofemoral nerve in the floor of the inguinal canal)
- Diagnostic block, prior to surgical dissection or neurolytic block (hazardous)
- Testicular pain, with or without history of trauma or surgery

TECHNIQUE
- Place the patient in the supine position.
- Produce a skin wheal with local anesthetic, 2 cm medial to the anterior superior iliac spine.
- Infiltrate all layers of muscle toward the umbilicus with an 1.5-inch, 25-gauge needle and 10 to 20 mL of 0.5% bupivacaine, for a distance of 10 cm.

EVALUATION OF BLOCK. Variable distribution of analgesia is noted in the medial thigh and groin, which should relieve the groin pain if the ilioinguinal nerve is involved.

7. Genitofemoral Nerve Block

INDICATION
- Groin or testicular pain, unrelieved by ilioinguinal block (lumbar sympathetic block is another reasonable treatment of testicular pain)

TECHNIQUE
- Place patient in supine position.
- Inject 5 mL 0.5% bupivacaine around the spermatic cord, at the base of the scrotum.

EVALUATION OF BLOCK. If pain relief occurs, but returns, the next option would be either to repeat the block as frequently as required or to do a cryoneurolysis or even rhizotomy of L1 and L2.

VIII. TRIGGER POINT INJECTIONS AND BOTOX

Trigger point injections are utilized to relieve pain associated with myofascial pain syndrome. This syndrome is characterized by spontaneous and evoked pain of affected muscles. It is commonly possible to palpate band-type muscle spasms, also known as trigger points, which trigger pain. These points are usually tender (also known as tender points). This syndrome can be either primary or secondary to other underlying diseases such facet, sacroiliac arthropathy, and disc herniation The reproduction of pain during injections into the muscle and relief of pain postinjection is the hallmark of this type of pain. Even though we routinely inject local anesthetics into the trigger points, some physicians use just dry needling, or steroids with or without the local anesthetics; some use normal saline.

TECHNIQUE. Inject 1 to 2 mL 0.25% bupivacaine, with or without 5 to 10 mg triamcinolone, into and around the trigger point, using a 25-gauge, 1.5-inch needle, and aspirating before injecting. Repeat as needed, and wherever required.

Patients who respond to trigger point injections may be good candidates for Botox treatment. The botulinum toxin type A is derived from the bacterium *Clostridium botulinum*. This bacterium produces a substance that blocks the release of acetylcholine and most likely decreases vesicle-dependent exocytosis of other neurotransmitters-neuropeptides. Blocked release of acetylcholine leads to muscle relaxation, improved muscle perfusion, and reduction of muscle spindle activity. It possibly inhibits cholinergic interneurons and diminishes central sensitization.

A typical dose of botulinum toxin type A is 25 to 50 units per muscle. A total dose of 300 units should not be exceeded per treatment session, although total doses of up to 800 units have shown to be safe. The toxic dose estimate is 3,000 units. The botulinum toxin type B has a similar mechanism of action and, when used, the doses should be higher in comparison to botulinum toxin type A. Most commonly injected muscles in the cervical area are the trapezius muscle, semispinalis capitis and cervicis, levator scapulae, and splenius capitis and cervicis. For the lower back, piriformis muscle, multifidus muscle, and, possibly, paraspinal muscles should be targeted. For best results, the midbelly of the muscle should be targeted instead of the actual trigger point for optimal results.

The botulinum toxin type A duration of action is up to 3 months. The efficacy of Botox treatment may diminish if injections are repeated more often than every 3 months. If treatments are performed less often, the effects of botulinum toxin type A may be potentiated. More studies are needed to fully support this treatment, but several studies support the use of Botox as opposed to placebo for myofascial pain.

IX. VERTEBROPLASTY

Percutaneous vertebroplasty is a relatively new procedure consisting of percutaneously injecting polymethylmethacrylate cement into vertebral bodies that are destabilized by osseous lesions or fractures, causing intractable pain. By reinforcing vertebral lesions, injected cement provides analgesia in these patients. The main indications for vertebroplasty are osteoporotic vertebral compression fractures, vertebral angiomas, and osteoporotic vertebral tumors. Recent clinical studies of vertebroplasty have shown good results.

TECHNIQUE

- The procedure is performed under fluoroscopic or CT scan guidance.
- Patient is placed in the prone position.
- An eleven-gauge bone marrow biopsy needle is directed through transpedicular approach into the vertebral body under local anesthesia.
- The depth of the needle is assured in lateral fluoroscopic views.
- An intraosseous venogram is then performed to ensure that the needle tip is not in a blood vessel.
- The cement is than injected under continuous fluoroscopic guidance.

SPECIAL COMPLICATIONS

- Leakage of cement into adjacent structures with neural damage due to mechanical compression and thermal necrosis may occur.

A high degree of technical expertise is needed to appropriately perform this procedure. Current research efforts are focused on designing improved bone cement that does not leak into unwanted areas and minimizes tissue damage.

X. ADDITIONAL DIAGNOSTIC AND THERAPEUTIC TECHNIQUES

Besides administering local anesthetics with or without steroids locally or regionally, one can administer local anesthetic (lidocaine) or adrenergic blockers systemically.

1. Intravenous Lidocaine Injection

Lidocaine is an amide local anesthetic and sodium channel blocker, which is given by controlled IV infusion to test the analgesic response and predict the possible efficacy of mexiletine (an oral sodium channel blocker). Although many positive responders demonstrate a good response to mexiletine, the true predictive value of this test is uncertain because it has not yet been shown that negative responders do not respond to mexiletine.

INDICATIONS
- Neuropathic pain syndromes, particularly with continuous or lancinating dysesthesias, for example, diabetic neuropathy, phantom limb pain, stump pain, and neuralgia.

PRETEST MANAGEMENT
- The patient is asked to eat lightly, before the procedure, and abstain for 4 hours immediately preceding the procedure.
- A baseline ECG and liver function tests (LFTs) are obtained. Myocardial conduction abnormalities (such as Wolff-Parkinson-White syndrome) are contraindications to this procedure. Abnormally elevated LFT results are contraindications to oral mexiletine.

SPECIAL COMPLICATIONS
- Cardiac arrhythmias
- Syncope
- Hypotension
- Ataxia
- Tremors
- Dizziness
- Nervousness
- Skin rash
- Visual changes
- Seizures
- Anaphylaxis/anaphylactic reaction

TECHNIQUE
- Blood pressure, ECG, and oxygen saturation are monitored continuously.
- Patient is supine on a bed, and an 18- or 20-gauge IV catheter is placed in an upper extremity.
- Preblock visual analog scale (VAS) pain rating is obtained. Pain must exist at the time of the test to be able to evaluate the efficacy of the infusion.
- 1 to 2 mg per kg lidocaine (without epinephrine) is injected over 10 to 15 minutes. Usually, 100 mg of lidocaine is injected for the average adult. If tinnitus, perioral numbness, metallic oral taste, and dizziness are experienced, injection speed should be reduced and restarted with resolution of the symptoms.

EVALUATION OF PROCEDURE
- VAS scores are obtained before, during, and after the infusion.
- A 50% or greater reduction in pain would suggest that a trial of oral mexiletine is worthwhile.
- Specificity of response can be tested by injecting 10 mL of normal saline prior to the IV lidocaine and by obtaining VAS scores.
- **Postinfusion**, the patient is observed for 30 minutes, in the sitting position, and then allowed to ambulate. If stable, the IV catheter is removed, and the patient is discharged.

2. Intravenous Phentolamine Infusion

Phentolamine is an α_1-adrenergic blocking agent, which is given intravenously as a test for sympathetically mediated pain. Because of lack of availability of phentolamine, the procedure is now rarely performed. However, it is the most specific test for diagnosis of SMP.

INDICATIONS
- Diagnosis, and occasional therapy for SMP
- Diagnosis and occasional therapy for SMP, when SB are contraindicated (e.g., anticoagulated patients, infection of needle entry site, etc.)

PRE-BLOCK MANAGEMENT
- Patients are requested to eat lightly up to 4 hours before the procedure.
- The patient is evaluated for cardiac disease or other conditions that may be affected by hypotension.

SPECIAL COMPLICATIONS
- Hypotension, mild to profound, possibly leading to hypoperfusion states
- Dizziness, lightheadedness
- Reflex tachycardia
- Syncope

TECHNIQUE
- With the patient in the supine position, ECG, blood pressure, and oxygen saturation monitors are placed.
- An 18- or 20-gauge IV catheter is placed.
- Baseline pain levels are recorded (VAS scores).
- A bolus of 500 mL lactated Ringer solution is administered via a continuous infusion. This solution helps counteract hypotension, and can act as a placebo test.
- Stimulus-independent pain evaluations (VAS scores), and stimulus-evoked pain evaluations (VAS, mechanical test, cold test, etc.) are performed and recorded.
- Propranolol, 2 mg intravenously, is administered to counteract reflex tachycardia.
- Phentolamine, 35 to 70 mg intravenously in 250-mL normal saline, is infused, over 20 minutes, without the patient's direct knowledge of initiation of the infusion.

EVALUATION OF PROCEDURE. Pain testing and vital signs are evaluated for another 30 minutes, before discharge. The data are used to indicate the presence of SMP, particularly if the pain is relieved. We have not found that a lack of pain relief definitively excludes the diagnosis, and either corroborative blocks or sympathetically independent pain may be considered.

POSTBLOCK MANAGEMENT

- Patients are observed for 30 minutes after the block, and somatosensory and pain evaluations are conducted.
- Patients are then allowed to sit up, and stand up, slowly as tolerated.
- If they are stable, they are discharged; if not, they are observed for as long as necessary, prior to discharge with an escort.

3. Intravenous Regional Sympathetic Blocks (Bier Blocks)

BACKGROUND. Intravenous regional sympathetic blocks are a treatment option for complex regional pain syndrome (CRPS) and SMP. As opposed to phentolamine infusion, these blocks lack specificity for diagnosis of SMP. Several medications can be used, including guanethidine, bretylium, labetalol, prazosin, clonidine, and reserpine. IV guanethidine and reserpine are not readily available in the United States. At MGH, we use the mixed α and β antagonist labetalol.

INDICATIONS

- Therapeutic sympathetic blockade of an upper or lower extremity
- Diagnostic blockade when patients refuse needle blocks, are on anticoagulants, or when needle blocks are contraindicated or have been unsuccessful

PRE BLOCK MANAGEMENT

- Patients are instructed to be NPO (nothing by mouth), up to 4 hours before the procedure.
- Baseline vital signs (i.e., ECG, blood pressure, and oxygen saturation) are obtained.

SPECIAL COMPLICATIONS

- Hypotension, mild to profound, particularly when deflating the pneumatic cuff, or with a leaking cuff
- Dizziness
- Ischemia or neuropathy in the affected limb, usually transient
- Orthostatic hypotension
- Syncope

TECHNIQUE

- Patient is placed in supine position. A 20- or 22-gauge IV catheter is placed in the affected extremity.
- Another 18- or 20-gauge IV catheter is placed in a nonaffected extremity for IV access and prehydration.
- The affected extremity is exsanguinated by elevating it, and tightly binding it with an elastic bandage (Esmarch bandage) from fingers to axilla.
- A pneumatic cuff is applied proximally, at a pressure of 250 mm Hg.
- A combination of 20 to 30 mg of labetalol and 100 mg of lidocaine is made into a 20-mL solution by adding normal saline, and injected into the affected upper extremity or 30 to 40 mg

of labetalol, and 200 mg of lidocaine are mixed into 35 mL solution with normal saline and injected into the affected lower extremity.
- The cuff's pressure is maintained at 250 mm Hg for 20 minutes, then either deflated slowly or intermittently deflated and reinflated over 5 to 10 minutes, while monitoring vital signs closely.

EVALUATION OF PROCEDURE
- Baseline (before procedure) and postprocedure pain evaluations are performed, including VAS score.
- A time course of the pain relief is noted because relief can range from hours to months.

XI. CONCLUSION

Interventional pain management is a rapidly growing field offering percutaneous, outpatient treatment options for many forms of chronic pain. The procedures most commonly used at the MGH Pain Center are described in this chapter. When used in carefully selected patients for specific indications, these procedures have excellent outcomes. Support from published trials continues to grow, and perhaps the greatest validation is that these procedures may obviate the need for more complex and more risky surgical interventions.

SUGGESTED READINGS

Bogduk N. International spinal injection society guidelines for the performance of spinal injection procedures. Part 1: zygapophysial joint blocks. *Clin J Pain* 1997;13(4):285–302.

Cluff R, Abdel-Kader M, Cohen S, et al. The technical aspects of epidural steroid injections: a national survey. *Anesth Analg* 2002; 95:403–408.

Fenton DS, Czervionke LF. *Image-guided spine intervention.* Philadelphia, PA: WB Saunders, 2003.

Pauza KJ, Howell S, Dreyfuss P, et al. A randomized, placebo-controlled trial of intradiscal electrothermal therapy for the treatment of discogenic low back pain. *Spine J* 2004;4(1):27–35.

Stojanovic MP, Vu T, Caneris O, et al. The role of fluoroscopy in cervical epidural steroid injections: an analysis of contrast dispersal patterns. *Spine* 2002;27(5):509–514.

Stojanovic MP, Zhou Y, Hord ED, et al. The single needle approach for multiple medial branch blocks: a new technique. *Clin J Pain* 2003;9(2):134–137.

Waldman SD. *Interventional pain management,* 2nd ed. Philadelphia, PA: WB Saunders, 2001.

13

Neuromodulation Techniques for the Treatment of Pain

Milan P. Stojanovic

Divinum est sedare dolorem—"It is divine to allay pain."
—*Galen, 129–199*

In recent years, complex interventions for pain control have become part of everyday practice in the pain clinic setting. Although more invasive than nerve blocks, these interventions have the advantage of not being neurodestructive. Unlike nerve ablation, these complex interventions may be reversible and therefore more appropriate for use in patients with nonmalignant pain. The clinical efficacy of these approaches has been widely documented in literature. In carefully selected patients, these interventions can reduce pain and suffering, increase functional status, decrease oral medication intake, and ensure early return to normal day-to-day activities. In comparison with more conservative measures for pain control, interventional treatments may appear costly. However, assuming that good outcome is achieved, the overall cost of interventions can be lower than that for conservative measures (as a result of decreased spending on medications and emergency room visits and fewer absences from work, etc.). It is important that the implementation of these interventions be integrated into a multidisciplinary treatment plan. Benefit from these procedures is achieved through careful evaluation of scientific evidence, good clinical judgment, and excellent technical skills.

I. SPINAL CORD STIMULATION FOR CHRONIC PAIN

Electrical stimulation for the treatment of pain was first documented in 600 BC; the process utilized electrical power from the torpedo fish. Renewed interest in pain medicine arose in 1967 when spinal cord stimulation (SCS) was introduced by Shealy et al. Their work was based on the Melzack and Wall "gate control" theory of pain. Initially, SCS implantation involved an open laminectomy. With advances in technology, SCS became minimally invasive, and is currently performed percutaneously. Further improvements in hardware design and patient selection have increased efficacy, with recent published success rates of 50% to 70%. As an alternative to SCS, peripheral nerve stimulation (PNS) can be performed in patients with localized neuropathic pain.

1. Mechanism of Action

The Melzack and Wall gate control theory of pain was the foundation for initial SCS trials. It was based on the idea that stimulation of A-β fibers closes the dorsal horn "gate" and reduces the nociceptive input from periphery. However, it seems that other mechanisms actually play a more important role. One proposed mechanism involves increased dorsal horn inhibitory action of neurotransmitters such as γ-amino butyric acid (GABA) and adenosine A-1 during SCS. Activation of descending analgesia pathways by serotonin and norepinephrine is another proposed mechanism. In patients with peripheral ischemic pain, the SCS may act by a combination of two mechanisms: suppression of sympathetic activity and suppression of a calcitonin gene–related peptide (CGRP). SCS also relieves angina in ischemic heart disease, probably via redistribution of the coronary blood flow.

2. Indications and Patient Selection

Patients with **complex regional pain syndrome (CRPS)** and patients with **extremity neuropathic pain** are the best candidates for SCS. Published reports reveal an excellent long-term success rate for SCS in patients with CRPS, with a reported efficacy of 50% to 91%, and a decrease in analgesic consumption by 50%. A recent study suggests that patients with good response to sympathetic block before SCS are more likely to have a positive response during their SCS trial and long-term pain relief after placement of a permanent SCS device. Phantom limb pain, stump pain, and spinal cord injury pain seem unresponsive to SCS. The likely explanation is that central nervous system (CNS) remapping, which may be critical to the development of these pain syndromes, is not affected by SCS. Diabetic neuropathy may respond well to SCS. However, the risk of infection in these patients is higher than in patients who do not have diabetes. The use of SCS in postherpetic neuralgia is controversial.

Patients with failed back surgery syndrome (FBSS) may respond well to SCS. It has been documented that patients with FBSS respond better to SCS than to a second operation. This applies in particular to low back pain (LBP) with a radiating component to the leg. In these patients, the chances of long-term success with SCS vary from 12% to 88%, with an average efficacy of 59%, as indicated by systematic review of literature. In addition, 25% of patients may return to work, 61% show an improvement in activities of daily living and 40% to 84% decrease consumption of analgesics. Opinion on axial LBP (pain limited only to the low back area) is divided. Some studies show that the dual lead system provides better pain relief for axial LBP than single lead stimulation does, whereas others find the opposite to be true.

Severe peripheral vascular disease is another indication for SCS. Patients with advanced peripheral vascular disease, who are not surgical candidates, respond well to SCS, with reported efficacy ranging from 60% to 100%. Besides providing pain relief, SCS promotes ulcer healing and potentially contributes to limb salvage.

Ischemic heart disease refractory to pharmacologic and surgical treatments may respond well to SCS, with reported efficacy rates of 60% to 80% several years after implantation. Patients with ischemic heart disease treated with SCS have demonstrated a reduction in anginal pain, decreased use of short-acting nitrates, and increased exercise capacity. SCS does not completely eliminate anginal pain but raises the anginal threshold. Fear of potential increase in myocardial damage does not seem to be justified.

New indications and techniques for PNS are emerging. Some patients with occipital neuralgia seem to respond well to PNS. In those cases, the stimulator lead is placed subcutaneously around the C1-C2 spinous process. In patients with pelvic pain (e.g., interstitial cystitis, pain of unknown origin), sacral placement of 2–4 SCS leads may provide adequate analgesia. Sacral placement also can be helpful in patients with impaired bladder control. Some cases of lumbar radiculopathy respond better to SCS lead placement directly through neural foramina (retrograde lead placement).

Infection, drug abuse, and severe psychiatric disease present major contraindications for SCS implantation. Before SCS implantation, a psychological evaluation of the patient is recommended.

3. Stimulator Trials

Before proceeding with permanent SCS implantation, a stimulation trial is warranted. The trial allows the patients to evaluate the SCS analgesic activity in their everyday surroundings. The criteria for a successful trial include at least a 50% reduction in pain, a decrease in analgesic intake, and significant functional improvement. The SCS trial is a minimally invasive procedure (similar to placing an epidural catheter) and can positively predict a long-term outcome in 50% to 70% of cases.

There is no consensus on the length of an SCS trial. The minimum trial time is 24 hours, although many centers perform 3- to 5-day trials. The beginning of a trial in the hospital setting allows for proper SCS adjustment, after which the patient is discharged home for several days of "home" trial. In cases of equivocal results, the trial time can be extended.

There are three technical approaches for SCS trial. In the first approach, the SCS lead is placed percutaneosly. After successful trial, the lead is removed and a new lead and an implantable pulse generator (IPG) are placed (on a separate occasion). Alternatively, the trial lead is tunneled and anchored via a surgical incision, which simplifies the final procedure and ensures that stimulation coverage remains the same during both the trial period and permanent implantation. The disadvantage of the second approach is the need for a second operative procedure for lead removal in case of an unsuccessful trial.

Percutaneous trial followed by lead placement via laminotomy is another, less frequently utilized, approach. In this case, wider electrodes are used in the permanent implantation, which may provide better coverage in certain patients, and are less prone to migration when compared to standard SCS leads.

4. Choice of Hardware

The hardware consists of the SCS lead, an extension cable, a power source, and a pulse generator. Lead design varies in the number of electrodes from four (Medtronic and ANS) to eight (ANS). The distance between the electrodes and the length of the leads also can differ. It is not clear whether an increased number of electrodes provides better coverage, but it might be beneficial in the event of lead migration. Leads with minimal space between electrodes (such as Medtronic Quad compact lead) are better suited for localized pain (such as foot pain) or for cases of isolated axial LBP. Many leads contain a removable stylet, which eases lead steering during implantation.

There are two types of pulse generators: (a) a completely implantable pulse generator (IPG) containing a battery, and (b) IPG powered externally through a radio frequency antenna applied to the skin. The IPG is more convenient and can be easily adjusted by the patient by using a small telemetry device. Patients can turn the stimulator on and off and can control the stimulation amplitude, frequency, and pulse width. A separate external programmer allows for more complex IPG reprogramming by the physician. If the stimulation is inadequate, the physician can change the polarity and the number of functioning electrodes to provide better coverage. Batteries have to be changed every 3 to 6 years, which requires a brief operative procedure. The battery life depends on the time the stimulator is used and the stimulation amplitude. The externally powered IPG is preferred in patients requiring higher amplitudes of stimulation.

5. Implantation Techniques

For lumbar lead placement the patient lies prone, and for cervical placement both prone and lateral decubitus positions are used. The skin is prepared and draped. Both trial and permanent implantation are performed under local anesthesia with light intravenous sedation. The most common entry sites for the lumbar area are T12-L1 or L1-L2 spinal interspaces, and for the cervical area, C7-T1. The physician identifies these interfaces with fluoroscopic guidance, making sure to obtain a true anteroposterior (AP) view. The true AP view is achieved by C-arm rotation until the spinous process is placed midline in relation to spinal pedicles.

For percutaneous SCS trial, the Tuohy needle entry site is at the level of the spinous process below the desired interspace. It is important to achieve a shallow entry angle or to use the alternate Piles needle. The needle tip should stay close to midline during insertion. As the needle is advanced, lateral fluoroscopic view can be obtained so the needle depth can be assessed. Once adequate depth is achieved, "loss of resistance" technique is used to identify the epidural space. At this point, the SCS lead is inserted in the epidural space under continuous fluoroscopic guidance. The curved stylet, or curved lead tip allows lead steering. During insertion and at final position, the lead tip should lie at the lateral border on the side where the pain is located. Once adequate lead position is obtained, the trial stimulation is performed. It is important that stimulation paresthesias provide 70% to 80% overlap with the location of the patient's pain. Adequate patient feedback during this stage is important. Maximal effort should be made to provide adequate pain coverage, because this optimizes the trial. Frequent lead repositioning might be needed during this stage. Once adequate coverage is achieved, the needle is removed under continuous fluoroscopy, ensuring no change in lead position. The lead is then taped to the skin.

Permanent stimulator placement technique is similar to that for the trial but is done in the operating room rather than in the pain clinic. Under local anesthesia and IV sedation, a skin incision is made along the cervical or lumbar insertion site. Tissue dissection is performed until lumbar fascia is encountered. The Tuohy needle and stimulator lead are then inserted as in the preceding text. Once adequate coverage is obtained, the Tuohy needle is removed under continuous fluoroscopic guidance and the SCS lead is anchored with sutures to the fascia and supraspinous ligament. The pocket for IPG is made in the gluteal or abdominal area. The SCS lead is than connected with the IPG through an extension cable tunneled through the skin. The skin and subcutaneous tissues are closed in layers.

Patients should avoid any vigorous activity for the first 6 to 8 weeks following permanent implantation to prevent lead migration and to allow for epidural scar tissue formation.

Lead Positioning

The SCS topographic coverage depends on the spinal level where the SCS lead tip is positioned. The following landmarks are only for orientation because interindividual variance can be considerable. Careful intraoperative mapping is needed for optimal coverage ("sweet spot placement").

Upper extremity: SCS lead tip at C2 through C5 level. The shoulder area can be difficult to cover (Fig. 1).
Foot: SCS lead tip at T11-L1 level (Fig. 2).
Lower extremity: SCS lead tip at T9-T10 level.
Low back: SCS lead tip at T8-T10 level; two parallel leads can be used.
Chest: SCS lead tip at T1-T2 level.
Occipital neuralgia: SCS lead placed around C1-C2 subcutaneously.
Pelvic pain: Multiple SCS leads placed retrogradely within the sacrum or through S2-S4 foramina.

6. Complications and Troubleshooting

(i) SCS Not Functioning or Inadequate Coverage

(a) Obtain AP and lateral fluoroscopic images of SCS lead tip to rule out lead migration.
(b) Image the IPG and all connections, and search for disconnection or breakage.
(c) Check the batteries by utilizing programmer.

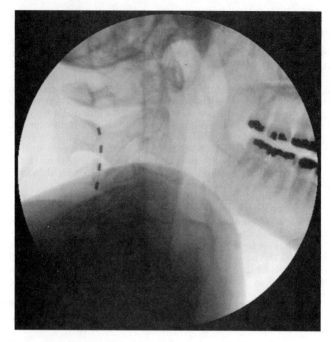

Figure 1. Spinal cord stimulation lead at the C2-C3 level as seen in lateral fluoroscopic view.

(d) Change amplitude and pulse width.
(e) If no response is observed to prior measures, reverse electrode polarity and change the activated electrodes.
(f) If adequate pain coverage cannot be obtained, measure the impedance of each electrode in relation to the IPG; the same impedance on two electrodes raises a possibility of a short circuit between the two electrodes.

Some mechanical failures might require surgical revision and replacement of affected SCS components.

(ii) Progressive Decrease in Stimulation Threshold

Consider intrathecal migration of the SCS lead. Lead migration can lead to serious complications such as spinal cord injury. Migration is most common in patients with considerable spinal canal stenosis. If stenosis is suspected, magnetic resonance imaging (MRI) of the targeted spinal level should be obtained before anticipated SCS lead placement.

(iii) SCS and Pacemakers

SCS devices can cause interference and inhibition of the cardiac pacemaker if used simultaneously. However, both devices can be used in the same patient if the following guidelines are followed: (a) both devices should be programmed in bipolar mode, (b) the

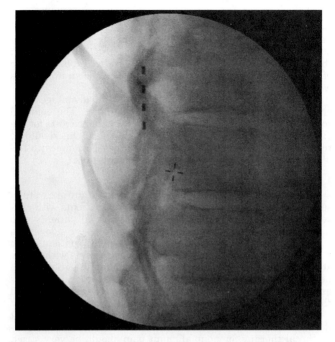

Figure 2.   **Spinal cord stimulation lead placed at thoracic spinal level as seen in lateral fluoroscopic view.**

SCS frequency should be set at 20 Hz, and (c) each SCS programming should be performed using continuous electrocardiograph (ECG) monitoring. A cardiology consultation should be obtained in these patients, and the manufacturer's recommendations should be closely followed.

The other most common SCS complications are hardware failure, lead migration, infection, skin irritation at the IPG site, and failure to provide pain relief. Bleeding at the IPG site (subcutaneous hematoma) is usually self-limiting and gradually reabsorbs in a few weeks. If infection occurs at the IPG insertion site, make sure to first aspirate the site before initiating antibiotic coverage and removing the hardware. SCS leads may be attracted into the magnetic field of MRI, and the manufacturer should always be consulted before MRI is undertaken.

II. CHRONIC INTRATHECAL THERAPY FOR CANCER AND NONMALIGNANT PAIN

Intrathecal drug delivery provides targeted delivery of medications and avoids side effects encountered by systemic administration. Drugs are delivered via a surgically implanted subcutaneous pump containing a reservoir for the medication. The pump is easily refilled every 2 to 4 months depending on the infusion rate.

Opioids are most commonly used, but other medications also can be employed. These include local anesthetics, clonidine, and baclofen, alone or in combination with opioids. Because numerous receptors involved in nociceptive transmission are located in the spinal cord, this approach seems to be very promising. The efficacy of intrathecal drug delivery has been shown in patients with malignant and nonmalignant pain.

The implanted intrathecal system has many advantages over epidural drug delivery via an external catheter. The epidural route can be more expensive because of maintenance costs for the external system and is less convenient; therefore, this should be reserved for short-term use only (<3 months). Patients with implanted pumps may safely undergo MRI procedures.

1. Patient Selection

Cancer pain responds well to intrathecal therapy in carefully selected patients. The following categories of patients with cancer might be considered for intrathecal trial: (a) patients who have failed oral or intravenous opioids due to severe side effects (i.e., nausea, vomiting, sedation, constipation), (b) patients with a life expectancy of more than 3 months, (c) patients without obstruction in cerebrospinal fluid (CSF) flow, and (d) patients with neuropathic cancer pain who do not respond to oral regimens and nerve blocks. The main contraindication for intrathecal therapy is infection.

Nonmalignant pain may respond to intrathecal therapy, but it should be considered as a last resort. Selection criteria for intrathecal therapy for nonmalignant pain should be very strict. Only patients who have failed nerve blocks, oral medications, physical therapy, and cognitive-behavioral programs and who have passed psychological evaluation should be considered for intrathecal trial.

2. Screening

Before considering implantation of intrathecal hardware, patients should undergo a trial procedure to better assess the odds of a favorable outcome. The actual trial procedure varies, and no consensus has been achieved on the best procedure. Before the trial, oral opioids are either discontinued or decreased substantially. It is important to monitor the patient for signs of respiratory depression during the trial. The most common screening methods are discussed in the following text.

Intrathecal trial is performed by implanting the temporary intrathecal catheter. Pediatric or standard epidural catheters can be used. After placement, the catheter is taped to the skin. The medication bolus is given first, followed by continuous infusion via an external infusion pump. The intrathecal opioid dose starts at 1/300th of the usual oral daily dose. The patient is kept in hospital (days or weeks) during which time the infusion rate is gradually increased. The longer the trial time, the greater the likelihood of decreased placebo response. Pain intensity, functional status, and use of breakthrough pain medications are monitored during the trial period.

Epidural trial is performed similarly. The epidural opioid daily dose is higher than the intrathecal dose, and is 1/30th of the daily oral dose.

One-time bolus is the simplest screening method. The intrathecal bolus of medication is given and the patient is monitored for 24 hours. The pain intensity, functional status, and use of breakthrough pain medications are monitored. Unlike the other methods, this method does not allow dose titration but can provide information on responsiveness to intrathecal opioids.

Side port catheter can be surgically implanted for a trial. Advantages include ease of adding an implanted infusion pump in case of a successful trial. However, the added risk of infection and the need to surgically remove the catheter in the case of a failed trial are disadvantages.

3. Hardware Selection

The two kinds of pumps that are most commonly used are: (a) battery-powered externally programmable pumps, and (b) nonprogrammable pumps, many of which are gas-driven. The amount of medication delivered by nonprogrammable pumps is dependent on drug concentration. Although externally programmable pumps offer the advantage of an adjustable infusion rate, continuous-rate pumps are cheaper and can be used in patients requiring less frequent rate adjustments.

4. Medication Selection and Dosage

Intrathecally administered medications should be preservative free. The most commonly used medication is morphine. Other opioids that are used include fentanyl, sufentanyl, hydromorphone, and meperidine. Opioid conversion dosage from other routes of administration is as follows: (a) intrathecal to epidural = 1:10; (b) intrathecal to intravenous = 1:100; (c) intrathecal to oral = 1:300. In opioid-naïve patients, morphine should be started at 0.2 mg/day and the dosage gradually increased. In opioid-tolerant patients, the initial intrathecal dose should be less than the conversion dose, whereas oral opioids should be used for breakthrough pain. Gradually, the intrathecal dose should be increased and breakthrough pain medications discontinued.

The addition of local anesthetics to intrathecal opioids may be useful for cancer and nonmalignant pain, with particular benefit in patients with neuropathic component of pain. A typical bupivacaine dosage range is 2 to 30 mg per day, although dosages of over 100 mg per day have been reported. α-Adrenergic agonists (e.g., clonidine and epinephrine) can be used in conjunction with opioids. Clonidine is now approved by the US Food and Drug Administration (FDA) for epidural administration and its intrathecal equivalent dosage is 50 to 900 μg per day. It should be carefully titrated because it can cause considerable hypotension (most severe in dosage range of 400 to 570 μg per day).

Other investigational drugs are used intrathecally, and their use is supported by excellent results in clinical trials. Somatostatin seems to be particularly beneficial for treatment of cancer pain. For neuropathic and nociceptive pain, investigational drugs include calcium channel blockers (SNX-111), acetylcholinesterase (neostigmine), NMDA receptor antagonist (ketamine), GABA-A receptor agonists (midazolam), and GABA-B receptor agonists (baclofen). Many other intrathecally administered analgesics have proven their efficacy in animal research, pending final testing in human trials.

5. Complications and Side Effects

Medication-related side effects and complications of neuraxial opiates include respiratory depression, pruritus, nausea, vomiting, urinary retention, reduced libido, edema with weight gain, and constipation. **Respiratory depression** can occur immediately following opioid administration or with several hours' delay; it is much more frequent in opioid-naïve patients. The factors increasing the risk for respiratory depression are advanced age, high opioid dose, and concomitant use of baclofen, benzodiazepines, and sedatives. Monitoring the vital signs and pulse oximetry are mandatory following initiation of intrathecal opioid infusion.

Pruritus, nausea, and vomiting usually occur with initiation of intrathecal opioid bolus administration and can precede the onset of pain relief. These side effects can be prevented by more gradual opioid dose increase. The incidence of **urinary retention** ranges from 40% to 80% and is not dose-dependent. It occurs most often in men with an already enlarged prostate. The cholinomimetic drugs, terazosin or carbachol, can be effective in treating urinary retention. **Hormonal abnormalities** are reported with intrathecal opioid administration. Serum concentrations of lipids, estrogens, androgens, and IGF-1, and 24-hour monitoring of urinary cortisol level should be done in these patients. There is 3% to 5% incidence of **decreased libido** in patients with intrathecal opioid therapy. Persistent decreased libido may require hormonal replacement. Approximately 5% to 10% of patients experience weight gain and edema, which is not dose-dependent.

Surgical complications include infection at pump insertion site, which may require complete hardware removal. Symptoms of infection are pain at insertion site, local increase in temperature, and edema. Antibiotics should be started after wound cultures (by aspiration) are obtained. **Seroma** at the insertion site is usually benign and does not require revision. Necrosis and skin perforations can also occur and should be surgically treated. **Meningitis** presents with stiff neck, fever, and meningeal signs. The CSF can be obtained from the pump for cultures and cell count. **Granuloma** formation at the catheter tip is a rare complication, potentially leading to cord compression. MRI of the spinal cord is indicated if neurologic symptoms occur in these patients. **Bleeding** at the pump site usually spontaneously resolves, although it can increase the incidence of infection. **Epidural hematoma** can lead to spinal cord compression. A **CSF leak** occurs after almost any intrathecal pump placement. However, if substantial, it can lead to severe **postdural puncture headache**. If conservative therapy fails, headache can be treated with an epidural blood patch. However, placement of the blood patch should be performed under fluoroscopic guidance to avoid the risk of intrathecal catheter damage.

Hardware complications most often involve the catheter and rarely the pump. **Catheter** kinking, disconnection, dislodgement, breaks, and migration can occur. The withdrawal symptoms and loss of analgesia are signs of inadequate drug delivery and warrant further investigation. Although the catheter is radiopaque and can be seen on fluoroscopy, it should be tested with nonionic contrast bolus. Before administering as a bolus, the medication should be aspirated from the catheter dead space to avoid overdose. This can be accomplished through the pump side port. If the pump does not have a side port, it should be emptied, filled by radiolabeled tracer, and imaged.

Pump failures also can occur. Torsion of the pump within the pocket with subsequent catheter kinking can be prevented by adequate pump anchoring. The most serious technique-related complication is drug overdose, which is caused by filling the pump through the side port. In case this occurs, CSF should be partially replaced with saline and the patient immediately transferred to the intensive care unit. Intrathecal naloxone should be administered. Other mechanical pump failures include battery depletion and internal pump failures. One should follow detailed manufacturer recommendations and testing protocols to rule out internal pump failure.

SELECTED READINGS

Hord D, Cohen S, Ahmed S, et al. The predictive value of sympathetic block for the success of spinal cord stimulation. *Neurosurgery* 2003;53(3):626–632; discussion 632–633.

Kemler MA, Barendse GAM, van Kleef M, et al. Spinal cord stimulation in patients with chronic reflex sympathetic dystrophy. *N Engl J Med* 2000;343(9):618–624.

North RB, Kidd DH, Zahurak M, et al. Spinal cord stimulation for chronic intractable pain: two decades' experience. *Neurosurgery* 1993;32:384–395.

Sheacy S, Mortimer JT, Reswick JB. Electrical inhibition of pain by stimulation of dorsal columns: a preliminary report. *Anesth Analg.* 1967;46:489–491.

Stojanovic M. Stimulation methods for neuropathic pain control. Current pain and headache review. *Current Science Inc* 2001;3(2):131–137.

Waldman SD. *Interventional pain management*, 2nd ed. Philadelphia, PA: WB Saunders, 2001.

Neurosurgical Pain Management

Ramin Amirnovin, G. Rees Cosgrove, and
Emad N. Eskandar

It is easier to find men who will volunteer to die, than to find those who are willing to endure pain with patience.
—*Julius Caesar*

I. GENERAL CONSIDERATIONS

1. Timing of Neurosurgical Interventions

All patients should undergo a reasonable trial of conservative therapy before any neurosurgical intervention is discussed. Specifically, oral analgesics, parenteral agents, and short-term anesthetic interventions (e.g., local blocks and temporary spinal infusion catheters) should be tried as preliminary treatments. Enhancing the quality of life of a patient with chronic pain is paramount, and when it is clear that the overall goals of pain management are not being met by less invasive treatment, surgical approaches should be considered. Early neurosurgical intervention can optimize function and can greatly improve pain control during the final months of life in patients with terminal cancer. Reserving surgical treatment for only the most debilitated patients reduces its functional benefit and increases the surgical risk. Unfortunately, there are no hard and fast rules about timing for surgical interventions, and individual clinical situations must be carefully assessed.

2. Augmentative Versus Ablative Procedures

Neurosurgical approaches to chronic pain are grouped into two categories: **augmentative** (where a device or substance is implanted) and **ablative** (where neural tissue is destroyed).

Augmentative techniques have the advantage of being reversible so that they can be discontinued if they prove ineffective, without loss of function. However, such procedures suffer from technical problems inherent in the infusion pump and stimulator systems. The patients undergoing these procedures also require more frequent follow-up visits. Ablative procedures are characterized by the finality of neural tissue destruction and, hence, the potential loss of function. Furthermore, most of these procedures are less successful in long-term pain control than augmentative methods are. By evaluating the patient's needs in the light of the risks and benefits, one can choose the proper type of procedure for a specific patient. For instance, in pain from malignancy, the patient's life span is limited, and, hence, a definitive ablative procedure may be more appropriate.

3. Scope of Neurosurgical Manipulations

Neurosurgical interventions for pain can be directed at the peripheral nerves, spinal cord, or the brain. When selecting an intervention, it is important to balance the potential benefit against the risk of loss of function. Also, the technical requirements of the procedure, postoperative management issues, and the general condition of the patient must be considered. Many pain complaints can be addressed by a neurosurgical intervention, but the important question is: At what cost?

4. Variability of Approach

Although algorithms exist for choosing specific procedures designed to relieve specific complaints, each patient merits careful evaluation before a procedure is suggested. This approach prevents unrealistic expectations, while maintaining flexibility in designing a course of therapy suited to the individual. A given neurosurgical procedure used to treat identical complaints in different patients can produce vastly different results. Hence, we caution against a rigid approach to neurosurgical intervention. A multidisciplinary approach to chronic pain is the best way to individualize treatment and optimize results.

II. APPROPRIATE SELECTION AND EVALUATION OF THE PATIENT WITH NEUROSURGICAL PAIN

1. Medical Workup and Treatment

Before considering any procedure for pain control, it is extremely important to exclude an underlying treatable medical condition. Unrecognized causative pathology or correctable structural lesions must be excluded before any functional neurosurgical procedure is undertaken.

All candidates for neurosurgery require the usual preoperative evaluations to ensure safety during anesthesia and surgery. Patients at high risk for surgery may be eager to undergo an intervention but may be unable to withstand the physiologic stress of surgery. Medical optimization of the preoperative status may require manipulations that are not in accord with a patient's wishes or with the approach of the care team. Such situations can be avoided in patients in whom it is difficult to control pain with a medical regimen by the early involvement of a neurosurgeon.

2. Malignant Versus Benign Pain

The common differentiation between pain of malignant and that of benign origin is clinically useful. In general, ablative approaches are more suitable for pain of malignant origin, when quality of life may be paramount. Ablative surgery for pain of benign origin, except for some specific conditions such as trigeminal neuralgia (TGN), is fraught with difficulties, especially when factors such as disability status, concurrent litigation, and psychosocial status dominate the clinical picture.

A second, more practical consideration is that patients who have benign pain and a normal life expectancy must be taken care of for decades after their surgical procedure. For example, the maintenance requirements for both the technical and emotional support of every patient can be important after implantation of chronic stimulators in the spinal canal or drug infusion systems. The maintenance requirements are not major considerations for patients with progressive malignant disease.

3. Multidisciplinary Team Approach

The comprehensive pain service, with its neurologic, anesthesiologic, psychiatric, nursing, and social service components, remains the best resource for ensuring optimal patient care. Neurosurgeons who elect to treat patients with chronic pain without this support network may find that the care of their patients is compromised. Similarly, the treatment of chronic pain is significantly hampered without the neurosurgeon's input. Early involvement of the neurosurgeon with patients who respond poorly to conservative measures, along with a careful evaluation of each patient's needs and status, and deliberate review of all nonsurgical and surgical options, will generally produce the best results.

II. SPECIFIC NEUROSURGICAL PROCEDURES

1. Ablative Procedures

In the past decade, most ablative procedures have been replaced by augmentative procedures. We only discuss the ablative procedures that are still in use.

(i) Peripheral Ablative Procedures

Peripheral nerve lesions in the extremities can result in **deafferentation pain**, but the procedure of choice for these **appendicular mononeuralgias** is chronic stimulation (as described in subsequent text) rather than ablation. In contrast, ablation provides good results for craniofacial pain syndromes, specifically TGN and glossopharyngeal neuralgia (GPN).

In treating TGN in an older or frail patient, the **ablation of the trigeminal nerve** yields acceptable results given the limited life-expectancy of this population. Three methods can be used to ablate the **trigeminal nerve**. The first two methods involve the percutaneous introduction of a needle (under fluoroscopic guidance) into the foramen ovale. Then, a heat-producing radiofrequency electrode or the injection of alcohol is used to produce a lesion on the trigeminal ganglion. These methods yield a 70% to 80% success rate at 6 years and a less impressive 30% success rate at 12 years. The third method of lesioning the trigeminal ganglion is by radiosurgery. Application of 80–Gy radiation to the proximal trigeminal nerve reportedly yields a success rate of 70% at 1 year, which declines to 56% by 5 years. Unlike the percutaneous radiofrequency or alcohol lesions, the effect of radiosurgery is not immediate, but rather takes 2 to 6 months to occur. The ablative procedures for TGN share a low rate of **anesthesia dolorosa** (pain despite sensory loss), which is the most common complication. For younger, less frail patients, microvascular decompression (MVD) can provide a higher long-term success rate (see subsequent text).

Currently, the first-line therapy for GPN is MVD, but, in patients in whom this fails, a craniotomy is occasionally performed for **sectioning of cranial nerve IX (glossopharyngeal) and the upper division of X (vagus)**. Outcomes have not been systematically studied because the procedure is rarely performed.

Dorsal rhizotomy (sectioning of the dorsal root) was one of the first operations used for pain control, and, although generally effective, it is also accompanied by sensory loss in the associated dermatome. Extensive dorsal root sectioning in an extremity leads to a useless limb and is not recommended. Partial or incomplete posterior rhizotomies have been employed for chronic pain of the thorax and painful spasticity, and have been especially useful in **occipital neuralgia**. The procedure provides pain control in 70% of the patients immediately after surgery, but only 28% of the patients receive long-term benefits. This difference is felt to be due to the poor localization of the involved nerve roots. Recent studies have confirmed that pain control can be improved by using the somatosensory evoked potentials (SSEP) during the procedure to guide lesioning of the correct dorsal root(s).

(ii) Spinal Cord Ablative Procedures

Deafferentation pain from brachial plexus root avulsion or spinal cord injury have been successfully treated with an open operation for **lesioning of the dorsal root entry zone** (DREZ). Small thermocoagulation lesions are made in the posterior spinal cord in the DREZ at multiple levels, interrupting nociceptive pathways in the Lissauer tract or destroying neurons of the **substantia gelatinosa**. Eighty percent of the patients achieve complete pain control immediately after the surgery, but only 60% of the patients have good pain control after 10 years. Patients with pain from spinal cord injury are relieved of the pain only at the level of injury. Pain below the level of cord injury is resistant to this procedure. Similarly, DREZ lesioning in phantom limb pain and postherpetic neuralgia has produced unsatisfactory results.

Bilateral pain, such as that seen with visceral pain from abdominal or pelvic tumors, was previously addressed by a *ventral* **commissural myelotomy**. Recent discovery of a distinct medial dorsal column pathway carrying pain from the viscera has led to a new, less risky procedure known as a **midline punctuate myelotomy**. In this open procedure, a lesion is made in the medial 2 mm of the dorsal columns bilaterally to a depth of 5 mm. Although only a handful of case reports exist, no major neurosurgical complications have been reported, and all patients have good pain control immediately after the procedure. Because the procedure has only been used in the malignant pain population, long-term follow-up is not available.

Interrupting the ascending **lateral spinothalamic tract** by either a percutaneous or an open **anterolateral cordotomy** has been used successfully for pain of malignant origin for many years. As with all ablations in the spinal cord, the risk for functional loss is real. Although almost all patients suffer a transient leg weakness from this procedure, only 5% of the patients have weakness in the leg after 1 month. Lower-extremity pain is most easily approached by open thoracic **cordotomy**, and bilateral lesions can be performed. Bilateral **cordotomy** increases the risk of neurologic deficits, especially autonomic disturbance. **Cordotomy** at the cervical levels above the diaphragmatic input on one side and below it on the other (i.e., C3 and C6) can avoid complex postoperative respiratory difficulties (Ondine curse). For reasons that are unclear, pain will often return 1 to 2 years after **cordotomy** of either type. Repeat **cordotomy** at a higher level can be performed, although this is rarely needed if the procedure is restricted to patients with a limited life expectancy.

(iii) Central Ablative Procedures

Given the technical advances of magnetic resonance imaging (MRI) and computerized tomographic (CT) imaging, accurate lesions of nociceptive pathways in the **mesencephalon, diencephalon**, and cortex are possible. The general approach to deep brain lesioning is similar to that of deep brain stimulation (see subsequent text). An electrode is stereotactically placed into the target site. The area is stimulated as the electrode position is adjusted. Once the desired effect is achieved, a lesion is created.

Lesioning the medial thalamus **(thalamotomy)** can provide unilateral or, in some cases, bilateral pain relief. However, long-term results are disappointing, and hence, **thalamotomy** is reserved for pain of malignant origin. A procedure for destroying the **cingulate** *gyrus* and the bundle in the frontal lobe **(cingulotomy)** also has been used in cases of diffuse chronic pain, malignant pain, or pain associated with depression. Approximately 50% of patients report good pain control after **cingulotomy**, but most have an early return of pain within several months. A recent report suggests that this recurrent pain eventually remits within a year and that 56% of patients are pain-free at a 9-year follow-up.

2. Augmentative Procedures

Augmentative procedures include the implantation of stimulating systems and chronic analgesic infusion systems. The stimulating systems are all similar in that they have an electrode in relation to the nerve, spinal cord, or deep brain, which is then stimulated by a subcutaneously implanted generator unit. All the augmentative procedures require more operative time than comparable ablative procedures. These procedures also require more follow-up visits to optimize the stimulation or infusion parameters.

(i) Peripheral Nerve Stimulation

Mononeuropathic pain is best treated by chronic stimulation, particularly when the pain is due to nerve injury. Peripheral nerve stimulation has been tried for other sources of pain (e.g., cancer and complex regional pain disorder), with only a 25% response rate. By contrast, 85% of patients with neuropathic pain from peripheral nerve injury will have good pain control by PNS. The implanted electrode is a sheet electrode, which is placed proximal to the site of nerve injury. Most surgeons perform a trial period of stimulation through an externalized lead before implantation of the permanent generator. The procedure has no major complications.

(ii) Spinal Cord Stimulation

Spinal cord stimulation is frequently used for treating chronic pain, particularly of nonmalignant origin, because of its reversibility. This technique remains popular despite the high cost of the hardware and its maintenance. Stimulators can be inserted percutaneously or during an open procedure. Unfortunately, no specific markers have emerged for the "best responders" to SCS. The major indications include failed back syndrome, neuropathic pain from peripheral nerve injury, complex regional pain syndrome, lower-extremity pain of vascular origin, and more recently, persistent angina pectoris (in end-stage coronary atherosclerosis). Although evidence suggests that SCS induces vasodilation by autonomic modulation (thereby causing pain relief in angina and peripheral vascular disease), its exact mechanism remains unclear. The immediate success rate for all indications except angina is 60% to 70%. Failure of pain control for patients without angina, when it occurs, is usually in the first year after surgery, but 50% of patients have good pain control at 7- and 15-year follow-up. Angina is immediately improved in 80% of patients, but long-term follow-up is not yet available. Spinal cord stimulation is described in more detail in Chapter 13.

(iii) Deep Brain Stimulation

Deep brain stimulation is only used by those who have an interest in the procedure and are committed to the treatment of patients by using stimulators. Under stereotactic MRI guidance, an electrode is introduced into either the **periventricular gray matter or the ventroposterolateral/ventroposteromedial (VPL/VPM) thalamic nuclei**. DBS works best for failed back syndrome, nociceptive pain states, and peripheral neuropathy, but it has *not* worked well for postherpetic neuralgia or for pain from thalamic or cord injury. Initially, relief is seen in 60% to 80% of patients, but only 50% of patients have long-term benefits. The best use of DBS is in treating chronic pain refractory to all other approaches in patients with a long life expectancy.

(iv) Motor Cortex Stimulation

Recent experimental results have shown that motor-sensory cortex stimulation (MCS) can inhibit nociceptive dorsal horn and brain stem neurons. These findings have inspired a new method of controlling pain. Motor cortex stimulation involves the placement of a sheet electrode on the surface of the **precentral gyrus**, using MRI and electrophysiological guidance. When used for central pain and trigeminal neuropathy, motor cortex stimulation is 40% to 70% effective. Unfortunately, there are currently no reliable outcome predictors; therefore the therapy should be reserved (as with DBS) for patients with pain refractory to all other approaches. Complications are similar to those of a minor craniotomy.

(v) Implantable Infusion Systems

The intrathecal infusion of opiate or local anesthetic solutions is an accepted and valuable treatment of cancer pain and selected patients with chronic nonterminal pain. An intrathecal catheter is introduced using a small superficial incision and the catheter is tunneled to the abdomen, where it is connected to a pump in a subcutaneous "pocket." The pumps can be programmed for complex patterns of infusion, and the infused mixture is replenished percutaneously. The pumps require battery changes approximately every 3 years, and mechanical failure of the system is common but not well quantified. The major complications include the risk of overdose and allergic reactions to the mixture. In patients with cancer, infusion systems provide an 80% success rate, but the long-term success for nonmalignant pain is uncertain. Because excellent pain relief in terminal illness is achieved from this minor surgery, the method is likely underused. This treatment option is described in more detail in Chapter 13.

3. Other Neurosurgical Interventions

(i) Microvascular Decompression

TGN, GPN, and hemifacial spasm are likely caused by nerve injury from vascular compression at the respective nerve's DREZ. The offending vessels for TGN and GPN are usually the **superior cerebellar artery** (SCA) and the **posterior inferior cerebellar artery** (PICA), respectively. In an MVD, a suboccipital craniotomy is used to move small vessels away from the DREZ of the appropriate cranial nerve and to place a Teflon sponge to maintain separation of the two structures. Immediate pain control can be achieved in as many as 80% patients for TGN and 95% for GPN. In a 10-year follow-up, the success rates were 70% for TGN and 80% for GPN. In experienced centers, 5% of patients will have cranial nerve **(trigeminal—V, glossopharyngeal—IX, or acoustic—VIII)** deficits, 1% to 2% will have cerebrospinal fluid (CSF) leaks, and less than 1% will have major complications (e.g., brain stem infarcts). Given the favorable outcomes, MVD has become the first-line therapy for refractory TGN and GPN. In patients who are too frail to undergo an MVD, a peripheral ablation procedure (see preceding text) is performed.

(ii) Sympathectomy

Complex regional pain syndromes are increasingly treated with spinal cord stimulation (see preceding text). **Sympathectomy** remains an alternative ablative option for frail patients or for those who do not respond to stimulation. **Sympathectomy** is now almost exclusively performed by anesthesiologists via percutaneous approaches. The T1 level should be avoided to prevent the complication of Horner syndrome. For specific cases, surgical **sympathectomy** may be necessary owing to technical difficulties. More than 90% of patients achieve a cure with **sympathectomy**. The major complications of the procedure are compensatory hyperhidrosis in 52% of patients and new neuropathic pain in 25%.

IV. SUMMARY AND CONCLUSIONS

Although the surgical treatment of chronic pain should always follow a reasonably exhaustive trial of conservative medical approaches, there is a role for surgical intervention in many patients with cancer and chronic pain. The neurosurgeon's participation in the overall treatment plan of the pain patient will provide an opportunity for surgical intervention early in the patient's course before the disease worsens or the frustration with lack of progress renders neurosurgical intervention difficult or impossible. A judicious approach by the referring pain specialist, as well as frank discussions with the patient, family, and care providers is likely to yield the best results for a patient who has not responded to medical management. Unfortunately, multiple factors and individual variability still render the surgical outcome for each patient somewhat difficult to predict.

As with all chronic pain patients, the entire multidisciplinary pain service should take responsibility for preoperative and postoperative care. No specific neurosurgical intervention will totally relieve persistent pain; it should only be considered as a single therapeutic option in an overall treatment plan. The management of chronic pain can be greatly improved by timely, selective neurosurgical intervention, and the intervention may provide an excellent quality of life in the face of intercurrent disease and chronic pain.

SELECTED READINGS

Becker R, Gatscher S, Sure U, et al. The punctate midline myelotomy concept for visceral cancer pain control—case report and review of the literature. *Acta Neurochir Suppl* 2002;79:77–78.

Burchiel KJ, ed. *Pain surgery*. New York: Thieme Medical Publishers, 1999.

Falci S, Best L, Bayles R, et al. Dorsal root entry zone microcoagulation for spinal cord injury–related central pain: operative intramedullary electrophysiological guidance and clinical outcome. *J Neurosurg* 2002;97:193–200.

Furlan AD, Mailis A, Papagapiou M, et al. Are we paying a high price for surgical sympathectomy? A systematic literature review of late complications causalgia: a meta-analysis of the literature. *J Pain* 2000;1:245–257.

Giller CA. The neurosurgical treatment of pain. *Arch Neurol* 2003; 60:1537–1540.

Gybels JM, Sweet WH. Neurosurgical treatment of persistent pain. In: Gildenberg PL, ed. *Pain and headache*, Vol. 11. Basel, Switzerland: Karger, 1989.

Hassantash SA, Afrakhteh M, Maier RV. Causalgia: a meta-analysis of the literature. *Arch Surg* 2003;138:1226–1231.

Hitotsumatsu T, Matsushima T, Inoue T. Microvascular decompression for treatment of trigeminal neuralgia, hemifacial spasm, and glossopharyngeal neuralgia: three surgical approach variations: technical note. *Neurosurgery* 2003;53:1436–1441; discussion 1442–1433.

Jessurun GA, DeJongste MJ, Blanksma PK. Current views on neurostimulation in the treatment of cardiac ischemic syndromes. *Pain* 1996;66:109–116.

Kemler MA, Barendse GA, van Kleef M, et al. Spinal cord stimulation in patients with chronic reflex sympathetic dystrophy. *N Engl J Med* 2000;343:618–624.

Kumar K, Toth C, Nath RK. Deep brain stimulation for intractable pain: a 15-year experience. *Neurosurgery* 1997;40:736–746.

Lahuerta J, Bowsher D, Lipton S, et al. Percutaneous cervical cordotomy: a review of 181 operations on 146 patients with a study on the location of "pain fibers" in the C-2 spinal cord segment of 29 cases. *J Neurosurg* 1994;80:975–985.

Levy RM. Deep brain stimulation for the treatment of intractable pain. *Neurosurg Clin N Am* 2003;14:389–399.

Long DM. The current status of electrical stimulation of the nervous system for the relief of chronic pain. *Surg Neurol* 1998;49:142–144.

Lopez BC, Hamlyn PJ, Zakrzewska JM. Systematic review of ablative neurosurgical techniques for the treatment of trigeminal neuralgia. *Neurosurgery* 2004;54:973–983.

Mailis A, Furlan A. Sympathectomy for neuropathic pain. *Cochrane Database Syst Rev* 2003(2):CD002918.

Meyerson BA. Neurosurgical approaches to pain treatment. *Acta Anaesthesiol Scand* 2001;45:1108–1113.

Patel A, Kassam A, Horowitz M, et al. Microvascular decompression in the management of glossopharyngeal neuralgia: analysis of 217 cases. *Neurosurgery* 2002;50:705–710.

Sampson JH, Grossi PM, Asaoka K, et al. Microvascular decompression for glossopharyngeal neuralgia: long-term effectiveness and complication avoidance. *Neurosurgery* 2004;54:884–890.

Schmidek HH, Sweet WH. *Operative neurosurgical techniques: indications, methods, and results*, 3rd ed. Philadelphia, PA: WB Saunders, 1995.

Stojanovic MP. Stimulation methods for neuropathic pain control. *Curr Pain Headache Rep* 2001;5:130–137.

Tasker RR. Neurosurgical and neuroaugmentative intervention. In: Patt RB, ed. *Cancer pain*. Philadelphia, PA: JB Lippincott Co, 1993.

Tasker RR. The recurrence of pain after neurosurgical procedures. *Qual Life Res* 1994;3:S43–S49.

Turner JA, Loeser JD, Bell KG. Spinal cord stimulation for chronic low back pain: a systematic literature synthesis. *Neurosurgery* 1995;37:1088–1095.

Wall PD, Melzack R. *Textbook of pain*. Edinburgh, UK: Churchill Livingstone, 1989.

Wilkinson HA, Davidson KM, Davidson RI. Bilateral anterior cingulotomy for chronic noncancer pain. *Neurosurgery* 1999;45:1129–1134.

Psychological Assessment and Behavioral Treatment of Chronic Pain

Ronald J. Kulich and Lainie Andrew

The pain of the mind is worse than the pain of the body.
—*Publilius Syrus, 1st century* BC

I. INTRODUCTION

The role of psychological factors in chronic pain is well established, and minimum standards of care require that physicians address psychosocial factors when managing chronic pain. The overall effectiveness of treatment is often determined by attention to psychosocial issues. Studies have demonstrated that early psychological intervention has a considerable effect on a patient's reported pain level, ability to cope, activity levels, return to work, and compliance with the medical regimen.

Although there is inherent wisdom in seeking early psychological or psychiatric consultation for complex chronic pain patients, the role of the primary or pain physician should not be underestimated. The treating physician can effectively reinforce positive mood, coping skills, function, and compliance with treatment. Alternatively, the naïve physician may unwittingly reinforce somatic overconcern, helplessness, disability, and lack of patient-perceived control over pain. Although participation of the psychologist or psychiatrist may be necessary, the role of the treating physician and other team members remains pivotal.

Comorbid psychological factors commonly addressed in the literature include anxiety, depression, somatic overconcern, sleep disorder, disability, and substance abuse. Although the exact incidence is debatable, it seems that psychiatric symptoms are present in 50% to 80% of patients with chronic pain. This rate is consistently higher than that reported in the general medical population. There is a growing body of literature supporting the existence of "vulnerabilities" or risk factors that result in a higher likelihood of developing disabling chronic pain. Premorbid vulnerabilities include a history of **major depression or anxiety disorder, somatoform disorder, substance use disorder, and post-traumatic stress disorder**. Poor employment history and job dissatisfaction also have been shown to be predictive of disabling chronic pain. Although the debate persists about the exact role of premorbid psychiatric symptoms in precipitating and maintaining chronic pain, there is little doubt that persistent pain, frustration with ineffective treatment, financial hardship caused by job loss, and other concomitant stressors substantially contribute to the development of psychological symptoms.

II. COMORBID PSYCHIATRIC SYMPTOMS AND DISEASE

1. Anxiety

Anxiety is the most common response to acute pain, and anxiety symptoms often persist when pain becomes chronic. Furthermore, anxiety serves to increase pain perception. Assessment of anxiety can be complicated by drug effects, including withdrawal from opioids or benzodiazepines. Anxiety symptoms commonly occur in specific situations related to fear of activity, injury, work, or social interaction. Although episodic disabling anxiety has been reported to occur in up to 80% of patients with chronic pain, base rates of anxiety in the general population are also high. It has been reported that, each day, primary care physicians see approximately one patient with an anxiety disorder and that approximately 30 million Americans suffer disabling anxiety symptoms.

Particular attention should be paid to patients with a diagnosis of **posttraumatic stress disorder**, a condition that often coexists with substance use disorders, depression, and personality disorder. Patients with early childhood abuse histories and/or histories of other serious emotional and physical trauma require formal psychological assessment to maximize adherence to treatment and to improve outcome.

2. Depression

Chronic pain and depression are commonly associated with each other, with a reported 50% incidence of major depression within 5 years of developing a chronic pain disorder. Mortality is high, and suicide has been reported in 10% to 15% of the patients who had prolonged pain and depression. Less severe symptoms of depression have been reported in 80% of the patients with chronic pain. Although it has been argued that studies overestimate depression in the chronic pain population because of an overlap in the symptoms of pain and depression, conservative estimates still exceed the rates in the general population. Investigations have failed to support arguments that improvement in depression necessarily results in improvement in the affective component of pain, but most practitioners agree that adequate assessment and aggressive treatment of depression benefits the patient with chronic pain.

3. Sleep Disorders

As with anxiety and depression, sleep disorder symptoms may have multiple causes, including drug side effects. Serious sleep disorders such as sleep apnea can result from a combination of weight gain and polypharmacy. Frequently, the patient complains of "pain waking me from sleep." However, as with depression, attempts to reduce pain often fail to ameliorate a functional sleep disorder. Depression, anxiety, and poor sleep habits remain the most common cause of sleep disorder in patients with chronic pain. The patient may nap throughout the day and may escape to the bedroom to "rest" during periods of severe pain. Spending many hours lying in bed "trying" to fall asleep complicates the problem, and the patient's typical sleep schedule remains disrupted by lack of a systematic daily schedule. The typical decrease in physical activity because of chronic pain further compromises sleep. Sleep medications, intended for short-term use, often make the situation worse. Sleep disorders have been shown to exacerbate musculoskeletal pain and contribute to affective disorder. Whether organic or functional, the nature of the sleep complaint requires thorough investigation. Even when sleep disorders are managed pharmacologically, they require concurrent aggressive behavioral treatment.

4. Somatization

Somatization presents another vexing problem for the physician treating pain. Although most patients may not meet formal psychiatric diagnostic criteria for **somatization disorder**, a thorough assessment may reveal other somatic symptoms dating back many years. Physicians sometimes restrict the focus of their evaluation to the primary presenting problem, often missing a history of multiple somatic complaints. In some cases, patients may intentionally minimize the complexity of their somatic history, whereas a thorough review may reveal a more complex picture. For example, review of the earlier record may reveal a history of fibromyalgia, irritable bowel syndrome, multiple whiplash injuries, noncardiac chest pain, chronic tension–type headache, and/or various pseudoneurologic symptoms reported to other physicians. The history of these complaints can predict a problematic treatment course.

It has been suggested that somatization or "symptom magnification" sometimes occurs because of visits to multiple health care providers who offer conflicting messages about the etiology of the patient's pain, as well as because of the frustration associated with multiple prior ineffectual treatment trials. The patient may report transient improvements with earlier treatments, with social reinforcement of complaints by family members or health care providers. Reports of improvement or deterioration may not be related to the actual effect of the intervention, whereas the physician may become unwittingly convinced that the treatment has been effective. The patient then seeks repeated trials of new treatments, with the patient and physician being reinforced after seeing transient gains with each effort. "Disease conviction," wherein the patients themselves maintain a steadfast commitment to maintaining their somatic preoccupation, is also described.

Another construct addressed in the literature is termed "catastrophizing," wherein the patient obsessively focuses on the myriad of possible negative factors associated with his or her physical condition. The patient with a marked somatic focus cannot accept that there may not be a physical "cure"; "acceptance" of symptoms, by contrast, may be associated with a positive outcome.

5. Malingering

The concept of "**malingering**" is different from somatization. In the case of malingering, the patient is intentionally feigning symptoms to achieve some gain, often financial gain. Malingering can coexist with documented physical and psychiatric conditions. Although physicians may attest to inconsistencies in the patient's examination or medical record, they do not always recognize intentional feigning of symptoms. Current evidence does not support the validity of certain strength testing devices and structured interview protocols that were developed in an attempt to identify malingering in the individuals with chronic pain. The validity of these tests in the individuals with chronic pain is questionable, and, currently, there are documented court cases challenging their use. Patients may lie to their physician, but the underlying factors are likely to be complex, and the correct response on the part of the physician is uncertain.

6. Personality Disorders

Although there are numerous types of personality disorders in the standard classification system, no psychiatric disorder presents a greater challenge to a pain physician than **borderline personality disorder**. Coexisting **substance abuse disorder, posttraumatic stress disorder**, and depression have been widely documented. Compliance issues often become a major theme of the relationship with the treating physician. Patients may loudly praise the skills of physician, whereas the accolades invariably change when the physician fails to meet the patient's perceived needs. The "relationship" between the physician and patient becomes the "problem," and the patient may respond with anger and with repeated requests for dose increases and changes in medication. The patients may attempt to enlist relatives and other health care providers to plead their case and arrive for unscheduled visits expecting to be rapidly accommodated. Complaints about other providers are commonplace, and there often is an effort to cause dissention among a treatment team. From a diagnostic perspective, these patients can be identified by their alternating displays of effusive praise for some providers and vehement complaints about the standards of care and medical ethics of others. Such patients are best managed by early clarification of the physician's circumscribed role and by deference to the primary care physician with respect to coordination of care. Interdisciplinary assessment may aid effective patient management. In addition, concurrent

CAGE-D

C   Have you ever thought you should CUT DOWN on your drinking
     or drug use?

A   Have you ever felt ANNOYED by others' criticism of your drinking
     or drug use?

G   Have you ever felt GUILTY about your drinking or drug use?

E   Do you have a morning EYE OPENER (start your day with
     alcohol or drugs)?

Figure 1.   Cage Questionnaire-D.

treatment by a psychologist or psychiatrist is often needed. In fact, these patients can be effectively treated in a structured psychiatric program, whereas a traditional pain center setting often fails to meet their needs.

7. Substance Abuse

Strong evidence supports the argument that current or past substance abuse predicts poor treatment outcome for a wide range of medical conditions, including chronic pain. Substance abuse occurs in the patients with chronic pain, with reported incidence of 3% to 19%. Studies employing toxic screening or other cross-validation assessments suggest a particularly high incidence in the patients with chronic pain. Physicians have been found to be particularly poor at assessing substance abuse and, therefore, may underestimate the problem. For example, a large study by the Center for Addiction and Substance Abuse found that only 16.9% of physicians were "very prepared" to spot illegal drug use and that only 30.2% were "very prepared" to spot prescription drug abuse. Furthermore, 46.6% of the physicians found it difficult to discuss prescription drug abuse. Forty-three percent of patients reported that their physician did not diagnose their substance abuse problem, 84.9% admitted lying to their physician, and 54.4% had difficulty discussing the issue because they did not want to stop using drugs or alcohol. In view of the poor performance of physicians in assessing substance abuse, formal substance abuse screening, including urine toxicology, should be considered a crucial component of the evaluation. Many pain physicians also employ self-report measures such as the four-item CAGE Questionnaire, which markedly improves their ability to identify the presence of a substance abuse. Figure 1 shows a modified version for assessing drug use. (See also Chapters 31 and 36 for questionnaires that assist in assessing substance abuse.)

III. PSYCHOLOGICAL ASSESSMENT

1. The Diagnostic Interview

The diagnostic interview is the basis of a thorough evaluation, although patient report is inherently flawed. Although there may be no intent to deceive, patients often report only what they consider important and what they believe the physician considers important. Accuracy can be improved by utilizing information from the past medical record. For example, a patient may provide more accurate information when a specific life event is referenced, such as asking the patient to describe a specific holiday. Table 1 lists recommended psychosocial content areas for inclusion in the evaluation.

Psychosocial histories are often cursory or neglected because of discomfort on the part of the clinician and patient, rather than time constraints. An explanation of the rationale for psychosocial questions can minimize patient anxiety. Patients are often relieved to acknowledge the serious impact of the pain on their lives. Some patients, however, become markedly defensive or confrontational with respect to discussion of psychosocial issues. In that case, the physician should persist in a matter-of-fact manner and should consider further consultation. Dealing with contention during an initial evaluation is preferable to confronting mediating psychosocial factors once treatment is underway.

Some practitioners prefer to conduct components of the initial diagnostic evaluation in the presence of a family member of the patient because the family members often provide additional information. An exception would be if spousal abuse were suspected. Family members should not, however, be used as interpreters, and professional interpreters should always be used if language is an issue.

Table 1.   Chronic pain interview content

Mental status including behavioral observation of pain behavior

Presenting pain complaints and other current/past somatic complaints

Precipitants and consequences of pain, for example, assistance from others, missed work

Prior treatments and patient's assessment of gain, attitudes toward earlier health care providers

Prior psychiatric Hx/substance abuse Hx including smoking, illicit drugs, compliance/problems with prescription drugs

Current anxiety symptoms including fear of activities or pain, Hx of severe emotional or physical trauma

Current depression symptoms including suicidal ideation and sleep disorder Sx

Recreational pursuits/activities of daily living

Work Hx including patient report job demands, periods of disability

Litigation including status of claims

Social supports including spouse support for activity or disability behavior

Patient expectations repain treatment and perception of his or her role

Hx, history; Sx, symptom.

The role of the family and social supporters cannot be underestimated. Although the level of social support generally predicts a positive outcome, the nature of family support can also seriously complicate treatment. Early studies demonstrated the effect of spouse attentiveness or "solicitousness" on pain complaints and pain behaviors and that the mere presence of a spouse can result in physiological changes. Some spouses unwittingly reinforce disability behavior by being oversolicitous about pain and disability complaints. A spouse may be more content to have the patient disabled and increasingly isolated because these changes give the spouse greater empowerment in the relationship. A family also may sabotage treatment by discouraging compliance and reinforcing worry about the patient's symptoms and related treatments. Determining a family's attitudes may help predict failure or may provide an opportunity to intervene to achieve treatment success.

2. Self-report Instruments

(i) Pain Ratings

Although early operant pain rehabilitation programs made the point of focusing on pain behavior and avoiding direct assessment of pain, most patients and pain clinicians still judge success by some measure of self-reported pain relief. The common standard has been the 10-point rating scale. More complex rating and classification strategies have been developed, with the McGill Pain Questionnaire being the most commonly cited. Although some question the utility of using instruments essentially designed for use in acute pain settings, clinicians are obliged to provide some assessment that can be quantified. Pain drawings also may provide another source of information, whereas these have been shown to be extremely poor instruments from a psychometric standpoint.

Unfortunately, pain ratings can be influenced by multiple factors, and some populations have particular difficulty understanding the numerical scales. Several safeguards can improve validity and reliability. First, the patient should be asked to offer a rating at the time of every visit. Reliability of pain ratings has been shown to improve in the older patients or in those patients with cognitive impairments when the request for a pain rating is repeated. Where possible, someone other than the treating physician should administer the rating scale to minimize bias. Finally, ratings should be supplemented by self-report questionnaires when possible because other variables such as quality of life may provide a more relevant picture of the patient's status.

(ii) Screening Questionnaires

Formal questionnaires should not be considered the exclusive realm of psychologists, and numerous sources review physician-administered questionnaires. These instruments are subject to the same biases and psychometric failings as unstructured interviews; nevertheless, they can be cost-effective by reducing clinician time and by improving diagnostic accuracy. Screening measures for depression are the most commonly used with chronic pain, whereas substance abuse screening items should routinely be used when chronic opioid therapy is pursued. Quality-of-life measures can provide a basis for judging treatment effectiveness. Instruments are face valid and provide a basis for fruitful discussion with the patient in treatment planning.

More complex instruments can be considered, although some require consultation by a psychologist. The Minnesota Multiphasic Personality Inventory-2 (MMPI-2) is the most commonly used self-report instrument of this type; particular care should be taken to use normative data from a chronic pain population when interpretations are made. Given this caveat, the MMPI has been shown to be a valuable test capable of predicting outcome after complex treatment interventions, particularly spine surgery. Table 2 offers a brief overview of several instruments.

Table 2.   Commonly used assessment instruments

Content	Questionnaire	Comment
Alcohol	CAGE	Brief, easily scored, inexpensive
Anxiety	Hamilton anxiety scale	Brief, clinician administered
Depression	Beck depression inventory	Brief, norms for chronic pain, inexpensive
Depression	CES-D scale	Brief, norms with multiple NIH-pain studies
Locus of control	Health locus of control	Brief, limited data on chronic pain
Personality disorder/ somatization/ depression/PTSD	Minnesota Multiphasic Personality Inventory, version 2	90+ minutes, reliability and predictive, validity data, expensive, requires psychologist
Quality of life	SF-36, SF-12	Up to 20 min, requires computer scoring, moderately expensive, includes disability score
Somatization	Patient health questionnaire	Brief, limited data on chronic pain

CAGE, Cut down, Annoyed, Guilty, Eye-opener; CES-D, Center for Epidemiologic Studies-Depression; NIH, National Institutes of Health; PTSD, Post-traumatic Stress Disorder; SF-36 and SF-12, Short Form-36 and Short Form-12.

3. Other Sources of Information

Other sources of information complete the evaluation, including a review of primary care records and phone contacts with other caregivers. Pharmacy records are available, as well as copies of other consultations, including independent medical examination reports and vocational counseling summaries. Standardized questionnaires also can be helpful.

4. Documenting Disability

Although we may be able to calculate a formal "rating" for physical or mental impairment, the construct of "disability" is inherently subjective. Various governmental agencies offer a range of definitions. The United States Social Security Act defines "disability" as an "inability to engage in any substantial gainful activity by reason of any medically determinable physical or mental impairment which can be expected to result in death or has lasted or can be expected to last for a continuous period of not less than 12 months." However, the patient with a "disabling" pain may be incapable of engaging in specific recreational or avocation pursuits. Activities of daily living may be impacted, with restrictions on sitting, walking, or lifting. Additionally, the patient may be disabled by concomitant symptoms, for example, fear of pain, problems with concentration, or cognitive effects from medications. When assessing the chronic pain patient, it is important to list specific self-reported limitations. For example, we may record the patient's report that he is unable to walk for more than 10 minutes, sit for more than 20 minutes, or lift a gallon of milk from the refrigerator. In addition to documenting self-reported disability, this information provides a basis for comparison when judging the effect of treatment interventions. The treating physician may employ standardized assessment instruments of functional status and "disability," such as the Short Form-36 (SF-36), because patients commonly underestimate their actual physical disability when queried in an interview setting.

Physicians are not obligated to provide written documentation in support of disability or work injury claims, although they often undertake this formal medicolegal role if they have expertise in the area of disability assessment.

IV. BEHAVIORAL TREATMENTS

The goals of psychologic therapies include reduction of pain, improvement in function, and reduction of concomitant symptoms such as depression, anxiety, sleep disorder, or perception of disability. Treatments may occur in a traditional one-on-one setting or in an interdisciplinary team setting in which clinicians systematically reinforce improved function and coping skills. Psychoeducational group programs are common in pain center settings, and outcome results are promising. Behavioral treatments are symptom specific and address discrete patient goals. There are multiple evidence-based reviews confirming the efficacy of behavioral treatments. Typical cognitive goals might include an increase in positive statements about managing pain, improved confidence, increased work activities, and improved affect. The patient's goals also may include developing relaxation skills and minimizing panic or anxiety during an exacerbation of pain. These skills can prevent dysfunctional behaviors such as escalating use of opioids, or spending increasing amounts of time doing nothing.

"Readiness for change" is recognized as a crucial point in the illness process when a patient elects to make adaptive change. The clinician's role is to assess the level of readiness and to assist the patient in a move from a "contemplative" stage to a more active and engaged stage. Determining what is working or not working in the patient's lifestyle and reinforcing behaviors that improve control over functional activity and pain accomplishes this.

1. Operant or "Functional Restoration" Approaches

Goal setting is often a frustrating and difficult challenge for the patient. The patient's tendency is to identify global, often overwhelming, goals. For example, the person disabled from work often has return to work as the only goal. In functional restoration programs, goals of treatment may include specific behaviors that are more rapidly achieved such as improved ability to carry groceries after a shopping trip or completion of specific tasks during a simulated work session. Often in a team, the clinician assists the patient to establish small achievable goals.

Patients' activity levels can vary wildly from virtually no activity on one day to frantic "catch-up" activity on another. This erratic activity schedule can increase the pain level and may reinforce the patient's belief that activity should be avoided. During this period of increased pain and "down time," patients' beliefs about disability becomes reinforced and fixed, their mood is negatively affected, and they perceive that the pain is controlling their life.

To counter this uneven activity level, a graded increase in activity has been formulated, formally known as **graded behavior change**. The patient begins a treatment program with a level of activity that is sustainable. Activity is based on a preset quota system, and pain-contingent activity is avoided. For example, the patient may start a program with 2 minutes of walking and increase the activity by 30-second intervals daily regardless of the pain level. Physical activities and exercises are often directed at full-body conditioning rather than at specific areas of injury. Patients reinforce their functional activity with positive "self-statements." They may chart their activity using a **daily scheduling diary**, with treatment team and family members reviewing and reinforcing their progress. This success gives the patient a greater sense of control and more ability to plan for social or occupational activities.

Formal operant or functional restoration approaches are usually initiated in an interdisciplinary outpatient setting. Formal operant programs convey the consistent message that the goal is not **pain relief**, but **pain acceptance**. There is a decided focus on improved function despite pain. Futile efforts to reduce pain are discouraged, and these are often termed "pain behaviors." These pain behaviors may include the use of PRN medications, ice, or relaxation strategies intended to provide comfort. Although rigid in their focus, programs of this sort have been shown to be successful in terms of getting patients back to work. Recent data on the construct of **pain acceptance** support this approach for appropriately selected patients. Patients are often frustrated by their earlier dealings with traditional health care providers and are said to be at their "medical endpoint"; they must be willing to jettison future medical diagnostic and treatment options.

2. Cognitive Approaches

Common cognitive variables associated with negative outcomes include "catastrophizing," fear avoidance, and helplessness. Catastrophizing is a belief that outcomes are negative and that situations are out of control. The patient may worry that something is medically wrong during each exacerbation of pain, may ruminate on the belief that the physician has "missed something," or may repeatedly rehearse potential negative outcomes from continued pain and treatment. The catastrophizing often extends to areas of the patient's life other than pain, such as worries about financial catastrophes, loss of social support, and other negative events. With respect to physical activities, fear avoidance invokes the patient's dysfunctional belief that certain activities lead to increased pain and injury. The clinician assists the patient to reconceptualize dysfunctional cognitions relating to activity, pain level, fear of injury, and many other concomitants of chronic pain. This effort often includes monitoring of dysfunctional thoughts with a written diary and rehearsal of positive statements about issues within the patient's control. Cognitive therapy interventions may directly target perceptions of pain, in contrast to traditional operant approaches in which "function" remains the preeminent goal and reports of pain are not addressed.

3. Relaxation Training and Biofeedback

Relaxation training is among the most commonly used behavioral techniques in pain center settings, and evidence-based reviews are supportive of this technique. Anxiety, pain, and functional sleep disorders have been effectively treated with relaxation training. The primary component of relaxation training is diaphragmatic breathing, a brief technique that can be applied across a range of settings. Patients also are typically taught more lengthy procedures such as progressive muscle relaxation or a passive relaxation. Progressive muscle relaxation involves tensing and relaxing specific muscle groups. During passive relaxation approaches, a patient is taught to allow each muscle group to relax, focusing on a sensation of relaxation. Passive relaxation approaches typically include intensive practice with imagery, and there is no isometric muscle exercise. Self-hypnosis procedures are a variant of the imagery approach, whereas the components of hypnosis vary widely across practitioners.

Cognitive components of relaxation training techniques have been shown to be particularly important, and recent research supports the finding that these cognitive factors are independent of placebo or suggestion. A combination of relaxation training and cognitive techniques has been shown to be effective in **functional sleep disorders**. The incidence of functional sleep disorder with chronic pain has been shown to be as high as 80%. Poor sleep habits are particularly common among patients presenting with chronic pain, and treatment includes structuring a regular sleeping and wake time. Daytime napping is discouraged and attention is paid to developing cues associated with relaxation and restful sleep.

Biofeedback assisted relaxation provides immediate physiologic input to a patient and therapist and confirms for patients that there is a physiologic response associated with their pain. Surface electromyography (sEMG) and temperature biofeedback are the most common modalities used in pain management, and the visual feedback displays the equivalent of muscle contraction for immediate viewing by the patient. Thermal biofeedback displays vasoconstriction/dilation and is most frequently used in the treatment of migraine or circulatory disorders such a Raynaud disease. As an adjunct to other behavioral, medical, or interventional pain treatment, biofeedback has been consistently shown to improve control over pain-related symptoms, although most studies pertain to headache and disorders of myofascial origin. There are possible contraindications of this technique with patients who display marked somatic focus. In these cases, patients are already acutely aware of their bodily functions, and additional close monitoring of symptoms can result in greater somatization and distress. Distraction strategies and operant approaches may offer a better alternative for such patients.

4. Vocational Counseling

Return to work remains a goal for many patients, as well as for employers, insurance carriers, and society in general. Some patients have a job waiting, whereas others are unlikely candidates for return to work because of many physical and psychosocial factors. Rehabilitation counseling is a specialized field that requires a master's degree or doctoral-level training, and clinicians are certified to provide these services. The activities of these counselors may include vocational interest and aptitude testing, conducting a "motivational analysis" to determine the patient's readiness for work, job-site evaluation, or placement for specific training or jobs. Adjustment counseling is the mainstay of treatment, assisting the patient in matching realistic goals with their functional abilities. Treatment is generally short term and goal-oriented. Workers' compensation administrative rules often mandate these services and require payment by insurance carriers. The services are also available through state unemployment agencies. Although interdisciplinary pain programs offered this type of counseling in the past, changes in funding have produced a shift, and many certified rehabilitation counselors now work directly for insurance carriers. Although rehabilitation counselors remain a valuable resource, caution is always needed when the incentives of the insurance carrier may conflict with the needs of the patient.

V. SPECIALIZED THERAPIES FOR COMORBID CONDITIONS

The therapies discussed in the preceding text are intended to address the more common comorbid psychological conditions in patients with chronic pain. However, patients with severe psychiatric illness may require more aggressive treatment. In some cases, it may be necessary to complete an intensive psychiatric program before entry into a pain program. Drug treatment is combined with intensive behavioral interventions such as **dialectical behavioral therapy**. Results are promising for chronic depression, posttraumatic stress disorder, and the personality disorders. The structure and intensity of these programs often precludes integration into a pain management setting. Similarly, when substance abuse is the primary problem, it may be necessary for the patient to enter an intensive focused psychiatric treatment program addressing the substance abuse before the pain can usefully be addressed. Successful treatment of substance abuse disorders enhances the likelihood of a positive outcome for pain treatment. Short-term behavioral interventions in a pain unit may still be required.

Smoking cessation and weight loss present a special dilemma in pain management settings. Although both conditions are amenable to pharmacotherapy, behavioral interventions have been the mainstay of treatment of these conditions. There is no question that both conditions have a considerable impact on pain, yet there has been debate about whether they should be addressed within a pain facility setting. Studies suggest that patients with pain show increased depression after rapid smoking cessation, and it has been argued that smoking cessation programs should be delayed until after completion of pain treatment. By contrast, when there is a direct medical impact, a patient may be required to complete a smoking cessation program before being considered for interventions such as spine surgery or the placement of an implantable device. We suggest that a smoking cessation service be made available to all patients, with appropriate counseling aimed at addressing the patient's individual needs.

As in the case of smoking cessation, conflicting arguments also arise over weight loss programs, and the situation becomes more complex considering that some pain medications may produce weight gain. Although weight gain is often a serious concern for patients, pain physicians commonly dismiss such concerns. Diet and weight counseling are included in some interdisciplinary settings, but formal behavioral weight loss programs have not been included traditionally within pain facility settings. Rehabilitation programs report mixed results with regard to weight loss, complicated by the fact that a desired improvement in physical function may be associated with weight gain, or failure to lose weight, because of an increase in muscle mass. Rather than offering an additional complex program with increased demands on the patient, we encourage the maintenance of a structured rehabilitative program that postpones dealing with long-term weight-directed lifestyle changes until after pain and function improve. We also encourage greater physician sensitivity to patients' concerns about the effect of pain medication on their weight.

VI. CONCLUSION

Psychosocial assessment remains a critical component of the chronic pain evaluation. Although the consulting psychologist or psychiatrist may be critical in complex clinical cases, the pain physician has a vital role in the psychosocial assessment of chronic pain. Similarly, the principles of behavioral management are not meant to be restricted to psychologists. The pain physician also can have a positive effect on patient behavior and substantially improve clinical outcomes by means of behavioral interventions.

SELECTED READINGS

Karjainen K, Malmivaara A, van Tulder M, et al. Multidisciplinary biopsychosocial rehabilitation for subacute low back pain among working age adults. *Cochrane Database Syst Rev* 2003;(2):CD002193.

Keefe FJ, Rumble ME, Scipio CD, et al. Psychological aspects of persistent pain: current state of the science. *J Pain* 2004;5(4):185–211.

Kulich RJ, Baker WK. Psychological evaluation in the management of chronic pain and disability. Current review of pain. *Curr Sci* 1997; 1:116–125.

NIH (National Institutes of Health) Technology Assessment Panel on integration of behavioral and relaxation approaches into the treatment of chronic pain and insomnia. *JAMA* 1996;276(4):313–318.

Sullivan MJ, Stanish WD. Psychologically based occupational rehabilitation: the pain-disability prevention program. *Clin J Pain* 2003; 19(2):97–104.

Turk D, Melzack R. *Handbook of pain assessment*, 2nd ed. New York: Guilford Press, 2001.

Turk DC, Gatchel RJ, eds. *Psychological approaches to pain management: a practitioner's handbook*. New York: Guilford Press, 2002.

Physical Therapy

Theresa H. Michel and Harriët Wittink

Life begins on the other side of despair.
—*Jean-Paul Sartre, 1905–1980*

The goal of physical therapy is to restore or improve function and to prevent disability. Referral to physical therapy is appropriate when pain impairs a patient's optimal functional ability or inhibits a patient's independence in activities of daily living, or when physical rehabilitation is a necessary component of treating the underlying cause of pain. The physician supplies a diagnosis and communicates any precautions, thereby allowing the physical therapist to use clinical judgment in designing an appropriate treatment program. Because patients may choose to see a physical therapist first, before a medical diagnosis is made, physical therapists perform screening, as well as a comprehensive assessment and a treatment plan based on this assessment. Referrals are made to appropriate medical practitioners. Physicians who refer to the physical therapist may make an "evaluate and treat" order that is a reasonable means of requesting a physical therapist to see a patient. In all cases, the key is collaboration and integration of component therapies between the physician and the physical therapist.

Physical therapists attempt to identify the relation between pathology, impairment, functional limitation, and disability to direct treatment appropriately. In acute pain, a clear relation exists between nociception, perceived pain, and impairment; therefore, treatment will focus on the elimination of pain. As a result, impairments are diminished, functional ability is restored, and disability is prevented. In patients with chronic pain, however, the relation between pain and disability is unclear. Treatment that solely addresses elimination of pain in patients with chronic pain will likely fail to alter the illness and disability behavior. Instead, treatment addresses function in spite of pain and promotes independence at a level of tolerance.

I. PHYSICAL THERAPY EVALUATION

Physical therapists are trained to assess physical impairments such as flexibility, strength, and endurance, as well as activity limitations. Through an interview and physical examination, most of the information needed to develop an appropriate treatment plan should be obtained. Although the physical therapist's interview and examination closely resemble those of other health care providers, observation of the patient's movement patterns and willingness to move are specific to the physical therapy examination. Transitional movements are observed when the patient sits, stands, walks, or climbs onto a plinth. Important diagnostic features include quality of motion, which can be distorted and erratic, and dysfunctional movement patterns including muscle guarding and pain behaviors.

Because patients' self-report of their functional ability has been shown to be influenced by mood, evaluation is supplemented by functional tests. Functional testing helps compare the patient's perception of what they are able to do with what they are actually capable of doing. Some functional tests that have been applied to the patients with chronic pain include the 5-minute walk test (distance in meters walked in 5 minutes), the number of stairs climbed in 1 minute, and the stand-up test (the number of times a patient can stand up from a sitting down position in 1 minute). A functional capacity evaluation (FCE) is usually performed to determine the patient's physical capacity to perform work. The assessment includes the patient's ability to lift weights from the floor to the waist and from the waist to overhead, carry, crawl, squat, sit, stand, walk, climb stairs, and push and pull weights. Aerobic fitness may be determined from a bicycle or treadmill test. Aerobic fitness represents the capacity to transport oxygen and generate energy and is part of the measure of a person's work capacity. An FCE is always somewhat subjective because it can only document how much a patient is willing to do on a given day.

II. PHYSICAL THERAPY INTERVENTION

Physical therapy treatment should have an observable endpoint associated with (a) restoration of optimal physical functioning; (b) reduction of the impact of pain on the patient's life, that is, reduced disability; (c) resolution of treatable impairments that interfere with normal function; (d) prevention of future occurrences; and (e) improvement of the patients' knowledge of independent pain management. Components of physical therapy intervention for pain are as follows:

- Education/self management techniques.
- Pain treatment or management for which active modalities (i.e., exercise) or passive modalities (i.e., massage, joint mobilization, electrotherapy, heat, and cold) can be used.

1. Education and Self-Management

Perhaps the most important goal in educating patients and teaching them self-management techniques is increased self-reliance. Many patients report feeling helpless and hopeless and cannot understand why they have pain. Increased self-reliance increases patients' participation in the intervention process and leads to better outcomes. Educating patients on their diagnosis and pathology is helpful in reducing fear and eliminating catastrophizing. It is important that the patient agrees with the goals of treatment. For example, if a patient feels that the only helpful treatment is medication, then chances of a successful outcome from physical therapy intervention are slim. When patients understand their pathology and agree with the goals of intervention, they are more likely to be compliant with the intervention offered.

It is helpful to teach patients self-massage and techniques for applying heat or cold as an active pain-control modality whether they have acute or chronic pain. For self-massage, patients can use a cane or umbrella handle to press against a trigger point and apply ischemic pressure or they can be taught to slowly rotate two tennis balls around a painful area. Heat and cold packs in all sizes are commonly available through pharmacies.

2. Pain Treatment or Management

(i) Active Modalities

Active modalities can be subdivided into three categories: (a) stretching exercise, (b) strengthening exercise, and (c) endurance exercise.

STRETCHING EXERCISE. The purpose of stretching is to regain normal flexibility around joints to allow patients to function in their optimal position. Muscle imbalance can be a precipitating factor in the development of both trigger points (TPs) and joint pain and therefore must be addressed. Numerous observations have been made about the fact that certain muscles respond to a given situation (e.g., pain and impaired afferentation by a joint) with tightness and shortening, whereas others respond by inhibition and weakness. Muscle responses seem to follow some typical rules; therefore, development of tightness and/or weakness may be considered as a systematic and characteristic deviation to the functional performance of these muscles. The final result of this deviation is a general imbalance within the whole muscular system. With an imbalance, a changed sequence of activation of the muscle in the movement pattern occurs. This change can further spiral the patient into a continuous cycle of weakness, tightness, abnormal movement patterns, and pain. Because tight muscles are thought to inhibit their antagonists, stretching muscles indirectly helps to restore strength.

Changes in muscle function play an important role in many painful conditions of the motor system and constitute an integral part of postural defects in general. Postural adjustments are the body's strategy in maintaining the center of gravity of the whole body. An increase in any one spinal curve must be compensated by a proportionate increase or decrease in the other curves. Fine muscle coordination is needed to prevent damage to a joint, especially during fast movement. Thus, balanced muscle coordination may be the best protection of our osteoarticular system. Treatment consists of stretching the short musculature and strengthening the weak muscles. Normal posture will be sought, resulting in normal bone alignment and normalized stresses across the joints. Restoration of normal muscle balance results in the following:

- Decreased repetitive microtrauma through normalization of biomechanical forces
- Normalization of reciprocal action muscles
- Restoration of normal flexibility (normal range of motion)

Passive stretching exercise is used in the treatment of TPs. An active TP is associated with spontaneous pain at rest or with motion that stretches or overloads the muscle. Specific to a TP is referred pain and the "jump sign." The pattern of referred pain from

TPs and associated phenomena is relatively constant and predictable and does not follow a dermatomal pattern or nerve root distribution. TPs and their referral patterns are described in detail in the classic works by Travell and Simons. Passive stretching is combined with spray and stretch techniques, which employ the use of a vapocoolant spray and stretching of the involved muscle to render the TPs inactive. The spraying is thought to reduce the pain of the stretch tension by blocking reflex muscle spasm initiated by autogenous stretch reflexes.

STRENGTHENING EXERCISE. Directly increasing muscle strength is achieved by high-intensity, short-duration exercise. Neuronal adaptation occurs first by an increase in the efficiency in recruiting motor neurons, followed by an increase in myofibrillar protein level after about 6 weeks of exercise. Increased muscle strength will help patients perform functional tasks such as lifting and carrying; it may also be helpful in decreasing pain perception. Increasing strength has been shown to decrease neck pain.

ENDURANCE EXERCISE. Endurance exercise is the term used for two types of exercise:

- Exercise targeted to increase maximal aerobic power or cardiovascular capacity by exercising patients at 65% to 80% of their maximal heart rate, usually by treadmill walking, biking, or any form of dynamic exercise of large muscle groups. Work and functional tasks such as walking, climbing stairs, repetitive lifting, fighting fires, carrying loads, scaling walls and running, such as is necessary for police or fire fighting work, have a substantial aerobic endurance component. Many tasks are defined by their energy cost, as expressed in oxygen consumption or metabolic equivalents (METs). Patients need a maximum aerobic power high enough to perform functional tasks (work) without excessive fatigue.
- Exercise (low intensity, long duration) is targeted to increase the aerobic capacity of a specific muscle so that the muscle can sustain both a single contraction and many repetitions of a motion for prolonged periods without fatiguing. This improved capacity improves neuromotor control and coordination, thereby preventing injury to passive structures during prolonged activities. Physical forces provide important stimuli to tissues for the development and maintenance of homeostasis. Endurance exercise of specific muscles is associated not only with increased capillary density of that muscle but also with increased strength of muscle, bone, and tendons. It results in thicker, stronger ligaments that maintain their compliance and flexibility and that are stronger at the bone–ligament–bone complex. This type of treatment is therefore essential in the management of sprains and strains of ligaments and of tendonitis. Synovial fluid lubricates the ligamentous structures of joints and provides nourishment to cartilage, menisci, and ligaments. Repetitive motion enhances this transsynovial nutrient flow. In the spine, the health of the joints depends largely on repeated low-stress movements. The intervertebral joints and the facet joints require movement for the proper transfer of fluid and nutrients across the joint surfaces. In the same way, the intervertebral

disc depends largely on movement for its nutrition. Endurance exercise therefore improves the body's ability to withstand repetitive physical forces and muscle fatigue. Because most functional tasks are repetitive in nature, most patients have a greater need of increased endurance than of increased strength. Lack of trunk muscle endurance plays an important role in chronic back pain. Jette and Jette (1996) showed that endurance exercise is associated with better outcomes in the treatment of patients with chronic back pain. Guidelines for the treatment of chronic back pain advocate the use of exercise and the avoidance of passive modalities.

Aerobic exercise is thought to have beneficial effects on pain perception and mood. It appears that pain inhibition through exercise can be mediated through the opioid and the nonopioid systems. Analgesic effects of exercise have been found at submaximal workloads of around 63% of Vo_{2max}. Rhythmic exercise stimulates the A-δ or group III afferents arising from muscle. Histologically, A-δ or group III afferents are a prominent group of fine myelinated fibers located in skeletal muscle nerves. More recent investigations indicate that these afferents respond to muscle stretch and contraction with low-frequency discharge. These afferents have been termed "**ergoreceptors,**" and it has been proposed that rhythmic exercise activates the ergoreceptors, which then activate the descending pain modulating systems.

Moderate aerobic exercise has been shown to be effective in the treatment of mild to moderate forms of depression and anxiety, which can be a powerful aide in the treatment of patients with chronic pain. Some groups of patients with chronic pain may have a dysfunctional perception of exercise-induced fatigue, with a lowering of pain thresholds instead of the normal elevation in pain thresholds found in healthy subjects after moderate exercise.

Exercise, in general, should be focused on regaining physical function. For that reason, exercises should imitate functional movements. Weight-bearing exercise helps reduce osteoporosis and is the treatment of choice in chronic complex regional pain syndrome (CRPS). Patients with CRPS are loath to use their affected body segment because any light touch stimulus will cause severe pain. A hand or a foot held in a protective posture but not put to any use will exhibit shortened muscles and tendons (e.g., foot plantar flexion and inversion). Functional activities are initiated, often beginning with reflexively provoked action, such as catching or kicking a ball or catching one's balance after perturbation. Functional progress is made through gait training using a mirror to promote symmetrical motion or through correcting improperly used muscles, restoring normal muscle length and postural alignment, and working on strength and endurance to balance muscle groups around major joints. Treatment can be made more tolerable with the assistance of lumbar sympathetic blocks, if there is sympathetic mediation of pain present.

(ii) Passive Modalities and Physical Agents

Physical agents commonly used in physical therapy are electrical stimulation ranging from low volt to high volt, ultrasound, heat, and cold.

Electrical stimulation is most commonly used for pain reduction, edema, muscle spasm, and stimulation of muscle contraction. For each type of neural tissue, there is an optimum frequency at which the maximum response will be elicited, namely, 0 to 5 Hz–sympathetic nerves, 10 to 150 Hz–parasympathetic nerves and 10 to 50 Hz–motor nerves. Iontophoresis involves the transmission of medication through the skin by means of electrical stimulation. Lidocaine and dextromethorphan are the commonly used medications for the treatment of pain and local inflammation such as in any kind of tendonitis. Transcutaneous electrical nerve stimulations (TENS) was developed on the basis of Melzack and Wall gate control theory. High-frequency stimulation is thought to stimulate A-β fibers, "closing the gate," whereas low-frequency stimulation is thought to activate the pain-inhibiting descending pathways. TENS, both high and low frequency, reduces pain and improves the range of motion in patients with chronic back pain. TENS is also effective in the treatment of migraine and tension-type headache.

- **Ultrasound** is a form of mechanotherapy. Ultrasound has both thermal and nonthermal effects. The thermal effects include increased blood flow, increased extensibility of collagenous tissues, decreased pain, and muscle spasm. The nonthermal effects of ultrasound include cavitation and micro streaming, which results in mast cell degranulation, altered cell membrane function, increased intracellular levels of calcium, and stimulation of fibroblast activity. This process results in an increase in protein synthesis, vascular permeability, angiogenesis, and the tensile strength of collagen. Sonation, therefore, may be beneficial in treatment when limitation of range of motion is caused by contractures of ligamentous and/or capsular tissues, to accelerate inflammatory processes, thereby decreasing edema associated with subsequent pain relief and wound treatment.
- **Local heat and cold** have varied applications. The local topical effects of heat are vasodilatation and local erythema, decreased fast fiber sensation, and, with prolonged exposure, decreased slow nerve fiber sensation. The electrical resistance of the skin is reduced as well. Superficial heat is used to increase circulation, reduce pain, and promote relaxation. Local cooling produces an intense vasoconstriction followed by periods of vasodilatation. Prolonged cooling decreases nerve fiber conduction. Cold is used in acute injuries to decrease swelling and pain, in chronic forms of musculoskeletal pain for pain relief, and in spastic muscle to reduce muscle tone. From clinical observation, most patients with neuropathic pain have difficulty in tolerating cold and report that it increases their pain.
- **Joint mobilization** is a technique used to improve joint mobility when the ligamentous and capsular structures limit passive range of motion. A variety of pathologic mechanisms can be involved in joint contracture development–immobilization, joint trauma, sepsis, degenerative processes, and a variety of disturbances that result in mechanical incongruity of the joint surfaces. A lesion of the capsule will give rise to limitation of capsular mobility. This decreased

mobility will limit the patient's active and passive range of motion and cause pain with movement. Treatment will be directed to restoration of normal capsular mobility and therefore to normal range of motion. Joint mobilization can restore normal capsular extensibility by applying carefully directed forces across the articular surfaces. All collagenous tissues rely heavily on movement to ensure adequate nutrition and respond to loading, as does bone. When not stretching the tissues, joint mobilization can be used to decrease pain by stimulating the type I and II mechanoreceptors. Joint mobilization is usually combined with ultrasound or heat because this is thought to make the tissue more extensible, the treatment being thereby more effective. Several studies have pointed out the immediate or short-term symptomatic reduction of pain after spinal manipulation and/or mobilization in patients with low back pain of less than a month's duration. Long-term results, however, were comparable for both the experimental and control groups in most studies.

- **Soft tissue mobilization** includes massage, passive stretching, and myofascial techniques such as myofascial release and craniosacral therapy. Massage can provide symptomatic relief by reducing pain through increasing local circulation and by stimulating A-β fibers. Trigger point massage in combination with passive stretching is thought to inhibit TPs in muscle, thereby reducing muscle pain. A special form of massage is called "**desensitization.**" Desensitization techniques such as tapping, stroking, and massaging the skin are used in the treatment of patients with CRPS to increase their tolerance of touch to the allodynic area. Patients are instructed to wear gloves or socks with progressively rough inside surfaces in addition. Massage therapy (MT) has been found to be effective in the treatment of subacute and chronic low back pain. A recent meta-analysis found that single applications of MT reduced state anxiety, blood pressure, and heart rate but not negative mood, immediate assessment of pain, and cortisol level. Multiple applications reduced delayed assessment of pain. Reductions of trait anxiety and depression were MTs' largest effects, with a course of treatment providing benefits similar in magnitude to those of psychotherapy.

III. PATIENTS WITH CHRONIC PAIN

Treating pain in nonterminal patients is a challenge and ideally should be accomplished in a team format. These patients often present with pain complaints that seem out of proportion with the objective findings and are completely disabled because of their pain, often in their work life as well as in their social and recreational lives. Patients with chronic pain usually present with primary as well as secondary impairments. The primary impairments are the result of the original injury and may or may not be treatable by physical therapy. The secondary impairments are the consequence of the patients' response to the initial injury with self-immobilization. Lack of exercise, poor body alignment, shortening and weakening of the joint structures, and overguarding of the injured part of the body result in a weakened physical condition, which can make normal daily activities more difficult, uncomfortable, and stressful. As a result, the patient's pain and suffering increase. These patients are commonly depressed as well, thereby further spiraling into a cycle of disuse, pain, and impairment. The impairments resulting from disuse are readily addressed by an aggressive exercise program composed of stretching, cardiovascular conditioning, strength and endurance training, and behavioral modification tailored to the patient's individual needs.

Behavioral modification approaches are an important part of treatment and include ignoring pain behavior, education on the "hurt not harm" principle, exposure to feared activities, and quota-based exercise. Patients are often afraid that they will harm themselves by becoming more active. To address this fear, a quota-based exercise approach is used. The patient is made to progress systematically, thereby learning that increased activity does not result in an equal increase in pain. Strong emphasis is placed on self-management techniques for pain because chronic pain is a long-term condition that patients will need to manage on their own.

Although exercise programs are tailored to patients' individual needs, they commonly include the following:

- Aerobic exercise: bike, treadmill, at 65% to 80% of predicted maximal heart rate
- Stretching exercises for shortened musculature
- Endurance exercise for the major postural muscles
- Coordination/stabilization exercises of spine and major weight-bearing joints and the muscles surrounding them
- Mobilizing exercise for the total body and for joints in functional patterns

Physical therapy goals for these patients are to increase function, decrease disability, establish effective pain coping and management skills, and decrease health care utilization in the long term. To achieve these goals, it is best that the physical therapist work within a team including behavioral therapists, occupational therapists, social workers, and physicians.

IV. CONCLUSION

The key to the success of physical therapy in the treatment of pain is the incorporation of physical therapy into a comprehensive treatment plan. Although physical therapy helps restore function, the therapy may be less effective if the pain is not optimally controlled by medical or interventional treatment (thereby impeding any improvement in physical function). Equally, attention to psychological well-being is important because physical therapy may not be successful if the patient approaches it in a negative state of mind or in a state of severe depression. Physical therapy is a vital component of multimodal pain management, and physical therapists are important members of the pain team.

SELECTED READINGS

Gurevich M, Kohn P, Davis C. Exercise induced analgesia and the role of reactivity in pain sensitivity. *J Sports Med* 1994;12:549–559.

Harding VR, Williams AC, Richardson PH, et al. The development of a battery of measures for assessing physical functioning of chronic pain patients. *Pain* 1994;25:367–375.

Hays KF. *Working it out. Using exercise in psychotherapy*. Washington, DC: American Psychological Association, 1999.

Jette DU, Jette AM. Physical therapy and health outcomes in patients with spinal impairments. *Phys Ther* 1996:76:930–945.

Lundberg T. Pain physiology and principles of treatment. *Scand Journal of Rehab Med* 1995:32(Suppl.):13–41.

Moyer CA, Rounds J, Hannum JW. A meta-analysis of massage therapy research. *Psychol Bull* 2004;130(1):3–18.

Shutty MS, DeGood DE, Tuttle DH. Chronic pain patients' beliefs about their pain and treatment outcomes. *Arch Phys Med Rehabil* 1990;71:128.

Thoren P, Floras J, Hoffman P, et al. Endorphins and exercise: physiological mechanisms and clinical implications. *Med Sci Sports Exerc* 1990;22(4):417–428.

Travell JG, Simons DG. *Myofascial pain and dysfunction: the trigger point manuals*. Baltimore, MD: Williams & Wilkins, 1983.

Whiteside A, Hansen S, Chandhuri A. Exercise lowers pain threshold in chronic fatigue syndrome. *Pain* 2004;109(3):417–428.

Wittink H, Michel T. Physical therapy: evaluation and treatment of chronic pain patients. In: Aronoff GM, ed. *Evaluation and treatment of chronic pain*, 3rd ed. Baltimore, MD: Williams & Wilkins, 1999.

Wittink H, Michel T, eds. *Chronic pain management for physical therapists*, 2nd ed. Boston, MA: Butterworth-Heineman, 2002.

Physiatric Treatment of Pain

Joseph F. Audette and Allison Bailey

What is needed most in architecture today is the very thing that is needed most in life—integrity. Just as it is needed in a human being, so integrity is the deepest quality in a building. . . . Integrity is not something to be put on and taken off like a garment. Integrity is a quality within and of the man himself. . . . It cannot be changed by any other person either, or by the exterior pressures of any outward circumstances; integrity cannot change except from within because it is that in you which is you— and due to which you will try to live your life . . . in the best possible way. To build a man or building from within is always difficult . . .

—*Frank Lloyd Wright from The Natural House, 1954*

Physical medicine and rehabilitation is one of the medical specialties that evaluates and treats patients with chronic pain. The primary focus of treatment is to restore structural integrity and maximize function, vocational viability, and community integration rather than to focus solely on eliminating pain. To initiate a successful treatment plan, the physical and psychologic obstacles to functional normalization must be identified and treated with the same aggressiveness that we use to identify and treat the cause of nociception and pain. As a corollary to this, we want to assess the extent to which our patients have been conditioned to be helpless and passive in the face of their chronic condition. Our goal is to determine the patient's residual functional capacity as well as his or her potential for further functional restoration and to provide the patient the opportunity to regain an internal locus of control to become active in their own rehabilitation.

I. PHYSIATRIC ASSESSMENT

1. History

(i) Medical/Surgical History

In addition to a standard medical and surgical history, special attention is given to determining the extent to which historic factors may have an impact on future function. The following are typical scenarios that may be encountered with a patient with chronic pain:

- A history of multiple prior surgical or other interventional procedures indicates a poor prognosis. Such a history suggests that the patient has been a passive participant in the therapeutic process, depending on external sources to "cure" the condition despite repeated failures.
- Multiple physical traumas such as frequent fractures and motor vehicle accidents may suggest a substance abuse history, which, if still active, would clearly interfere with any treatment plan. This type of history also may be a clue to potential characterologic disorders.
- Psychological trauma related directly to the original injury can be just as debilitating as the physical trauma. Questions relating psychological trauma to physical trauma should be asked: Does the patient have bad dreams associated with the trauma? Is the sleep disturbance due to the patient's thoughts rather than their pain? When **posttraumatic stress disorder** is suspected, a full psychological assessment is needed.
- The sleep history is extremely important in chronic pain and should be elucidated in detail. Issues of nighttime restlessness and nonrestorative sleep due to pain or racing thoughts, poor sleep hygiene, daytime napping, and inappropriate use of medication for sleep, if not addressed, will interfere with recovery. Sleep disturbance indicates that the prognosis for functional recovery is poor, and aggressive treatment should be a primary goal.
- Contraindications or limitations to a full functional restoration treatment plan should be determined. Special consideration should be given to the following:
  - Cardiopulmonary history, which may affect therapeutic conditioning and medication trials.
  - Internal fixation with hardware or implantation of devices such as pumps or stimulators may have a structural impact on range of motion of specific joints and may influence rehabilitation. In most cases, however, erroneous limiting beliefs about the functional implications of the hardware or devices are present in the patient and should be corrected. For example, a history of spinal fusion does not mean that a patient is permanently disabled, and to avoid confusion, the patient should be informed of this during the assessment.
  - Severe psychological or motivational impairments should be identified and treated before any pain rehabilitation is initiated.
  - Severe learning disabilities or cognitive impairments such as those occurring with traumatic brain injuries may limit the patient's ability to comply with a treatment program.

(ii) Pharmacologic History

The ways in which patients take their medication is just as important as what they take. Frequent use of short-acting analgesics can encourage learned helplessness and passivity about self-management of pain and may imply that the patient has no internal resources to cope with normal fluctuations in pain intensity. As a correlate to this, it is important to determine whether patients use any other nonpharmacologic approaches to pain management such as distraction, relaxation, ice, heat, and stretching. Assess whether there is large affective component to the painful sensations and the use of medications by the words the patient uses to describe his or her symptoms. Analgesics are often used to relieve emotional distress more than to treat nociceptive pain. Sustained release formulations or agents with a long half-life are much less likely to treat emotional distress rather than nociceptive pain. Assess whether there is a functional improvement in addition to pain relief while using analgesics. In other words, does the patient **do more** if he or she is in less pain? This assessment can help determine whether a patient truly benefits from a medication.

(iii) History of Prior Treatments

In addition to determining what interventional treatments have been performed, the patient's attitudes about these treatments should be explored. Overuse of interventional approaches can lead to passivity and learned helplessness in the face of chronic pain and should be avoided. The nature of prior physical rehabilitation should be determined. There are two broad categories: **passive**, or modality-driven and hands-on treatments, versus **active**, or patient-driven, participatory treatments. An active approach is preferable in a chronic situation and should be ordered if the patient has not taken this approach. If patients have failed an active rehabilitation program, it is important to determine the cause. Patients who are fearful of increased pain during treatment or who believe that they are at risk of harm because of the pain will often require active psychological treatment in conjunction with continued active therapy to address this issue. Some increase in pain, initially, is unavoidable in an active functional restoration process. Often, appropriate therapeutic injections and medications can be used to ameliorate the pain to help encourage more active participation in the rehabilitation process. Medications or invasive treatments alone are unlikely to improve function in a chronic situation.

(iv) History of Prior and Present Function

An accurate assessment of a patient's functional status can be difficult to ascertain in a medical interview. Specifically asking "What can't you do?" rather than "What can you do?" can often make it easier to pinpoint the patient's functional limitations. If patients don't give details, assess the status of major functional domains such as self-care, household chores, shopping, driving, and, if relevant, work. Determine the patient's level of function prior to the onset of the pain syndrome; this will help set the goals of treatment. If it seems unreasonable to return a patient to his or her former functional status on the basis of the clinical presentation, vocational counseling may be indicated. However, do not assume that because other doctors, including surgeons, have reinforced the patient's disability, they are right. Numerous studies have shown that even after spinal surgery, patients can return to their former work capacity if motivated to do so. Determine the drive time to the office visit to better assess a patient's sitting tolerance. Always ask about the patient's leisure and avocational activities. This information may help determine inconsistencies with reported functional intolerances and may also give clues about possible anergia and depression.

(v) Psychosocial History

It is important to assess the patient's emotional support system. Will the patient's home environment interfere with treatment or be supportive of treatment? Emotional traumas, either as a child or as an adult, can have a negative impact on prognosis, and appropriate psychologic assessment should be instituted if there is evidence of these historic factors. Depression is a common comorbid problem in chronic pain and should not require any alterations in the treatment plan other than the inclusion of psychiatric assessment and management. In the case of severe psychomotor retardation or mania, however, mental health stabilization would be required before any other pain treatments are initiated. A similar approach should be taken if Axis II pathology, such as sociopathic behavior, severe narcissistic personality disorder, or borderline personality disorder, is suspected. Readiness to change or motivation can be assessed. If the patient has realistic goals and plans that do not depend on the complete elimination of pain, the readiness to change is a positive indicator of treatment success.

(vi) Home and Environment

Family history of disability can be a negative prognostic indicator. If there are strong role models of disabled family members, the patient's perception of these family members may help predict the patient's potential for functional recovery. Ongoing litigation can interfere with instituting a successful treatment plan. Probe what the patient's thoughts are about the case and ask if returning the patient to their former functional status would have negative legal or financial repercussions. In some cases, it is best to put treatment on hold until the litigation is settled. Financial status should be assessed because this may be a barrier to treatment. At times, financial duress also can be a motivator.

2. Physical Assessment

(i) Structural Assessment

Structural assessment is an essential component of a physiatric physical examination both for diagnostic and functional purposes. Pain—and, in particular, chronic pain—causes considerable alteration in body mechanics. Even when the principal nociceptor involved has been successfully treated, pain perpetuation and continued disability can often occur if normal structure, strength, and physical conditioning have not been restored.

(ii) Gait

Antalgic gaits are common in patients with chronic pain. Pain behaviors can be seen during this phase of assessment. Use of assistive devices, except in the older patients, is usually a sign of illness behavior and is rarely necessary for safety. A compensated Trendelenberg gait is a sign of hip abductor weakness, due either to true neurologic weakness (rare) or to reflex inhibition of the hip abductor caused by sacroiliac (SI) joint inflammation from hip joint disease. A vaulting gait over one leg may indicate leg length discrepancy, which puts stress on postural structures and may be a perpetuating factor in spinal pain syndromes.

(iii) Spine

Congenital scoliosis can be distinguished from a functional or acquired scoliosis by forward flexion of the spine bringing out the rotatory component of congenital scoliosis, indicated by a hump sign in the thoracic region (Adams test). Acquired scoliosis is due to asymmetric muscle shortening of spinal extensors and lateral flexors. This asymmetric muscle shortening will often cause a **cross pattern** of pain, with discomfort on the ipsilateral side of the shortened muscles in the low back and on the contralateral side in the scapular and cervical regions. Regardless of the cause, if not addressed in physical rehabilitation, acquired scoliosis will be a cause of pain perpetuation. **Apparent short leg syndrome (ASLS)**, best seen with patient lying supine, is caused by muscle shortening of the hip rotators, such as the gluteus medius and piriformis, and is commonly associated with sacral joint dysfunction and inflammation. As opposed to a congenital or **true** leg length discrepancy, the short leg with ASLS will be more externally rotated while supine because of the contraction of the hip external rotators. In such cases, use of a lift in the shoe would be contraindicated and could exacerbate the problem. Thoracic kyphosis with forward thrusted head, extended cervical spine, and internally rotated shoulders is common with pain syndromes in the midback, head, and neck. This condition puts the patient at risk for myofascial pain and muscular nerve entrapment syndromes at the occipito-cervical junction and anatomic thoracic inlet.

II. PHYSIATRIC ASSESSMENT AND TREATMENT OF SPECIFIC PAIN SYNDROMES

1. Myofascial Pain

Myofascial pain syndrome (MPS) is a common, yet under-recognized, cause of chronic pain. Failure to recognize this cause of pain and disability can lead to frustration for both the caregiver and the patient because of treatment failures and inappropriate use of other interventional treatments.

According to the *Integrated Theory,* the pain associated with MPS is thought to be due to the firing of both low-threshold Group III and high-threshold Group IV muscle nociceptive afferents. These nociceptors are believed to be activated by pH changes in the muscle caused by transient ischemia. This theory, however, does not explain why many individuals without pain also have taut muscle bands, called latent trigger points, that would fit the criteria for MPS, except that they lack pain at rest. One explanation is that the pain associated with an active trigger points depends on segmental central sensitization at the level of the spinal cord, which can lead both to the abnormal muscle irritability or the phenomenon of the twitch response and to pain at rest.

A **myofascial trigger point (MTrP)** is the common endpoint of any chronic irritation to muscle tissue. Muscle tissue is extremely reactive to joint and nerve irritation in related structures and often provides the primary nociceptive signal. Some of the pain syndromes in which the pain experienced by the patient is due to MPS are listed here:

- Structural deviations in posture lead to chronic strain of postural muscles and MTrPs
- Facet inflammation and dysfunction leads to regional MTrPs, which are common following motor vehicle accidents (MVAs) with extension injuries
- Chronic radiculopathies can lead to MTrPs in the myotome of the affected root
- Lumbar or cervical spondylosis
- Joint inflammation in shoulder, SI joint, and hip, leading to MTrPs in the muscles that control the joint motion

MPS can mimic a number of other clinical conditions, making diagnosis by history alone difficult. Table 1 lists some diagnoses and the associated muscles involved. The physical examination of MTrPs should extend beyond identifying of point tenderness over a muscle. Many conditions will have positive point tenderness over a muscle without being an MTrP, such as myositis, polymyalgia rheumatica, fibromyalgia, muscle spasm, and focal dystonias. With proper training, good interrater reliability has been found if the following diagnostic methods are used:

- Cross fiber, snapping palpation eliciting a local twitch response (LTR)
- **Recognizable** pain with deep palpation
- Pain with passive stretch or resisted contraction of affected muscle group

Table 1.   Clinical presentations of myofascial pain

Clinical Condition	Muscles Involved with MTrPs
Tension headaches	Upper trapezius, splenius capitis, semispinalis, scalenes, SCM
TMJ	Masseter, temporalis, SCM
Cervical radiculopathy	Upper trapezius, scalenes, levator scapula, teres minor
Thoracic back pain	Lower trapezius, rhomboids, serratus anterior and posterior
Lumbar back pain	Quadratus lumborum, gluteus medius, ileopsoas
Lumbar radiculopathy	Gluteus medius and piriformis
Greater trochanter bursitis	Gluteus medius and piriformis without sciatic entrapment
Coccygodynia	Piriformis and gemelli without sciatic entrapment
Biceps tendinitis	Pectoralis minor, biceps, subscapularis
Rotator cuff tendinitis	Supra- and infraspinatus, teres minor, latissimus dorsi

MTrPs, myofascial trigger points; SCM, sternocleidomastoid; TMJ, temporomandibular joint.

- Loss of passive range of motion (PROM) in appropriate joint controlled by affected muscle group
- Sustained dermatographia over MTrP due to histamine release
- Characteristic referral pattern of pain with sustained pressure over MTrP

2. Fibromyalgia

Fibromyalgia can be distinguished from MPS by the diffuseness of the tender points that may or may not be trigger points. These points are symmetrically distributed and will affect both upper and lower parts of the body in fibromyalgia but not in MPS. In addition, history-related factors, such as sleep disturbance, depression, chronic fatigue, irritable bowel, dysmenorrhea, cystitis, and chronic sinusitis, are more commonly found in fibromyalgia. Fibromyalgia is a systemic, not a localized, disease.

Because pain from fibromyalgia generally cannot be eliminated, treatment should focus exclusively on functional restoration. In general, use of both the low-dose tricyclic antidepressants (TCAs) at night and the newer antidepressants such as the selective serotonin norepinephrine reuptake inhibitors (SSNRIs), such as venlafaxine or duloxetine, during the day may be helpful. Tramadol has also been shown in randomized trials to be superior to antiinflammatory medications for the treatment of pain in fibromyalgia. Pharmacologic treatment should be combined with skilled relaxation training and other cognitive and behavioral techniques to modulate pain. Although the use of opioids in fibromyalgia has some proponents, in general, there is a risk of poor functional outcome and worsening depression and fatigue. In a randomized trial comparing IV ketamine to morphine and lidocaine, only ketamine had a significant positive effect on pain intensity, pressure pain, and exercise endurance.

To avoid pain exacerbation, patients undergoing physical rehabilitation should focus on flexibility and conditioning rather than aggressive strengthening. Invasive procedures should be avoided unless there is a co-morbid condition such as a radiculopathy or joint effusion that would have a reasonable probability of responding.

3. Back and Neck Pain

(i) Waddell Signs

Spinal pain syndromes are among the most common presenting problems in pain clinics and can be complicated by issues of secondary gain and excessive illness behavior. The Waddell signs are not evidence of malingering but rather signs of disease affirmation, conviction, and psychological distress (see Table 2).

(ii) Selected Syndromes to Rule out

- Cervical facet syndrome: Cervical facet syndrome is often associated with MTrPs in specific zone of occipital region (C34), neck (C45, C56) and scapular region (C67, T12, T23, and down). Positive local pain with the Spurling test (extension and rotation of neck with compression).

Table 2. Waddell signs

	Normal Illness Behavior	Abnormal Illness Behavior
Assessment Methods		
Pain drawing	Localized with appropriate neuroanatomical features	Magnified, covering diffuse regions of body
Pain adjectives	Sensory	Affective, evaluative
Symptoms		
Pain	Localized	Whole leg pain
Numbness	Dermatomal	Whole leg
Weakness	Myotomal	Whole leg giving way
Time pattern	Varies with time	Never free of pain
Response to treatment	Variable benefit	Intolerance of treatments Frequent ER visits
Signs		
Tenderness	Localized	Superficial, nonanatomical
Axial loading	No lumbar pain	Lumbar pain
Straight leg raise	Limited on distraction	Improves with distraction
Sensory	Dermatomal	Regional
Motor	Myotomal	Jerky, give away weakness
Tenderness	Appropriate pain	Overreaction

ER, emergency room.
From Waddell G, Pilowsky I, Bond MR, et al. Clinical assessment and interpretation of abnormal illness behaviour in low back pain. *Pain* 1989;39:41–53, with permission.

- Lumbar facet syndrome: Lumbar facet syndrome is characterized by increased pain with extension, less pain with flexion, or increased pain with extension together with rotation. Occasionally, the pain is referred to anterior thigh.
- SI joint dysfunction: Pain can radiate to groin or to the sciatic nerve distribution. Increased pain is observed with Patrick test, compression test, and Yoeman test. With the patient lying supine, shortening and external rotation of the leg can be observed. Pain on palpation over posterior superior iliac spine (PSIS) is observed when the patient is lying prone.

III. PHYSIATRIC TREATMENT OF PAIN

1. Physical and Occupational Therapy Referral

The type of physical therapy (PT) referral depends on the conditions found on the basis of the assessment phase of the evaluation.

Four major referral options should be considered in a chronic pain state depending on the following patient characteristic subtypes:

(i) Chronic Pain Without Major Functional Impairments or Psychological Factors

Refer to PT with the goal of correcting structural deviations seen on examination, improving strength of postural muscles, increasing aerobic conditioning, and learning a home exercise program. Emphasize an active program rather than a passive, modality-based treatment. Teach the patient to self-administer heat and cold to manage pain, self-massage with tennis balls, and use desensitization techniques to deactivate nerve injury if present.

(ii) Chronic Pain (Not Spine Related) with Major Functional Impairments but No Major Psychological Factors

Refer to PT, with the same goals mentioned, in the preceding text. Refer to an occupational therapist (OT) with a pain specialty. The goals are to work on functional adaptations, increase awareness of coping and pacing strategies to prevent pain flare-ups with activity, educate that pain in the chronic state is no longer a signal to avoid movement or activity, and teach the patient muscle tension reduction techniques to prevent the effects of physiologic arousal and anxiety on pain perception.

(iii) Chronic Pain (Spine Related) With Major Functional Impairments but No Major Psychologic Factors

Refer the patient to quota-based spine rehabilitation program in case of chronic pain (spine related) with major functional impairments but no major psychologic factors. The treatment team often consists of only a physician, a physical therapist and a PT aide or assistant. The goals of such an approach are to restore tissue integrity, dynamic spine strength, endurance, and flexibility while immersed in a system of behavioral modification based on the Fordyce model. The patient receives overt rewards for meeting the physical quotas set by the system, and all pain complaints and illness behavior are completely ignored. Unlike most standard PT, this system does not allow the patient's symptoms to limit progression (see Table 3).

(iv) Chronic Pain (Both Spine and Non–Spine Related) with Major Functional and Psychologic Impairments

In case of chronic pain (both spine and non–spine related) with major functional and psychologic impairments, the patients must be referred to the multidisciplinary functional restoration program. The treatment team is more robust, involving a physician, a psychologist, and often a psychiatrist along with both PT and OT services. Treatment is still goal based but can be more individualized and is not limited to treatment of spine pathology (see Table 4).

2. Therapeutic Injections

The techniques of various invasive approaches are described in other sections of this handbook. When utilized by a physiatrist, the invasive technique is never used as the sole method of treatment of a painful condition but rather as an adjunct to allow the patient to

Table 3. Goals of quota-based system

Rehabilitation Task	Goal
Flexibility	100 degrees of lumbar flexion 25 degrees of lumbar extension Straight leg raise of 75 degrees
Strength	Trunk extension and flexion strength 100%–120% of ideal body weight. Functional lift from floor 40%–50% of ideal body weight.
Conditioning	Heart rate 80% of age determined target Work load greater than 6,000 Kg-m/9, minute(s)

From Rainville J, Sobel JB, Banco RJ, et al. Low back and cervical spine disorders. *Orthop Clin North Am* 1996;27(4):729–746, with permission.

Table 4. Details of services offered in functional restoration program

Rehabilitation Task	Detail
Physical	Treatment approach not specific to spinal pathology, more flexible Goals set in conjunction with patient's input not imposed by quotas Emphasis placed on education and self-management of pain Work simulation activities individualized to patient return to work goals
Cognitive	Counseling on sleep hygiene Counseling on social, environmental, and psychological barriers Behavioral approach applied to address fears, passivity, kinesiophobia Relaxation, muscle tension reduction, reduction of physiologic arousal
Medical	Pharmacologic management of sleep disturbance and mood disorder Medication education and optimization of pharmacologic regimen Oversight of goal accomplishment, medical limitations addressed Therapeutic injections given to assist in reaching functional goals

better participate in the process of functional restoration. Many physiatrists will have training in spine injection techniques, including epidural, facet, and SI joint, as well as in other joint injection techniques, such as those for the knee, shoulder, ankle, wrist, and digits, which are addressed in this section. Injection techniques for myofascial pain vary widely; however, recently, there have been studies providing better practice guidance in this area. Ultimately, any therapeutic injection requires giving thought to the various factors that led to the tissue damage and irritation and should be done in conjunction with the appropriate noninvasive treatments mentioned earlier to help prevent recurrence and patient passivity in the face of illness.

Trigger Point Injections:

There are four major methods of injection. Typically, a 25- to 27-gauge needle 1.5 to 2 inches long is adequate, although some prefer larger-bore needles such as 20 or 22 gauge when mechanically disrupting muscle tissue in a taut band. When using local anesthetic, the volume and type used varies greatly, but generally 1 to 10 mL of either 0.5% lidocaine or 0.25% bupivacaine is adequate depending on muscle size and technique. Lidocaine is less myotoxic than bupivacaine, and there is no advantage to using higher concentrations of anesthetic. Several techniques are employed:

- Injection with local anesthetic and steroid solution
- Injection with local anesthetic or alone
- Injection with local anesthetic or normal saline accompanied by vigorous repeated needling or probing of the needle into the taut band (an LTR in the muscle with needling is often produced)
- Dry needling either with a standard needle mentioned above or with an acupuncture needle (32 to 34 gauge), with overt attempt to elicit the LTR

Scientific guidance about which technique is superior is still lacking. Biopsy of muscle tissue with trigger points has not shown evidence of inflammation. Clinical studies have not shown additional benefit from using steroids and their use is not necessary for therapeutic effect.

Botulinum toxin type A (Botox) injections into trigger points currently are being studied in many centers. Botulinum toxin type A binds irreversibly to the presynaptic motor endplate and prevents release of acetylcholine leading to chemical denervation. This technique essentially puts the muscle to rest for up to 2 to 6 months until axon terminals sprout and form new synaptic connections with the muscle. Some advocate its use in with chronic MTrPs. Further research is needed to prove its long-term efficacy over other less expensive techniques.

3. Pharmacologic Management

Certain patients with chronic pain are unlikely to benefit greatly from invasive measures. In such cases, the appropriate use of medication can help achieve the functional goals set in rehabilitation. The goals of medication are to restore sleep, modulate pain without causing excessive dependence or dysfunction, and to stabilize mood. Medications used for fibromyalgia are often also effective for MPS.

IV CONCLUSION

In summary, the goal of assessment and treatment from a physiatric point of view is to determine the appropriate clinical resources necessary to return patients to their former functional capacity. A combination of rehabilitation, psychological, pharmacologic, and invasive resources is often needed, and in this situation, a physiatrist will often act as a team leader with physical therapist and OT as well as mental health professionals to ensure a cohesive multidisciplinary treatment plan. Ultimately, we want to enable patients to find the internal resources to regain the lost integrity that chronic pain causes, and although this can be the most difficult endeavor, the rewards of succeeding with a challenging patient cannot be underestimated.

SELECTED READINGS

Audette JF, Wang F, Smith H. Bilateral activation of motor unit potentials with unilateral needle stimulation of active myofascial trigger points. *Am J Phys Med Rehabil* 2004;83(5):368–374.

Chesire WP, Abashian SW, Mann JD, et al. Botulinum toxin in the treatment of myofascial pain syndrome. *Pain* 1994;59:65–69.

Chu J. Dry needling in myofascial pain related to lumbosacral radiculopathy. *Eur J Phys Med Rehabil* 1995;5(4):106.

Fishbain DA, Goldberg M, Meagher BR, et al. Male and female chronic pain patients categorized by DSM-III psychiatric diagnostic criteria. *Pain* 1986;26:181–197.

Fukui S, Ohseto K, Shiotani M, et al. Referred pain distribution of the cervical zygapophyseal joints and cervical dorsal rami. *Pain* 1996;68:79–83.

Gerwin RD, Shannon S, Hong CZ, et al. Interrater reliability in myofascial trigger point examination. *Pain* 1997;69:65–73.

Han S, Han SC, Harrison P, et al. Myofascial pain syndrome and trigger-point management. *Reg Anesth* 1997;22(1):89–99.

Hong CZ. Lidocaine injection vs dry needling to myofascial trigger points. *Am J Phys Med Rehabil* 1994;74(4):256.

Hong CZ, Torigoe Y, Yu J, et al. The localized twitch response in responsive taut bands of rabbit skeletal muscle fibers are related to the reflexes at spinal cord level. *J Musculoskeletal Pain* 1995;3(1):15–32.

Mense S. Review article: nociception from skeletal muscle in relation to clinical muscle pain. *Pain* 1993;54:241–289.

Rainville J, Sobel JB, Banco RJ, et al. Low back and cervical spine disorders. *Orthop Clin North Am* 1996;27(4):729–746.

Simons D, Travell J. *Myofascial pain and dysfunction: the trigger point manual*, 2nd ed., Vol. 1. Baltimore, MD: Williams & Wilkins, 1999.

Waddell G, Pilowsky I, Bond MR, et al. Clinical assessment and interpretation of abnormal illness behaviour in low back pain. *Pain* 1989;39:41–53.

Acupuncture

Jasmin M. Field, Lucy L. Chen, and May C. M. Pian-Smith

In any path of study, knowledge never comes entirely at once but piecemeal. Truth presents herself in fragmentary form, and we put pieces together.
—*R. Abbe*

I. INTRODUCTION

Acupuncture is an ancient healing tradition that originated in China more than 3,000 years ago. It has evolved into many different types (e.g., traditional Chinese medicine, five elements theory, Korean hand acupuncture, scalp or ear acupuncture, Japanese acupuncture, and French energetics system) and has been practiced all over the world. Over the last few decades, acupuncture has gained increasing popularity and has come under increasing scrutiny in Europe and America, beginning in the 1970s in the United States. Since then, because of increasing support by the governments of the respective countries, substantial clinical/laboratory investigation, and strong consumer demand, there has been vast progress in the Western understanding and practice of acupuncture.

A number of specific events contributed to the current interest in and the integration of Chinese medical practice. In 1996, the U.S. Food and Drug Administration (FDA) changed the classification of acupuncture needles from experimental to medical equipment, subjecting their marketing and use to the same strict quality control standards applied to medical needles, syringes, and surgical scalpels. In 1997, the National Institutes of Health (NIH) convened a Consensus Development Conference on Acupuncture, acknowledging that acupuncture was widely practiced by thousands of physicians, dentists, acupuncturists, and other practitioners for relief from or prevention of pain and for various other health conditions. The NIH Office of Alternative Medicine (OAM) later expanded and was renamed the National Center for Complementary and Alternative Medicine (NCCAM). NCCAM currently funds research projects relating to acupuncture use for multiple medical and pain conditions.

The United States has seen an increasing demand for and acceptance of complementary therapies. It has become incumbent on health care practitioners to have knowledge of treatment alternatives to conventional medicine and to understand associated clinical implications. In a national survey published in the *Journal of the American Medical Association* (*JAMA*) in 1998, Eisenberg et al. found that the number of visits to alternative therapy centers was twice that of visits to primary care physicians and that the money spent on complementary and alternative medicine (CAM) was nearly equal to out-of-pocket expenditures for conventional care.

Most medical schools in the United States have included subjects on integrated medicine. Third-party reimbursements for alternative therapies also have increased with patient demand. With health care costs in the United States exceeding $1.7 trillion in 2003, health insurance providers have begun to emphasize preventative measures, particularly in the face of a rapidly aging population. CAM espouses a more holistic, purposeful effort toward maintaining health, contrasting with conventional medicine's interventional approach toward management of disease. CAM will therefore likely play a vital role in minimizing costs and in improving patient health and satisfaction.

II. METHODS AND TRADITIONS

According to traditional Chinese medicine, *qi* (pronounced "chee") is the life force or energy that flows through all living things and influences health on physical, mental, emotional, and spiritual levels. Any imbalance (deficiency or excess) or blockage of *qi* is thought to cause disease or pain. Acupuncture treats disorders by influencing the flow of *qi,* thereby restoring the normal balance of organ systems. In human beings, *qi* is thought to flow through the body along specific pathways called meridians. There are 12 major meridians named after organ systems, and eight minor meridians, which run vertically along each side of the body (bilateral pairs share the same name).

Depending on the particular school of thought on acupuncture, there are between 600 and 2,000 acupuncture points on the human body. For example, microsystem acupuncture such as auricular acupuncture or Korean hand acupuncture uses several extra points outside the traditional meridians. Points in the ear, hand, foot, or scalp correspond to organs throughout the body.

Acupuncture involves insertion of very fine needles in the skin at specific points in order to promote health and restore proper function of the body. Acupuncture points are usually chosen on the basis of the practitioner's assessment of the particular imbalance that needs to be restored. Points can be stimulated to add or dissipate energy, or to *tonify* (strengthen or restore) a particular organ system. Traditional diagnostic techniques for acupuncture include methods of evaluation such as looking at the patient's tongue for shape, color, texture, and smell, or feeling radial and ulnar pulses for information about the entire body.

Several sizes of needles are available. Needles can be manipulated in many ways—often by rotating the needle in specific directions or by applying electricity. The sensation of *deqi*—an aching, warm, or tingling sensation at the insertion site noted by the patient, which usually corresponds to the practitioner feeling the needle "catching" in the muscle—is thought to be necessary for therapeutic effect.

Electroacupuncture (EA) is commonly practiced in Europe and America and uses electrical impulses conducted through needles for enhanced stimulation of acupuncture points. Different frequencies of electricity have been shown to have distinct effects and mechanisms of action. Percutaneous electrical nerve stimulation (PENS) is a modified form of acupuncture that is practiced in many pain clinics. PENS points are chosen in a dermatomal distribution associated with pain symptoms. Transcutaneous electrical nerve stimulation (TENS) is modified acupressure in the same distribution as PENS.

Related techniques include moxibustion (burning of herbs to apply heat near acupuncture points), acupressure and reflexology (stimulation of points without penetration of the skin with needles), and cupping (heat creates a partial vacuum in small jars, which are used to stimulate points with suction). Other variations employ stimulation of acupuncture points using laser and ultrasound.

III. COMPLICATIONS AND SIDE EFFECTS

In the hands of a skilled practitioner, complications associated with acupuncture are actually rare, and usually mild. The most commonly reported complication is bruising or bleeding. (Note that there are no specific guidelines on anticoagulation therapy and acupuncture.) A second, less common side effect of acupuncture and related treatments is a transient vasovagal response, which resolves quickly and completely with repositioning of the patient.

Since 1965, there has been a handful of case reports in the literature about severe complications and exceedingly rare fatal reactions associated with acupuncture, although many reported cases were not proven to be causative. When present, serious side effects have generally occurred in older, more debilitated patients, or in the hands of less skilled practitioners, and include pneumo/hemothorax, pericardial effusion, pericardial tamponade, infective endocarditis, intraabdominal and intramuscular abscess, peroneal nerve palsy, and mycobacteriosis and other infections.

Although acupuncture is clearly considered to be safe, it is important to remember that it is not always entirely benign. In Europe and America, a large segment of the patient population who may benefit from acupuncture—that is, those intolerant to medications or those who failed other therapies because of fragility, debilitation, or comorbidities—are also at highest risk for acupuncture complications.

IV. SCIENTIFIC BASIS

Since the introduction of CAM into conventional medicine in the 1970s, there has been a great deal of laboratory research on the "scientific" basis of acupuncture's effects. There is now a considerable amount of data supporting the efficacy of acupuncture for painful syndromes. Mechanisms involving the central nervous system, peripheral nerves, endorphins, and monoamine neurotransmitters are clearly involved. Different means of acupuncture stimulation (depending on the location of the needle, its relation to the site of pain, and the manner in which the needle is manually or electrically stimulated) elicit different mechanisms of pain inhibition.

1. Central Nervous System

In the most widely accepted acupuncture model, needling of nerve fibers in the muscle sends impulses that activate the spinal cord, midbrain, and hypothalamus–pituitary system.

- The spinal cord site uses enkephalin and dynorphin to block incoming messages during electroacupuncture at a low frequency (2 to 4 Hz). Other neurotransmitters (e.g., GABA) are stimulated with high-frequency (50 to 500 Hz) acupuncture.
- The midbrain uses enkephalin to activate the raphe descending system, which inhibits the transmission of spinal cord pain through the synergistic effects of serotonin and norepinephrine. Another midbrain circuit bypasses the endorphin-mediated steps during high-frequency electroacupuncture.
- At the hypothalamus–pituitary level, the pituitary releases β-endorphin into the blood and cerebrospinal fluid (CFS) to produce distant analgesia. The hypothalamus sends long axons to the midbrain and activates descending analgesia via β-endorphin. This center is activated only with low-frequency (not high-frequency) electroacupuncture.

2. Endogenous Opioid Peptides

The following findings from several laboratories support the role of endorphins and a humorally mediated mechanism of some forms of electroacupuncture:

- The effects of acupuncture are not immediate; analgesia occurs after a 20- to 30-minute induction period, as might be expected in a humorally mediated mechanism.
- Analgesia persists for 1 to 2 hours after cessation of acupuncture.
- Naloxone and other opioid antagonists inhibit acupuncture analgesia.
- Animals genetically deficient in opioid receptors or endorphins show poor acupuncture analgesia.
- Endorphin levels in blood and CSF rise during acupuncture.
- Substances that inhibit endorphin enzymatic degradation enhance acupuncture effects.
- Acupuncture analgesia can be passed from one animal to a second animal via CSF transfer or via cross-circulation of blood between the two animals. This effect is blocked by naloxone given to **either** animal.

3. Neurotransmitters

During high-frequency electroacupuncture, other neurotransmitters (e.g., serotonin and norepinephrine) act as mediators. This observation is supported by the following findings:

- With high-frequency EA, there is rapid onset of analgesia, without a long induction period.

- When lesions are made in areas of the brain rich in serotonin-releasing cells (e.g., the raphe magnus of the brainstem and medial medulla oblongata) acupuncture-induced analgesia is abolished.
- Agents that block biosynthesis of serotonin (e.g., p-chlorophenylalanine) block acupuncture analgesia.
- Agents that block serotonin receptors block acupuncture.
- Analgesia is enhanced when serotonin levels are increased.
- Norepinephrine is implicated as a mediator in studies demonstrating suppression of EA effects via inhibition of the descending adrenergic system with yohimbine and phentolamine.

4. Nitric Oxide

New research suggests that electroacupuncture induces upregulation of neuronal nitric oxide/NADPH diaphorase expression in the gracile nucleus in rats. L-arginine-derived nitric oxide then mediates acupuncture signals through dorsal medulla–thalamic pathways. This may play a major role in central autonomic regulation of somatosympathetic reflex activities, which contribute to acupuncture effects in somatic and visceral pain processing, and cardiovascular regulation.

5. Functional Magnetic Resonance Imaging

Functional magnetic resonance imaging (fMRI) signals are thought to reflect changes in metabolic activity via observation of changes in blood flow. Changes in oxygenated blood flow to specific areas of the brain indicate which anatomic areas of the brain are activated or deactivated during mental states and activities such as electroacupuncture. Most fMRI techniques involve no exposure to radioactive materials, therefore images can be safely taken frequently and for longer duration, providing for improved statistical evaluation. Functional MRI is faster and allows visualization of smaller structures in greater detail than positron emission tomography (PET) or single photon emission computerized tomography (SPECT) scans. Several recent studies have reported use of fMRI for imaging effects of acupuncture in the brain. These studies suggest that acupuncture needling modulates the hypothalamic–limbic system and subcortical structures. Further studies are underway to correlate signal changes with changes in pain thresholds.

V. EVIDENCE BASE

In 2002, the World Health Organization (WHO) published a summary and review of all clinical trials through the year 1999 and determined four categories of disorders treated by acupuncture. The first category includes conditions for which acupuncture has been shown to be an effective treatment (through controlled trials):

- Allergies
- Biliary colic
- Depression
- Dysentery

- Dysmenorrhea
- Epigastritis
- Facial pain
- Headache
- Essential hypertension
- Primary hypotension
- Induction of labor
- Knee pain
- Leucopenia
- Low back pain
- Malposition of fetus
- Morning sickness
- Nausea and vomiting
- Neck pain
- Dental pain
- Periarthritis of the shoulder
- Postoperative pain
- Renal colic
- Rheumatoid arthritis
- Sciatica
- Sprain
- Stroke
- Tennis elbow

Other categories include conditions for which acupuncture (by credentialed practitioners) is recommended, especially when conventional therapies have failed, even though trials provide only limited support of its effectiveness.

Although there is still controversy about the strength of scientific support for acupuncture, there have been many recent advances, particularly in relation to acupuncture, in the treatment of pain. It is becoming evident that data may be limited more by study design and nonstandardized practices than by treatment effect. Many convincing studies on acupuncture have been published since the latest metaanalyses, reviews, and government health agency statements. Generalized conclusions are still challenging because of the variation in acupuncture points selected and in techniques used for a given clinical condition, variation in the mode of needle stimulation, in treatment duration and intervals between treatments, and perhaps even in the attempted translation of Eastern culture to Western. True blinding of the patient is difficult, and of the treating acupuncturist, impossible. Nonspecific needling (i.e., not at recognized acupuncture sites or at non–site-specific points for the disease in question) can elicit responses that may be similar to responses to active treatment, thereby skewing results and making interpretation difficult. Placebo effect cannot be excluded. Studies often have low power because blinded trials must include acupuncture-naïve patients. But study designs have improved, and new technologies for creating controls and placebos seem promising.

Several developments in study techniques and equipment have occurred over the last several years. A placebo or "sham needle," designed to make the patient feel that the skin is being punctured, was developed in 1998. The needle shaft disappears inside itself and adheres to the skin via a small plastic ring (which is then added to real acupuncture needles for study groups). In two reports by Sator-Katzenschlager et al., electroacupuncture delivered through a miniature ear-stimulator was found to be effective in alleviating chronic back and neck pain; separately, the device was found to be a good tool for the masking of study participants, in that 90% to 97% of the sham group (with no actual electricity delivered by the device) thought they were actually in the experimental group.

Acupuncture points now can be localized using an electronic microvoltmeter, which measures the potential difference between two electrodes loaded on springs at a calibrated pressure to determine and "electrodermal response." This technique is now commonly utilized for standardizing randomized controlled trials and has been validated by comparison to manual identification of acupuncture points under fMRI.

Two recent studies on low back pain illustrate the shortcomings and inconsistencies involved in developing and interpreting acupuncture trials. Leibing et al. studied 131 outpatients receiving physiotherapy for 12 weeks and randomized them to three groups: physiotherapy alone, physiotherapy with sham acupuncture, or physiotherapy with real acupuncture. Each noncontrol group had 20 sessions over 12 weeks, for 30 minutes each, at fixed (predetermined to be relevant), standardized acupoints. Real acupuncture was better than physiotherapy alone for pain intensity ($p = 0.000$), disability ($p = 0.000$), and psychological distress ($p = 0.020$), but when it was compared to sham acupuncture, only the psychologic effects were significant ($p < 0.04$). Leibing et al. concluded that traditional acupuncture had a predominant placebo effect on low back pain. Molsberger et al. conducted a similar, though underpowered and prematurely concluded, trial involving 186 inpatients receiving orthopaedic treatments. Patients were randomized to orthopaedic treatment controls, orthopaedic treatment plus sham acupuncture using the minimal acupuncture technique described in the preceding text, and orthopaedic plus manual acupuncture (no EA) at sites specific to the patient's symptoms. These investigators found true acupuncture to be significantly better than both sham ($p < 0.00003$) and control ($p < 0.00001$) at 3 months, but directly after treatment was complete, the difference between acupuncture versus sham was significant ($p = 0.013$), whereas acupuncture versus control was not significant ($p > 0.05$). These results, therefore, seem to directly contradict those of Liebing et al.

VI. CONCLUSION

Acupuncture has become increasingly popular in Europe and America as people have become more familiar with the customs and cultures of China and as the healing qualities of acupuncture therapies become more established in Western understanding. Acupuncture has a long history of success in the China, but we are still investigating its scientific basis, how it interacts with conventional therapies, how effective it is in Western patients, and how to best integrate acupuncture into current Western practices. There are many new studies detailing the efficacy, safety, and proposed mechanisms of acupuncture. Although some of the data remain controversial, clinical trials and the technologies to support them continue to improve.

SELECTED READINGS

Barnes P, Powell-Griner E, McFann K, et al. CDC Advance Data Report 343. *Complementary and alternative medicine use among adults: United States*. NCCAM Press Release, 2002. Available at: www.nccam.nih.gov. Accessed May 27, 2004.

Eisenberg DM, Davis RB, Ettner SL, et al. Trends in alternative medicine use in the United States, 1990–1997, results of a follow-up national survey. *JAMA* 1998;280(18):1569–1575.

Kleinhenz J, Streitberger K, Windeler J, et al. Randomized clinical trial comparing the effects of acupuncture and a newly designed placebo needle in rotator cuff tendonitis. *Pain* 1999;83:235–241.

Leibing E, Leonhardt U, Kostter G, et al. Acupuncture treatment of chronic low-back pain–a randomized, blinded, placebo-controlled trial with 9 month follow-up. *Pain* 2002;96:189–196.

Melchart D, Weidenhammer W, Streng A, et al. Prospective investigation of adverse effects of acupuncture in 97,733 patients. *Arch Intern Med* 2004;164(1):104–105.

Molsberger AF, Mau J, Pawelec DB, et al. Does acupuncture improve the orthopedic management of chronic low back pain–a randomized, blinded, controlled trial with 3 month follow-up. *Pain* 2002;99:579–587.

National Center for Complementary and Alternative Medicine (NCCAM). Available at: www.nccam.nih.gov. Accessed 2005.

Pian-Smith MCM, Pham LH, Smith FWK Jr. Neurophysiologic basis of acupuncture. In: Gellman H, ed. *Acupuncture for treatment for musculoskeletal pain: a textbook for orthopaedics anesthesia and rehabilitation*. Langhorne, PA: Gordon and Breach Science publishers, 2001.

World Health Organization. Acupuncture: review and analysis of reports on controlled clinical trials, 2002. Available at: http://www.who.int/medicines/library/trm/acupuncture/clinicreportsacupuncture.shtml. Accessed 2005.

Chronic Pain Rehabilitation

Elizabeth Loder and Patricia W. McAlary

Like an alarm bell stuck in the "on" position . . . such is chronic benign pain.
—*Bruce Smoller and Brian Schulman*

I. THE SCOPE OF THE PROBLEM

Despite steady improvements in the treatment of pain, there remains a group of patients whose recovery is minimal, although they have been subjected to concerted attempts at appropriate therapy. Unrelieved pain is associated with severe impairment of physical, psychological, and social well-being. Unemployment, reduced physical activity, and sleep disruption associated with chronic pain may lead to a downward spiral of physical inactivity, decreased socialization, altered sleep-wake cycles, and medication overuse. Once entrenched, these maladaptive behavior patterns are difficult to reverse. Secondary depression and medication overuse may develop, along with family dysfunction and poor work performance. Patients with chronic pain are five times more likely than the general population to use medical services, and 58% of patients with chronic pain have anxiety or depression that can further complicate their treatment.

The development of **chronic pain syndrome** (see Table 1), in which patients develop disability out of proportion to the underlying disease, with associated behavioral abnormalities, requires multidisciplinary treatment. The treatment philosophy, which must be accepted by the patient and family, shifts from cure to management. Medication reduction, increased "uptime" and regular physical exercise, involvement in hobbies or return to work, and psychological intervention all help the patient to return to some semblance of normal living, despite the persistence of pain.

Optimal management of chronic pain must address not only the initiating physical pathology but also the social and psychological sequelae that accompany the pain and contribute to poor quality of life. Specialized outpatient pain rehabilitation programs that

Table 1.   Characteristics of patients with chronic pain syndrome

- Demanding, angry, skeptical (of help)
- Doctor shopping ("fix me")
- Somatizing; dependency on health care system—often for multiple medical problems
- Preoccupation with pain
- Marked pain behavior
- Passive–dependent personality traits
- Caretaker—meets needs of others at own expense
- Denial of emotional or family conflicts
- Major disruption in multiple areas of life
- Feelings of isolation and loneliness
- Lack of insight into self-defeating behavior patterns
- Use of pain as a symbolic means of communication
- May be conscious or unconscious of secondary gain

From Aronoff GM. Psychological aspects of nonmalignant chronic pain: a multidisciplinary approach. *Res Staff Physician* 1984;3, with permission.

provide coordinated, multidisciplinary care can be helpful. Inpatient treatment may be necessary for patients with impaired mobility or advanced debilitation, for those whose severe medication overuse requires special tapering from opioid or barbiturate drugs, and for those with associated medical or psychiatric morbidity that precludes outpatient treatment.

1. The Pathologic Nature of Chronic Pain

Chronic pain differs from acute pain in that the former is a pathologic state that is of no benefit to the individual, unlike acute (physiologic) pain, which arises in response to injury or inflammation and protects the individual from further injury. Acute pain is time-limited and resolves as healing takes place. Chronic pain, by contrast, is caused by changes in the nervous system that are not reversible (nerve injury, sensitization, new fiber growth, reorganization, etc.), and is unremitting and extremely difficult to treat. Standard acute pain treatments [nonsteriodal antiinflammatory drugs (NSAIDs) and opioids] have only limited efficacy in treating chronic pain. Moreover the pain, muscle guarding, and decreased activity that serve a useful purpose in acute pain become counterproductive in chronic pain. Avoiding activity no longer serves the purpose of protecting healing tissues from further injury, but instead leads to deconditioning. Patients tend to respond to chronic pain in the same way that they respond to acute pain, but the response is dysfunctional and paradoxically promotes worsening rather than improvement.

II. GENERAL PRINCIPLES OF CHRONIC PAIN TREATMENT

In nearly all cases, multidisciplinary treatment rather than medical treatment alone is required to reverse the complex behavior patterns that develop as a result of chronic pain. When it is not possible to eliminate pain, emphasis shifts from efforts directed solely at pain relief, whatever the cost, toward efforts to maximize the patient's ability to function despite the pain. It is important that this change in philosophy is accepted and understood by the patient, his or her family, and the physician.

It is often hard for patients (or families) to reach the point at which they are ready to embrace a treatment model that emphasizes management and coping but does not promise a cure. They feel compelled to seek additional medical opinions or treatment options before accepting the rehabilitation approach. Physicians may contribute to the problem when they focus only on the specialty treatments they are trained to provide. Prolonged searches for a "cure" can be counterproductive and can expose the patient to further harm from aggressive surgical, medical, or alternative treatments. Tactful discussion between the physician and the patients and their families can help make clear that rehabilitation does not mean giving up on efforts to improve the underlying problem or simply learning to live with the pain.

III. EVALUATION OF THE PATIENT

1. History and Examination

A thorough physical examination is essential to identify sources of pain and to reassure the patient that the pain problem is taken seriously. A history of the pain problem, as well as a detailed review of previous medical records documenting treatment trials, reasons for treatment failures, and the timing of interventions is helpful. Information on specific dosages and length of pharmacologic treatment trials helps the physician assess the adequacy of previous treatments. Whenever possible, the physician should review the original test results [e.g., computerized tomography (CT) scans and magnetic resonance imaging (MRI)] rather than relying on summary information in medical records. Access to comprehensive records may be difficult to obtain, in which case patients or family members can participate by obtaining and organizing this information.

During the initial evaluation, special attention should be paid to the emotional context of the pain problem and its meaning in the patient's life. For example, pain resulting from an injury-causing event in which others were killed or injured, or from what is perceived as a botched surgical procedure, will be difficult to treat without paying attention to the psychologic aspects. Likewise, a history of repeated adversarial or unsatisfactory interactions with multiple health professionals should prompt consideration of the presence of personality or other psychiatric disorders that could complicate treatment. Speaking directly with previous or current caregivers can provide invaluable insight into patterns of self-defeating behavior or other reasons for treatment failure.

2. Pain Intensity and Impact

Patient complaints of pain, functional disability, medication use or overuse, and comorbid psychiatric and medical illnesses must be taken into account to develop an appropriate, individualized treatment plan. In the treatment of chronic pain, ratings of functional ability are more useful than conventional 0 to 10 pain rating scales in gauging the impact of pain and in deciding the type of treatment. A 0 to 3 scale is often employed, with 0 indicating no impact of pain on ability to function, and 1, 2, and 3 representing minimal, moderate, and severe impairment of function by pain, respectively. The use of obsessive or overly detailed pain charts is discouraged (unless they are needed to judge specific interventions) because it encourages somatic preoccupation and attention to pain. In most chronic pain treatment plans, pain behaviors such as grimacing, sighing, or rubbing affected body parts are discouraged because they draw the attention to the pain rather than reinforcing productive "well" behaviors (see Table 2).

Information should be obtained on the impact of pain and pain treatment on the patient's functioning in social, family, and occupational or school settings. It is helpful to ask patients to describe a typical day's schedule and activities, and what would be different if they were not in pain. Disability and financial status and involvement with workers' compensation or the legal system are factors that can influence pain presentation and may also have a bearing on treatment. Education and work history can be important, especially if the pain results from a work-related injury.

Detailed information on sleep disturbance, alterations in sleep–wake cycles, and depression or anxiety should be obtained. Psychiatric or personality disorders exacerbate chronic pain and should be identified and treated. A family history of psychiatric illness or disability may also contribute to the pain. Finally, family beliefs about the patient's condition and the family's role in the pain problem (e.g., "enabling" or overly solicitous behavior, anger, or neglect) should be determined.

Table 2. Pain and well behaviors

Pain behaviors
- Pain talk, focus, and verbal complaints
- Grimacing
- Moaning, groaning, and crying
- Shifting position, guarded movement, limp
- Quiet and withdrawn
- Self-neglect and self-denial
- Blaming attitude
- Avoids self-help groups

Well behaviors
- Takes responsibility for own actions
- Understands own limits and strengths
- Sets realistic goals
- Exercises regularly
- Practices pain-reducing techniques
- Appropriate assertive behavior
- Positive attitude
- Seeks out group support

From Hayes JL, McAlary PW, Popovsky BE, et al. Alteration in comfort: a nursing challenge. In: Aronoff G, ed. *Evaluation and treatment of chronic pain*, 2nd ed. Philadelphia, PA: Williams and Wilkins, 1992, with permission.

3. Attitudes Toward Pain

Patients who believe that they can help control or manage their pain are often referred to as having an **internal locus of control**. In contrast, patients who feel dependent on physicians, the health care system, or medications to control their pain often are referred to as having an **external locus of control**. Successful adaptation to chronic pain is more likely in patients with an internal locus of control. Treatment efforts should aim to reinforce a patient's belief in his or her ability to affect pain levels. Efforts to involve the patient in treatment and to create a sense of control should be a part of all aspects of chronic pain treatment. Self-management strategies, such as those outlined in Table 3, help deemphasize the pattern of reliance on medications, procedures, and other passive treatments.

IV. TREATMENT

The effects of unrelieved pain are pervasive, and rehabilitation demands coordinated, multidisciplinary treatment. Patients are encouraged to set functional goals during the initial evaluation, and regular meetings of the treatment team should occur to assess progress toward these goals, share information, and refine treatment plans. Appropriate functional goals should be realistic, achievable, and under the control of the patient.

A specialized inpatient or outpatient treatment program provides a team of appropriately trained personnel to coordinate an intensive, synergistic treatment plan. Early, targeted intervention for patients whose pain is not improving is helpful and ultimately cost-effective. All too often, however, early, intensive intervention for chronic pain is precluded by factors such as lack of insurance coverage, so that only the most refractory patients (whose outcomes are actually substantially poorer) receive such treatment.

1. Group Therapy

A variety of topics and skills can be taught effectively to patients with chronic pain in a group setting. Group meetings offer

Table 3.   Examples of independent pain control techniques

Ice massage/cold packs
Hot packs
TENS
Acupressure
Self-massage, use of *theracane*
Whirlpool baths/showers
Exercise
Distraction
Meditation/relaxation/biofeedback
Self-hypnosis/imagery
Music therapy
Humor
Therapeutic touch
Pain diaries and journals
Rest periods

TENS, transcutaneous electrical nerve stimulation.

support and reinforcement of adaptive behaviors through group feedback and discussion. In all cases, the group must be carefully supervised to ensure positive educational experiences. Family education, postural reeducation and movement, stress management skills, substance abuse information, life skills training, and other topics are appropriate for group teaching. The therapeutic milieu is an essential component of both outpatient and inpatient pain programs and is helpful in reducing the isolation and lack of social understanding encountered by patients with chronic pain.

2. Individual Components of a Chronic Pain Treatment Program

The following components of chronic pain treatment are useful in nearly every case. Certain patients with less complicated presentations may require only some of these interventions.

(i) Medication Reduction and Optimization

The use of medication in chronic pain is best viewed as one component of the patient's overall management plan. Medication alone is unlikely to be effective in dealing with the problem, and its importance should be placed in perspective. An important aspect of treatment is a thorough, thoughtful review of medications with the dual goal of eliminating unnecessary medications and ensuring that patients have had adequate trials of disease-specific treatments. Because the causes of chronic pain are heterogeneous, it is important to carefully ascertain, through retrials of treatments if necessary, that patients have had appropriate trials of treatments known to be helpful for their particular condition.

Many medications that provide short-term relief from symptoms can cause long-term complications that interfere with successful treatment. Medications prescribed for sleep, muscle spasm, and anxiety belong to this category. The use of these medications over a prolonged period can cause sedation, poor concentration, and emotional detachment, which can impede the ability to function. Patients also come to rely on the sedative and psychoactive effects of medications in modulating emotional as well as physical pain. In many cases, although medications no longer help, patients and physicians are reluctant to discontinue them, fearing that things might get worse if they are stopped.

The decision to use long-acting or maintenance opioids must be made on an individual basis. Many patients with chronic pain will show improved function and decreased pain when treated with these medications. Unfortunately, a subset of patients who experience inadequate pain relief continue to take increasing doses without satisfactory response, deteriorate functionally, and possibly display drug-seeking or addictive behavior. Recent evidence that prolonged exposure to high doses of opioids may lead to opioid-induced abnormal pain sensitivity provides one explanation for this apparent paradox. As a general principle, patients with chronic pain are only offered long-acting opioids. Short-acting opioids are more likely to produce a "high" and pose a higher risk of addiction. Patients who come to associate an altered sensorium with pain relief may regard alternative therapies (including long-acting opioids) as less than optimally effective. A patient's insistence on only short-acting opioids is a marker of possible addiction.

Increasing evidence suggests that chronic opioid use may paradoxically worsen pain, by producing opioid-induced hyperalgesia or other central nervous system changes.

(ii) Physical Reconditioning

By avoiding activities that aggravate or produce pain, nearly all patients with chronic, unrelieved pain develop some measure of physical deconditioning. Their decreased activity level generally results in a downward spiral of physical inactivity and reduced capacity for exercise that exacerbates pain, rather than diminishing it. Physical therapy supervision of a gradual program of reconditioning and therapeutic exercise is the cornerstone of successful rehabilitation. The roles and contributions of therapists in a multidisciplinary pain team vary according to the needs of the patient and the interests and expertise of the therapists. A system that allows therapists to have a flexible role and the ability to treat in conjunction with other disciplines provides optimal results.

Physical therapy is aimed at increasing patients' use of independent pain management modalities such as self-massage, heat and cold, and transcutaneous electrical nerve stimulation (TENS). Physical therapy modalities such as massage or ultrasound that are passive and do not foster independence are less useful in chronic pain treatment.

An important focus of physical therapy is improved aerobic and functional capacities. Patients with chronic pain may have failed prior physical therapy regimens in which they may have been encouraged to discontinue activity with the onset of pain. A major challenge for the physical therapist working with these patients is to educate them that hurt does not always mean harm. It is advisable to begin with short, easy sessions, increasing duration and intensity in small increments and to use a realistic, quota-based program that encourages a gradual increase in exercise tolerance. With this approach, patients quickly come to understand that some of their pain may be caused by previous inappropriate use of assistive devices, muscle weakness, and muscle guarding. A physical therapist with experience in the treatment of chronic pain will be able to develop an appropriate program for patients with chronic pain.

Exercise not only improves physical functioning but also reduces pain levels, has a beneficial impact on depression and feelings of self-worth, and helps restore a normal sleep–wake cycle. Exercises aimed at improving postural tension, body mechanics, and muscle imbalance also can have a beneficial impact on pain and function.

(iii) Occupational Therapy

The impact of pain on daily life can be severe. Patients may be limited in their ability to perform basic self-care activities such as bathing, and dressing, or find it difficult to prepare meals, perform housekeeping chores, or shop for groceries. Occupational therapists help patients incorporate effective pain control strategies into activities of everyday life. Specific strategies can include goal-setting, group programs, pacing techniques, assertive communication, the use of appropriate body mechanics during everyday activities, and assistive devices or environmental modifications to support independent function.

Activity levels in patients with chronic pain often closely mirror pain levels; patients remain in bed or do very little on days when their pain is particularly severe and then compensate with intense overactivity on days when their pain is better. This drastic swing in activity levels leads to a sense of frustration in the patient and makes it difficult for him or her to participate reliably in work, social, and school activities. Occupational therapists can work with patients to identify such patterns and to concentrate on pacing techniques. These techniques emphasize avoidance of large swings in activity levels and encourage frequent breaks in activity regardless of pain levels, as well as regular use of active pain control techniques to prevent pain escalation. They also include scheduling the use of hot and cold packs and relaxation strategies as part of the patient's daily routine. Scheduled use of ice massage, self-massage (often facilitated by the use of inexpensive devices such as **theracanes** that allow massage of distant body parts without undue stretching or straining), TENS, or hot packs can enhance the effectiveness of other therapeutic and pharmacologic interventions. Use of these strategies and progress toward desired activities and goals can be monitored through graphs or charts. As progress occurs, particularly if it is without large increases in pain, patients are able to directly observe the benefits. Patients also can be "rewarded" for pain self-management practices by incorporating pleasurable activities into these routines.

(iv) Nonpharmacologic Pain Control Techniques

Biofeedback, self-hypnosis, and other relaxation strategies are useful adjuncts to chronic pain treatments. Such treatments often reduce, although may not eliminate, the use of pain medication and improve a patient's sense of control over pain. These strategies are most effective when used preemptively on a regular basis; their effectiveness decreases once pain is established. Many of these techniques are taught by psychologists, who can at the same time identify counterproductive and maladaptive behavior patterns. Patients often benefit from cognitive-behavioral therapy aimed at altering beliefs and ideas about pain and improving coping mechanisms. Patient motivation is also a target of such treatment because it alters coping behavior and is an important factor in how well patients learn to manage pain.

(v) Psychiatric and Psychologic Intervention

Psychiatric disorders can complicate the management of chronic pain. Patients with premorbid psychiatric disorders cope less well with chronic pain, and unrelieved chronic pain can trigger the development of psychiatric disorders, particularly depression. Psychiatric evaluation is therefore essential for all patients with debilitating chronic pain. Appropriate management of identified disorders will improve the patient's ability to cope with chronic pain and to comply with treatment. Psychiatric oversight of the many psychoactive medications used in the chronic pain population is also important.

A history of prior physical, sexual, or emotional abuse or trauma is common in patients with chronic pain. Recent work suggests that early trauma may produce permanent changes in the functioning of the hypothalamic–pituitary axis and in the response to later painful events. The identification of a history of trauma has important treatment implications and should be sought in all patients with disabling chronic pain. Patients with a history of a traumatic childhood with unmet dependence needs; early adult responsibilities; or physical, emotional, or sexual abuse are often less able to cope with pain. These patients may have coped well before the onset of pain, but the development of a pain problem can provide an unconscious but socially acceptable way to ask to be taken care of.

Patients with chronic pain may deny family or relationship stressors, blaming all life disruption on their pain and consciously or unconsciously using pain as a way to avoid unpleasant or unwanted obligations in many areas. For this reason, a careful review of social and family relationships is helpful. An assessment of mood and suicidal potential is also important because chronic pain is a risk factor for both suicide and suicide attempts.

(vi) Family Intervention

Perhaps the most neglected aspect of chronic pain is its impact on family members and on other elements of a patient's social support network. Chronic pain in one member of a family commonly causes shifts in family roles and functions. Spouses or children may take over aspects of the patient's role, such as housework, shopping, or wage earning. Family and friends may inadvertently support or encourage further disability and dependency through enabling, oversolicitous behavior. Alternatively, they may gradually become impatient with the patient's disability and withdraw from the relationship, further isolating the patient from emotional and social support. It is important to recognize that, in many cases, the family and the social network of the patient gradually adapts to the presence of an ill member, and the patient may be relegated to the designated sick role in the family. Family dynamics then act to perpetuate and reinforce pain behavior and illness roles. Once established, these maladaptive family behaviors can be difficult to change. Inattention to these family patterns places patients at high risk for relapse after rehabilitation. Family-treatment team meetings or groups aimed at teaching family and social supports the principles and philosophy of pain management improve outcomes and reduce relapse.

(vii) Return to Productive Activities

Many patients believe that the presence of chronic pain means that they cannot or should not participate in occupational, social, or academic activities. They fear aggravation of their pain or worry that overexertion will cause permanent physical harm. In fact, participation in appropriate work, school, and social activities is generally therapeutic for patients with chronic illness. In most patients with chronic pain, the benefits of social interaction, regular sleep–wake cycles, and self-esteem that productive activities promote far exceed any drawbacks. In general, patients should be encouraged to remain as active as possible. Decisions by the treatment team to support disability status, withdrawal from school, or the avoidance of social activities or hobbies should be very carefully considered. Although the intention—relieving the patient of an activity, which may seem to aggravate pain—is laudable, very often, discontinuation of such activities does not improve the pain and leads to further isolation, depression, and reinforcement of the sick role. In most cases, it is preferable to have a vocational counselor or other treatment team member help the patient develop realistic plans for return to activity that can be implemented over time. Job descriptions should be carefully reviewed and genuine medical contraindications to certain activities or work demands incorporated into any return-to-work or other plans.

(viii) Follow-up

Chronic pain can be managed but not cured; most patients will require careful and regular multidisciplinary follow-up indefinitely. Unfortunately, this is often not understood by third-party payers, and treatment resources are limited. Periodic review of medication regimens, attention to psychosocial aspects of the patient's situation, and careful evaluation of the progression of any underlying disease are all-important in chronic pain. A strong physician–patient relationship is therapeutic and can help keep the patient from further iatrogenic harm. A physician whom the patient has come to know and trust, and who shows sincere interest in the patient's well-being over time, is in the best position to help the patient consider the advantages and disadvantages of any new or alternative treatment options.

V. MEASURING THE BENEFITS OF TREATMENT

The benefits of chronic pain treatment are reflected by a patient's return to a more normal, less pain-focused life, rather than by a reduction in pain level. These benefits can be assessed by measuring decreased use of the health care system (i.e., fewer emergency room visits and acute medical and psychiatric admissions; decreased physician office visits, and decreased polypharmacy), return to productive activities (not just paid work), decreased pain-related depression, improved sleep, and resumption of normal family and social relationships. A tool frequently used to measure pain program outcomes is the SF-36, a standardized measure of health-related quality of life, which produces measures of physical role and social well-being.

VI. CONCLUSION

Chronic pain rehabilitation programs provide an opportunity for patients with chronic pain to take a completely different approach to their pain problem. Most of these patients have had multiple treatments, sometimes from many different treatment centers in an attempt to relieve their pain. The rehabilitation approach will, for the first time, take a broad look at the patient's situation (physical, medical, psychological, social, educational, etc.) and set up an intensive program that will address all aspects of the pain. The program will teach the patient how to manage and live with pain and how to live as normal a life as possible.

A list of rehabilitation programs can be obtained from the Commission of the Accreditation of Rehabilitation Facilities (CARF) (see Appendix II).

SELECTED READINGS

Allen M, Giles G. Occupational therapy in the treatment of patients with chronic pain. *Br J Occup Ther* 1986.

Ballantyne JC, Mao J. Opioid therapy for chronic pain. *N Engl J Med* 2003;349:1943–1953.

Bogduk N, Mersey H, ed. *Classification of chronic pain, descriptors of chronic pain syndromes and definitions of pain terms*, 2nd ed. Seattle, WA: IASP Press, 1994.

Jamison R. Psychological factors in chronic pain. *J Back Musculoskel Rehab* 1996;7:79–95.

Jensen MP, Nielson WR, Kerns RD. Toward the development of a motivational model of pain self-management. *Pain* 2003;4:477–492.

National Occupational Therapy Pain Association. Available at: www.notpa.org.uk/home.shtml. Accessed 2005.

20

Radiotherapy and Radiopharmaceuticals for Cancer Pain

Thomas F. DeLaney

The report of my death was an exaggeration.
—*Note to London correspondent of the New York Journal, June 1897, by Mark Twain*

I. GENERAL PRINCIPLES

Pain is a frequent complication of cancer. It can be a presenting symptom of the disease, a sign of local recurrence of tumor after prior treatment, or a symptom of metastatic disease. Palliative radiation therapy became a mainstay of nonsurgical cancer treatment soon after the discovery of x-rays. Radiation, delivered by external beam, implantation (placement of radioactive sources within the tumor), or systemic radiopharmaceutical can be effective in the management of cancer pain. Radiation therapy can relieve pain related to either metastatic disease or symptoms from local extension of primary disease. This chapter focuses on the treatment of pain related to metastatic disease. It is worth emphasizing that radiation therapy can complement analgesic drug or other therapies and may enhance their effectiveness because this therapy directly targets the cause of pain.

In principle, ionizing radiation is delivered to the tumor with the intent of reducing or eliminating viable cancer cells while maintaining normal tissue integrity. It is most commonly given as megavoltage external beam photons produced by a linear accelerator. Electrons, which have a more limited range in tissue defined by their energy, also can be produced by linear accelerators and can be very useful in the treatment of superficial tumors, with the additional benefit of sparing normal tissues below the tumor. Systemically administered radiopharmaceuticals, such as strontium-89 (^{89}Sr) or samarium-153 (^{153}Sm), have a role in the treatment of patients with symptomatic metastatic disease involving multiple bones, whereas iodine-131 (^{131}I) is appropriate for the treatment of patients with metastatic thyroid cancers that are iodine avid. Brachytherapy (implantation of radioactive sources into tumor) is a useful mode of radiation delivery because of the physical advantage of very high radiation doses applied to the tumor compared to the surrounding normal tissue and the biologic advantage of low dose rate (which differentially spares the normal tissue). Brachytherapy is usually used in the management of the primary tumor; it is less commonly used for palliation of metastatic disease.

External beam radiation is prescribed by absorbed radiation dose (the SI unit is the Gray; 1 Gy is equal to 100 rads) per unit volume in a selected field. The total dose, the number of daily fraction, and the volume of tissue irradiated are determined by considering the needs and the likely benefit for each patient.

II. INDICATIONS FOR RADIATION THERAPY

The primary indications for radiotherapy in the management of cancer pain are listed in Table 1. These indications include bone pain from metastases (with or without pathologic fracture), spinal cord compression, tumor infiltration of nerve plexus, blockage of hollow viscera, and reduction in space-occupying lesions (particularly cerebral metastases). Radiotherapy also can be very useful in palliation of bleeding from tumors, cough or dyspnea secondary to tumor invading bronchus, and superior vena cava syndrome.

When making decisions about the use of radiation therapy, physicians should consider the type of neoplasm, the relative effectiveness of available treatment modalities, the patient's prior treatment, and the extent of his or her disease (i.e., single or limited versus multiple metastatic sites), as well as the patient's performance status, length of expected survival, and bone marrow reserve.

Table 1.   Indications for palliative radiation therapy

Pain relief
Bone pain
Nerve root and soft-tissue infiltration

Control of bleeding
Hemoptysis
Vaginal bleeding
Hematuria
Rectal bleeding

Control of fungation and ulceration

Dyspnea
Tumor obstructing trachea or bronchus

Oncologic emergencies
Spinal cord compression
Cerebral metastases causing raised intracranial pressure
Superior vena cava syndrome

Relief of blockage of hollow viscera

Shrinkage of tumor masses
Causing symptoms by virtue of site or space occupancy

From Ashby M. The role of radiotherapy in palliative care. *J Pain Symptom Manage* 1991;6:380–388, with permission.

The efforts of the radiation oncologist should be closely coordinated with those of other physicians and health care personnel. Patients with particularly difficult pain problems may benefit from presentation at a tumor board or other appropriate multidisciplinary conference to allow for input and discussion among the varying specialists with expertise in the management of cancer pain.

III. GOALS OF PALLIATIVE TREATMENT

The intent of palliative treatment is rapid and durable pain relief. Ideally such treatment should maintain symptom control for the remainder of the patient's life, with minimal associated morbidity. Radiation therapy can arrest local tumor growth that might otherwise lead to intractable pain, cord compression, airway obstruction, uncontrolled bleeding, or pathologic fracture. For some patients, the resultant elimination of or reduction in the need for narcotic pain medications can improve quality of life. Reduction in pain also can improve ambulation.

Treatment should be tailored to the patient's clinical condition and overall prognosis. Patients with good performance status and with a limited burden of metastatic disease near crucial structures such as the spinal cord or brachial plexus may benefit from radiation treatment programs that give a higher total radiation dose delivered in multiple fractions. Although such a program may require more initial visits to the radiotherapy clinic, it is likely to result in more durable palliation in the patient with a longer life expectancy. In contrast, patients with widely metastatic disease and limited life expectancy should be considered for rapid, limited-fraction treatment courses.

IV. RADIATION THERAPY FOR TREATMENT OF BONE METASTASES

For a single site or a limited number of sites of bone metastases, external beam radiation therapy is appropriate and may relieve symptoms for an extended period. For patients with symptomatic bone metastases at multiple sites, it is more appropriate to institute analgesics along with available systemic chemotherapy or endocrine therapy and bisphosphonates. If symptoms persist, consider systemic radiopharmaceuticals, localized external radiotherapy to the most symptomatic areas, or hemibody irradiation.

Most patients referred for palliation of metastatic bone pain have the most frequently occurring types of primary tumors, namely, breast, prostate, or lung tumors. Eighty to 90% of these patients experience pain relief following radiation therapy, with 50% of these patients obtaining complete relief. Most patients experience some pain relief within 10 to 14 days after the start of therapy. Seventy percent of patients have pain relief by 2 weeks after the completion of treatment; 90% have relief within 1 to 3 months. Pain relief after radiation therapy is durable in 55% to 70% of patients.

Although it has been assumed that tumor shrinkage is responsible for pain relief in this setting, the exact mechanism of pain relief is poorly understood; patients often experience pain relief at radiation doses that are well below that is necessary to induce a complete regression of the tumor.

Several small studies did not report any clear differences in overall response rates among patients with different tumor histologies. However, a large, randomized radiation therapy oncology group (RTOG) study that looked at different radiation fractionation schemes reported a higher percentage of complete pain relief in patients with breast and prostate primaries compared to patients with lung and other types of primary tumors. Sites of metastases do not correlate with the degree of pain relief. Severe and frequent pain indicates a poor prognosis. A sudden increase in pain during treatment should raise concerns about a pathologic fracture, and appropriate radiographs and orthopaedic evaluation should be performed.

Radiation affects both tumor cell and adjacent normal osteoclasts and osteoblasts. The presence of tumor, however, is a greater threat to the structural integrity of bone than the adverse effects of radiation on bone healing. Bone reossification will often occur following tumor eradication. There was recalcification of 78% of osteolytic lesions treated in one study and another 16% showed no further progression after radiation therapy.

Evaluation of patients with bone metastases includes bone scintigraphy, which is more sensitive than skeletal radiography except in patients with purely lytic (osteoclastic) disease such as myeloma. Bone scintigraphy also will detect many initially asymptomatic metastases; some of which may subsequently become symptomatic. Abnormal areas on bone scan in long bones should be examined by skeletal radiographs to determine whether there are areas of advanced lytic disease that should be radiated or orthopaedically stabilized to prevent pathologic fracture. Lytic lesions that are greater than 2.5 cm in size in weight-bearing bones or that have lysis of greater than 50% of cortical bone may require orthopaedic fixation. Magnetic resonance imaging (MRI) should be used in patients with bone pain in whom the bone scans and radiographs are normal. MRI of the spine is appropriate in patients with suspected spinal cord compression. In such patients, at least a sagittal midline scout view of the entire spine also should be obtained to rule out the occasional second site of spinal cord compression.

The radiation therapy ports are planned using data from the history and physical examination, bone scan, skeletal films, computerized tomography (CT) scans and/or MRI scans, and review of any prior radiation therapy fields. Soft-tissue masses, most often associated with bone metastases to the vertebral bodies or pelvis, must be included in the radiotherapy fields. The distribution of bone marrow must be considered, especially in patients receiving chemotherapy.

There has been considerable debate about the optimal total dose, fraction size, and duration of treatment of metastatic lesions in bone. In patients with metastatic cancer in whom life expectancy is limited, quick and effective treatment with minimal morbidity is desired. One of the most commonly employed fractionation schemes, 3,000 cGy in 10 fractions over 2 weeks, has been compared in a number of recent studies to shorter treatment schedules. A randomized RTOG study assigned 759 patients to one of five treatment schedules that ranged from 4 days to 3 weeks in overall duration: 500 cGy in 4 fractions, 300 cGy in 5 fractions, 400 cGy in 5 fractions, 300 cGy in 10 fractions, or 270 cGy in 15 fractions. No significant difference was seen in the response. An independent reanalysis of the data, however, noted that the protracted fractionation schemes were more likely to provide complete relief and cessation of opioid intake. In other randomized trials, there is no clear advantage for the longer, multiple-fraction regimens when compared to shorter or single-course regimens. Three large European randomized studies compared 800 cGy in one fraction with 3,000 cGy in 10 fractions (Royal Marsden Hospital, 288 patients), with 2,000 cGy in 5 fractions or 3,000 cGy in 10 fractions (Bone Pain Trial Working Party, 765 patients), or with 2,400 cGy in 6 fractions (Dutch Bone Metastasis Study, 1,171 patients). No difference was seen with respect to pain relief, time to its achievement, duration of relief, or toxicity. Retreatment was given more frequently in the single-fraction arms, which may in part be related to physician willingness to reirradiate an area that had received the lower prior radiation dose. A large randomized trial was recently completed by the cooperative clinical trials group, the RTOG. This trial compared 800 cGy in one fraction with 3,000 cGy in 10 fractions for patients with pain from bone metastases from prostate or breast cancer. Nine hundred and forty-nine patients were enrolled between 1998 and 2002, of whom 898 were eligible and analyzable. Patients who were entered into the trial were expected to have a life expectancy of greater than 3 months and had no prior surgery or radiotherapy to the affected site. They were stratified according to single or multiple sites of pain, weight-bearing versus non-weight–bearing bone, the severity of pain score, and whether they were receiving bisphosphonates. Pain relief and reduction in narcotic usage were similar between the two fractionation schemes, with 15% and 18% of patients experiencing complete relief in the single and multiple fraction arms respectively; partial responses were seen in 50% and 48% respectively. Pain relief was similar whether or not the patient was on bisphosphonates. At 3 months, 33% of patients no longer required narcotic medications. Acute toxicity was mild, although a slightly higher rate of 17% grade 2 to 4 acute toxicity was seen in the group receiving 30 Gy compared with 10% when 8 Gy was given, P <0.0001.

The following are guidelines for treatment fractionation. It is expedient to give single-fraction irradiation to the debilitated patient with a very short life expectancy. Single large fractions, however, to some sites such as the abdomen and brain may not be well tolerated acutely. Hence, each radiation oncologist must consider the site of disease, the patient's performance status and social situation, and any normal tissue in the treatment field when deciding on a treatment regimen. Patients with one or few sites of metastases who have a good performance status and a primary disease that responds well to systemic therapy may live for many years after irradiation for bone pain. Large fractions that are known to produce more late effects in normal tissue must be used with considerable caution in these patients, especially when radiation fields include the brain, spinal cord, kidneys, or major portions of the liver or bowel. At the same time, it should be taken into account that these patients may survive long enough to have problems with recurrent tumor in involved bone sites that have not been radiated to sufficiently high doses. Patients with bone metastases producing spinal cord compression are not suitable for single-fraction treatment because of the obvious neurologic risks of recurrent tumor in this site.

It has been difficult to demonstrate a clear dose–response relationship in treatment of bone metastases, often because the groups studied have been heterogeneous, with different histologies and survival times after treatment. Arcangeli and colleagues from Italy reported a significantly higher frequency of complete pain relief with higher radiation doses. They reported complete pain relief rates of 81%, 65%, and 46% with doses of 40 to 46 Gy in 20 to 23 fractions over 5 to 5.5 weeks, 30 to 36 Gy in 10 to 12 fractions over 2 to 2.3 weeks, and 8 to 28 Gy in 1 to 4 consecutive fractions. Hence, in patients with good performance status, limited metastatic disease, and long expected survival after palliative irradiation, doses greater than 4,000 cGy with conventional fractionation are recommended. For patients whose expected survival is short, a high dose is less important because they will not live long enough to manifest recurrent tumor.

V. HEMIBODY IRRADIATION

Sequential hemibody irradiation has been utilized for patients with diffuse, widely disseminated bone metastases. The irradiation is designed to avoid repeated trips to the hospital for multiple courses of irradiation in such patients. It results in complete relief of pain in 21% of patients and partial relief in 77% of patients; most of those treated have had breast, prostate, or lung cancer. Pain control is achieved rapidly, with improvement noted within 2 days among half of the patients experiencing pain relief. Kuban reported good palliation with hemibody irradiation in patients with disseminated prostate cancer. Palliative effects were maintained until death in 82% of the patients treated to the upper half of the body and 67% of patients treated to the lower half of the body.

For hemibody radiation, 600 cGy of irradiation is delivered to the upper hemibody and 800 cGy to the lower hemibody. Patients treated for metastases of the upper body are usually hospitalized for a day, hydrated, and premedicated with antiemetics and corticosteroids. Patients subjected to midbody and lower body therapies are premedicated as outpatients in order to minimize nausea and vomiting.

In one large study of hemibody irradiation by the RTOG, there were no fatalities related to treatment. Treatment to the lower and midbody were well tolerated, with severe nausea and vomiting, diarrhea, or hematologic toxicity occurring in 2%, 6%, and 8% of patients, respectively. Upper body treatment with partial lung shielding induced severe nausea and vomiting, fever, or hematologic toxicity in 15%, 4%, and 32% of the patients, respectively. Hematologic complications are worse in patients who have received prior chemotherapy or who receive the treatment with low peripheral blood counts. A group from Memorial Sloan–Kettering has reported that fractionated hemibody irradiation (2,500 to 3,000 cGy in 9 to 10 fractions) yields more durable pain relief without any increase in complications.

VI. SYSTEMIC RADIOISOTOPES

Several systemically administered radiopharmaceuticals have been used to palliate pain caused by multiple osseous metastases. ^{131}I can provide pain relief in patients with well-differentiated thyroid carcinoma, with bone scan evidence of response in 53% of patients. ^{89}Sr, samarium-153-ethylenediaminetetramethylene-phosphonate (^{153}Sm-EDTMP), and rhenium-186-HEDP are used to treat patients with sclerotic metastases (metastatic prostate cancer and other selected cases). These agents have an onset of response that usually occurs during the first week of therapy and lasts for 3 to 4 months.

Patient selection is important. Relative indications include bone metastases causing pain that is not controlled by analgesics or that arises in a patient intolerant to narcotics, absence of soft tissue masses, osteoblastic lesions, multiple metastatic sites, and tumor that is refractory to hormonal treatment or chemotherapy. Because of the limited penetration of the β-emissions delivered by systemic radioisotopes, patients with spinal cord compression are not appropriate for radioisotope therapy and should be treated with external beam radiation. Because these agents can depress the marrow and are cleared by the kidneys, severe thrombocytopenia, neutropenia, and renal impairment are also relative contraindications. Urinary incontinence presents a radiation safety hazard and is also a contraindication. These agents can be used when the patient has already had localized radiation therapy to a painful site.

^{89}Sr is a bone-seeking calcium analog incorporated by osteoblasts into new bone. It is a β (electron) emitter with a 1.46 MeV maximum energy, a physical half-life of 50.6 days, and a 4 to 6 mm range in tissue. It has no considerable γ-emissions, so it cannot be imaged. Patients release very little radioactivity into the environment and therefore most can be treated as outpatients. Unbound ^{89}Sr is eliminated in the urine within 2 days. Strontium-89 has been well studied in prostate or breast cancer but can be used for osteoblastic metastases from other primaries. Moderate or greater pain relief has been documented in approximately 80% of prostate and breast cancer, with complete relief in approximately 10% to 30%. Pain relief is not usually seen until 2 to 3 weeks after injection. The recommended dose of ^{89}Sr is approximately 4 mCi (60 to 80 μCi per kg). Strontium can be retained in metastatic bone for up to 90 days. The dose delivered to tumor depends on disease burden; it is estimated to be 800 to 2,000 cGy in patients with diffuse disease versus 3,000 to 10,000 cGy with limited or moderate tumor burden.

When evaluated in a placebo-controlled phase III trial as an adjuvant therapy in patients treated with external beam radiation, ^{89}Sr did not affect the degree of pain relief at the index lesion, but a greater proportion of patients in the ^{89}Sr group were able to discontinue analgesics (17.1% versus 2.4%), remained free of new painful bone metastases at 3 months (58.7% versus 34%), and had a longer time to further radiation therapy (35.3 versus 20.3 weeks).

Toxicities that can result from ^{89}Sr include thrombocytopenia, neutropenia, and hemorrhage. In the adjuvant trial cited in the preceding text, grade 3 thrombocytopenia was seen in 22.4% and grade 4 in 10.4% of the ^{89}Sr group, resulting in the need for platelet transfusions in 5.2%. This result compares with 1.7% grade 3 and 1.7% grade 4 thrombocytopenia in the placebo group, which did not require any platelet transfusions. Hemorrhage occurred in 14.9% of the patients treated with ^{89}Sr and 5.2% of the control patients. Grade 3 neutropenia was seen in 10.4% and grade 4 in 1.5% of the patients in the ^{89}Sr arm and in none of the control patients. Occasionally a patient will have a flare-up of pain several days after administration. This occurrence may be associated with a favorable treatment response according to some investigators. Some patients have reported a flushing sensation, often facial, but this is self-limited.

Samarium-153-EDTMP is a therapeutic agent composed of radioactive [153]Sm and a tetraphosphonate chelator, EDTMP. It has recently been approved for use as a systemic radiopharmaceutical. The recommended dose is 1 mCi per kg. The agent has an affinity for bone and accumulates in osteoblastic regions of bone. Its physical half-life of 1.9 days results in higher rates of dose delivery than ^{89}Sr, which typically translates into more rapid onset of action and more rapidly reversible toxicity. Its 0.81-MeV maximum energy β-emission is lower than that of ^{89}Sr, yielding lower penetration in tissue of 2 to 3 mm and theoretically less marrow toxicity. It also has a γ-emission, which allows for imaging with gamma camera to document the accumulation of isotope at affected sites. Treatment efficacy seems similar to that of ^{89}Sr, with approximately half its reported risk of marrow toxicity.

Rhenium-136-etidronate is a combined β- and γ-emitter, with a maximum β-emission of 1.07 keV. It has a 9% emission of γ-rays of 137 keV, which are suitable for imaging as well. -Rhenium-136-etidronate, with its relatively short physical half-life of 3.8 days, may produce a faster onset of pain relief and a higher dose rate than are possible for radionuclides with a longer half-life. In addition, [186]Re-etidronate is suitable for repetitive treatment, provided the interval between treatments is sufficient.

A randomized phase III trial assigned 152 men with hormone-refractory prostate cancer and painful bone metastases to treatment with 1 mCi per kg radioactive [153]Sm versus nonradioactive [152]Sm lexidronam complexes. The radioactive isotope had positive effects on measures of pain relief compared with placebo within 1 to 2 weeks. Reductions in opioid use were recorded at weeks 3 and 4. Mild, transient bone marrow suppression was the only adverse event associated with [153]Sm-lexidronam administration. The mean nadir white blood cell and platelet count (3 to 4 weeks after treatment) was 3,800 per μL and 127,000 per μL, respectively. Counts recovered to baseline after approximately 8 weeks. No grade 4 decreases in either platelets or white bloods cells were documented. A similar randomized trial with [186]Re-etidronate demonstrated a therapeutic advantage when compared to placebo in a similar patient population.

VII. CONCLUSION

It is important for pain specialists treating patients with pain from cancer to remember the powerful effects of radiation therapy in reducing pain and in treating various other symptoms (see Table 1). Radiation is not only an effective way to shrink the primary tumor but also an effective therapy for soft-tissue metastases and widespread bone metastases. Radiation therapy can be palliative as well as curative. A good working relationship between pain physicians and radiation oncologists contributes greatly to the effective management of cancer pain.

SELECTED READINGS

Anderson PR, Coia L. Fractionation and outcomes with palliative radiation therapy. *Semin Radiat Oncol* 2000;10:191–199.

Arcangeli G, Giovinazzo G, Saracino B, et al. Radiation therapy in the management of symptomatic bone metastases: The effect of total dose and histology on pain relief and response duration. *Int J Radiat Oncol Biol Phys* 1998;42:1119–1126.

Ashby M. The role of radiotherapy in palliative care. *J Pain Symptom Manage* 1991;6:380–388.

Hartsell WF, Scott CB, Bruner DW, et al. Randomized trial of short- versus long-course radiotherapy for palliation of painful bone metastases. *J Natl Cancer Inst* 2005;97:798–804.

Janjan N. Bone metastases: approaches to management. *Semin Oncol* 2001;4(Suppl. 11):28–34.

Kuban DA, Delbridge T, el-Mahdi AM, Schellhammer PF. Half-body irradiation for treatment of widely-metastatic adenocarcinoma of the prostate. *J Urol* 1989; 141:572–574.

McEwan AJB. Use of radionuclides for the palliation of bone metastases. *Semin Radiat Oncol* 2000;10:103–114.

McQuay HJ, Collins SL, Carroll D, et al. Radiotherapy for the palliation of painful bone metastases. *Cochrane Database Syst Rev* 2000;(2): CD001793 .

Pandit-Taskar N, Batraki M, Divgi CR. Radiopharmaceutical therapy for palliation of bone pain from osseous metastases. *J Nucl Med* 2004;45:1358–1365.

Ratanatharathorn V, Powers WE, Moss W, et al. Bone metastasis: review and critical analysis of random allocation trials of local field treatment. *Int J Radiat Oncol Biol Phys* 1999;44:1–18.

Rose CM, Kagan AR. The final report of the expert panel for the Radiation Oncology Bone Metastasis Work Group of the American College of Radiation Oncology. *Int J Radiat Oncol Biol Phys* 1998; 40:1117–1124.

V

Acute Pain

21

Postoperative Pain in Adults

Jane C. Ballantyne and Elizabeth Ryder

Rich the treasure, Sweet the pleasure
Sweet is pleasure after pain
For all the happiness man can gain
Is not in pleasure, but in rest from pain.
—*John Dryden, 1631–1700*

Thirty years ago, patients were encouraged to rest for days, even weeks, after surgery. Postoperative hospital stay was longer, feeding was delayed, patients were not expected to get out of bed, and analgesia was needed only for pain at rest. Since then, the concept of accelerated recovery, whereby normal physiologic function is restored as rapidly as possible, has replaced the idea that rest is best. Patients are encouraged to mobilize, take oral fluids, eat, and return home as rapidly as possible. Multiple trials confirm that accelerated recovery is associated with improved surgical outcome. Optimal pain control is an integral component of accelerated recovery; and paradoxically, although opioids are the most effective analgesics available, postoperative pain management is now based on multimodal analgesia and opioid sparing. Opioid side effects that delay recovery, particularly sedation and decreased bowel mobility, are therefore minimized. Multimodal analgesia also makes sense because acute pain is an integrated process mediated by a range of transmitters and neural pathways, so it seems rational to target analgesics to a number of different processes. Present-day postoperative pain management involves using a number of different approaches, embracing modern technology (e.g., microprocessor-controlled pumps, refined catheters, other infusion technologies) and, most important, optimizing pain relief by listening to patients' complaints of pain.

I. PRINCIPLES OF POSTOPERATIVE PAIN MANAGEMENT

1. Psychologic Preparation

Patients who are carefully prepared for the experience of surgery and postoperative pain are markedly less anxious and easier to treat postoperatively. Patients need reassurance. If they have never had surgery before, they should be told what to expect. They should be aware that some degree of postoperative pain is inevitable, and that their doctors and nurses will work with them to treat it. Patients should also be familiar with the chosen pain assessment method and the need to assess pain on a regular basis. They should be told about the choices for postoperative pain management, and these options should be discussed during their preoperative visit.

2. Assessing Pain

A policy of regular assessment is important because it draws attention to the existence of pain and prompts improved treatment. Assessments of pain severity, analgesic side effects, and markers of recovery are the tools by which analgesic regimens can be tailored to need. The method used does not need to be elaborate; in fact, it is preferable to use rudimentary scales such as the 0 to 10 verbal analog scale (VAS). It is standard practice at Massachusetts General Hospital (MGH) to record pain scales on the vital signs chart (the so-called **fifth vital sign**) as well as in the patient's medical record. Regular pain assessment has become part of standard care in hospitals and other health care facilities throughout the United States, and the Joint Commission on Accreditation of Healthcare Organizations (JCAHO) has developed new standards for both pain assessment and pain management (see Appendix II for Web address).

3. Preemptive Analgesia

The concept of preemptive analgesia was born from the observation in animals that changes occur in the central nervous system (CNS) secondary to peripheral injury and inflammation. The term **central sensitization** embraces a number of different and complex neurobiologic changes that arise after peripheral injury and ultimately increase pain sensitivity. It seemed rational, then, that an analgesic intervention that reduced pain transmission to the CNS might prevent central sensitization, thereby reducing postinjury or postoperative pain. In animal models of injury, preemptive analgesic interventions such as neural blockade and high-dose opioid treatment convincingly reduce postinjury pain sensitivity. Yet in human studies, preemptive analgesia has not been consistently effective, and to date, preemptive analgesia does not seem to have much clinical utility.

More recently, it was established that the N-methyl-d-aspartate (NMDA) receptor plays an important role in the development of central sensitization. Clinical preemptive analgesia studies now focus on using NMDA receptor antagonists to reduce central sensitization, and real benefits have been demonstrated. Unfortunately, none of the currently available NMDA antagonists (ketamine, dextromethorphan, and amantadine) are ideal and their use is limited by either side effects or poor efficacy. Studies are now focused on dose finding to optimize current drugs, and on a search for better NMDA antagonists.

A different but related phenomenon is that of central sensitization that is already present at the time of surgery, as it occurs in chronic pain syndromes. The question here is whether the treatment of central sensitization before surgery, notably before an amputation, can reduce postamputation pain, particularly phantom pain. In 1988, when Bach et al. demonstrated a statistically significant difference in the occurrence of phantom limb pain between patients treated for 72 hours preamputation with epidural blockade and those who did not receive preoperative epidural therapy, his findings were hailed as strong validation of the concept of preemptive analgesia. Yet what these investigators really did, if anything, was eliminate any central sensitization that existed before the surgery, rather than prevent the onset of central sensitization after the incision. Bach's results have never been reproduced, despite attempts to replicate his findings. Therefore, one must be cautious about recommending preamputation epidurals at present. However, the idea of being able to reduce phantom pain by means of perioperative neuromodulation remains attractive, and further research is needed, particularly into methods of reducing phantom pain with NMDA antagonists.

II. SPECIAL POPULATIONS

1. The Elderly

Older individuals often appear stoical, and it is not clear whether they have a different threshold for pain, whether past experience has altered their attitude toward pain or whether they truly do not feel pain to the same extent as younger adults. It is tempting to undertreat pain in older individuals because they do not always communicate pain clearly. Moreover, they may not metabolize drugs efficiently, which is an additional concern, especially when using opioids. Older individuals are more likely to become sedated and confused when given opioids, and are at increased risk of sedation and confusion when sleep deprived and outside their normal environment. Often the best approach is the simplest. For severe pain, small, intermittent doses of IV morphine (2 to 6 mg every 4 hours) or the equivalent should be used. Epidural therapy can be helpful and circumvents the use of systemic opioids, although even epidural fentanyl can cause confusion in older patients.

2. The Mentally and Physically Disabled

These patients present a challenge because they may be unable to communicate the status of their pain clearly. As with the very young, effective pain management with the very old may require time and patience to be spent learning what patients are experiencing and how best to help them. Vital signs, behavioral cues, positioning, muscle guarding, and grimacing may be the only guiding factors at first. The cooperation of those who normally care for these patients is indispensable. Although drugs are metabolized normally in most of these patients, individuals with baseline breathing difficulties may be more sensitive to the respiratory depressant effects of opioids.

3. Substance Abusers and Drug Addicts

Patients with a history of past or present substance abuse may be difficult to manage during an acute pain episode. The behavioral factors that make inpatient management difficult are compounded because opioids do not work well in patients who have become opioid-tolerant. It is often difficult to determine whether opioid-seeking behavior is due to inadequate pain control or to addictive behavior. The medical staff may become exasperated, thereby compromising patient care. These patients should be given the benefit of optimal control of acute pain, while detoxification should be postponed until the acute pain has resolved. It is helpful to work closely with addiction specialists, including psychiatrists and social workers, to prepare the patients for discharge and possible rehabilitation.

It is important to obtain a history of "recreational drug use," both past and present. The information may be unreliable but should at least be sought. It should be ascertained whether the patient is in withdrawal, and if so, the withdrawal should be treated. Large doses of opioids may be needed to avoid withdrawal and treat pain. Even patients who abuse substances such as alcohol, cocaine, and marijuana may exhibit some degree of cross-tolerance with opioids, thus requiring higher than normal opioid doses. Patients on methadone maintenance should continue their preadmission dose, or this should be converted to an alternative opioid or mode of delivery, and additional opioid prescribed as needed. Patient-controlled analgesia (PCA) is an effective modality for drug abusers, because it provides an element of control and lessens the anxiety associated with trying to obtain additional medication.

Opioid analgesia can usefully be supplemented with nonopioid treatments such as nonsteroidal antiinflammatory drugs (NSAIDs), epidurals, local nerve blocks and anxiolytics. Alpha-agonists such as clonidine may be useful because they provide analgesia and reverse symptoms of withdrawal. Other treatments for withdrawal include benzodiazepines and neuroleptics, in addition to supportive measures.

4. Intensive Care Patients

Patients admitted to intensive care form a special population because, in many cases, they are unable to communicate, either because of severe illness or because they are ventilated, sedated, and sometimes even paralyzed. It is important to treat pain in these patients in order to reduce the anxiety associated with pain and inability to communicate pain. When it is impossible to assess pain, as in heavily sedated or unconscious patients, it is reasonable to assess analgesic requirements on the basis of the amount of surgical or other trauma the patient has undergone. Patients on a ventilator can be treated with higher than normal doses of opioids (if desired) because there is no risk of respiratory depression. Continuous infusion is the most frequently chosen mode of delivery. Fentanyl or hydromorphone may be preferred to morphine in patients with renal insufficiency who tend to accumulate the active morphine metabolite morphine-6-glucuronide. Methadone may also be useful for prolonged intensive care unit (ICU) stays because there is less risk of developing tolerance than with other opioids. It has recently been found beneficial to use the α_2 agonist dexmedetomidine for ICU sedation, not only because of its hypnotic effects but also because of its analgesic synergy with opioids (opioid sparing). It may also help minimize withdrawal symptoms during weaning from opioids.

Alert or ICU patients who are breathing on their own can be treated for pain like patients in other units, with the proviso that severely ill patients may handle drugs inefficiently. Epidurals are useful even in patients on a ventilator, and they ease weaning from ventilation.

III. TREATMENT OPTIONS

1. Nonsteroidal Antiinflammatory Drugs

NSAIDs are useful as sole analgesics for mild to moderate pain, and useful alternatives or adjuncts to opioid therapy and regional analgesia. Because they act by a unique mechanism, mostly in the periphery (not in the CNS), their action complements that of other analgesic therapies. Their analgesic effect is secondary to their antiinflammatory effect, which in turn is due to prostaglandin inhibition. Prostaglandin inhibition is also responsible for their chief side effects—gastritis, platelet dysfunction, and renal damage. NSAIDs are contraindicated in patients with a history of peptic ulcer disease, gastritis, or NSAID intolerance, with renal dysfunction (creatinine >1.5), and with bleeding diatheses. Many surgeons prefer not to use NSAIDs in the immediate postoperative period for patients who have undergone renal or liver surgery, grafts, muscle flap procedures, or bone fusions, since they may increase bleeding or impede healing. The newer **coxibs** seem to be relatively free of gastrointestinal (GI) effects and are platelet sparing, but the incidence of other side effects is similar to that of the standard NSAIDs. The exact role of **coxibs** in the management of acute pain is still being evaluated.

Ketorolac is a potent NSAID (equipotent with morphine), with a chief indication for acute pain. It is the only NSAID analgesic available for parenteral use in the United States. It is expensive (approximately 20 times more costly than morphine), and because its potency extends to its side effects, its use is restricted to 5 days (manufacturers' recommendation). Ketorolac can also be used to supplement epidural analgesia, particularly when the epidural does not cover the whole surgical area, for example, after thoracotomy.

The NSAIDs are described in more detail in Chapter 8.

2. Systemic Opioids

Systemic opioid therapy has long been the conventional treatment approach for postoperative pain, and is the standard by which other treatments are measured. This does not make it inferior to other pain treatments. In fact, systemic opioid therapy (either oral or parenteral) remains the primary treatment used for patients experiencing moderate to severe acute pain. No new treatment has entirely replaced the opioids, yet newer accelerated recovery protocols demand an alternative to opioids as the sole analgesic because opioid side effects (nausea, sedation, reduced bowel mobility) interfere with the goal of rapid resumption of normal physiologic functions (eating, drinking, urinating, defecating, walking, coughing). Today's standard is to use multimodal analgesia, opioids being an important component, whereas the regime also aims to minimize opioid use.

Routes of opioid administration and their indications are summarized in Table 1. The oral route is the simplest and used for patients who are prescribed nothing by mouth (NPO). The rectal route is not popular in the United States. The intramuscular and subcutaneous routes are rarely chosen because it is considered unnecessary to subject patients to painful injections. Judiciously administered intravenous opioids (i.e., given as small boluses while monitoring pain level, respiratory effort, and alertness) are safe and preferable. The intravenous route is also ideal for PCA, which is discussed in the subsequent text. Most postoperative patients receive bolus administration of opioids, which allows for ready titration of dose according to need. Continuous intravenous or subcutaneous therapy is sometimes useful—for example, in patients on ventilators. Oral administration is resumed as soon as oral intake is reestablished. The short-term use of long-acting opioids is sometimes helpful.

Commonly used opioids and their doses are summarized in Table 2. Morphine is the opioid of choice at the MGH. Dose ranges are usually prescribed so that nurses can select specific doses that best meet the patients' needs. Morphine is a simple agonist at μ, κ, and δ receptors, and its actions are not complicated by partial agonism or mixed agonism/antagonism. Its effects and side effects are well known and understood. Morphine may be contraindicated in patients with biliary spasm because it is believed that it can worsen the spasm, but this issue is still under debate. Other opioids are used when patients express a preference for another drug, when they are either "allergic" to or report significant side effects from morphine, or when morphine does not appear to be effective. Hydromorphone is a useful alternative to morphine, and may be associated with less dizziness, nausea, and light-headedness in some patients. For many years, meperidine was popular for treating acute pain, but it is no longer used as first-line treatment because of its known toxicity (excitatory effects in the CNS due to the metabolite normeperidine).

The side effects of opioid drugs limit their use. Respiratory depression is a true risk, and patients receiving opioids should be closely watched, especially at the start of treatment. Monitoring for adequacy of ventilation includes observing the patients' state of arousal, respiratory rate, including depth and pattern of breathing, as well as color (skin and mucous membranes). Pulse oximeters and respiratory monitors can be helpful, especially

Table 1. Methods for achieving pain control

Intervention	Comments
NSAIDs	
Oral (alone)	Effective for mild to moderate pain. Begin preop. Relatively contraindicated in patients with history of peptic-ulcer or renal disease and risk of or actual coagulopathy. May mask fever.
Oral (adjunct to opioid)	Potentiating effect resulting in opioid sparing. Cautions as mentioned in preceding text.
Parenteral (ketorolac)	Effective for moderate to severe pain. Expensive. Useful where opioids contraindicated, especially to avoid respiratory depression and sedation. Cautions as in preceding text.
OPIOIDS	
Oral	As effective as parenteral in appropriate doses. Use as soon as oral medication is tolerated.
IM	Has been the standard parenteral route, but injections painful and absorption unreliable. Hence, avoid this route when possible.
SQ	Preferable to IM for low-volume continuous infusion. Injections painful and absorption unreliable. Avoid this route for long-term repeated dosing.
IV	Parenteral route of choice after major surgery. Suitable for titrated bolus or continuous administration (including PCA), but requires monitoring. Significant risk of respiratory depression with inappropriate dosing.
PCA	IV or SQ routes recommended. Good, steady level of analgesia. Popular with patients but requires special infusion pumps and staff education. Cautions as for IV opioids (preceding text).
Epidural and intrathecal	When suitable, provides good analgesia. Expensive if infusion pumps employed. Significant risk of respiratory depression, sometimes delayed in onset. Requires careful monitoring.
LOCAL ANESTHETICS	
Epidural and intrathecal	Limited indications. Expensive if infusion pumps employed. Effective regional analgesia. Opioid sparing. Addition of opioid to local anesthetic may improve analgesia. Risk of hypotension, weakness, numbness.

Table 1.   *Continued*

Intervention	Comments
Peripheral block	Limited indications. Limited duration unless catheters employed. Effective regional analgesia. Opioid sparing.
TENS	Effective in reducing pain and improving physical function. Requires skilled personnel and special equipment. Useful as an adjunct to drug therapy.
EDUCATION/ INSTRUCTION	Effective for reduction of pain. Should include procedural information and instruction aimed at reducing activity-related pain Requires staff time.

NSAIDs, nonsteroidal antiinflammatory drugs; IM, intramuscularly; SQ, subcutaneously; IV, intravenous; PCA, patient-controlled analgesia; TENS, transcutaneous electrical nerve stimulation.

during periods of high risk, for example, during early recovery. Severe respiratory depression should be treated with small intravenous boluses of naloxone (Narcan). If naloxone is given too quickly, severe agitation, and in extreme cases, flash pulmonary edema secondary to aggressive respiratory effort, may result. The ampule of naloxone (0.4 mg) can be diluted in saline in a 10 mL syringe and then 2 to 3 mL can be given every minute as needed. After naloxone reversal, patients should continue to be closely monitored because naloxone's duration of action is only approximately 20 minutes, and the effects of the agonist may outlast this. Naloxone will reverse opioid effects quite rapidly; so if the patient does not respond, one should consider alternative causes of the respiratory compromise.

Other opioid-related side effects are not dangerous but they can interfere with treatment success. Some side effects can be effectively treated without adjusting the opioid dose—nausea with antiemetics, pruritus with antihistamines, and constipation with laxatives (postoperative ileus should not be treated with laxatives) (Table 2). Sometimes it is necessary to decrease the dose, change the opioid, or even stop it. Other causes of side effects should always be considered, for example, nausea could be caused by anesthetics, antibiotics, or by the surgery itself.

The opioids are described more fully in Chapter 9.

3. Patient-controlled Analgesia

In many institutions, including MGH, PCA is the standard therapy for postoperative pain. PCA is the self-administration of analgesics (usually via the intravenous route) by patients instructed in the use of a device specifically designed for that purpose. The goal of PCA is to provide doses of analgesic immediately

Table 2. **Analgesics and related drugs: dosage examples for adults**

Generic Name	Proprietary Name	Oral Dose (mg)	Parenteral Dose (mg)
Nonsteroidal antiinflammatory agents			
Acetaminophen[a][b]	Tylenol	500–1000 q3–4h	
Ibuprofen+	Motrin, Advil	200–800 q6h	
Ketorolac	Toradol		30(load) + 15 –30q6h
Naproxen	Naprosyn	250–500 q12h	
Celecoxib	Celebrex	100–200 q12h	
Opioids			
Butorphanol	Stadol		2–4 q3–4h
Codeine		15–60 q4–6h	30–60 q4–6h
Hydromorphone	Dilaudid	2–4 q4–6h	2–4 q4–6h
Meperidine	Demerol	50–150 q3–4h	100–150 q2–3h
Methadone	Dolophine	2.5–10 q6–8h	2.5–10 q6–8h
Morphine+		10–20 q2–3h	5–10 q3–4h
Morphine SR	MS Contin, Oramorph, Kadian	15–30 q12h	
Nalbuphine	Nubain		5–10 q4–6h
Naloxone (antagonist)	Narcan (also in Percocet, Percodan)	5–10 q3–4h	0.2–1.2 bolus
Oxycodone		10–20 q12h	
Oxycodone SR	OxyContin		
Antiemetics, major tranquilizers			
Droperidol	Inapsine	5–15 q8h	1.25–5 q6h
Metoclopramide	Reglan	10 tid	10 q6h
Ondansetron	Zofran		4 q4–8h
Prochlorperazine	Compazine	5–10 tid	5–10 q4–6h
Antihistamines, anxiolytics			
Diphenhydramine	Benadryl	25 q4h	
Hydroxyzine	Vistaril	50–100 qid	25–100 qid
Lorazepam	Ativan	0.5–2 q6–8h	0.5–2 q6–8h
Laxatives			
Senna	Senokot	1–2 tab tid	
Docusate	Colace	100 tid	

Dosages and intervals are initial estimates for an average 70-kg adult and may need to be adjusted according to the individual patient's weight, preference, or tolerance.

This list is not comprehensive. Other classes of drugs not listed may be beneficial in postoperative pain for individual cases.

[a]Acetaminophen is not antiinflammatory but is efficacious in acute pain.

[b]Also available as suppository.

based on the demand of the patient. The use of portable micro-computer-controlled infusion pumps allows this dosing to be achieved quickly and easily (literally at the touch of a button); therefore small, frequent, and easily titratable doses can be given. This approach avoids the extreme swings in plasma levels and in efficacy and side effects associated with the larger, less frequent doses used during standard therapy. Other advantages of PCA are the inherent safety of using small doses and the fact that obtunded patients will not press for additional doses, and the preference of most patients for techniques that offer a sense of control. An exception to the general safety of PCA is its use by older and confused individuals, who, despite early obtundation (or maybe because of it), will sometimes overdose themselves. Studies show that patients vary widely in their physical need for opioids, and PCA accommodates a wide range of analgesic needs. With standard PCA orders, patients can receive anywhere between 0 to 10 mg of IV morphine each hour.

Nurse-controlled boluses may be needed at the start of treatment, because patients are often sedated by residual anesthesia and incapable of using PCA properly. It is tempting to think that once patients are connected to PCA pumps, they do not need further pain assessment or treatment, but if pain is neglected in the early postoperative period, it may be more difficult to treat later. Individualizing the PCA settings and frequently assessing patients' analgesia levels are critical during the first 24 hours following surgery. The MGH PCA orders are shown in Figure 1. They include an alternative treatment should the intravenous route fail, as well as general guidelines for dosing and monitoring. Morphine continues to be the drug of choice for PCA, with hydromorphone used when morphine has failed or is contraindicated. Meperidine can also be used, but, as discussed in preceding text, it has limited indications.

The success of PCA depends first and foremost on patient selection. Patients who are too old, too confused, too young, or unable to control the button or who do not want the treatment are not suitable candidates. Ideally, patients should be educated before surgery about PCA and the concept of self-dosing. Teaching points include expectations for pain relief, informing patients of their active role in pain management (both in pain reports and medication management), elimination of fears and misconceptions about opioids, including fear of addiction, and fear of overmedication.

4. Adjuncts

(i) Neuropathic Pain Medications

The neuropathic pain medications include anticonvulsants, antidepressants, and systemic local anesthetics. These drugs are described in Chapters 10 and 11. Although the utility of these drugs for chronic pain is well established, they are not used for acute pain. Early studies in acute pain patients have demonstrated clinically relevant efficacy, and the area is ripe

Massachusetts General Hospital
PCA Order Sheet

DOCTORS' ORDER SHEET

Date	Req Area
	PATIENT IDENTIFICATION AREA

	Monitoring
1. Date: Time:	
2. Drug: (check one) ☐ Morphine 1mg/ml ☐ Hydromorphone (Dilaudid) 0.5mg/ml	1. Record baseline HR, BP, RR.
	2. Record HR, BP, RR 15 minutes after ending
3. Orders for Pump Settings (May refer to guideline - below right)	initial bolus infusion loading dose.
Demand Dose from _____ ml to _____ ml	3. Record RR, analgesia, and sedation levels every 4
Start Dose at _____ ml	hours (refer to Scoring Guide below).
Delay Time _____ minutes	If vital signs, mental status, or sedation problems appear,
Basal Rate _____ ml/hr 7A-11P	record RR and BP every 1 hour or more often until stable.
_____ ml/hr 11P-7A, pm	4. Discontinue PCA and call House Officer for:
Hour Limit ≤ _____ ml/hr	HR < _____ SBP < _____ RR < _____
4. Bolus Loading Dose:	Increasing lethargy.
_____ ml every 5 minutes until patient	5. Prior to pump availability, if patient reports a pain level
comfortable. Maximum total loading dose	≥ 5 (on the 0-10 scale), initiate orders in #6 (in left column)
_____ ml. Notify HO if patient remains	until PCA pump started.
uncomfortable after completing maximum bolus dose.	6. Call floor pharmacist for special problems.

5. Infuse D5W at KVO via Y set if no maintenance	Guidelines for standard starting doses:	Morphine	Hydromorphone
IV solution ordered.	Demand Dose	0.5 - 2ml	0.2 - 1ml
	Delay	6 min.	10 min.
6. In the event of pump failure or nonpatent IV,	Basal	0 - 0.5ml	0ml
	Hour Limit	≤ 20ml	≤ 6ml
administer drug _____ , _____ mg,	Start with: Dose/Delay time/Basal Rate	1/6/0	0.5/10/0

	PATIENT-CONTROLLED ANALGESIA SCORING GUIDE
IM every _____ hr., pm, pain.	PAIN LEVEL:	Use a range from 0 - 10 where: 0 = "no pain" and 10 = "worst pain imaginable"
	SEDATION LEVEL:	1 = wide awake 2 = drowsy 3 = dozing 4 = awakens when aroused 5 = asleep
Doctor's Signature _____	VERBAL RESPONSE:	5 = oriented and converses 4 = disoriented and converses 3 = inappropriate words 2 = incomprehensible sounds 1 = no response

Figure 1.   Patient-controlled analgesia (PCA) order sheet.

for further study now that we recognize the value of multimodal analgesia.

(ii) N-Methyl-D-Aspartate Receptor Antagonists

NMDA receptor antagonists reduce central sensitization, hyperalgesia, and opioid tolerance. The theoretical attractions of NMDA receptor antagonist treatment of acute pain are obvious—they could reduce postoperative and postsurgical chronic pain by reducing central sensitization, and they could reduce opioid requirements and tolerance. Yet no completely satisfactory regime has emerged that provides a useful effect without unacceptable side effects. This is largely because currently available NMDA antagonists (ketamine, dextromethorphan, and amantadine) have disruptive side effects, or are not sufficiently effective. Efforts are still underway to establish dosing regimes that might optimize the use of existing drugs, and further studies are assessing new antagonists that may prove useful.

(iii) α_2 Agonists

Although the perioperative use of systemic α_2 agonists (oral or transdermal) has been advocated for blood pressure control and for analgesia, the analgesic effect has not proved satisfactory. However, neuraxial clonidine is effective, and is used as an adjunct to neuraxial local anesthetics and opioids (see subsequent text).

5. Epidural Analgesia

For certain well-chosen indications, a functioning epidural produces superior pain relief, and is known to improve surgical outcome (see Table 3). However, a considerable degree of technical expertise is needed to place epidural catheters and, even in the best hands, the treatment can fail. Thus, a promise of superb pain relief is not always fulfilled. Because it involves carefully and blindly locating the epidural space (see Fig. 2), epidural placement and management is time-consuming and labor-intensive. Nevertheless, both surgeons and anesthesiologists at MGH are sufficiently convinced of the positive benefits of epidural analgesia to offer the treatment to all our patients in whom it is indicated, being careful to explain both its risks and its benefits. A description of the technique of epidural catheter placement can be found in Chapter 12.

(i) Indications

Epidurals are recommended for postoperative pain primarily for the following indications (discussion of when to use epidurals intraoperatively is beyond the scope of this chapter):

- Patients having thoracic or abdominal surgery
- Patients having lower limb surgery in whom early mobilization is important (early active or passive mobilization)
- Patients having lower body vascular procedures in whom a sympathetic block is desirable

Table 3.   Known benefits of postoperative epidural analgesia

Superior analgesia
Improved pulmonary function
Better graft survival after lower limb vascular procedures
Increased bowel mobility, associated with shorter hospital stay
Fewer cardiac ischemic events
Shorter recuperation after joint surgery, associated with early
    aggressive mobilization

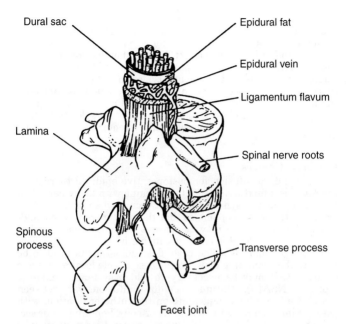

Dural sac
Epidural fat
Epidural vein
Ligamentum flavum
Lamina
Spinal nerve roots
Spinous process
Transverse process
Facet joint

Figure 2.   Anatomy of the epidural space.

- Patients who are not anticoagulated or in whom anticoagulation is not planned in the immediate postoperative period
- Patients with compromised cardiac or pulmonary function

(ii) Contraindications

Contraindications to epidural placement are the following:

- Patient refusal
- Coagulopathy
- Concurrent or planned treatment with low-molecular-weight heparin or with potent antiplatelet agents
- Bacteremia
- Local infection at epidural insertion site
- Spine pathology (relative contraindication)

(iii) Management Principles

The management of epidural catheters should always be under the direct supervision of anesthesiologists. Patients should be seen daily to ensure that catheters and medications are working effectively. Pain reports should be satisfactory, and side effects such as pruritus, sedation, and changes in sensation or motor function should be carefully evaluated. Catheters and their insertion sites should be inspected for migration, integrity of the dressings and inflammation or back tenderness. Anesthesia personnel should make changes to the analgesic regime and administer specific medications as necessary. At the end of treatment, the anesthesia team should be responsible for removing the catheter and ensuring that it is removed intact. Nurses should be properly educated before they care for patients with epidural catheters. Important teaching points include typical medication doses and concentrations, anticoagulation issues, assessment parameters, the normal appearance of the catheter and catheter site, operation of the infusion pumps, common medication side effects that can be treated by them, and side effects requiring a call to the physician in charge.

(iv) Drug Choices

The standard infusion for postoperative epidural therapy at the MGH is a mixture of 0.1% bupivacaine with 20 μg per mL of hydromorphone. A synergistic effect occurs when one combines local anesthetic with opioid, so that the mixture optimizes analgesia. However, there may be reasons to remove one or other component (e.g., local anesthetic causing hypotension, or opioid causing pruritus), in which case, dose adjustments need to be made to the remaining drug. In the case of sole local anesthetic treatment, it may be necessary to add a systemic analgesic (opioid or NSAID). Continuous epidural infusions vary between 4 and 8 mL per hour depending on the catheter location, with possible infusion rates up to 20 mL per hour. Fentanyl is our second choice of epidural opioid, and is reserved for patients who are sensitive to opioid effects (e.g., the very young and the very old). Because of its lipophilicity, fentanyl tends to bind locally to spinal cord receptors, rather than spread with cerebrospinal fluid (CSF) movement. The analgesic effect of fentanyl localizes to the level of epidural insertion, whereas hydromorphone and morphine (the least lipophilic of the opioids) produce better spread, but a greater risk of delayed respiratory depression secondary to the spread of drug to higher centers in the CNS. Standard epidural orders include: infusion dose ranges for nurses to titrate based on the patient's report, orders for alternative treatments should the epidural fail, and orders for the treatment of adverse side effects (see Fig. 3).

The addition of clonidine to the local anesthetic and opioid has been found to significantly improve the quality and duration of neuraxial analgesia. The effect is mediated by descending modulatory pathways to the spinal dorsal horn. Despite neuraxial administration, systemic side effects (hypotension, bradycardia, and sedation) can occur. Dose finding studies are still underway, and the therapeutic window for useful analgesia without side effects seems to be narrow. A reasonable regime uses a 1 to 2 μg per kg bolus followed by 0.4 μg/kg/hour.

(v) Management of Inadequate Analgesia

The best way to ensure that an epidural catheter is well positioned is to establish an anesthetic level using local anesthetic. Testing can be attempted at any stage, but it should be remembered that: (a) responses are less reliable in a patient who is in the early stages of recovery after anesthesia, and (b) a bolus injection

Massachusetts General Hospital

Epidural Order Sheet

DOCTORS' ORDER SHEET

UNIT NO.
NAME

Date:
Patient's age:
Patient's weight:
Drug allergies:

Pain service page number is 27246 (PAIN)

(See guide on the back of this sheet for scales of pain level, sedation level, verbal response and motor strength)

1. **Prepared epidural mixture:**
   - ☐ bupivacaine 0.1%, dilaudid 0.02 mg/cc
   - ☐ bupivacaine 0.25%, dilaudid 0.02 mg/cc
   - ☐ bupivacaine 0.1%, morphine 0.05 mg/cc
   - ☐ bupivacaine 0.1%, fentanyl 2 μg/cc
   - ☐ bupivacaine 0.1%
   - ☐ bupivacaine 0.25%

2. **Rate and range**
   initial rate ________ cc/hr
   titrate within the range ________ – ________ cc/hr

3. **Backup orders**
   For respiratory depression give Narcan 0.1 mg, repeated q 5 mins to a maximum of 0.4 mg if necessary

   If epidural fails for any reason, stop the epidural infusion, call the Pain Service, and give:
   DRUG: ________
   DOSE: ________ mg IV q 5 minutes until comfortable
   MAXIMUM DOSE: ________ mg
   Monitor vital signs q 5 mins x 3 after bolus doses

   For PCA (use only when directed to by the Pain Service):
   DRUG/CONCENTRATION ________ / ________ mg/cc
   BOLUS DOSE ________ cc
   BOLUS LOCK-OUT ________ minutes
   RATE 7am - 11pm ________ cc
   11pm - 7am ________ cc
   HOURLY LIMIT ________ cc

Signature: ________________ MD

82658 8/98

1. **Epidural management**
   A. 15 minutes after a bolus dose, initiation of infusion, or an increase in rate:
   - record HR and BP
   - record verbal response and motor strength
   - record RR q 1° x 4
   - record pain and sedation levels q 1° x 4 if patient is awake

   B. At steady state (ie > 4 hrs after a bolus dose, initiation of infusion, or an increase in rate:
   - record RR q 2°
   - record HR and BP q 4°
   - record pain and sedation levels, verbal and motor responses q 4° if patient is awake

2. **For the following side effects, call the Pain Service:**
   RR < 10, HR < 50, SBP < 90
   nausea, vomiting, itching, urinary retention

3. **For RR < 8, call the Pain Service, and:**
   1. if the patient is obtunded, give O_2
   2. stop the epidural infusion
   3. give Narcan 0.1 mg q 5 mins, to a maximum of 0.4 mg, if necessary
   4. monitor O_2 saturation, if necessary

NO SYSTEMIC OPIATES OR SEDATIVES UNLESS ORDERED BY THE PAIN SERVICE

IN THE CASE OF PROBLEMS CALL THE PAIN SERVICE, PAGE # 27246 (PAIN)

In an emergency, if unable to contact the Pain Service, call anesthesia in the operating room, 6-8995 or 6-8910

Figure 3. Epidural order sheet.

can produce hypotension and so it is necessary to be in a monitored situation. If a patient undergoes surgery under combined epidural/general anesthesia, catheter function should be tested preoperatively. Another surprisingly helpful test is to inject 5 to 7 mL of the analgesic infusion (i.e., low-dose local anesthetic), in which case no special monitoring is needed because the low-dose anesthetic is unlikely to produce hypotension. If the catheter is well positioned, analgesia should be noticeably improved by the injection.

Once good catheter function is established, several approaches to improve analgesia can be taken. A bolus injection can be given (as described earlier), if it has not already been given. The infusion rate can be titrated upward, as tolerated. Systemic analgesics can be given. NSAIDs are useful adjuncts to epidural analgesia, especially when the epidural level does not cover the area of surgical pain, as when the incision is high, or when pain is referred outside the epidural area (as in shoulder pain associated with chest tubes and diaphragmatic irritation). Systemic opioids (including PCA) can also be added, but, in this case, it is our practice to remove the opioid from the epidural mix to avoid possible overdose.

(vi) Patient-Controlled Epidural Analgesia

Patient-controlled epidural analgesia (PCEA) has become a standard of care in many institutions around the country. Allowing patients to gain control is one great advantage to PCEA. One must consider the lipophilicity of the opioid used, the onset of action and the duration of pain relief when prescribing demand doses and lockout intervals. The PCEA dosing for the standard MGH epidural mix (0.1% bupivacaine with 20 μg per cc hydromorphone) is 2 mL bolus every 20 minutes (lockout), with basal infusion 4 to 6 mL per hour.

(vii) Side Effects

Most side effects (see Table 4) are alleviated by either lowering the infusion rate, or by changing the drug or dose. Pruritus is a common side effect of neuraxial opioid and usually responds well to antihistamine treatment. The mixed agonist/antagonist nalbuphine (Nubain) (5 to 10 mg IV, 4 to 6 hourly) also works well, as does low-dose naloxone infusion.

Contrary to popular belief, nausea rarely occurs because opioid doses are low. Gut mobility is in fact improved by epidural therapy.

Urinary retention may occur, especially when lumbar catheters are used, so we tend to continue Foley catheters until the epidural is out.

Unilateral lower extremity numbness with occasional weakness or motor block is a side effect of the local anesthetic. This usually occurs when the epidural catheter tip has migrated along a nerve root and the local anesthetic is concentrated in one area. Pulling the catheter back, or lowering the infusion rate, often rectifies the problem. However, one should always remain vigilant and continue to watch for more serious complications.

(viii) Complications

The most common complications are failed block/analgesia, and postdural puncture headache (PDPH) (see Table 5). Both are considered benign, although they may be devastating to patients who have committed to an epidural in order to optimize their

Table 4.   Common side effects of epidural analgesia

Opioid	Local anesthetic
Pruritus	Hypotension
Sedation	Mild sensory/motor changes
Dizziness	Urinary retention
Urinary retention	

Table 5. Epidural complications

Common	Failed block/analgesia
	Postdural puncture headache
Rare	Skin infection
	Epidural hematoma or abscess
Extremely rare	Anterior spinal artery syndrome
	Transverse myelitis
	Meningitis

surgical experience. The incidence of these common complications is difficult to establish because reports vary, and the occurrences likely vary according to reporting and practice habits. Failed block/analgesia rate was 15% in an MGH survey, whereas PDPH may occur in up to 86% patients after accidental dural puncture (rate 0.16% to 1.3%). The incidence of other self-limiting neurologic complications such as radicular pain and peripheral nerve lesions is difficult to determine, because these occurrences are rarely reported.

Of far greater concern is permanent neurologic injury, including paraplegia, which may be caused by epidural hematoma or abscess, even when these are diagnosed and treated in a timely manner. A rash of reports of epidural hematoma occurring after neuraxial interventions in patients receiving low-molecular-weight heparin (LMWH) alerted us to the dangers of breaching the epidural space in patients receiving highly effective thrombosis prophylaxis. More problems followed when chronic treatment with potent and long-acting antiplatelet agents, such as clopidogrel, became more widespread. The use of activated protein C, our current best agent for severe sepsis, also precludes the use of neuraxial blockade. Given the rapidity with which new agents enter practice, and the lag time before the extent of a problem can be assessed, we are left with a great deal of uncertainty about the safety of neuraxial procedures. To make the judgment even more difficult, one of the major reasons that older studies showed a benefit to spinals and epidurals in terms of serious morbidity, was their ability to reduce thromboembolism. This benefit may no longer apply in an era of improved pharmacologic thromboprophylaxis.

Epidural abscess occurs less often than epidural hematoma but may be equally catastrophic, and can cause permanent and serious neurologic injury, even death. The mortality of spinal abscess can be as high as 18%. The incidence of epidural abscess secondary to neuraxial blockade is estimated at 1 in 250,000 in healthy patients but 1 in 2,000 in diabetic or immunocompromised patients.

Other serious complications such as anterior spinal artery syndrome, transverse myelitis, and meningitis have been reported, but are extremely rare.

PDPH is thought to be the result of a small CSF leak secondary to accidental dural puncture. Typically, there is a delay in onset of the headache (approximately 24 hours), so that the complication tends to manifest itself on the first postoperative day.

Because PDPH tends to worsen on sitting up, and particularly on walking, and to improve on lying down, it may not present itself until the patients get out of bed for the first time after surgery. Other characteristics of the headache are that it tends to occur at the back of the head (occiput) and neck, and produces a tight, pulling, and throbbing sensation. Conservative management consists of bed rest (up to bathroom only), plenty of fluids (IV or oral) and headache medication (NSAIDs, acetaminophen, caffeine, and theophylline all work well). If there is no resolution, or if conservative measures are contraindicated, a blood patch is recommended. This consists of an epidural injection of 20 mL of the patient's own blood (drawn under sterile conditions), and is thought to close the dural puncture. The exact mechanism by which an epidural blood patch works is uncertain, but is probably either a pressure effect, or a laying down of clot or fibrosis onto the puncture site.

Epidural hematoma and abscess can have a variable presentation, but the cardinal signs of impending spinal cord compression are sensory and motor changes in the lower extremity (often bilateral), and pain in the back. In the case of lesions in the sacral canal, cardinal signs are changes in bladder and bowel function, and absence of pain. If there is any reason for concern, the first response should be to discontinue the epidural infusion, and possibly remove the epidural catheter, especially if there is evidence of infection at the skin (if there are coagulation issues, it may be better to leave the catheter until they are resolved; see in subsequent text). Although minimal sensory changes are common and may be benign, prolonged motor changes that do not resolve on discontinuing the epidural infusion are always worrying, as is back pain. If there is no resolution after simple measures, a magnetic resonance imaging (MRI) should be ordered and the involvement of neurology sought. Early intervention is the key to preventing disastrous complications, and early surgical decompression usually results in complete resolution. Without these measures, spinal cord compression, and later paraplegia, may develop.

(ix) Anticoagulation and Epidurals

The incidence of epidural hematoma after neuraxial injection, catheter placement, or catheter removal has been estimated to be 1:190,000, with many of the reported cases being associated with anticoagulant use. Unfortunately, the literature has little information about the risk of epidural hematoma and specific anticoagulants, especially the latest generation of anticoagulants and antiplatelet drugs. Published guidelines are based on the known pharmacology of the drugs, as well as clinical evidence from case reports (anecdotal and published). Epidural bleeding is known to occur secondary to single shot neuraxial techniques as well as neuraxial catheter insertion and removal, so that recommendations are needed for the start and end of neuraxial therapy, as well as for starting anticoagulant therapy after neuraxial instrumentation or catheter removal.

The American Society of Regional Anesthesia and Pain Medicine (ASRA) periodically issues consensus guidelines on the use of neuraxial interventions in patients receiving thromboprophylaxis (see Appendix II for Web address). MGH guidelines are based on ASRA's recommendations, and summarized in Table 6.

The NSAIDs and low-dose subcutaneous standard heparin are not considered a risk. High-dose infusions of standard (unfractionated)

Table 6.   Guidelines for epidural placement and removal during anticoagulant therapy

Drug	Monitoring	Time After Last Dose Before Placing or Removing Catheter	Time After Placing or Removing Catheter Before Restarting Medication
Warfarin	INR (<1.5)	Check INR if treatment >24 h	Same day
NSAID, ASA	No significant risk		
Thrombolytics	None	10 d	10 d
SC heparin	No significant risk		
IV heparin	PTT	2–4 h	1 h
LMWH	Anti-Xa (however, not predictive of risk of bleeding)		
Low dose Dalteparin (Fragmin) (<5,000 U qd) Enoxaparin (Lovenox) (<60 mg qd)		12 h	2 h
High dose Bid dosing		>24 h	2 h
Ticlopidine (Ticlid)	None	14 d	24 h
Clopidogrel (Plavix)	None	7 d[a]	24 h
Abciximab (Reopro)	None	48 h	12 h
Tirofiban (Aggrastat)	None	8 h	4 h
Eptifibatide (Integrilin)	None	8 h	4 h

INR, international normalized ratio; NSAID, nonsteroidal antiinflammatory drug; ASA, acetylsalicylic acid; IV, intravenous; PTT, partial thromboplastin time; LMWH, low molecular weight heparin.
Regional anesthesia is contraindicated in patients receiving fondaparinux (Arixtra).
[a]After a single dose, catheter can be removed within 24–48 h. If this window is missed, it is necessary to wait 7 d before catheter removal.

heparin are relatively easy to handle because their effects are predictable. The partial thromboplastin time (PTT) usually returns to within satisfactory range of normal 2 to 3 hours after discontinuation, at which point epidurals can be placed or removed.

In the case of warfarin prophylaxis, international normalized ratio (INR) should ideally be less than 1.5 before placing or removing a catheter. However, it should not be necessary to give fresh frozen plasma (FFP) or keep a patient in the hospital in order to remove an epidural catheter when the INR is static (which sometimes occurs in severely ill patients); the risks of both these interventions are higher than the risk of bleeding as a result of catheter removal.

European once-daily (low-dose) dosing regimes for LMWH were associated with less problematic epidural bleeding than U.S. twice-daily (high-dose) regimes. Low-dose regimes are now also used in the United States, and ASRA recommends different precautions for high-dose versus low-dose regimes (Table 6). There is no practical test of LMWH activity (the anti-Xa level is not a reliable predictor of the risk of bleeding, and is available only on a limited basis); prothrombin time (PT), INR, and PTT values do not reflect LMWH activity.

Clopidogrel (Plavix) use is associated with a high incidence of surgical bleeding and epidural hematoma (anecdotal reports). These problems were particularly obvious when this drug was first used, and the effect on bleeding, and slow reversal of this effect, were not appreciated. The current recommendation is that regional anesthesia is contraindicated for 7 days after termination of treatment with clopidogrel [14 days after ticlopidine (Ticlid)]. The newer antiplatelet drugs seem less prone to increase surgical bleeding, but, as already mentioned, we rely on anecdotal evidence for perioperative events, and sometimes anecdotal evidence is misleading. Regional techniques should not be conducted in patients receiving fondaparinux (Arixtra).

6. Single Shot Neuraxial Morphine

Neuraxial morphine is safe provided dosing is reasonable and patients are appropriately monitored. A single shot of morphine into the epidural space (1 to 4 mg) or intrathecal space (0.1 to 0.4 mg) can provide prolonged analgesia (up to 24 hours), but carries a risk of delayed respiratory depression. Morphine is poorly lipophilic, tends to stay in CSF once there, and is subject to CSF flow with passage to higher centers including the respiratory center. At the same time, the fact that morphine tends to remain in CSF is the reason that it produces excellent selective spinal analgesia (i.e., good spread to spinal cord receptors). Single shot neuraxial morphine is an excellent means of providing analgesia when there is no epidural catheter. Patients should be monitored in the same way as those receiving epidural opioid infusions (Fig. 3). PCA can be used to provide supplementary analgesia, but for safety, only demand doses are used rather than continuous infusions.

7. Intraoperative Neural Blockade

Nerve blocks performed before or during surgery provide excellent pain control during the early postoperative period. Infiltration of wounds with local anesthetics by surgeons can also contribute significantly to the control of early postoperative pain. Intraoperative neural blockade can reduce postoperative analgesic requirements and, in some cases, eliminate the need for postoperative analgesia. Intraoperative nerve blocks are particularly useful in children, who tolerate analgesics poorly and in whom pain is particularly distressing.

8. Prolonged Neural Blockade—Use of Catheters

Neural blockade can be prolonged beyond the life of the chosen local anesthetic by using continuous infusions via catheters. Neural cryotherapy and direct severance of nerves were used to prolong nerve blockade, but these practices are no longer recommended because they are known to result in an unacceptably high incidence of chronic pain. Continuous analgesic/anesthetic infusions can be administered at various sites, offer a safer alternative to neuraxial techniques, and are particularly useful when active mobilization is needed. It is useful to infuse analgesics into the brachial plexus after shoulder or hand surgery, and into the femoral sheath after knee surgery. It may also be helpful to infuse them into joints after joint surgery as well as into wounds.

Pumps for use at home have recently been developed (e.g., the Pain Buster Pain Management System) for infusing into joints and wounds. Local anesthetics and opioids have been used. Patients seem enthusiastic about these pumps, but they are still considered investigational because they have not been shown to improve pain or reduce systemic analgesic used in trials to date.

By contrast, infusions of local anesthetics via brachial and lumbar plexus catheters have established efficacy. Patients must be hospitalized, at least while the treatment is stabilized. Bupivacaine 0.1% at 10 to 20 mL per hour is used initially. If that is not effective, a higher concentration (0.25%) can be used, and/or a bolus injection of 20 mL of 0.25% to 0.375% bupivacaine can be tried. Bolus injection is also useful before physical therapy. Patients may also use supplemental analgesics. Occasionally patients can be allowed to go home with a plexus catheter, either with a home pump, or reserving the catheter for injection before physical therapy sessions.

9. Transcutaneous Electrical Nerve Stimulation

Transcutaneous electrical nerve stimulation (TENS) is useful for reducing postoperative pain in selected patients. The device consists of a series of electrodes that are placed on the site of the pain (either side of the surgical incision in the case of postoperative pain) through which a low-voltage electrical stimulus is passed. The treatment is based on the gate-control theory of pain by Melzack and Wall. Randomized, controlled trials have confirmed its efficacy in postoperative pain compared with controls (no TENS), but no better than sham TENS (electrodes with no current). Sham TENS is better than no TENS, suggesting there is a strong placebo effect. TENS does not stand up against drug therapies as a sole treatment of anything other than mild postoperative pain, but it may be useful for reducing analgesic requirements and possibly for improving pulmonary function in selected patients.

10. Behavioral Therapy

The goal of behavioral therapy is to provide patients with a sense of control over their pain. All patients benefit from being well prepared psychologically for the experience of surgery and postoperative pain. Simple relaxation strategies and imagery can help those patients who find such interventions appealing, and do not need to be complex to be effective. Simple strategies, such as brief jaw relaxation, music-assisted relaxation, and recall of peaceful images, can reduce anxiety and analgesic requirements. They take only a few minutes to teach, although they may require continual practice and reinforcement. Patients who wish to learn simple relaxation exercises can be given a brochure describing the exercises. Therapeutic touch is another popular method and is particularly helpful when postoperative pain is refractory to other modalities. Elaborate behavioral therapy techniques (e.g., biofeedback or counseling), have no place in the treatment of acute postoperative pain, unless the pain is likely to be prolonged or to recur.

IV. CONCLUSION

Postoperative pain has often been inadequately treated in the past, in part because of complacency, and in part because of fear of analgesic side effects. But today's patients expect better pain control and are better educated about their options. Effective postoperative pain management involves adherence to certain basic principles. First and foremost, pain must be assessed regularly and systematically so that pain treatment can be modified according to need. Pain scores should be documented so that the pain course is apparent to all caregivers. Pain that is treated preemptively or controlled early is easier to manage than established or severe pain. In this respect, treatment during the intraoperative and early postoperative periods is essential. Patients should be involved in their treatment and be educated about their surgery and the options available for treating postoperative pain. The actual choice of treatment is of secondary importance, as long as the principles of postoperative pain management are adhered to.

SELECTED READINGS

Bach S, Noreng MF, Tjellden NU. Phantom limb pain in amputees during the first 12 months following limb amputation, after preoperative lumbar epidural blockade. *Pain* 1988;33:297–301.

Ballantyne JC, Carr DB, DeFerranti S, et al. The comparative effects of postoperative analgesic therapies on pulmonary outcome: cumulative meta-analyses of randomized, controlled trials. *Anesth Analg* 1998;86(3):598–612.

Ballantyne JC, Carwood C. Optimal postoperative analgesia. In: Fleisher LA, ed. *Evidence-Based Practice of Anesthesiology.* Philadelphia, PA: WB Saunders, 2004:449–457.

Ballantyne JC, Kupelnick B, McPeek B, et al. Does the evidence support the use of spinal and epidurals for surgery? *J Clin Anesth* 2005 (*in press*).

Ballantyne JC, McKenna J, Ryder E. Epidural analgesia–experience of 5,628 patients in a large teaching hospital derived through audit. *Int J Acute Pain* 2003;4:89–97.

Carr DB. Acute pain management: operative or medical procedures and trauma. *Clinical Practice Guideline*. Rockville, MD. AHCPR Publication No 92-0032: Agency for Health Care Policy and Research, Public Health Service, U.S. Department of Health and Human Services, 1992.

Cousins M. Power I acute and postoperative pain. In: Wall PD, Melzak R, eds. *Textbook of Pain*, 4th ed. Edinburgh: Churchill Livingstone, 1999:447–491.

Horlocker TT, Wedel DJ. Spinal and epidural blockade and perioperative low molecular weight heparin: smooth sailing on the Titanic. *Anesth Analg* 1998;86(6):1153–1156.

Mao J. Opioid-induced abnormal pain sensitivity: implications in clinical opioid therapy. *Pain* 2002;100:213–217.

Postoperative Pain in Children

Lucy L. Chen and Jane C. Ballantyne

Charm ache with air, and agony with words.
—*William Shakespeare, 1564–1616*

It has only been over the last two decades that pain relief in children has become an area of major concern. Recent research clearly shows that neonates and infants are in fact sensitive to pain and that pain elicits physiologic, sometimes deleterious responses in them in much the same way as adults. Moreover, such research shows that traumatic pain experiences can psychologically scar young children and make them fearful for a long time because they are not mature enough to be able to rationalize their experiences.

There are many differences between adults and children that make pain treatment in children a particular challenge: (a) it is not as easy to assess pain in children as it is in adults; (b) children, particularly neonates and infants, do not metabolize drugs as well as adults; (c) children hate needles; (d) epidural catheters are technically more difficult to place and more difficult to maintain in children; and (e) the sight of a child in pain is particularly distressing, especially to the parents. This chapter discusses general issues about postoperative pain management in children.

I. PLANNING FOR POSTOPERATIVE ANALGESIA

The intraoperative and postoperative anesthesia and analgesia plan should be made before the surgery. Children and their parents should be told honestly what to expect and be reassured that everything will be done to alleviate any pain or discomfort. It is often helpful to find out how the child copes with pain and distress, how he or she communicates pain (e.g., "boo–boo," "hurt," "sore"), and whether the child relies on special blankets, toys, or other means for comfort and reassurance. If the child has had surgery before, then the following questions apply:

- What was the past pain experience of the child?
- What medications were used in the past, and did they work well?

- Were nonpharmacologic techniques used and did they work well?
- What coping techniques were beneficial?

If patient-controlled analgesia (PCA) is used, it is helpful to teach the child and the parents the principles of PCA or to explain regional anesthetic techniques if they are chosen. The parents and child should be intimately involved in the evaluation, management, and decision making whenever possible.

II. ASSESSING ACUTE PAIN IN INFANTS AND CHILDREN

Pain assessment is the key to effective pain management. Consistent assessment must occur regularly and the same scale and format must be used for each assessment so as not to confuse the child or parents. In neonates and infants, clinical judgment alone is often used, whereas simple assessment tools are useful in older children. Broadly, there are three stages of a child's development, each of which requires a different means of pain assessment.

1. Infants, Neonates, and Children Aged 4 Years and Younger

Infants and neonates clearly cannot report their pain. However, children as young as 18 months can indicate their pain and give a location, although they cannot specify pain intensity before about 3 years of age. At the age of 3 years, they can give a gross indication, such as "no pain," "a little pain," or "a lot of pain," but their reports are not always reliable. The parents' impression is often the best indicator in these very young patients. Nurses and doctors need to listen to the parents, as well as use objective measures of pain. The following behavioral and physiologic responses can be used as a measure of pain in young children, particularly those who are non-communicating, although the signs may not be specific to pain:

- Crying, screaming, moaning, whimpering
- Facial expression (e.g., grimacing, furrowed brow)
- Posture, tone, guarding, thrashing, touching painful area
- Palmar sweating
- Sleep pattern
- Respiratory rate and pattern
- Heart rate and blood pressure

Several systematic and validated measurement tools could be used, such as CRIES (developed by Krechel and Bildner in 1995), that utilize various combinations of physiologic and behavioral indicators of pain, although their use is not often warranted in cases of acute pain. The principles of pain assessment in very young children and issues of the nervous system and cognitive development are described in Chapter 33.

2. Children Aged 4 to 8 Years

Assuming that the young children (from 4 years to 8 years) have normal development, they can provide reliable self-reports of pain using assessment tools designed for young children, such as the FACES pain-rating scale (see Chapter 6, Fig. 1), by communicating through their parents, or through direct communication with doctors and nurses. Simple numeric scales using age-appropriate language may be helpful at the upper end of this age range.

3. Children Older Than 7 Years

Children older than 7 years who understand the concept of numeric order can use verbal numeric scales or visual analog scales such as those used in adults (see Chapter 6).

III. TREATMENT CHOICES

When choosing treatment options for both procedural and postoperative pain for children, the following considerations should be kept in mind:

- Drug conjugation in the liver is the predominant method of metabolism for most analgesics. Neonates, having an immature cytochrome P450 system, will conjugate drugs slowly.
- Renal clearance of drugs and their metabolites is usually adequate at 2 weeks after birth. Before this, the clearance of many drugs may be delayed, necessitating an increase in dosing intervals.
- Because of the increase in total body water concentration in neonates, water-soluble drugs have a larger volume of distribution.
- Neonates have less plasma protein binding, resulting in increased free drug concentration.

In general, these pharmacokinetic factors mean that lower per-kilogram doses are needed in neonates and infants, but sometimes at increased dosing intervals. However, the effects of immaturity are complex and some drugs may actually be needed in larger doses because of differences in drug sensitivity and distribution. There is no substitute for using pediatric drug tables when prescribing drugs for young children.

1. Acetaminophen and Nonsteroidal Antiinflammatory Drugs

Acetaminophen and nonsteroidal antiinflammatory drugs (NSAIDs) are effective for mild to moderate pain or as adjuncts to opioid and regional analgesia. Such drugs offer the advantages of not being associated with respiratory depression and being relatively free of side effects. Pediatric dosing for these drugs is presented in Table 1.

(i) Acetaminophen

Acetaminophen has only minimal antiinflammatory effects because its effects are mainly central. In patients who have a history of asthma or an increased risk of gastrointestinal (GI) mucosal insult or renal insufficiency, acetaminophen is favored over NSAIDs. Acetaminophen is available in many formulations, including tablets, capsules, syrups, suspensions, and suppositories. It is also included in many compound analgesics (Tylenol no. 3, Percocet, Vicodin, Ultracet, etc.). The intravenous (IV) form of acetaminophen (Paracetamol) is available in Europe but not in the United States. Rapid absorption without first-pass liver metabolism makes the rectal route useful in children.

(ii) Nonsteroidal Antiinflammatory Drugs

Currently used NSAIDs do not cross the blood–brain barrier in appreciable amounts; therefore their effects are mainly peripheral.

Table 1. Pediatric dosing of commonly used nonsteroidal antiinflammatory drugs (NSAIDs) and acetaminophen

Drug	Dose	Comments
Acetaminophen (PO and PR)	10–15 mg/kg q4h	Lacks the peripheral antiinflammatory activity of other NSAIDs. Doses up to 30–40 mg/kg can be given PO or PR for severe pain; maximum daily dose is 100 mg/kg
Aspirin	10–15 mg/kg q4h	Limited usage in children because of its association with Reye syndrome
Ibuprofen	4–10 mg/kg q6–8h	Available as several proprietary and generic drugs; also available as oral suspension
Naproxen	5 mg/kg q12h	Also available as oral liquid
Ketorolac (IV)	0.5 mg/kg q6–8h	Potent and injectable; usage limited by side effects; should not be used for more than 5 d

Note: Doses are for oral use unless otherwise stated.
PO, by mouth; PR, by way of the rectum; NSAIDs, nonsteroidal antiinflammatory drugs; IV, intravenous.

The use of NSAIDs is associated with well-recognized side effects including gastritis, possible GI bleeding, platelet dysfunction, and renal dysfunction. These side effects limit their use after major surgery and in certain patients (e.g., those with renal disease or coagulopathies).

Aspirin (acetylsalicylic acid) currently has very limited use in children and in infants because of its recognized association with Reye syndrome. The most widely used NSAID is ibuprofen, available in a number of formulations including an oral suspension and chewable tablets appropriate for use in children and infants. Dosages of 5 to 10 mg per kg every 4 hours up to a daily maximum of 40 mg per kg may be used either as needed or preferably around the clock for 48 to 72 hours. Other NSAIDs used in the treatment of children include naproxen, indomethacin, tolmetin, diclofenac, ketoprofen, and ketorolac. Of these, only ketorolac, at doses up to 0.5 mg per kg, is approved in the United States for parenteral and oral administration for the treatment of pain. Ketorolac can be useful for treating postoperative pain when the oral route cannot be used, when opioids are poorly tolerated, or when additional analgesia is needed. IV indomethacin is used to treat patent ductus arteriosus but has virtually no application in the treatment of pain. Indomethacin suppositories may be useful occasionally.

The newer selective cyclooxygenase (COX-2) inhibitors are less likely to cause GI side effects because they selectively inhibit the inducible COX-2, sparing the constitutive enzyme (COX-1), particularly in the GI tract. They may be useful as an alternative to standard NSAIDs when there is concern about the GI effects from NSAIDs, although studies regarding the use of these drugs in children and infants have not yet been completed.

2. Opioids

Opioids are the most commonly prescribed analgesics and are potent and effective in the treatment of moderate to severe pain. These drugs are fully described in Chapter 9. Opioids can be used safely in children with appropriate monitoring, dosing regimens, and techniques of administration.

(i) Pharmacokinetics

Opioids are metabolized differently in children at different ages. In newborns and infants, the pharmacokinetic factors described in the preceding text indicate that lower per-kilogram doses are needed than in older children, although the larger volume of distribution of these drugs may mean that a relatively large loading dose (given under controlled conditions) may be needed. Neonates and premature infants are extremely sensitive to the respiratory depressant effects of opioids, and respiratory depression may occur at doses that do not even produce analgesia. Infants are also at an increased risk of apnea following a rapid bolus dose because of the rapid peak dose to the brain. The half-life of morphine in neonates is 6 to 8 hours and about 10 hours in premature infants (compared to 2 hours in adults), necessitating markedly lower infusion rates than in older individuals. As children grow, morphine clearance rapidly approaches the adult level, and in adolescents it is actually greater than that in adults. Recommended opioid doses for children are presented in Table 2.

Table 2.   Recommended starting doses for opioids in children weighing <50 kg

Drug	Oral	Parenteral
Morphine	0.3 mg/kg q3–4h	0.05–1 mg/kg q3–4h
Codeine	0.5–1 mg/kg q3–4h	Not used
Hydromorphone	0.03–0.06 mg/kg q3–4h	0.015 mg/kg q3–4h
Oxycodone	0.05–0.1 mg/kg q3–4h	Not available
Hydrocodone	0.05–0.1 mg/kg q3–4h	Not available
Meperidine	1–3 mg/kg	1 mg/kg
Methadone	0.1–0.2 mg/kg	0.05–0.1 mg/kg
Fentanyl	15–20 μg/kg ("lollipop")	0.5–1 μg/kg

Equianalgesic doses are listed in Appendix VII.

(ii) Choice of Opioids

Morphine is commonly the drug of choice in infants and in children. Because of the associated histamine release with morphine, hydromorphone or fentanyl may be used in patients with asthma. Codeine, oxycodone, and morphine are the opioids most commonly chosen for oral administration in children.

(iii) Route of Administration

Opioids can be given parenterally, orally, rectally, transdermally, transmucosally, or neuraxially. In the immediate postoperative period, the IV route (via an indwelling catheter) is most commonly chosen. If there is no IV in place, the rectal route may be useful.

a) PARENTERAL. The IV route is the parenteral route of choice. Drugs can be given either intermittently or through a continuous infusion. Intermittent boluses are used if pain gets out of control or when there is a need for analgesia for anticipating noxious stimulation such as dressing changes. PCA is used when children are old enough to use this technique. Nurse-controlled analgesia (NCA) via a PCA pump is also an option.

Continuous Intravenous Infusion. Continuous IV infusions are used in young children (<5 to 7 years) with moderate to severe pain, when they are not able to use PCA, in order to maintain steady plasma drug levels and stable analgesia. A loading dose of the drug is commonly given to reach a steady state before the infusion. Careful monitoring of vital signs and special monitors are sometimes necessary to prevent excessive sedation and respiratory depression. This precaution is particularly important in neonates and in all spontaneously breathing children. If pain cannot be controlled with infusion, the rate of infusion may be increased. However, the rate of infusion **should not be repeatedly and rapidly increased**; accelerating the infusion rate is a common misstep that frequently causes potentially dangerous respiratory depression.

Morphine is the most commonly used opioid for continuous infusions. Analgesic levels are usually obtained after a loading dose of 10 to 100 μg per kg of morphine, and an infusion at 10 to 30 $\mu g/kg/hour$ is then started. Recommended infusion rates vary according to age and severity of pain (see Table 3). In some circumstances, it may be desirable to use a different opioid. The Massachusetts General Hospital (MGH) standard orders for continuous opioid infusions are shown in Figure 1.

Patient-Controlled Analgesia. PCA is used in older children (>5 years old) at MGH when they understand how to use it. The principles of PCA are explained in Chapter 21. It is sometimes appropriate to allow parents or nurses to operate the infusion pump or other delivery device for the child, but caution should be exercised. Before allowing parents to participate, the prescribing physician should be absolutely certain that the parents understand the principles of PCA, and, in particular, that they should not press the button unless the child is awake and is requesting analgesia for pain. Standard MGH PCA orders are shown in Chapter 21, Figure 1. Table 4 presents a PCA dosing guideline for morphine, hydromorphone, and fentanyl.

Table 3.   Guidelines for continuous intravenous infusion of morphine

Population	Pain Level	Morphine µg/kg/h
Preterm neonate	Severe	5–10
	Moderate	2–5
	Mild	0–2
Term neonate	Severe	10–20
	Moderate	5–10
	Mild	0–5
Older infant	Severe	15–30
	Moderate	10–20
	Mild	0–10

Adapted from Yaster M, Krane EJ, Kaplan RF, eds. *Pediatric pain management and sedation handbook*. St. Louis, MO: Mosby, 1997:199, with permission.

Massachusetts General Hospital

Pediatric Continuous Intravenous Analgesia

DOCTORS' ORDER SHEET

UNIT NO.
NAME

Date:
Patient's age:
Patient's weight:
Drug allergies:

Pain Service page number is 27246 (2-PAIN)

(See guide on the back of this sheet for scales of pain level and sedation level)

1. **Discontinue previous pain medications.**

2. **No systemic narcotics to be given except by order of the Pain Service.**

3. **Drug (check one):**
   ☐ morphine 0.2 mg/cc
   ☐ morphine 1 mg/cc
   ☐ _____

4. **Initial bolus loading does (if needed):**
   _____ cc (_____ mg) every _____ minutes, prn until patient is comfortable.
   Maximum total loading dose:
   _____ cc (_____ mg)

5. **Infusion rate:**
   (a) For Abbott (APMII) pump, select PCA mode 1: "Continuous Only"
   (b) Range ____ - ____ cc/hr (____ - ____ mg/hr)
   (c) Start at: _____ cc/hr (_____ mg/hr)

6. **For respiratory depression:**
   (a) Discontinue infusion
   (b) Narcan 2µ g/kg, repeated q 5 mins x 2 if necessary, maximum 6 µ g/kg
   (c) Administer oxygen by facemask (4L/min), if necessary

8. **In the event of pump failure or non-patent IV:**
   _____, ____ mg SQ/IM q _____ hr prn for pain

Signature: _____ MD

MONITORING

1. Record baseline HR, BP and RA (respiratory assessment of rate and depth) 15 and 30 minutes after initial bolus loading dose.

2. Record RA q 2 hrly and analgesic and sedation scores q 4 hrly

3. Page the Pain Service for:
   (a) Inadequate analgesia
   (b) Respiratory depression (RR < _____)
   (c) Excessive sedation
   (d) Mental status change
   (e) Change in vital signs
       HR <
       SBP < ____

IN THE CASE OF PROBLEMS CALL THE PAIN SERVICE, PAGE # 27246 (2-PAIN)

In an emergency, if unable to contact the Pain Service, call anesthesia in the operating room, 6-8995 or 6-8910

I3418 2/99

Figure 1.   MGH pediatric continuous intravenous (IV) morphine order sheet.

Table 4. Guidelines for patient-controlled analgesia (PCA) dosing

Drug	Bolus dose (μg/kg)	Lockout (min)	Basal rate (μg/kg/h)	Hourly limit (mg/kg)
Morphine	10–30	6–10	10–30	0.1–0.15
Hydromorphone	3–5	6–10	3–5	0.015–0.02
Fentanyl	0.25–0.5	10	0.15	0.005

Adapted from Yaster M, Krane EJ, Kaplan RF, eds. *Pediatric pain management and sedation handbook*. St. Louis, MO: Mosby, 1997:100, with permission.

b) ORAL. The oral route is used when the pain is mild to moderate. Either pure opioid or an opioid combination can be chosen. Codeine, oxycodone, morphine elixir, acetaminophen with codeine (Tylenol no. 3), and oxycodone with acetaminophen (Percocet) are all useful in children. Recommended doses can be found in Table 2. Morphine and hydromorphone are available as suppositories and may be useful when the oral and IV routes are not available. Rectal doses are the same as oral doses.

c) TRANSDERMAL. A transdermal fentanyl patch is available for the treatment of moderate to severe pain, but this has limited application in infants and children. The lowest available dose is 25 μg per hour; therefore, the patch is not suitable for children weighing less than 25 kg or for those requiring a low dose (i.e., those who have not yet developed a tolerance to opioids). The patch has a long onset time and a long elimination half-life, and therefore it is not suitable when rapid titration is needed. Occasionally, the patch is useful in children undergoing surgery who have already become opioid tolerant because of preexisting cancer or chronic pain.

d) TRANSMUCOSAL. Transmucosal administration of fentanyl is effective for acute pain relief. Fentanyl Oralet (fentanyl in a sugar matrix—"fentanyl lollipop") is absorbed through the buccal mucosa when the child sucks on the lollipop. It is usually absorbed into the systemic circulation in 10 to 20 minutes, and it is more effective than oral/gastric intestinal administration because it bypasses the first-pass hepatic metabolism. Fentanyl Oralet has been approved for use in children for premedication before surgery, certain procedures (lumbar puncture, bone marrow aspiration, etc.), and breakthrough pain for patients with cancer pain. A suitable dose is 10 to 15 μg per kg (25% to 33% absorption rate), and its effects last approximately 2 hours. If excessive sedation is noted, the lollipop should be removed from the child's mouth immediately. In children, the Fentanyl Oralet should only be used under direct medical supervision, with suitable monitoring in place. (The only exception would be opioid-tolerant children treated at home during terminal illness.)

e) NEURAXIAL. Opioids given intrathecally or epidurally provide analgesia that is both effective and relatively free of side effects because much smaller doses are used. Hydromorphone and fentanyl are used at the MGH. Differences among opioids when administered neuraxially are described in Chapter 21. As a general principle, an epidural dose is 1/10th of an IV dose, whereas an intrathecal (spinal) dose is 1/100th of an IV dose.

f) NOVEL ROUTES OF ADMINISTRATION. Recently, several alternative routes have been described for adults and, possibly, for children. For example, intranasal administration of fentanyl, sufentanyl, and butorphanol has been used for relieving postoperative pain after myringotomy. Unfortunately, there are few studies supporting novel opioid delivery systems in children.

3. Regional Anesthesia and Analgesia

Regional and local anesthetic techniques are often used in children and provide the advantages of prolonged analgesia extending into the postoperative period and reduced distress and opioid requirement. Infants and young children appear to be relatively resistant to the hemodynamic and respiratory effects of epidural or spinal blockade so that the techniques are generally safe. Catheters may be utilized to even further extend the use of regional analgesia. The most common regional technique used in children is the epidural technique, using low-dose local anesthetics with or without opioids. This technique blocks C-fibers specifically and spares sensory and motor nerves so that patients can move normally. Opioids have a predominant spinal effect due to a large number of spinal cord opioid receptors.

(i) Epidural Analgesia

For a description of epidural analgesia in adults, see Chapter 21. Many of the principles in adults also apply to children and are not repeated here. In small children, epidural catheters are technically more difficult to place because of the difference in anatomy between children and adults, and these catheters are more difficult to maintain because of the challenges of preventing catheter migration or disconnection caused by movement, of protecting the catheter from the diaper contamination, and of maintaining catheter patency when small catheters are used. Single-shot epidurals, including caudals, are very useful in children and provide excellent analgesia during the early postoperative phase. For a single shot caudal injection, we give 0.3 to 1 mL per kg of 0.125% to 0.25% bupivacaine, sometimes with the addition of 2 to 4 μg per kg clonidine, which provides additional analgesia with minimal risk of hypotension (see clonidine in Appendix VII).

a) INDICATIONS. At the MGH, postoperative epidural catheter treatments are reserved for children undergoing thoracic, abdominal, or lower-limb procedures that are expected to produce severe pain. Single-shot techniques provide useful analgesia after surgical procedures of the torso, pelvis, and lower limbs, including hernia repair, circumcision, tendon lengthening, and clubfoot release. The caudal route is most commonly selected for single-shot epidural injections.

b) CONTRAINDICATIONS
- Patient or parent refusal
- Coagulopathy

- Bacteremia
- Local infection at the epidural insertion site
- Spine pathology, neurologic deficit, raised intracranial pressure (relative contraindications)

c) BENEFITS

- Superior analgesia with clear sensory and motor function
- Opioid sparing and decreased risk of respiratory depression
- Increased bowel mobility
- Decreased bladder spasm after urologic surgery

d) DISADVANTAGES AND RISKS

- This technique poses the risk of local anesthetic toxicity.
- If opioids are used, respiratory depression can occur.
- Urinary retention is common. Pruritus may be a problem in up to 30% of patients. Nausea occurs rarely in this population.
- Catheter migration may occur, resulting in intrathecal, intravascular, or extradural placement. Indications of catheter migration include sudden increase in block density, blood in catheter, or failure to provide analgesia.
- Although rare, epidural hematoma and abscess may occur. Particular caution should be used when a child has a history of coagulopathy or is receiving anticoagulant therapy. Practitioners should be familiar with the guideline for neuraxial analgesia from the American Society of Regional Anesthesia and Pain Medicine (ASRA) (see Appendix II for Website address). Careful monitoring of neurologic function and patient status is imperative to detect early signs of adverse events.

e) EPIDURAL PLACEMENT IN CHILDREN

Anatomic Differences. In infants, the level of the spinal cord and dural sac are continuously changing up to 1 year of age (see Table 5). The relation of the line between iliac crests to the spinal cord level changes as follows: in the neonate the line is at spinal cord level L5-S1, in an older child at L5, and in an adult at L4-L5. It is also useful to know the depth of the epidural space in children, especially because the ligaments are less dense than in adults and provide a different feel. A useful formula to approximate depth (in mm) of the epidural space from the skin in children is as follows:

Infant: depth (mm) = 1.5 × weight in kilograms
Child: depth (mm) = 1 × weight in kilograms   (22.1)

Techniques. A needle or catheter may be placed in epidural space at the appropriate dermatomal level to inject or infuse

Table 5.   Age differences in spinal cord anatomy

Age	Dural Sac Ending	Spinal Cord Ending
Full-term neonate	S3-S4	L4
6 mo	S2	L2-L3
1 y	S1	L1

local anesthetics, opioids, or other medications. Threading a catheter within the epidural space is easier in children than in adults. For caudal epidural injections the needle is inserted between the sacral cornuae at the base of the sacrum. A catheter can be threaded through the caudal canal to the lumbar or thoracic epidural space, if desired. Because most pediatric epidural catheter placement is performed under general anesthesia, it is common practice to place epidurals at the caudal or lumbar (not thoracic) level so as to avoid spinal cord injury.

f) MANAGING EPIDURAL INFUSIONS

Choice of Medication. Epidural opioids are avoided or used with caution in infants and children at risk (e.g., those with pulmonary dysfunction or developmental delay or those infants who have a high risk of respiratory depression or apnea or were born prematurely). The selection of epidural infusion solution and its dose are summarized in Table 6. When initial bolus is needed, the following is acceptable practice in MGH: 0.05 mL/kg/spinal segment using either 1% lidocaine or 0.125% to 0.25% bupivacaine, not to exceed a dose of 5 mg per kg of lidocaine or 2.5 mg per kg of bupivacaine.

General Care. The standard of care when providing epidural analgesia for children is similar to that for adults. This protocol consists of the following:

- 24-hour pain service coverage for patients receiving epidural analgesia
- Ventilatory status monitored and recorded hourly
- Vital signs monitored and recorded every 4 hours
- Daily pain service evaluation for pain control satisfaction, side effects, and neurologic status
- Daily examination of the catheter site for signs of inflammation or infection

Table 6.   Epidural infusion solution choice and doses

Drug	Recommend Use	Dose
0.1% Bupivacaine	Neonate, <3 mo	0.2–0.25 mg/kg/h
	>3 mo	0.4–0.5 mg/kg/h
0.1% Bupivacaine with Fentanyl 2 μg/mL	3 mo to 5 y	Cath tip below T10: 0.2–0.3 mL/kg/h Cath tip above T10: 0.1–0.2 mL/kg/h
0.1% Bupivacaine with hydromorphone 10–20 μg/mL	>5 y	Cath tip below T10: 0.2–0.3 mL/kg/h Cath tip above T10: 0.2–0.3 mL/kg/h

- Children younger than 6 months should be considered at risk of respiratory depression and a low threshold should be set for more intensive monitoring
- Heels padded to prevent pressure sores
- No systemic opioids should be given while the patient is receiving epidural opioids. But if there is a need to cover the pain area that the epidural infusion could not cover, the opioid could be removed from the epidural infusion solution and be given intravenously.

g) TREATMENT OF SIDE EFFECTS AND COMPLICATIONS. Local anesthetic toxicity is rare in the postoperative setting. If it occurs, it should be treated as described in Chapter 37. The abnormal neurologic examination may indicate a residual block from surgery, migration of the catheter to one side or one nerve root, catheter irritation, or the more sinister possibility of impending epidural hematoma or abscess. In most cases (other than epidural hematoma or abscess), recovery will occur when the rate of infusion is reduced or held, the catheter is pulled back, or the treatment is stopped.

The cardinal signs of epidural hematoma or abscess are back pain and sensory/motor neurologic deficits. These symptoms and signs should always prompt withdrawal of treatment, close neurologic monitoring, and possible investigation with magnetic resonance imaging (MRI). An appropriate and timely intervention, including surgery, is crucial because patients may suffer permanent neurologic damage if the surgical decompression is not performed in time.

Other side effects from epidural opioid include pruritus, nausea and vomiting, urinary retention, and respiratory depression. Treatment is summarized in Table 7. Respiratory depression is the most serious of these complications. Treatment involves administering oxygen; providing ventilatory support, if necessary; stopping of the epidural infusion; and administering naloxone ($2\ \mu g$ per kg, IV). It is also possible that catheter migration could have occurred, resulting in an intrathecal infusion.

Table 7. Adjuncts to treatment of acute pain in pediatric patients

Drug	Indication	Dose
Naloxone	Respiratory depression	$2\ \mu g/kg$
Naloxone	Pruritus	$0.5–1\ \mu g/kg$
Benadryl (diphenhydramine)	Pruritus	$0.5\ mg/kg$
Nalbuphine	Pruritus	$10–20\ \mu g/kg$
Ondansetron	Nausea	$0.1\ mg/kg$
Metoclopromide	Nausea	$0.1–0.2\ mg/kg$

(ii) Spinals

Spinal anesthesia and analgesia are most commonly used in neonates for surgical operation. The L4-L5 space is often chosen. For neonates, the doses of local anesthetics used are relatively higher than those for an older child or an adult. The duration of action is also shorter in children than in older patients. Hyperbaric bupivacaine and tetracaine are the most commonly used agents. The use of a single injection of an opioid [most commonly, preservative-free morphine sulfate (Duramorph) 2 to 10 μg per kg] into the spinal fluid prolongs the analgesia (12 to 24 hours or more) and is reserved for children older than 5 years. Because delayed respiratory depression is liable to occur, close monitoring of the respiratory function status is required for up to 24 to 36 hours after the injection.

Other Techniques

Peripheral nerve blocks provide anesthesia and analgesia in the early postoperative period for children. It includes ilioinguinal, femoral, penile, brachial plexus, and lumbar plexus blocks. EMLA cream (a eutectic mixture of local anesthetics—lidocaine and prilocaine) has been proven to be useful in children to benumb the skin before needling, and even to provide postoperative pain relief (e.g., after circumcision). Other topical local anesthetic preparations are occasionally useful (e.g., lidocaine gel for mucous membranes).

4. Nonpharmacologic Techniques

Nonpharmacologic techniques are adjuncts to analgesic medications to help ease a child's discomfort or anxiety level associated with pain. These techniques work best when the patient and his or her family are introduced to the particular technique and if they are actively participate.

Cognitive Approaches

Education has been shown to be effective in children, especially when preoperative teaching has been conducted.

Distraction may be useful in all age groups, but it needs to be age specific. Attention is focused on stimuli other than the pain sensation. The stimuli must be interesting to the patient; consistent with the developmental level, energy level, and capability of the child; and stimulating to major sensory modalities (i.e., hearing, vision, touch, and movements). Some examples for specific ages are as follows:

- Toddler/Preschooler: blowing bubbles, singing, music cassettes, pop-ups, or "I Spy" books
- School-aged/Adolescent: music or story via headset, singing or tapping rhythm, or conversation

Cutaneous Stimulation

Massage or rubbing the skin may be very soothing but is generally not recommended for premature and full-term neonates. The application of heat or cold is often useful in localized pain.

Transcutaneous electric nerve stimulation (TENS) can also be used (see Chapter 16).

Guided Imagery

Guided imagery uses a patient's own imagination to develop sensory images to decrease pain, thereby making pain more acceptable or changing pain into a different sensation. Examples are throwing pain away like a snowball, blowing pain away, or imagining pain medication traveling through the body to relieve the pain.

Relaxation

These techniques are used to decrease anxiety and skeletal muscle tension, potentially relieving some of the mental and physical effects of pain. Techniques include breathing exercises, progressive relaxation, remembering past peaceful experiences, and using pacifiers and stroking in infants and toddlers.

Acupuncture

Acupuncture has shown good effects for treating postoperative nausea and vomiting in children. However, the utility of acupuncture for children and adolescents with acute postoperative pain has not been established.

IV. CONCLUSION

Improvements in pain management in infants and children play an integral role in advancing the medical care of children. Further progress in education, research, and knowledge will allow us to apply those lessons learned in the adults to the care of young patients. It is incumbent upon all caregivers to consider pain and analgesia at every juncture in the care of sick children.

SELECTED READINGS

Ashburn M, Rice L, eds. *Management of pain.* New York: Churchill Livingstone, 1998.

Berde CB, Sethna NF, Levin L, et al. Regional analgesia on pediatric medial and surgical wards. *Intensive Care Med* 1989;15(1):S40–S43.

Carr DB. Acute pain management: operative or medical procedures and trauma. *Clinical practice guideline.* AHCPR Pub No. 92-0032. Rockville, MD: Agency for Health Care Policy and Research, Public Health Service, U.S. Department of Health and Human Services, 1992.

Dalens B, ed. *Regional anesthesia in infants, children, and adolescents.* Baltimore, MD: Williams & Wilkins, 1995.

Deshpande JK, Tobias JD. *The pediatric pain handbook.* St. Louis, MO: Mosby, 1996.

Golianu B, Krane EJ, Galloway KS, et al. Pediatric acute pain management. *Pediatr Clin North Am* 2000;47(3),559–87.

Krechel SW, Bildner J. CRIES: a new neonatal postoperative pain measurement score. Initial testing of validity and reliability. *Paediatr Anaesth* 1995;5:53–61.

Lloyd-Thomas AR. Pain management in paediatric patients. *Br J Anaesth* 1990;64(1):85–104.

McKenzie I, Gaukroger P, Ragg P, et al., eds. *Manual of acute pain management in children*. Melbourne, FL: Churchill Livingstone, 1997.

Schechter NL, Berde CB, Yaster M, eds. *Pain in infant, children, and adolescents*, 2nd ed. Philadelphia, PA: Lippincott Williams & Wilkins, 2003.

Zwass M, Polaner D, Berde C. Postoperative pain management. In: Cote CJ, Todres ID, Ryan JF, et al., eds. *A practice of anesthesia for infants and children*. Philadelphia, PA: WB Saunders, 2001.

Pain in Burn Patients

Salahadin Abdi and Bucknam McPeek

There is physical pain, there is mental pain and scarring. You can see the outside, but what a lot of people don't see is that we are truly burned on the inside as well.
—*Burn survivor*

More than 2 million burn injuries occur annually in the United States, of which thermal burns are the most prevalent; chemical and electrical burns occur less commonly. Approximately 1 in 20 patients with burn injuries require extended hospitalization. Burn injury results in both physical and psychological distress, and pain is a major component of both. In fact, burns are among the most painful of all injuries. Pain evaluation and treatment are important aspects of the care of patients inflicted with burn injuries.

The management of acute and chronic pain from burn injuries is challenging and may require input from an experienced pain specialist. A careful pain management plan will help circumvent potential hazards in these often critically ill and psychologically disturbed patients. It is important to be attentive to the specific type of pain the patient is experiencing and to the risks of pain treatment in relation to the pathophysiology of the injured patient. The likelihood of developing chronic pain and life-long suffering (e.g., chronic pain, posttraumatic stress disorder) can be reduced by appropriate and aggressive acute pain management techniques, with meticulous attention to psychological and social factors. The purpose of this chapter is to outline the essential issues so that proper planning and care can be provided.

I. TYPES OF BURN INJURY

The extent of a burn injury is measured as percentage of body surface area burned. Burns vary in depth from superficial to full thickness, with a possibility of massive destruction of muscle or bone in the latter.

by erythema, and involves only the epidermis. There is usually only mild to moderate discomfort, and healing occurs within a week.

Second-degree burns are deeper, partial-thickness injuries that destroy the epidermis and variable amounts of dermis, as well as epidermal appendages. Second-degree burns are extremely painful. Most of the pain is caused by the damage of sensory nociceptive receptors that are preferentially sensitive to tissue damage. In addition to direct damage from the burn, second-degree burns damage the protective layer of skin and expose the normally protected nerve endings. These lesions heal slowly, with some tissue contraction, nerve regeneration, and the occasional need for skin grafting.

Third-degree burns destroy the skin completely. These burns are, by definition, of full thickness. Regions of third-degree burns may be painless after the initial injury for a period because of destruction of the cutaneous nociceptors. Although the central part of the initial wound may be insensate, painful areas of second-degree injury surround almost every third-degree burn. These areas heal by epidermal regeneration because some of the epidermal appendages remain intact. This healing process can be painful. With inadequate cleansing and debridement, a surface pseudomembrane that consists of wound exudate and necrotic eschar accumulates. As long as the eschar and pseudomembrane exist, the center of a third-degree burn is painless. The eschar is usually removed surgically because the unremoved eschar and membrane serve as a nidus of infection (the major life-threatening factor in burn injury). It is important to emphasize that patients with third-degree burns suffer severe pain and need treatment despite some areas of their burn being insensate.

II. TYPES OF BURN PAIN

There are two categories of pain:

- **Procedural pain (incidental/evoked pain):** This refers to pain experienced during or after wound care, stent removal, dressing change, physical therapy, or other treatments. This type of pain is usually short-lasting but of great intensity. Debridement usually requires general anesthesia. It is helpful to administer an adequate and appropriately timed dose of a narcotic analgesic and or benzodiazepine before beginning any procedure.
- **Background pain (spontaneous/resting/constant pain):** Background pain is the pain experienced by the patient while at rest. This type of pain is usually dull and continuous and is of lower intensity. Nevertheless, this low-intensity pain should be controlled, otherwise it may prime patients to experience more pain, as well as increase their anxiety, particularly about procedures. Background pain is best treated with opioids (or alternative analgesics) administered on a regular, rather than on an as-needed, basis.

In addition, there are two temporal components of burn pain, acute and chronic. In the acute postburn state, the most severe pain results from therapeutic procedures such as dressing changes.

Background pain may persist for weeks to months or even years. Pain related to burn injury might worsen with time because of several factors, including increased anxiety and depression, continuing sleep disturbance, and deconditioning and regeneration of nerve endings (possible neuroma formation, known as postburn neuralgia). Chronic pain may result from contractures, nerve injury (neuropathic pain), or nerve and tissue damage subsequent to surgical procedures.

III. TREATMENT OF ACUTE BURN PAIN

The main treatment goal for serious burns is the removal of necrotic tissue and other sources of infection; this requires cleaning the burn area by debridement or surgical excision. Microorganisms that release exotoxins and endotoxins exacerbate the inflammation already present in burns and quickly colonize retained necrotic tissue. After removal of necrotic tissue by cleaning or surgical excision, the next step is to promote coverage of the open wound wherever possible by a skin graft from unburned areas of the patient's own body. In large burns, autologous skin grafts or artificial skin can provide temporary coverage.

Patients suffer continual shifts from mild to moderate background discomfort to excruciating pain associated with treatments such as burn dressing changes, manual debridement of open wounds, and physical therapy. In addition, there are frequent surgical operations, excisions of eschar, and harvesting of large areas of normal skin for grafting (also a source of pain). Burn dressing changes and debridements may occur twice a day, physical therapy once or twice a day, and surgical interventions several times a week. Because of the variation in the intensity of pain from hour to hour or even from minute to minute, treatment of patients with acute pain from burn injuries requires repeated assessments and titration of analgesic drugs. Patients typically require increasing amounts of opioid medication to control pain during these procedures as they develop tolerance to the opioid (Chapter 9).

The interpretation and assessment of pain behavior in these patients can be very difficult. The pain is often compounded by anxiety. Giving the patient a role in his or her pain management helps alleviate the anxiety. An honest explanation about procedure-related pain and how it can be relieved is a necessary prerequisite for developing a treatment plan with the patient. The following are treatment options for burn-related pain.

1. Acetaminophen

Acetaminophen is a weak analgesic and antipyretic. It is used as the first-line treatment of minor burns but can also be used as an adjunct to opioids for major burns. Because this drug mainly acts centrally, it is not associated with the typical side effects of the nonsteroidal antiinflammatory drug (NSAID) that are produced by the latter's prostaglandin inhibition in the periphery. Acetaminophen is not useful for long-term pain management because of its toxic and accumulative effects on the liver. See Chapter 8 for a full description.

2. Nonsteroidal Antiinflammatory Drugs

NSAIDs reduce inflammation and pain. They may be used as sole analgesics for mild to moderate pain or as adjuncts to more potent analgesics. Side effects, specifically gastrointestinal (GI) bleeding, may limit their use in seriously burned patients who are particularly susceptible to GI bleeding. If used, prophylaxis should be given with a prostaglandin analog (e.g., misoprostol) or H2 blockers (e.g., ranitidine) (Caution: **Do not** give high doses of NSAIDs as a substitute for opioids for the management of procedural pain). A full description of the NSAIDs and their uses is provided in Chapter 8.

3. Opioids

Opioids are the mainstay of treatment used for severe acute pain. Various routes of administration have been described and tested in patients with burn injuries. Morphine is the most widely used drug in burn centers. Hydromorphone (Dilaudid) is useful in patients who have intolerable side effects from morphine or in those who are sensitive to morphine. Meperidine is not recommended because of the toxicity of its metabolite, normeperidine. Continuous fentanyl infusion tends to cause a rapid development of tolerance, which leads to a high dose requirement. However, bolus fentanyl administration is sometimes useful for procedures such as burn dressing changes. It should be remembered that high-dose fentanyl can produce chest wall rigidity and should not be used in self-ventilating patients in whom muscle relaxants cannot be used to overcome the rigidity. Methadone can also be used and has the advantage of N-methyl-D-aspartate (NMDA) receptor antagonist activity, which, theoretically at least, could be important in the prevention of neuropathic pain. In patients who are fed enterally, a bowel regimen should be initiated at the start of opioid therapy. Chapter 9 provides a complete description of the opioids and their uses.

For most patients with burn injuries, the best mode of administration of opioids is probably intravenous patient-controlled analgesia (PCA) (see Chapter 21). This technique allows patients to self-administer the drug, usually morphine or hydromorphone. PCA eliminates the dependency of patients on nurses and provides immediate relief when needed. Most patients, even children as young as 6 or 7 years, learn to control their pain using PCA. Younger children, or adults who cannot push a button, may require a continuous infusion of opioid at least during the acute phase. The onset of analgesia after an intravenous morphine bolus is approximately 6 to 10 minutes, so patients can pretreat themselves or be pretreated by a physician or nurse before painful therapeutic procedures. When patients have substantial background pain, they may require a basal infusion in addition to demand doses.

4. Ketamine

Ketamine is an atypical anesthetic and potent analgesic that is an NMDA receptor antagonist and induces a "dissociative" anesthetic state. It can be used for both anesthesia and analgesia in patients with burn injuries. The main advantages of ketamine use over opioid treatment are the preservation of spontaneous ventilation and airway reflexes and the stimulation of the cardiovascular system secondary to an induced catecholamine release.

Ketamine anesthesia is commonly associated with unpleasant postanesthesia phenomena, such as vivid nightmares and hallucinations, which can be minimized by the concomitant use of a benzodiazepine. These effects are rarely associated with the subanesthetic doses that are used for analgesia. Ketamine should be used with an antisialogogue such as atropine or glycopyrrolate.

5. Antihistamines

Antihistamines are used in the burn center for the management of anxiety, itching, and pain (adjunctive effect). These drugs potentiate opioid analgesia and are particularly useful for their antipruritic effect, given that the pruritus in patients with burn injuries is sometimes worse than the pain, especially during the healing phase of the injury. They are also useful to promote sleep and relieve anxiety.

6. Clonidine

Clonidine has both analgesic and sedative actions. It has been reported to be useful in treating patients with pain caused by burn injury that is inadequately controlled with opioids. Clonidine can counterbalance the sympathetic stimulation of ketamine by reducing sympathetic outflow and can be added to ketamine when this is being used by intravenous infusion.

7. Regional Anesthesia

Regional anesthetics can be used for analgesia or even for anesthesia if the burn wound is limited and is accessible for a regional anesthesia technique. Epidural and spinal anesthesia/analgesia are relatively contraindicated in seriously ill patients with hypotension and/or sepsis.

8. General Anesthesia

General anesthesia is sometimes needed for minor procedures if the pain is severe and cannot be adequately and safely controlled in the awake patient.

IV. TREATMENT OF CHRONIC BURN PAIN

The pain experience for patients with burn injuries unfortunately does not necessarily end after the acute phase, and many patients will continue to have chronic pain even after complete wound healing. It is sometimes necessary to use long-term opioid therapy to maintain a reasonable level of comfort for these unfortunate patients, and it may be necessary to add adjuvant pain medications for the specific treatment of neuropathic pain. As already stated, the NSAIDs and acetaminophen are less suitable for long-term pain therapy. Issues of opioid therapy in chronic nonterminal pain (CNTP) are discussed in Chapter 30. A description of neuropathic pain and its treatment can be found in Chapter 25. The most intractable cases should be referred to a pain clinic. Many of these patients need nonpharmacologic as well as pharmacologic treatment, and a multidisciplinary approach (including behavioral therapy, physical therapy, and occupational therapy) is optimal.

V. NONPHARMACOLOGIC TREATMENTS FOR BURN PAIN

Patients with burn injuries need psychological support in both the acute and chronic phases of burn treatment. Burn survivors frequently have fear, depression, nightmares, and hallucinations. Psychosocial support is as necessary as pharmacologic intervention (e.g., anxiolytic and antidepressants). Burn injury results not only in short-term changes and severe acute pain but also in chronic pain, long-term changes in health status, and often distressing permanent disfigurement. There are many psychological interventions that can be helpful to patients with burn injuries, including hypnosis, relaxation, and biofeedback. These techniques are described in Chapter 15.

VI. CONCLUSION

In summary, the pain experienced by patients with burn injuries is often excruciating and unrelenting and is an unwelcome accompaniment to an already devastating injury. The management of pain in these patients can be extremely challenging and demands expertise and experience. It is important to choose the right modality (or combination of modalities) with the aim of adequately controlling background, as well as procedural, pain. It is equally important to consider the psychological aspects of the pain and to provide psychosocial, as well as pharmacologic, support. An interdisciplinary team approach is the key to successful pain management.

SELECTED READINGS

Atchinson NE, Osgood PF, Carr DB, et al. Pain during burn dressing change in children: relationship to burn area, depth, and analgesic regimens. *Pain* 1991;47:41–45.

Carr DB, Osgood PF, Szyfelbein SK. Treatment of pain in acutely burned children. In: Schechter NL, Berde CB, Yaster M, eds. *Pain in infants, children, and adolescents.* Baltimore, MD: Williams & Wilkins, 1993.

Choiniere M, Auger FA, Latarjet J. Visual analogue thermometer: a valid and useful instrument for measuring pain in burned patients. *Burns* 1994;20:229–235.

Choiniere M, Grenier R, Paquette C. Patient-controlled analgesia: a double-blind study in burn patients. *Anesthesia* 1992;47:467–472.

Dauber A, Carr DB, Breslau A. *Burn survivors' pain experiences: a questionnaire-based survey.* Presented at the 7th World Congress on Pain. Paris: International Association for the Study of Pain, 1993.

Herman RA, Veng-Pedersen P, Miotto J, et al. Pharmacokinetics of morphine sulfate in patients with burns. *Burn Care Rehabil* 1994; 15:95–103.

Kariya N, Shindoh M, Nishi S, et al. Oral clonidine for sedation and analgesia in a burn patient. *J Clin Anesth* 1998;10:514–517.

Lyons B, Casey W, Doherty P, et al. Pain relief with low-dose intravenous clonidine in a child with severe burns. *Intensive Care Med* 1996;22:249–251.

Osgood PF, Szyfelbein SK. Management of pain. In: Martyn JAJ, ed. *Acute management of the burned patient.* Philadelphia, PA: WB Saunders, 1990.

Perry S, Heidrich G. Management of pain during debridement: a survey of U.S. burn units. *Pain* 1982;13:267–280.

24

Pain Management in Sickle Cell Disease

Jatinder Gill

Pain is not just a symptom demanding our compassion; it can be an aggressive disease that damages the nervous system.
—*Gary Bennett*

Sickle cell disease is an inherited hemoglobinopathy primarily affecting individuals descended from inhabitants of equatorial Africa and of areas around the Mediterranean Sea, in Saudi Arabia, and in some parts of India. It is a debilitating chronic multisystem disease with variable phenotypic expression. Acute pain is often the first symptom of sickle cell disease and the most common reason that patients seek medical attention.

One third of the patients experience a benign course, one third have two to six hospital admissions for pain per year, and one third have more than six pain-related hospitalizations per year. Hospital personnel often develop a bias about the genuineness of the painful crises in the third group of patients, especially because pain is a subjective sensation. It is, however, this group that is most in need of medical help. The extreme variability in severity of the clinical phenotype of sickle cell disease remains unexplained and probably relates to genetic, microvascular, rheologic, and hematologic factors.

I. PATHOPHYSIOLOGY

Hemoglobin S (HbS) has a tendency to polymerize when deoxygenated, but the polymerized form rapidly reverts with oxygenation. Repeated cycles of polymerization cause oxidative damage to red cell membranes and lead to irreversibly sickled cells, adhesion of the cells to the endothelium of the vessel, and vascular occlusion. The resultant hypoxia causes further sickling and starts a vicious cycle, leading to tissue infarction and pain. Increased intramedullary pressure secondary to inflammation and necrosis within the bone is an important cause of the pain. Sickling seems to correlate directly with high hemoglobin levels and neutrophil counts and indirectly with fetal hemoglobin (HbF) values.

II. CLINICAL FEATURES AND CONTEMPORARY MANAGEMENT

Sickle cell disease is a multisystem disease. Infants and children are at risk for overwhelming infection from encapsulated bacteria such as pneumococcus. The function of the spleen is impaired, thus depressing immune response. Penicillin prophylaxis, vaccination, and a high index of suspicion are advocated. Meningitis, bacterial pneumonias, cholecystitis, and osteomyelitis are common in adults.

Patients with sickle cell disease are chronically anemic, and profound anemia may occur in the presence of splenic sequestration, exaggerated hemolysis, or aplastic crisis, and may require transfusion. Folic acid supplementation is required to support high turnover rates of bone marrow cells.

Neurologic complications caused by cerebrovascular occlusion occur in up to 25% of patients. Monthly transfusion programs are recommended for children to prevent recurrent strokes. Primary prevention using magnetic resonance imaging (MRI) and transcranial Doppler screening, and initiation of transfusion programs for at-risk patients are recommended.

These patients often have restrictive lung disease, hypoxemia, and pulmonary hypertension, probably secondary to earlier pulmonary occlusions and infarctions. They are at risk for acute chest syndrome, with infection usually caused by atypical agents. Acute chest syndrome has a high mortality rate and requires treatment in the intensive care unit (ICU) setting. A high index of suspicion is required in patients presenting with chest pain and fever, especially in the presence of hypoxemia.

Hepatobiliary complications are common, with up to 70% of patients demonstrating gallstones. Many patients eventually need a cholecystectomy. Hepatic dysfunction may relate to transfusion-associated iron overload or infection. Hyperbilirubinemia secondary to benign cholestasis (no fever or pain) should be differentiated from hepatic crisis that presents with fever, pain, abnormal liver function tests, and hepatic failure.

Poor medullary flow in the kidneys leads to papillary infarctions, hematuria, and renal tubular acidosis. In addition, patients may develop glomerular dysfunction. Proximal tubular dysfunction may lead to hyperuricemia, especially with heavy analgesic use. Some patients eventually develop chronic renal failure.

Proliferative sickle cell retinopathy with the potential of bleeding, leading to blindness, should be treated with laser photocoagulation. Occlusion of the central retinal artery requires immediate transfusion.

Priapism develops in many individuals and, if prolonged, may lead to impotence. If a patient responds poorly to conservative treatment for 12 hours, exchange transfusions, corporal aspiration, use of a-adrenergic agents, and even surgical creation of a fistula may be required to prevent impotence. Hormonal or vasoconstrictive preventive therapy may be needed.

Osteonecrosis may occur, leading to vertebral fractures or necrosis of femoral head, and can be acutely painful. Major reconstructive surgery may be required in patients with advanced disease of the joints who fail to rehabilitate. Bone marrow infarction can be differentiated from osteomyelitis by scans. Arthritis may result from periarticular infarction or from gout. Nonsteriodal antiinflammatory drugs (NSAIDs) are useful adjuncts in patients with bone pains.

Chronic bilateral leg ulcers are common over the shins. In addition to causing chronic pain, these ulcers also may lead to osteomyelitis and septicemia. Subdermal vascular occlusions can cause chronic myofascial pain.

The mean life expectancy in sickle cell disease is approximately 42 years in men and approximately 48 years in women. Patients with severe disease and multiple crises tend to have a shorter life span.

III. ACUTE PAIN CRISIS

Despite the multiple problems associated with sickle cell disease, the most common reason for these patients to be hospitalized is for an acute pain crisis requiring aggressive inpatient management. The usual precipitants are exposure to cold, dehydration, alcohol intake, infections, stress, and menstruation. In more than half the cases, there is no clear cause.

Approximately 5% of patients account for one third of hospital admissions, and, regrettably, caregiver hostility toward this group of patients is common. It is important to remember that these are the patients who tend to die young, and hence pain is a direct marker for mortality. The incidence of pain is highest in young male adults.

Pain typically affects one region of the body. Common sites of pain include the back, bilateral large joints, chest, sternum, ribs, and the abdomen. In children, the smaller joints of the hand and feet may be involved. Fever is present in about half the patients. Patients usually are able to tell whether a new crisis feels like a typical crisis or not.

The etiology of the pain is probably related to ischemia of the tissue undergoing infarction and an increase in intramedullary pressure due to inflammation. The pain in sickle cell disease is often described as excruciating, commonly rating more than nine on the visual analog scale. The importance of ruling out any catastrophic events requires maintaining a high degree of suspicion for acute chest syndrome in a patient with acute chest pain, for osteomyelitis or septic arthritis in a patient with bone or joint pain, or for acute abdomen in a patient with abdominal pain. Furthermore, a work-up may be needed on the basis of the index of suspicion, for example, chest films in a patient with dyspnea and with chest pain or diagnostic aspiration of an acutely tender joint. A good history and a physical examination, together with a review of previous admissions, are indispensable.

1. Management of Mild Vasoocclusive Crisis

Old admission records, previous treatments, complications of the disease, and baseline pain medications are very helpful in directing the treatment. Once it has been established that the patient does not require emergent investigation or intervention, aggressive hydration and pain treatment should be instituted.

Pain treatment should not be withheld during this initial phase. Fluids may be taken by mouth or given intravenously. Opioid medication may be given by mouth if tolerated, but the intravenous (IV) route is usually preferable, at least in the initial period. For oral use, oxycodone, hydromorphone, or morphine are good choices. NSAIDs are useful for bone pain and should be used if no contraindications exist. With NSAIDs, a fixed-dose regimen is preferable to an as-needed regime.

If the patient can be stabilized he or she may be discharged home with a tapering supply of oral opioids. Failure to adequately manage pain is likely to result in readmission; therefore, it is important that the patient be provided with an adequate supply of analgesics. If the pain does not diminish or if the patient has other symptoms such as fever or severe nausea, a longer hospital stay may be required.

2. Hospital Management of Painful Sickle Cell Crisis

(i) Opioids

The pain experienced during a sickle cell crisis is described as excruciating, and opioids are often the first-line treatment. There is no benefit to first trying alternative analgesics in the acute stage. Adjuncts may, however, be used simultaneously.

The care team must take a patient's reports of pain seriously and must administer medications in a timely manner. Doing so encourages the patient to trust the care team, and also prevents undue suffering.

a) ROUTE OF ADMINISTRATION.   Opioids may be given orally if tolerated, but in most situations parenteral narcotics are needed in the initial stages. In patients with chronic pain using opioids on a long-term basis, the baseline (chronically used) medications can be continued to provide continuous background analgesia and can be supplemented with the regimen chosen to treat the acute episode. Alternatively, the patient's ongoing analgesic dosage can be administered intravenously after calculating the equivalent IV dosage and can also be supplemented with additional medication to manage the acute pain. Transdermal fentanyl can be used in later stages of the crisis, but in the initial acute episode, the slow onset of analgesia and difficulty with titration make this delivery method a poor choice.

Formerly, these patients were treated with intramuscular (IM) injections of meperidine and hydroxyzine. However, in the light of an improved understanding of meperidine toxicity and the ease with which IV therapy can be used, there is very little rationale for continuing to recommend this treatment. IM injections should probably be reserved for situations where there is no IV access, or before IV access is obtained. IM injections are painful and may lead to myositis and abscesses; in addition, the rate of drug absorption is unpredictable.

IV narcotics can be given by continuous infusion, by nurse-administered bolus injection or by using a patient-controlled analgesia (PCA) pump. PCA is a very attractive option in the acute management of sickle cell crisis, and probably the treatment of choice. Unfortunately, PCA is not widely available and may not be an option in some settings. Patients can be maintained on a safe low basal rate of opioid, especially at night, and demand doses can be titrated to comfort and safety.

b) CHOICE OF OPIOID. Morphine and hydromorphone are the first-line agents. Hydromorphone may be preferred in patients with renal dysfunction because morphine-6-glucuronide, an active metabolite of morphine, may accumulate if renal failure occurs. Meperidine is no longer used as a first-line opioid (see Chapter 9) and is reserved for patients who cannot tolerate other opioids. In these patients, it is reasonable to consider using meperidine, but due caution should be exercised with regard to its known toxicity, especially in patients with renal involvement and seizure disorder, and its potential for producing addiction.

Opioids often give rise to adverse side effects such as nausea, itching, and sedation. Different medications and dosing intervals may be tried to get the best match in terms of side effect profile. Side effects should be treated with appropriate medications such antiemetics and psychostimulants (see Chapter 9 for a full description of the opioid drugs).

c) WEANING. The typical crisis lasts for approximately 4 to 7 days and its course often is unpredictable. However, some patients with typical crisis may repeat the course of their last crisis. As pain eases, the demand for analgesics and reports of pain decrease. At this point, the patient may be switched to an oral regimen. The total IV dose used by the patient over the last 24 hours is measured and then converted to an equivalent oral dose (approximately 1:3 ratio, see Appendix VII). Other routes also could be chosen at this point, including rectal and transdermal. The dosage is gradually reduced as tolerated. For a successful change from parenteral to oral narcotics, it is crucial that a plan is formulated for the patient on an individual basis and that adequate amount of medications are prescribed. Prompt attention to the patient's reports of pain at this juncture will go a long way toward successful weaning.

d) TOLERANCE AND ADDICTION. Opioid tolerance is a recognized but poorly understood phenomenon. It usually develops over weeks, but tolerance can also arise rapidly when the patient receives high doses during an acute episode. Once tolerance develops, the analgesic effects of these medications, as well as their sedative and respiratory-depressant effects, diminish. Therefore, these patients may require high doses of opioids to achieve adequate pain control. The increased dosage requirements of opioid-tolerant patients should not be interpreted as addiction.

Patients with sickle cell disease also are at risk for withdrawal if their narcotic regimen is abruptly discontinued. Reducing the opioid dose by no more than 20% per day prevents withdrawal in most individuals. If a withdrawal syndrome does occur, it can be reversed by reintroducing the opioid at 25% to 40% of the original dose.

Addiction refers to a situation in which a medication is used primarily for its mind-altering effects and not for its intended analgesic effect. Addiction is a behavioral problem, characterized by maladaptive drug-seeking behavior, which is distinct from the opioid seeking of patients in pain (see Chapter 35). It has been clearly shown that patients with sickle cell disease are no more prone to addiction than any other group of patients. The incidence of addiction in the opioid-treated population as a whole, and in the population with sickle cell disease, ranges from 3% to 19%. However, wrongly assuming that patients with sickle cell disease develop addiction plays a negative role in effectively treating their pain.

A patient with an addiction provides a challenge in pain management. On the one hand, the need for the opioid medication is clear, but, on the other hand, the patient is likely to abuse his or her medication. Management should be centered on recognizing and accepting the addiction problem and on providing structured, consistent care, preferably with input from addiction or psychiatric specialists. The aim should be to manage the pain and addiction concurrently, without compromising one or the other unduly. Acute pain crisis is not the time for initiating detoxification measures.

(ii) Antiinflammatory Drugs

NSAIDs are useful and commonly used in the treatment of acute crisis, as well as for chronic bone pain. NSAIDs effectively supplement opioid analgesia because of their peripheral rather than central mechanism of action.

Important side effects include decreased platelet adhesiveness (risk of bleeding), renal dysfunction, and gastritis. Ketorolac is available for short-term IV use. During acute pain episodes, these medications are more effective if prescribed as fixed doses and not on as-needed basis, although, for safety reasons, the as-needed basis is preferred for long-term use (see Chapter 8).

The use of steroids is controversial. These drugs may decrease the duration of the episode but can also lead to rebound crises. Furthermore, the use of steroids is complicated by several severe side effects. Hence, steroids are not among the first line of drugs in the management of acute crisis.

(iii) Epidural Analgesia

Epidural analgesia is an effective modality for the treatment of pain below the midthoracic region. Although it provides excellent regional analgesia, it is not commonly used because adequate analgesia can often be provided by noninterventional techniques. If the pain is widespread, it may not be covered by epidural medication. In a patient with severe pain not responding to parenteral analgesics, epidural anesthesia can be an excellent alternative. Patients at risk for acute chest syndrome may benefit from epidural analgesia by minimizing systemic medication, respiratory depression, and sedation. Ventilation may be aided with the provision of better analgesia.

(iv) Adjunctive Medications

Antihistamines such as hydroxyzine (Vistaril) and diphenhydramine (Benadryl) are commonly used in patients with sickle cell disease who are experiencing pruritus. These medications have been shown to potentiate the analgesic effects of opioids and also increase their sedating effects.

Overall, nausea and vomiting are less of a problem in patients with sickle cell disease than in patients with cancer. This problem is often treated with medications such as droperidol, metoclopramide, prochlorperazine, scopolamine, and ondansetron. Ondansetron is a good choice for a patient who is sedated, because the drug is free of sedating effects.

Benzodiazepines are used for many reasons in patients with sickle cell disease. These drugs may be used for anxiolysis, sleep induction, myoclonus, and muscle spasm, and seizure disorders. Judicious use of these adjuncts is appropriate during an acute episode. They may produce excessive sedation and render the patient unable to properly use PCA. The sedation also limits the amount of opioid that can safely be administered. Alprazolam may induce episodes of mania, hypomania, hostility, and anger.

Analeptics such as methylphenidate (Ritalin) occasionally may be useful in patients who experience excessive sedation from opioid use.

(v) Other Measures

Analgesia and fluid replacement form the cornerstone of the management of acute sickle cell crisis. Fluids may be replenished parenterally or enterally. Although fever is not uncommon during an acute sickle cell crisis, its presence should nevertheless prompt a search for an infective source. These patients remain vulnerable to infection, and the appropriate cultures should be performed. Antibiotics may be used when clinical suspicion for infection is strong or in the presence of objective data.

Blood transfusion is restricted to complicated situations such as acute chest syndrome, stroke, and a severe prolonged attack, or in cases of frequent recurring episodes. Hemoglobin level of less than 5 g per dL or a decrease of more than 2 g per dL below the baseline may be an indication for transfusion. A higher hematocrit reading alone may indicate that the patient is predisposed to an acute crisis. Exchange transfusions may be required in the setting of severe, prolonged attack in a patient with stable hematocrit.

Supplemental oxygen has not been shown to be of any benefit in reducing the pain or the duration of the crisis. This lack of benefit probably relates to the fact that sickle cell crisis is a vaso-occlusive crisis that has already occurred. Oxygen is, however, essential in a patient with hypoxemia.

(vi) Prevention of Recurrent Crises

Patients should be advised about lifestyle; avoidance of extremes of temperature, exercise, and alcohol may decrease the frequency of these episodes. Patients should be advised to decrease or abstain from smoking, to drink enough fluids on warm days, to wear warm clothing on cold days, and to seek early treatment of infections. Medical treatments such as hydroxyurea can considerably lower the incidence of painful crises.

IV. MANAGEMENT OF CHRONIC PAIN

1. Etiology

Some patients with sickle cell disease experience chronic pain secondary to multiple causes, as described in subsequent text.

Their lives revolve around this all-pervasive pain as they go from physician to physician in search of better treatment. Constant pain can eventually lead to psychopathology, and these patients are at greater risk for depression. In addition, they have poor prospects for fruitful employment because of the disease-induced physical and emotional impediments. In general, their socioeconomic status is poor at baseline and further complicates their successful rehabilitation.

These patients tend to be labeled as drug seekers and difficult patients. It is not difficult to appreciate the reasons for chronic pain in these patients. In most patients, the pain is of nociceptive origin and is due to diverse causes such as chronic leg ulcers, avascular necrosis of the femur and the humerus, vertebral fractures, chronic osteomyelitis, arthropathies, and recurrent vasoocclusive crises.

Neuropathic pain has also been reported, although rarely, in patients with sickle cell disease. The apparent low incidence of neuropathic pain in this population may arise because the nociceptive component predominates, and the neuropathic component therefore goes unrecognized. The rich and complex interconnecting blood supply of the nerves may protect the patients from infarction during a vasoocclusive crisis. Mental nerve involvement with numbness of the cheek has been most often described in patients with sickle cell disease.

As with neuropathic pain, reports of myofascial pain and fibromyalgia are rare in this group. This observation may again represent the fact that the predominant nociceptive component overshadows other components.

2. Medications

Because most of the pain in patients with sickle cell disease is of nociceptive origin, NSAIDs and opioids are the mainstay of treatment. Whenever possible, medications should be prescribed by a single clinic where care is consolidated. Long-term opioid narcotics should be administered using the same principles as for other nonterminal chronic pain conditions (see Chapter 30). Titration of medications, changes in the choice of the opioid, and concerns with tolerance and dependence are issues that are best addressed by a single physician or group of physicians. Many patients with sickle cell disease are successfully treated with nonopioid analgesics or with minimal or weak opioids.

There is paucity in the literature about the utility of neuropathic pain medications in patients with sickle cell disease. Anecdotal reports of beneficial effects of tricyclic antidepressants and anticonvulsants warrant trials of these medications in select patients in combination with other medications. Some conditions such as priapism, seizure disorder, and urine retention in patients with sickle cell disease may contraindicate the use of tricyclics.

Laxatives, antihistaminics, and antiemetics may be required to manage the side effects of medications.

3. Nonpharmacologic Interventions

Education goes a long way in helping patients cope with their disease and in encouraging treatment compliance. Reasonable expectations, knowledge of medications, therapeutic goals, and what to expect from the provider should be clearly explained. Counterirritant measures such as transcutaneous electric nerve stimulation (TENS), massage, and heat may be beneficial in select patients. Intensive physical therapy in a patient with a painful degenerative joint disease helps ameliorate pain. Biofeedback, coping mechanisms, distraction, and motivation are all valuable adjuncts. Patients with sickle cell disease are poor candidates for interventional pain therapies.

V. NEW THERAPIES

Hydroxyurea has been shown to reduce the incidence of acute crises by 50% and is likely to be more commonly used in the future. Its long-term effects are not clear and therefore warrant close monitoring. Although sickle cell crisis may primarily be related to polymerization of the abnormal hemoglobin, there is increasing focus on microcirculation, vascular endothelium, red cell membrane, and abnormalities in coagulation. Newer drugs targeting these areas are being developed and tested. Low levels of nitric oxide (NO) may be involved in the pathogenesis of sickling. Studies using NO and L-arginine supplementation show early promise. The results of allogenic bone marrow transplantation are improving, and the treatment is becoming increasingly accepted for children with symptoms of the disease. Gene therapy also seems promising, although this promise remains elusive.

VI. CONCLUSION

Sickle cell disease is a chronic multisystem disease that subjects a patient to a life of misery and pain. Many of these patients are socioeconomically disadvantaged, lack good health coverage, and have poor support systems.

Appreciation of the excruciating pain that these patients experience and prompt treatment based on the patient report are the essence of their pain management. These patients do not have a higher potential for addiction, and pain medications should not be withheld for such concerns. Treatment of a challenging patient requires tolerance and clear communication. Contact should be established with a physician who knows the patient well.

At the very least, these individuals need to be treated with respect, compassion, and patience.

SELECTED READINGS

Ballas SK. *Sickle cell pain.* Seattle, WA: IASP Press, 1998.

Serjeant GR. Sickle-cell disease. *Lancet* 1997;350:725–730.

Vijay V, Cavenagh JD, Yate P. The anaesthetist's role in acute sickle cell crisis. *Br J Anaesth* 1998;80:820–828.

Yale SH, Nagib N, Guthrie T. Approach to the vasoocclusive crisis in adults with sickle cell disease. *Am Fam Physician* 2000;61: 1349–1356.

Yaster M, Kost-Byerly S, Maxwell LG. The management of pain in sickle cell disease. *Pediatr Clin North Am* 2000;47:699–710.

VI

Chronic Pain

Neuropathic Pain Syndromes

Dennis Dey and Anne Louise Oaklander

It is evidently impossible to transmit the impression of pain by teaching, since it is only known to those who have experienced it. Moreover, we are ignorant of each type of pain before we have felt it.
—*Galen, 129–199*

Neuropathic (or neuralgic) pain is always caused by injury to the pain-sensing portions of the nervous system, although many such injuries do not cause chronic pain. The hallmark of neuropathic pain is that it occurs or persists in the absence of tissue injury or inflammation, and therefore, it lacks the protective benefits of acute pain. Chronic pathologic pain without recovery is more devastating than pain that accompanies tissue injury and resolves with healing. Also, this "invisible pain" often creates a psychological burden because family members and medical providers cannot see an objective correlate. Mutual trust and communication between patient and caregivers must be established for effective care.

Neuropathic pain ensues when pain-processing (nociceptive) neurons generate action potentials despite the absence of tissue injury. Normally, neurons fire only when activated by tissue-damaging stimuli (e.g., high heat, cutting, or inflammation). Neuropathic pain is therefore a nociceptive hallucination analogous to the sensory hallucinations that can occur after damage to other sensory systems (e.g., tinnitus after hearing loss). Unfortunately, the precise location of such misfiring is often unknown, or it may occur at multiple levels of the nervous system, making it difficult to treat the pain. Any type of neural injury—whether from trauma, infection, or inflammation—or biochemical imbalance can produce neuralgic pain, and interruptions any-where along the pain pathways, from the nerve endings in the skin to the somatosensory cortices, will suffice. The most common clinical feature is chronic pain paradoxically colocalizing with decreased sensory function. Other neurologic symptoms, such as motor or autonomic disturbances, are common but may go unrecognized. Because there are no objective diagnostic tests for this condition, a careful history and physical examination remain the most important diagnostic tools.

I. CLINICAL PRESENTATION

1. Pain and Sensory Abnormalities

The clinical spectrum of neuropathic pain ranges from barely noticeable to severely disabling. One or more of the following symptoms are present in neuropathic pain patients regardless of etiology, mechanism, and location of neural injury:

- Ongoing (or stimulus-independent) chronic pain described as "burning," "aching," "crushing," or "gnawing"
- Abnormal stimulus-evoked pain, especially after mechanical stimuli
- Brief lancinating pains described as brief, severe jolts of pain, sometimes called "electrical" or "lightning pains"; these can be spontaneous or can be evoked by a stimulus; this type of pain does not occur without neural injury and is near-pathognomonic for the neuralgias

The relative importance of these different types of pain varies across diseases and even within the same patient at different times. For instance, trigeminal neuralgia is known for severe lancinating pains, which can be provoked by an innocuous stimulation of a trigger zone on the face. However, questioning will reveal that most patients have also experienced the other features of neuropathic pain at some point.

Perturbations of somatosensory function (see Fig. 1) are also characteristic of neuropathic pain. The most common feature is **numbness**, or hypoaesthesia. Paradoxically, patients may report decreased sensation in the same area where they experience maximum pain or they may be unaware of their sensory deficit until it is elicited during examination. Pain thresholds can be lowered—**hyperalgesia**—or raised—**hypoalgesia Paresthesias**, sometimes described as a pins-and-needles feeling, are positive sensory phenomena suggestive of neuropathic pain. Patients may also use the word **numbness** to describe paresthesias, so the terminology may require clarification. Some patients report **allodynia** or pain from innocuous stimuli, such as light touch. Mechanical allodynia is most common, and some patients go to extreme lengths to avoid having their neuropathic area touched (see Fig. 2). Pain can be caused by contact with clothing or bedsheet or even by a breeze. Patients with trigeminal neuralgia may not be able to shave areas of their face, and intraoral allodynia can interfere with eating and cause weight loss or malnutrition. Some women with postherpetic neuralgia (PHN) on the torso are unable to wear a brassiere, and some patients with distal painful neuropathies hang their feet over

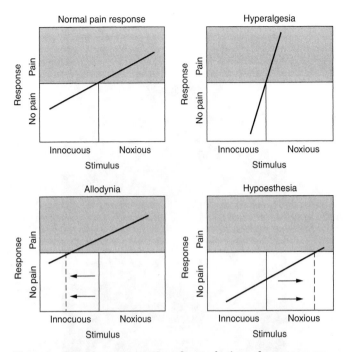

Figure 1. Graphic representation of perturbations of somatosensory function associated with pathologic pain states.

the edge of their bed to avoid the bedclothes. Many patients describe worsening of their pain in cold weather. This may reflect a component of **cold allodynia. Warmth allodynia** prompts some patients to carry ice bags or fans to continually cool the painful area. Quantitative sensory testing has not revealed a consistent pattern of sensory abnormalities that characterizes neuropathic pain.

Some of these symptoms occur in acute and inflammatory/ nociceptive pain (e.g., sunburn). This observation suggests that acute pain may have a neuropathic component. However, if the neurons are normal, these symptoms remit once the tissue injury heals, whereas in case of neuropathic pain they persist.

2. Other Clinical Features

Because different types of neurons mingle closely within the central and peripheral nervous systems, the damage affecting nociceptive neurons often affects other neural systems as well. Patients whose motor pathways are damaged can have abnormalities of muscle tone, bulk, and strength. The presence of objective motor signs or an abnormal electromyogram (EMG) can be helpful in making the diagnosis of neuropathic rather than nociceptive pain. However, because the nociceptive neurons are not tested, a normal EMG does not rule out neuropathic pain. Increased tone in the affected area is suggestive of a central

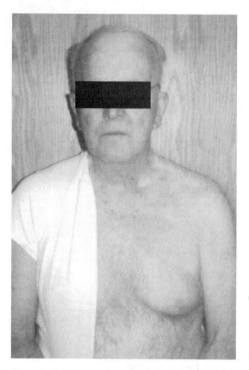

Figure 2. Some patients go to extreme lengths to avoid having their neuropathic area touched. This man has postherpetic neuralgia (PHN) and has cut his shirt in half because of allodynia.

lesion, such as that from stroke; in contrast, peripheral lesions, such as compressive radiculopathies or nerve injuries, can reduce tone. Dystonias, or sustained pathologic cocontraction of agonist and antagonist muscles, are increasingly recognized as a component of complex regional pain syndrome (CRPS). It remains unclear whether these abnormal movements reflect peripheral motor damage from the inciting trauma or whether they are caused by secondary abnormalities in the spinal cord or brain. Sometimes, only minor motor symptoms, such as a tendency to develop muscle cramps, are present. Of course, disuse of a painful limb can cause secondary motor changes (e.g., contractures) as well. Occasionally, the motor damage is primary and pain is secondary to the abnormal muscle contractions, as in the focal, segmental, or generalized primary dystonic syndromes.

Autonomic abnormalities are common and are characteristic in several neuralgias because most peripheral nociceptive neurons have efferent autonomic functions as well as afferent actions. Therefore, autonomic abnormalities are to be expected when these neurons are damaged. Damage to these axons produces changes in color and temperature in the affected tissues and can cause swelling because of abnormal leakage of intravascular fluid. These effects can exacerbate pain. Small-fiber neuropathies are an underrecognized cause of pedal edema. Trigeminal neuralgias are an underrecognized cause of chronic rhinorrhea. Similarly, animal studies have shown clearly that the growth of skin, hair, nails, and other cutaneous structures becomes abnormal if innervation is disrupted. Damage to the autonomic neurons that innervate more centrally located areas can produce symptoms such as orthostatic hypotension, impotence, delayed gastric emptying, abnormal sweating and thermoregulation, and difficulties with elimination. Occasionally, cardiac arrhythmias may become clinically significant after central or peripheral lesions.

II. MECHANISMS OF NEUROPATHIC PAIN

Neuropathic pain is generated by electrical hyperactivity of neurons along the pain pathways. The sensory pathway consists of at least three neurons, and **lesions anywhere along the pathway** can lead to neuropathic pain. Changes in expression of neuronal ion channels and receptors, synaptic connectivity, and anatomy all contribute to neuropathic pain (neural plasticity). Although **functional changes** are related to repetitive painful input into the nociceptive system (central sensitization), neuropathic pain is also associated with **anatomical changes**. Severe degeneration of peripheral nociceptive neurons has been shown in at least two types of neuralgias, PHN after shingles and peripheral small-fiber neuropathies. Loss of inhibitory spinal interneurons and growth of touch fibers into the pain pathway may occur as well. In phantom limb pain, cortical sensory neurons that have lost their input from the periphery may connect to neighboring nerve cells and lead to bizarre phenomena such as the evocation of phantom hand pain by touching the subject's mouth.

Increasingly, it has been recognized that nearby nonneuronal cells, including both neural support cells and immunocytes, secrete factors that alter the **local macromolecular milieu** and that modulate nociceptive signal processing. Finally, **limbic** and **cognitive circuits** influence the capacity of the brain to "listen to" incoming nociceptive signals. Acute pain, even when severe, can be suppressed in the presence of other more urgent concerns, such as fight or flight; however, chronic pain can be amplified by emotional states such as anxiety and depression. The impetus for unraveling the complex mechanisms of neuropathic pain is the hope of developing new treatments and of using existing medications to target pain and related symptoms more precisely. Detailed discussion of pain pathways and pain mechanisms can be found in Chapter 1.

III. SPECIFIC NEUROPATHIC PAIN SYNDROMES

1. Peripheral Syndromes

(i) Generalized Painful Polyneuropathies

Most neuralgias originate from peripheral nerve injury. Bilateral pain, usually, but not always, starting in both feet and spreading proximally, usually indicates the presence of a length-dependent polyneuropathy. These polyneuropathies can be classified by etiology, distribution, and pathology. Some are specific to the type of axon involved, but many affect more than one type of axon (e.g., sensory-motor polyneuropathy). Motor symptoms typically include weakness and affect the distal muscles, often the extensor groups. Sensory disturbances can be classified by examination with pin, heat or cold, and vibratory stimuli. The distribution of neuropathies can be symmetrical or asymmetrical, multifocal or focal. In the polyneuropathies, neuronal dysfunction is first reported in the extremities, the distal portions of the longest axons. Often, the earliest symptoms are those of the autonomic and small-fiber sensory modalities. The diagnostic evaluation includes a thorough history to ascertain the etiology, including questions regarding systemic illnesses, injuries, nutritional deficiencies, family history, and toxin exposure. Lists of recommended diagnostic tests are available at www.neuroskinbiopsy.mgh.harvard.edu. Painful sensory neuropathies have been associated with systemic disorders such as human immunodeficiency virus (HIV) infection, diabetes mellitus, alcohol abuse, hepatitis, malignant cancers, monoclonal gammopathies (IgG, IgA, and IgM), rheumatoid arthritis, collagen vascular disease, and amyloidosis. Inherited neuropathies, such as the hereditary sensory and autonomic neuropathies (HSAN), can also cause neuropathic pain. HSAN-1 is the most common characterized HSAN seen in the United States. In severe neuropathies, there can also be complete absence of pain sensation with devastating consequences (mutilation secondary to repetitive and unnoticed trauma). This observation shows the vital importance of an intact pain response. Affected children or carriers of Fabry disease can develop painful inherited sensory neuropathy associated with loss of almost all nociceptive nerve endings in the skin. Some painful small-fiber neuropathies of unknown cause (idiopathic) are present in multiple family members and likely have genetic causes that await investigation. Other acquired neuropathies are those associated with exposure to toxins such as heavy metals or to drugs, such as anticancer, antituberculosis, and antiretroviral agents.

In the United States, the most common cause of painful neuropathies is glucose intolerance. It has become clear in recent years that neuropathy can be one of the earliest manifestations of diabetes and can even precede the development of serum abnormalities that are used to classify patients as having diabetes. Two-hour glucose tolerance testing has been shown to be a more sensitive method of detecting abnormalities of glucose metabolism in patients with neuropathy than tests of fasting plasma glucose levels or measurements of hemoglobin A1c. Diabetes causes several types of neuralgia, but those involving small fibers are most common. A patient with diabetic small-fiber neuropathy presents with "burning feet" and autonomic features including impaired thermoregulation and sweat production. Neuropathy and vascular insufficiency are the main risk factors for foot ulcers and amputation. In painful diabetic polyneuropathy, both myelinated and unmyelinated fibers can degenerate. Demyelination can be present as well. Endoneural vascular resistance, insufficient neurotrophic support, and autoimmune inflammation may all contribute to nerve damage. Diabetes mellitus also causes other types of neuropathies, including proximal motor neuropathies due to intraneural vasculitis (diabetic amyotrophy), autonomic neuropathies, and vulnerability to compressive lesions; acute painful neuropathies from nerve ischemia, hypoglycemic neuropathy, treatment-induced neuropathy; and distal motor neuropathies. Patients with multifocal neuropathies (mononeuropathy multiplex) develop local loss of function in several peripheral nerves. Systemic lupus erythematosus, rheumatoid arthritis, cholesterol emboli, and polyarteritis nodosa, as well as diabetes mellitus, also can cause this pattern. The pathologic basis of these syndromes is nerve infarction from vasculitis. Prognosis for recovery is favorable if the underlying cause of infarction can be treated.

(ii) Painful Mononeuropathies

Isolated focal peripheral nerve lesions are most often due to trauma. Although unintentional injuries are probably the most common cause, iatrogenic injuries from surgery or needle-stick are an underappreciated close second. Because a proportion of injuries occur on the job, or from participation in sports, these patients are likely to be young and in their most productive years, and are often male. Nerve injuries may not be diagnosed at the time of the initial accident because they are not visible on x-ray, and medical attention usually focuses on more obvious injuries. Clinicians should evaluate these patients with the aid of a handbook that demonstrates the individual nerve territories. Stewart's textbook *Focal Peripheral Neuropathies* is an invaluable resource. It may be helpful to refer patients with difficult-to-diagnose syndromes to a neurologist or neurosurgeon with subspecialty training in peripheral nerve injury. Nerve lesions affecting predominantly sensory neurons and producing pain as the major symptom are less likely to be diagnosed than those that produce frank motor deficit as well. Delays in diagnosis can be unfortunate because patients with some types of peripheral nerve injuries benefit from early surgical nerve repair. Furthermore, failure to diagnose a nerve injury can result in repeated surgeries if the pain is erroneously attributed to other causes. Nerve injuries in patients without a history of trauma or surgery are usually the result of internal entrapment, compression, or nerve ischemia. Chronic nerve entrapment injury can be associated with rheumatic disease, diabetes mellitus, uremia, hypothyroidism, repetitive use, or malnutrition, or rarely occur in otherwise healthy individuals.

The hallmark of nerve injuries is the tendency for the worst pain to occur primarily in the distribution of a particular peripheral nerve or branch. The most useful aid to diagnosis is to ask patients to draw an outline around the area where their pain and sensory abnormalities are most severe. Often, the outlined area will correspond to the territory of a specific nerve or branch. However, the pain can spread outside traditional nerve territories. For instance, C-fibers trifurcate within the substantia gelatinosa on entry to the spinal cord and send collateral axons approximately two segments up and down the cord, thus enabling lesions of single nerves to produce widespread effects. Also, loss of afferent input into the spinal cord appears to cause ectopic axonal sprouting that serves to enlarge the receptive fields of spinal pain-processing neurons. Interestingly, some patients will develop bilateral "mirror image" pain after unilateral injury. Animal studies have confirmed that nerve injuries to one limb can induce structural changes in axons of the "mirror image" territory in the contralateral limb. It is not yet clear if and how this produces neuropathic pain.

A common focal neuropathy is the **carpal tunnel syndrome**. This causes pain and, in severe cases, weakness of the median-innervated thumb and forefinger. Another common painful entrapment is **meralgia paresthetica,** which presents as superficial pain along the anterior thigh. It is due to entrapment of branches of the lateral femoral cutaneous nerve as they pass beneath the inguinal ligament. It can be worsened by obesity or pregnancy. Saphenous nerve injury can produce pain in the knee joint and/or medial surface of the lower leg in patients who have undergone knee surgery or arthroscopy or have suffered an injury. Routine venipuncture at the antecubital fossa has been demonstrated to occasionally injure the medial or lateral cutaneous nerves of the forearm. Virtually any nerve, branch, or twig containing sensory neurons can be entrapped or damaged with resultant neuropathic pain in a minority of patients.

(iii) Painful Neuronopathies Including Shingles

Other injuries are centered on the neuronal cell body. For somatosensory neurons, these are in the dorsal root ganglia or in the trigeminal (Gasserian) ganglion for axons innervating the face. Sensory neuronopathies rarely reflect paraneoplastic syndromes or Sjögren disease. In two thirds of patients with paraneoplastic syndromes, sensory neuronopathy precedes the discovery of the malignancy. An important clue that points to a neuronal rather than an axonal process is that the first manifestations may not be distal only (in the feet) as is usual with axonopathies. The onset is usually rapid and associated with burning dysesthesias or paresthesias. Areflexia can ultimately result from this syndrome because of loss of the afferent limb of the monosynaptic reflex.

In the United States, acute herpes zoster infection (shingles) is by far the most common sensory neuronopathy. It means that 20% of people will develop shingles in their lifetime. A proportion of patients with shingles will be left with PHN. Both shingles and PHN disproportionately affect the older patients. Fifty percent of patients older than 70 years with shingles will experience long-lasting PHN. Suppression of cell-mediated immunity often associated with advancing age or concurrent medical illness permits latent varicella zoster virus (VZV) to erupt into shingles. The unilateral dermatomal distribution and vesicular rash are the clinical signatures of varicella zoster viral reactivation in the dorsal root ganglia. The thoracic segments are the most commonly affected. The next most common site is the ophthalmic division of the trigeminal nerve. The pain is described as burning and is often associated with itching or lancinating pain. PHN is defined as the persistence of pain 3 to 4 months after onset of rash. Over time, the distribution of pain symptoms can widen to involve adjacent dermatomes. Shingles is so common that it causes neuropathic pain syndromes affecting every area of the body including the limbs and genitals. Shingles can cause motor and autonomic abnormalities as well, and adjunctive therapies may be needed. PHN can rarely be present after shingles without a visible rash (*zoster sine herpete*).

Acute infection produces a mixed inflammatory/nociceptive and neuropathic pain syndrome. Early treatment (within 72 hours of rash onset) with antiviral medications (acyclovir, famcyclovir, or valacyclovir) shortens and lessens the symptoms of zoster, and decreases the risk of subsequent PHN by about one half. There are almost no side effects of oral antiviral medications, so they should be used in virtually all patients with shingles, and administration of these medications should be instituted as soon as possible. Early and aggressive pain control might help decrease the risk of long-term PHN. Rarely, other options, such as addition of corticosteroids or placement of thoracic epidural catheters, can assist the management of severe acute shingles pain. Patients with shingles near the eye require ophthalmologic consultation because intraocular complications can ensue and can cause vision loss if not optimally treated. Evidence from examination of nerve endings within skin biopsies taken after shingles suggests that most patients with PHN have severe loss of cutaneous innervation, especially nociceptive innervation, in the affected skin.

(iv) Amputation

Neuropathic pain can be a major problem following amputation. Although the problem has been best described in regard to limb amputation, neuropathic pain can occur after a wide variety of amputations, including mastectomy, and removal of visceral organs such as the rectum. Several mechanisms can contribute. Stump pain can be due to nerve injury, tissue trauma, infection, or vascular insufficiency. Sectioned nerves can form painful neuromas—tangles of axonal sprouts that have not found a distal nerve stump, and are entrapped in connective tissue. Mechanical stimulation of the neuromas can trigger severe pain.

Occasionally, nerve injury pain remits as the hypersensitive axon sprouts reach their end-organ target. This process can take months or longer because of the slow rate of axonal growth (about 1 mm per day at best). Regrowth after nerve injury can be mapped by tracing the location of Tinel sign (painful paresthesias elicited with percussion over the hypersensitive ends of regenerating axons).

Phantom pain, in contrast, is perceived distal to the site of the amputation. Pain is only one of many phantom sensations that can be experienced by amputees. Patients in pain before their amputation, for example, from infection or injury, may experience precise memories of their earlier pain. Phantom sensations are thought to result from spontaneous electrical activity in central sensory neurons that are deprived of their normal afferent input. Treatment options are similar to those for other neuropathic pain syndromes but are often less successful.

(v) Trigeminal and Other Cranial Neuralgias

Most commonly, cranial neuralgias arise from peripheral lesions that affect the peripheral axons or cell bodies; however, clinically indistinguishable syndromes can develop with central lesions of the cranial nerve nuclei and central axons that descend through the brainstem. Cranial neuralgias can occur as a result of strokes, multiple sclerosis, or compression, most commonly by meningiomas; therefore, patients with new unexplained onset need imaging of the brain. The peak onset of trigeminal neuralgia is in patients older than 50 years. Classic versions of this syndrome are marked by brief episodes of lancinating pain, usually in the territory of the second or third divisions of the trigeminal nerve. Touch or chewing can often trigger the pain. New onset of this syndrome in a young adult (under 30 years) raises suspicion of multiple sclerosis. This suspicion is even more of a concern if the symptoms are bilateral.

Neuralgias of the sensory division of the facial nerve have been best described in the Ramsay Hunt syndrome, in which shingles affects the ear. Vesicles (and pain) usually develop within the outer ear canal and can spread to the cheek. The eighth cranial nerve and other cranial nerves or the brainstem can also be affected by spread of infection or inflammation through this tight-packed space.

Glossopharyngeal neuralgia, due to lesions of the somatosensory component of the ninth cranial nerve, produces neuropathic pain in the back of the throat or behind the angle of the jaw. Associated motor damage can produce difficulties of speech or swallowing. These syndromes are described in more detail in Chapter 29.

2. Central Syndromes

Neuropathic pain of central origin was originally described after thalamic stroke by Dejerine and Roussey. However, any type of central nervous system (CNS) lesion, including demyelinating, vascular, infectious, inflammatory, and traumatic, can produce pain as long as it is located in the central pain-processing pathways of the spinal cord or the brain. An unusual feature of central pain is that onset can be delayed by weeks, months, and occasionally up to 2 years after a temporally well-defined insult such as a stroke. This may reflect the slower rate of Wallerian degeneration and myelin clearance within the CNS than in the peripheral nervous system.

(i) Spinal Cord

Traumatic spinal cord injury (SCI) and demyelinating diseases such as multiple sclerosis are the two most common causes of spinal cord neuropathic pain. Syringomyelia, spinal cord tumors, vascular malformations, and ischemia are other lesions that can produce pain. Chronic painful dysesthetic limb and visceral pain develop in more than one third of patients with SCI and 10% of these patients characterize their pain as severely disabling. SCI pain is a complex mix of (a) peripheral pain from damage to incoming nerve roots, (b) central pain from internal cord damage, (c) visceral pain from distension, and (d) orthopaedic pain from bone or joint injury or instability. In more than half of the patients the onset is within 6 months of the initial injury. SCI pain is variously described as: "burning," "shooting," and "crushing." Demyelination of the cervical and thoracic cord is common in multiple sclerosis and can produce lancinating pain in radicular distribution or episodes of burning pain.

Syringomyelia and syringobulbia are cavities that develop within the spinal cord or lower brainstem. They can be congenital or a consequence of trauma or tumor within the spinal cord. These cavities typically produce bilateral neuropathic symptoms. These symptoms primarily affect the body segments innervated by the damaged area of cord because incoming pain axons cross close to the central canal (anterior commissure) near the level where they enter the cord. Ascending or descending tracts carrying information from other body areas travel in the lateral margins of the cord are less affected by these centrally located cavities. Pain is a common and early symptom of these syndromes.

(ii) Brain

Any brain lesion involving the sensory pathway can lead to neuropathic pain, but stroke is the most common etiology. Up to 6% of strokes are associated with chronic pain that limits rehabilitation and contributes to the development of poststroke depression. Well-known stroke syndromes that commonly produce pain include internal capsule or thalamic-region strokes and the lateral medullary infarction syndrome of Wallenberg. The anatomical localization of the pain reflects the part of the pain pathway that has been damaged. Thalamic-region syndromes can involve part or all of the contralateral hemi-body. Wallenberg syndrome (due to vertebral or posterior inferior cerebellar artery occlusion) produces pain and sensory loss on the ipsilateral face (due to disruption of descending trigeminal axons) and contralateral body (due to disruption of ascending spinothalamic tract fibers that decussated in the spinal cord).

The most common description is "burning" similar to that reported by patients with multiple sclerosis, postcordotomy dysesthesia, and syringomyelia. Poststroke pain has several characteristic features:

- The region of most intense pain encompasses only a portion of the total territory of sensory deficits.
- Functional recovery is poorest in the regions of most severe pain.
- Thermal perception and sensation to pin are more commonly affected than light touch.

IV. DIAGNOSTIC EVALUATION OF PATIENTS WITH NEUROPATHIC PAIN

1. History

Neuropathic pain is a clinical syndrome that requires a specific diagnosis. The history is the most helpful diagnostic tool. The success of the evaluation rests on the clinician's ability and willingness to validate and evaluate the patient's pain. Rarely, the pain is reversible, and determining the etiology can help lead to a cure. The pain assessment integrates the following points: onset, location, temporal profile, pain quality, pace of progression, severity and associated disability, aggravating and alleviating factors, response to past treatments, habits, and coping skills.

History of prior medical conditions and injuries (including iatrogenic ones) often reveals the diagnosis. Detailed information about previously attempted treatments should be obtained to help determine future options. Psychological assessment is important. Unrelieved pain can contribute to or unmask psychiatric disorders such as depression, anxiety, panic disorder, and posttraumatic stress disorder. History should include an inventory of mood symptoms and consideration of affective signs since many patients will need evaluation and treatment of depression at some time.

2. Examination

A targeted medical and musculoskeletal exam can provide important information. Several neurologic conditions (e.g., neurofibromatosis and shingles) affect the skin and the nervous system, so a thorough examination of the undressed patient can be helpful. Features such as skin temperature or the presence of edema or discoloration can provide clues about the location of nervous system involvement and the severity of the condition. The positioning of an extremity or use of clothing to protect a limb from physical contact reveals much about the patient's complaint. As with all components of the exam, the absence of findings does not disprove the presence of a pain condition.

The mental status examination should be performed in every instance because it can reveal depression, anxiety, or sedative side effects of medications. The cranial nerve examination should be detailed if the patient has a problem affecting the head or neck. The motor examination should be detailed in the area that is painful because it can aid in localization and diagnosis. Alterations in muscle tone and bulk, as well as strength should be documented. Functional testing of strength, such as by examining gait, is helpful as well. All relevant deep tendon reflexes should be elicited because these can provide clues about the presence of either a peripheral (if decreased) or a central (if increased) lesion.

The neurologic sensory examination can be normal or abnormal. Surprisingly, sensory function is sometimes relatively preserved, even in the face of considerable neuronal damage or degeneration. Sensory abnormalities do not always fit neatly into discrete modalities such as pinprick or temperature sensation. For this reason, it is crucial to test several different modalities in a given territory. The patients should be allowed to describe the sensory experience using their own terms. It can be useful to have the patient use marking pens to outline their regions of abnormality or discomfort; this aids in localization. Normal areas should be examined first to establish a baseline, and the patient should be queried as to how sensation in areas of interest compares. Subsequent questions can establish the characteristics by severity and deviations from normal. As always, the behavior accompanying the patient's answers provides helpful context. It is important to also evaluate positive sensory signs including allodynia, hyperpathia, and hyperalgesia. **These findings are the most specific for neuropathic pain syndromes.** Allodynia can be tested mechanically by brushing the affected area with a cotton swab and with a thermal stimulus such as a cool metal reflex hammer or tuning fork. In contrast, to test hyperalgesia, a normally painful stimulus (usually a pin) is applied; an exaggerated pain response is consistent with a positive result.

3. Diagnostic Testing

Magnetic resonance imaging (MRI) or computerized tomography (CT) is indicated for localization of cranial and spinal cord lesions causing central pain syndromes. Increased T2 signal will persist after a stroke or demyelination, active demyelinating plaques, and many brain tumors enhance with contrast. CT scan of the head will often reveal a hypodense neuroanatomic correlate after some time. For radicular pain syndromes ("pinched nerves"), CT myelogram is still the most sensitive imaging modality for bony stenosis affecting the nerve roots. MRI of the spinal cord is valuable when the exam and history are suggestive of a sensory level and an inflammatory cord lesion is likely or edema, secondary to compression, is suspected. Specific MRI and magnetic resonance angiography (MRA) studies [e.g., constructive interference in steady state (CISS) sequences] have been shown to be especially useful in detecting the presence of a blood vessel impinging on the trigeminal ganglion. Such a finding may suggest microvascular decompression be considered for definitive treatment.

Nerve conduction studies (NCS) and EMG provide physiologic information about the sensory and motor components of peripheral nerves. Most neuropathic pain syndromes are mediated by small diameter C and Aδ fibers, which are not recorded with these tests so their value in the evaluation of neuropathic pain syndromes is limited. In short, they are helpful if abnormal, but do not exclude nerve injury if normal. Also, the sensory nerve action potentials (SNAP) can have normal amplitudes in patients with neuropathic syndromes of radicular origin because the causative lesion is proximal to the dorsal root ganglion. Unfortunately, normal electrophysiologic studies still lead some practitioners to conclude that patients cannot have an organic cause for their complaints. Acute inflammatory demyelinating polyneuropathy (AIDP; also known as Guillain-Barré syndrome) produces slowing of conduction velocities, prolongation of the distal motor latencies, conduction block, and temporal dispersion on NCS. The neuropathic pain associated with AIDP, however, is often in the low back due to demyelination of the sensory nerve roots.

Local anesthetic nerve blocks can be useful diagnostic tools, particularly if electrophysiologic studies are either not helpful or not feasible. Temporary relief of pain from a local anesthetic injection near a particular nerve or spinal root can help localize injury to a particular nerve or nerve segment in mononeuropathies and entrapments. Nerve blocks usually do not provide long-term pain relief.

Modern histologic examination of nociceptive axons, especially with quantitation, joins electrophysiologic recording as a useful diagnostic test for peripheral neuropathies. The older method of removal of a segment of the sural nerve for light and electron microscopic analysis is the most definitive test for evaluating neuropathies of various causes. However, sural nerve biopsies cannot be repeated, are only useful for lesions that affect the sural nerve, and are quite invasive (occasionally causing neuromas, infections, and other clinical problems). For patients with pain as their primary symptom, or for suspected neuropathy patients with normal EMGs and NCSs, sural nerve biopsies are being replaced by histologic examination of sensory nerve endings in punch biopsies of skin from the affected area, or the removal of epidermis only from suction skin blisters. Immunohistochemical markers against PGP9.5 allow preferential visualization of the nerve endings as they course through the skin. In the epidermis, which is predominantly innervated by free nociceptive nerve endings, quantitation of the density of nerve endings is performed at specialized centers including Massachusetts General Hospital (MGH). Skin biopsy studies have almost universally shown that chronic neuropathic pain is associated with profound loss of nociceptive nerve endings from painful areas of the skin.

Comprehensive evaluation of sensory function can be performed by administering well-characterized stimuli of known intensity and recording the patient's perceptions. This is called quantitative sensory testing (QST) and is described in Chapter 7. These psychophysical evaluations commonly are used in research laboratories studying pain and analgesia in humans and animals. Although these evaluations are of some use in clinical practice, considerable expertise and computerized thermal stimulators are required for a full evaluation. Screening with a specific von Frey monofilament of defined force can be useful to screen for loss of protective sensation. Although the results of QST are quantitative, they are nevertheless subjective.

There are currently no blood or body-fluid tests specific and sensitive for neuropathic pain. Nonetheless, in some cases, these tests can help identify potentially treatable conditions. Any patient with unexplained painful neuropathy should be tested for glucose intolerance using the more sensitive 2- or 3-hour glucose tolerance tests rather than relying on fasting glucose or levels of glycosylated hemoglobin. Sometimes, evaluation of markers for connective tissue disease is helpful. In polyradiculopathy, in which sensory symptoms are accompanied by weakness and areflexia at multiple levels, cerebrospinal fluid (CSF) protein and lymphocyte counts contribute to the diagnosis of inflammatory demyelinating polyneuropathy. In chronic sensory neuronopathies without a clear diagnosis, evaluation for paraneoplastic antibodies and basic screening for evidence of tumor may be indicated. When a sensory level is detected on neurologic examination, CSF samples may show evidence of inflammation.

V. TREATMENT OF NEUROPATHIC PAIN

Medical treatment is first-line therapy for neuropathic pain syndromes. The efficacy of drugs against neuropathic pain has been discovered serendipitously through clinical observation, usually after the drugs have been marketed for other indications. Although pain researchers and pharmaceutical companies search for new compounds with molecular specificity, most of the effective treatments in current clinical use have activity at multiple sites within the pain pathways.

The good news is that multiple medications have proven effective against neuropathic pain in randomized placebo-controlled clinical trials. The bad news is that none of these medications is effective in all patients, and we do not yet know how to predict who will be improved by which medication. Because of these limitations, it often is necessary to try several different medications before identifying the optimal agent and dosing schedule for a particular patient. This sequential process should be explained to the patient to ensure that their expectations for the extent and timing of relief are realistic. In general, the medication, or class of medications judged most likely to be effective should be tried first, raised to an adequate level, and monitored for efficacy and side effects. It is a common mistake to declare a medication ineffective without having titrated to a therapeutic dose. The four major classes of medications for treating neuropathic pain syndromes are tricyclic antidepressants (TCAs), anticonvulsants, opioid analgesics, and topical agents. A full description of dosing, side effects, and mechanisms can be found in Chapters 9, 10, and 11. Specific considerations for the use of opioids in chronic nonterminal pain are discussed in Chapter 30.

1. Tricyclic Antidepressants

Historically, the TCAs have been the mainstay of medical therapy for neuropathic pain. They are well studied and widely prescribed. There is strong evidence of efficacy in diabetic neuropathy and postherpetic neuralgia and they are effective for most neuropathic pain symptoms. Despite this, patients only rarely obtain complete relief and often are unable to tolerate the side effects of this class. Caution is needed in patients with cardiovascular disease, closed-angle glaucoma, and dementia.

Older patients or those on complicated regimens should begin at the lowest dose. Tolerability and degree of relief guide the process of weekly dose escalation in small increments. It is important to proceed slowly in the early phase of titration as the anticholinergic side effects (e.g., constipation, dry mouth, and confusion) may prompt susceptible patients to discontinue medication prematurely. Most patients experience pain relief in the range of 30 to 100 mg per day of desipramine or nortriptyline. If at the upper end of this range, significant relief is not attained, other therapies should be tried. Venlafaxine and duloxetine also inhibit serotonin and norepinephrine reuptake and may have fewer side effects than the TCAs; however, evidence of efficacy is not as strong as for TCAs.

2. Anticonvulsants

(i) Gabapentin and Pregabalin

The relatively benign side effect profile of gabapentin (Neurontin) has propelled it to a first-option treatment of neuropathic pain. Gabapentin has U.S. Food and Drug Administration (FDA) approval for the treatment of PHN. Efficacy has also been established for diabetic neuropathy, mixed neuropathic pain syndromes, Guillain-Barré syndrome, spinal cord injury, and phantom limb pain in randomized placebo-controlled trials. Unlike earlier anticonvulsants, gabapentin has few drug–drug interactions and there is less concern about serious side effects, although, rarely, leukopenia can occur and the drug can accumulate in patients with impaired kidney function. Recently, caution has been advised if gabapentin is used in children because of the potential for increased emotional lability. As with TCAs, the initial dose should be low and is preferably given at night. Most responders report significant relief after titrating to 1,800 mg to 3,600 mg per daily, divided in three doses. Dizziness and mild sedation are common. Edema of the extremities is the most frequent specific side effect.

Like gabapentin, pregabalin has been shown to have efficacy for PHN and diabetic neuropathy. The mechanism of action and side effect profiles of both drugs are similar.

(ii) Sodium-Channel Blockers

First-generation sodium-channel blocking anticonvulsant drugs, such as carbamazepine and phenytoin, have long been preferred drugs for the treatment of lancinating pain. This parsing of treatment by symptom has not been supported by more recent trials. The most effective use of these first-generation agents is in trigeminal neuralgia where carbamazepine markedly reduces pain in approximately 75% of patients. Considerable pain relief for patients with diabetic neuropathy has been demonstrated in controlled trials, but second-generation anticonvulsants (e.g., gabapentin) are favored because they have fewer side effects. Regardless of the diagnosis, the analgesic dose response varies greatly among patients.

For central pain syndromes, carbamazepine is generally effective in the dose range used for treatment of seizures. Blood count with liver and renal function should be monitored. Oxcarbazepine is a newer alternative to carbamazepine that has a lower incidence of hepatic and hematologic side effects. Lamotrigine has shown positive effects particularly in central as well as peripheral neuropathic pain but can rarely cause Stevens-Johnson syndrome.

3. Opioids

Although opioids traditionally were thought ineffective for neuropathic pain, they are an important alternative in patients who do not respond to other therapies, opioids are an important alternative. These agents may offer the most disabled patients relief when other drugs and modalities have been ineffective. The belief that opioids are ineffective in neuropathic pain has recently been refuted, and their efficacy for neuropathic pain has now been convincingly demonstrated in several randomized trials. The risk of addiction is a real, albeit sometimes exaggerated concern. Nonetheless, a personal history of substance abuse remains a relative contraindication to their use. Significant psychiatric comorbidity and a family history of substance abuse also increases the risk of aberrant use of opioids.

4. Topical Agents

The introduction of topical therapies in the forms of patches, creams, and gels is a promising advance. These are applied to painful skin and act locally at the peripheral sites of pain generation. The absence of systemic side effects and drug interactions, in most cases, make these treatments useful, especially in the geriatric population. Lidoderm, a topical formulation of 5% lidocaine, is approved for the treatment of PHN. Lidocaine gels, ointments, or sprays can be helpful for patients with pain affecting mucous membranes. They provide temporary analgesia to engage in specific activities such as chewing, defecation, sexual activity, or use of tampons or pads during menstrual periods. Systemic absorption is less predictable than with the 5% patch and serum levels may need to be monitored.

5. Adjunctive Treatments

The chronicity of neuropathic pain states creates significant disability. An interdisciplinary approach to the care of these patients should address the psychosocial burdens and functional impact of living with chronic pain.

Physical and occupational therapies may be indicated to address loss of strength, decreased range of motion, and abnormal muscle tone. Physical and occupational therapies maximize functional gains and minimize secondary problems from disuse. Functional imaging studies suggest that increased use and function of a painful extremity may help reverse abnormal brain activity as well.

Supportive psychotherapy is sometimes indicated for patient and family alike. Behavioral therapy encourages safely increasing physical activity. Cognitive approaches foster ways of thinking about pain that are less negative and self-defeating. Treatment with medication can improve reactive depression. Severely affected patients may be considered for electroconvulsive therapy.

Last, but not least, simple interventions such as placing a cardboard box under the covers of a patient with allodynia of the feet can improve sleep.

6. Invasive Treatment Options

(i) Implanted Neural Stimulators

Invasive methods of pain treatment should be considered for the management of neuropathic pain states refractory to medical therapy. This technique requires long-term commitment on the part of the patient and pain specialist. Serious surgical complications are rare but minor complications occur in up to one third of patients. Electrical stimulation of central or peripheral axons of primary afferent fibers offers the potential for dramatic relief of even long-lasting neuropathic pain. This is accomplished using implanted stimulators of the dorsal column of the spinal cord or of the injured peripheral nerve. The evidence supporting the use of dorsal column stimulators is not limited to neuropathic pain states and the mechanism of pain relief is not well understood. Chronic precentral and central motor cortex electrical stimulation for poststroke pain and deafferentation syndromes are used in the most advanced centers. Recent technical advances have been promising, but further clinical studies are needed. Peripheral stimulation of individual injured peripheral nerves is a technique with success rates significantly higher than most other medical and surgical options.

(ii) Implanted Intrathecal Infusion Pumps

The evidence for the efficacy of pumps administering morphine, hydromorphone, and baclofen is less conclusive and limited to case series. Their primary indication is for pain that clearly improves with opioid therapy in patients who are unable to tolerate oral opioid therapy due to adverse effects. Device related complications are common in the long run.

(iii) Decompressive Neurosurgery

Select patients with well-defined lesions may benefit from surgical exploration and decompression. Such treatment is well accepted for carpal tunnel syndrome, but unfortunately underutilized for patients with painful nerve compressions elsewhere. Pain relief after lysis of connective tissue bands compressing peripheral nerves has been described at multiple locations in the body. The relatively benign nature of these procedures, which do not involve cutting or injuring neural tissues, must be emphasized.

(iv) Ablative Neurosurgery

These procedures are rarely indicated, and are performed far less frequently now than in the past. Cutting nerves usually relieves pain only temporarily, if at all. These procedures, which should only be performed by those with neurosurgical training, are probably underutilized in the specific circumstance of patients with intractable pain from advanced disease and limited life expectancy. For them, the risks of damage to motor or autonomic pathways may be acceptable in order to achieve good pain control for their remaining time. Transection of the pain pathways of the spinal cord can be performed percutaneously by a skilled neurosurgeon using fluoroscopic guidance. Cutting nerves that innervate areas of neuropathic pains initially appears to be an attractive option, but a century of practice has shown this to be generally ineffective. Furthermore, it can in fact worsen neuropathic pain. Unfortunately, one still sees patients treated with neurectomies who develop complex, intractable neuropathic pain syndromes as a result.

(v) Neuromas

Neuromas can form after traumatic or surgical amputation. They consist of tangles of axonal sprouts that have not been able to find a distal nerve stump through which to reinnervate their target and are entrapped in connective tissue. Neuromas can be extremely sensitive to mechanical stimuli. Some neuromas benefit from surgical resection, with burial of the new proximal nerve stump in muscle or a deeper tissue where it is less likely to be jostled.

VI. CONCLUSION

Whereas neuropathic pain was considered a distinct entity associated with specific diagnoses such as diabetic peripheral neuropathy, postherpetic neuralgia, and trigeminal neuralgia, it is now understood to contribute to many chronic pain syndromes, including CRPS, cancer pain, and even chronic low back pain, due to associated changes in neuronal function and anatomy. It is perhaps the most challenging type of pain we treat in the pain clinic, and the most difficult to understand. It is a prominent focus of attention for clinicians and neuroscience researchers who together are attempting to unravel its mechanisms and improve the specificity and efficacy of its treatments. Neuropathic pain is an integral part of the practice of pain management, and it is worthy of an intensive effort to help its unfortunate victims and to overcome the shortcomings in its treatment.

SELECTED READINGS

Amato AA, Oaklander AL. Case records of the Massachusetts General Hospital. Weekly clinicopathological exercises. Case 16-2004. A 76-year-old woman with pain and numbness in the legs and feet. *N Engl J Med* 2004;350:2181–2189.

Devinsky O, Feldmann E. *Examination of the cranial and peripheral nerves.* New York: Churchill Livingstone, 1988.

Dworkin RH, Backonja M, Rowbotham MC, et al. Advances in neuropathic pain: diagnosis, mechanisms, and treatment recommendations. *Arch Neurol* 2003;60(11):1524–1534.

Stewart JD, ed. *Focal peripheral neuropathies*, 3rd ed. Philadelphia, PA: Lippincott Williams & Wilkins, 2000.

Woolf CJ. Dissecting out mechanisms responsible for peripheral neuropathic pain: implications for diagnosis and therapy. *Life Sci* 2004;74(21):2605–2610.

Complex Regional Pain Syndrome

Eugenia-Daniela Hord

Pain, whose unchecked and familiar speed Is howling, and keen shrieks day after day.
—*Percy Bysshe Shelley, 1792–1822*

In 1995, the International Association for the Study of Pain introduced the name Complex Regional Pain Syndrome (CRPS). Complex Regional Pain Syndrome I (CRPS I) and Complex Regional Pain Syndrome II (CRPS II) are new names for two classic neuropathic pain syndromes previously known as **reflex sympathetic dystrophy** and **causalgia**. The new terminology was suggested to avoid the misleading term "sympathetic," and to create uniform diagnostic criteria. Although there are still some dissenters, the new terminology is now largely accepted. CRPS I occurs without a definable nerve lesion, whereas CRPS II follows an identifiable major nerve lesion. On the basis of the presence or absence of the sympathetic component of pain, both types of CRPS can be divided further into sympathetically maintained pain (SMP) and sympathetically independent pain (SIP). A diagnostic sympathetic blockade can help distinguish SMP from SIP. These syndromes remain among the most fascinating and enigmatic of the pain syndromes.

I. HISTORY

The clinical syndrome we refer to as CRPS was scarcely mentioned in the medical literature before 1864 when Weir Mitchell, an American Civil War physician, described a syndrome consisting of burning pain, hyperesthesia, and trophic changes following nerve injury in the limbs of the soldiers. He named this pain syndrome **causalgia**.

Similar pain states were later documented in postsurgical patients, as well as in those with no clearly inciting cause. In the 1920s, Leriche, a French surgeon, established a link between the sympathetic nervous system and causalgia by demonstrating that sympathetic blockade or sympathectomy relieved the symptoms of many of his patients. Patients with no clear-cut peripheral nerve injury, or those with pain in more than one peripheral nerve distribution, had what became known as reflex sympathetic dystrophy, which is now called CRPS I.

In 1946, Evans devised the term **reflex sympathetic dystrophy** to describe a similar syndrome in patients with no obvious nerve damage. Since then, numerous attempts have been made to explain the pathophysiology behind these clinical features, and a host of different names have been used to describe them.

II. BASIC MECHANISMS

Numerous theories have been offered to explain the pathophysiology of CRPS, but the exact mechanisms remain unclear. Most theories postulate that sympathetic dysfunction plays a significant role in the development and maintenance of the syndromes. Indeed, CRPS and SMP are closely integrated. However, there are CRPS syndromes in which part or all of the pain appears to be SIP.

CRPS most likely involves both peripheral and central mechanisms. Peripherally, one observes events after nerve injury that herald long-term changes in neural processing. In animal models, persistent afferent small-fiber activity begins days to weeks after peripheral nerve ligation or section, and can be measured at the site of a developing neuroma as well as in the dorsal root ganglia. The neural sprouts at these sites have growth cones, which have mechanical and chemical sensitivities not possessed by the original neurons. These neural sprouts also may have increased numbers of sodium channels, leading to increased ionic conductance and hence increased spontaneous activity. There is also evidence of an abnormal coupling between sympathetic efferent and nociceptive afferent neurons (C-fibers and/or afferent somata within the dorsal root ganglia). It is hypothesized that a partial nerve lesion induces an up-regulation of functional α_2 adrenoceptors at the plasma membrane of nociceptive fibers. These mechanisms could be the pathologic pathway of SMP. Additionally, more recent evidence supports the involvement of neurogenic inflammation in the pathogenesis of edema, vasodilation, and sweating in CRPS.

Centrally, changes in the morphology of the spinal dorsal horn ipsilateral to a peripheral nerve injury may be secondary to intrinsic mechanisms arising in response to a chronic barrage of impulses, or in response to retrograde transport of chemical factors from the area of the lesion. The role of glutamate release in the spinal cord after peripheral nerve injury is being evaluated with growing interest. Increased spontaneous activity in the primary afferent neuron may be a factor leading to spinal cord glutamate release. The fact that some patients could have hemineglect further supports the involvement of the central nervous system in the pathogenesis of CRPS.

III. CLINICAL PRESENTATION

The initial signs and symptoms of CRPS may begin at the time of injury or may be delayed for weeks. Sometimes, the traumatic event cannot be identified. CRPS I occurs without a known nerve lesion, whereas CRPS II consists of the same signs and symptoms following an identifiable major nerve lesion. Because CRPS I and II have identical symptoms, it seems likely that the cause of CRPS I is also nerve injury but that the nerve injuries go undetected because they are partial, fascicular, or involve primarily small unmyelinated axons. These specific types of nerve lesions are notoriously difficult to diagnose by examination or electrodiagnostic studies.

CRPSs are characterized by pain, changes in cutaneous sensitivity, autonomic dysfunction, trophic changes, and motor dysfunction. Untreated CRPS was characterized by three stages: acute, dystrophic, and atrophic. However, the sequential progression is hard to identify now that most patients are treated and do not display the later stages of disease progression.

Spontaneous pain is present in the majority of the patients. It can be burning, sharp stabbing, electric shocklike aching, and the quality can vary in time. The pain appears disproportionate to the inciting event. Sensory changes are common CRPS and include allodynia and hyperalgesia. Sensory deficits also can be present.

Autonomic dysfunction manifests as edema, changes in sweating (hypo- or hyperhidrosis), skin color changes (red or pale), and skin temperature differences. These signs can vary from time to time, and may be reported despite not being obvious at the time of the examination.

Trophic changes are largely the result of disuse. They include changes in nail growth and aspect, skin changes (can be thin and shiny or thick), hair loss, or hypetrichosis (see Fig. 1). Bones are osteoporotic and joints may ankylose (see Fig. 2).

The motor dysfunction includes weakness and later atrophy. Dystonia and tremor are also described.

IV. DIAGNOSIS

Pain is the cardinal feature of CRPS, but there are also sensory changes, autonomic dysfunction, trophic changes, motor impairment, and psychological changes. The diagnosis is based on the

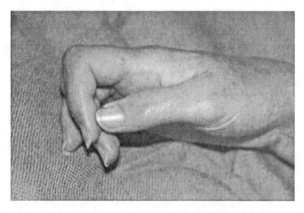

Figure 1.   The appearance of the hand in CRPS. The skin is smooth, glossy, tight, and cool, the overlying hair has fallen out, and the nails are severely brittle. The digits are thin and tapered. The joints are ankylosed.

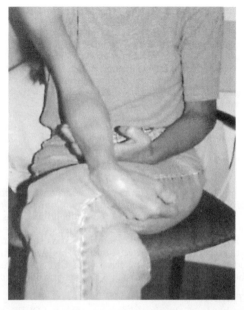

Figure 2. Woman with severely affected right arm. Muscle wasting is pronounced and there are flexion contractures.

whole clinical picture, with additional information from carefully performed and interpreted confirmatory tests to ascertain the presence or absence of SMP and autonomic dysfunction. These include diagnostic sympathetic blockade (e.g., stellate ganglion block, lumbar sympathetic block) and tests such as the quantitative pseudomotor axon reflex test, which allows a continuous hygrometric assessment of pseudomotor activity and is considered a good indicator of C-fiber function. Clinical experience suggests that early intervention, as well as early diagnosis, is helpful. Table 1 lists the common clinical features of CRPS used in the differential diagnosis of CRPS, and diagnostic criteria are listed in Table 2.

Table 1.   Common clinical features of CRPS

A recent or remote history of accidental or iatrogenic trauma
Pain that is burning, aching, or throbbing in nature
The presence of one or more of the following:
    Vasomotor/sudomotor disturbances
    Trophic changes
    Limb edema
    Cold sensitivity
    Muscle weakness or atrophy
    Pain relief after regional sympathetic blockade

Table 2.   IASP diagnostic criteria for CRPS

I	Initiating noxious event (trauma, infection, surgery, etc.)
II	Continuing pain, allodynia, or hyperalgesia with which the pain is disproportionate to any inciting event
III	Evidence at some time of edema, changes in skin blood flow, or abnormal sudomotor activity in the region of the pain
IV	Requires absence of an alternative explanation for the symptoms

Note: CRPS type I occurs without a known nerve lesion, whereas CRPS type II requires the presence of a known nerve lesion.
From Merskey H, Bogduk N. *Classification of chronic pain: pain syndromes and definitions of pain terms,* 2nd ed. Seattle, WA: IASP Press, 1994:40–43, with permission.

The diagnosis of CRPS requires the exclusion of confounding medical problems, as well as the evaluation of diagnostic criteria. The IASP criteria are acknowledged to be suboptimal, presumably because of continued uncertainty over the causes. But these criteria are the current consensus criteria, and should be used to standardize patients recruited into research studies. The IASP continues to clarify and refine the diagnostic criteria for CRPS, and hopefully this will help eliminate diagnostic and therapeutic dilemmas.

V. TREATMENT

Progress has been slow in refining treatment of CRPS. Because the condition is complex and incompletely understood, the treatment has been varied and formulated to address presumed pathophysiologic causes and to ameliorate specific symptoms. The common goal is functional restoration. Pharmacologic therapy as well as regional anesthetics and surgical interventions should be used in conjunction with physical therapy (PT). CRPS prognosis in adults is more guarded than in children. Most children with recent-onset CRPS will improve spontaneously and should be treated conservatively.

1. Physical Therapy

PT should be started as soon as a diagnosis is made, even a presumptive diagnosis. In cases in which PT has already been started (e.g., after surgery on the hand or foot, or after casting for a fracture), the pain may worsen as CRPS develops, but discontinuing PT will only make matters worse. PT should continue, but the approach may be altered. The major role of PT seems to be to treat the secondary complications such as decreased joint and tendon range of motion and subsequent atrophy. One randomized controlled study demonstrated that physical and, to a lesser extent, occupational therapies reduced pain and improved active mobility in recent-onset CRPS I. Mobilization of the affected limb is of paramount importance. Elevation, massage, and contrast bath also have been used. Often, the pain must be aggressively treated (as in subsequent text) in order to accomplish this. A gentle approach using heat, massage, vibration, and other mild stimuli will help to restore more normal sensory processing. Isometric strengthening should be followed by progressive stress-loading as tolerated. One must be careful when using medication or, in particular, regional anesthesia in conjunction with PT to avoid aggressive range of motion exercises and heavy loading of the affected limb. (Chapter 16 contains a full description of PT for patients with CRPS.)

2. Pharmacologic Treatments

Research into treatments has been gravely hindered by the loose definitions used, and there have been almost no multicenter, randomized, placebo-controlled trials. There are currently no medications approved by the U.S. Food and Drug Administration (FDA) for the treatment of CRPS.

In 1997, Kingery reviewed the controlled clinical trials for CRPS and peripheral neuropathic pain and concluded that the CRPS trials used fewer subjects and were usually of lesser quality (not placebo controlled, blinded, or analyzed with appropriate statistical tools) than the neuropathic pain trials. Here we describe medications proven effective for other types of neuropathic pain, even if not specifically tested on patients with CRPS.

(i) Neuropathic Pain Medications

TRICYCLIC ANTIDEPRESSANTS. TCAs are effective in treating neuropathic pain syndromes, including postherpetic neuralgia, diabetic neuropathy, and CRPS. These agents have independent analgesic effects but also can facilitate the treatment of pain by improving mood, sleep, and anxiety states. Few patients experience total relief, and usage is often limited by side effects. This should be considered when prescribing these drugs, particularly in the elderly. Refer to Chapter 11 for a full description of these drugs.

ANTICONVULSANTS. The anticonvulsants are a heterogeneous group of drugs, some of which have known efficacy for the treatment of neuropathic pain. Several anticonvulsants have been used successfully for CRPS, including phenytoin, carbamazepine, vaproic acid, and gabapentin. Gabapentin has advantages over older agents such as carbamazepine and phenytoin because of its better side-effect profile. Case reports and small series support the efficacy of gabapentin in adult and pediatric CRPS. Newer antiepileptic medications also may be effective, but randomized placebo-controlled clinical trials are lacking at the moment. The anticonvulsant drugs and their use in pain management are described in Chapter 10.

LOCAL ANESTHETICS. Mexiletine, a sodium channel blocker, originally was developed as an anticonvulsant, but until recently it has been used almost solely as a Class Ib antiarrhythmic. It is structurally similar to lidocaine and has been demonstrated to be useful in treating neuropathic pain states. Although few studies exist, it is generally felt that mexiletine may be useful in the treatment of CRPS.

Recently, transdermal lidocaine patches have been used successfully in areas of localized neuropathic pain with allodynia and hyperalgesia in postherpetic neuralgia. EMLA (eutectic mixture of local anesthetic) cream is a topical preparation containing both lidocaine and prilocaine. These topical lidocaine preparations appear to be useful in the treatment of localized areas of hyperesthesia associated with CRPS, but this efficacy has not been confirmed by trials (see Chapters 10 and 25).

(ii) Nonsteroidal Antiinflammatory Drugs

Nonsteriodal antiinflammatory drugs (NSAIDs) are not useful as sole pharmacologic therapy in CRPS because pain relief is generally inadequate, although they may be helpful during the early stages of the disease. They may occasionally be useful as adjunctive therapy, especially when there is joint and tendon involvement. The risks, benefits, and desirability of NSAIDs are discussed in Chapter 8.

(iii) Opioids

For many reasons, the use of opioids in neuropathic pain states is controversial. Formerly, neuropathic pain was considered to be unresponsive to opioids, although currently opioid responsiveness with a rightward shift of the dose response curve (indicating efficacy but at higher doses) is accepted. Although there are no well-controlled trials of opioid therapy in patients with CRPS, it appears that in certain patients opioid treatment can usefully improve pain. Therefore, for refractory pain, a trial of opioids may be warranted. Opioids should only be used as adjuncts to other treatments, and great care should be taken when prescribing for patients with a history of substance abuse or obvious risk factors for abuse (see Chapter 30).

(iv) Inhibitors of Osteoclast Activity

Some patients with CRPS have abnormalities of bone metabolism, including excess bone resorption in the affected area, although this is likely a secondary consequence of reduced mobility and/or loss of innervation to the bone. For this reason, inhibitors of osteoclast activity (e.g., bisphosphonates or regulators of bone metabolism like calcitonin) have been evaluated as treatments for recent-onset CRPS. There is also evidence of direct antihyperalgesic effects of some of these compounds. The mechanisms by which calcitonin and bisphosphonates control pain in early CRPS are unclear: bisphosphonates hinder the synthesis of prostaglandin E2, proteolytic enzymes, lactic acid, and pro-inflammatory cytokines; calcitonin inhibits the synthesis of proteolytic enzymes and lactic acid. None of these agents can be given orally; calcitonin is available as a nasal spray, and bisphosphonates usually are administered intravenously.

(v) Corticosteroids

Corticosteroids have been advocated for use in the early stages of CRPS. There is evidence that by decreasing inflammation they relieve pain and minimize ectopic electrical activity after nerve injury. Recent studies suggest there is a marked inflammatory component in the early stages of CRPS. Thus, if a patient has pain secondary to joint movement and trophic changes, a trial of corticosteroids with a reasonably rapid taper is recommended. Using this approach, one may avoid many of the undesirable side effects of steroids when evaluating and treating the inflammatory component of CRPS early in the disease.

(vi) Others

Lioresal (Baclofen) is a γ-aminobutyric acid-receptor (type B) agonist that increases the function of dorsal-horn interneurons that inhibit the output of projection neurons, including those transmitting pain signals via the spinothalamic tracts. For some time, it has been used successfully both orally and intrathecally for treatment of spasticity. Some patients with CRPS develop dystonia. Short-term efficacy of intrathecal baclofen for relieving CRPS spasticity was demonstrated in one recent study. Oral and intrathecal baclofen as a treatment of neuropathic pain independent of spasticity have been evaluated in preclinical and clinical studies. There is some evidence for efficacy in treating CRPS pain, even in patients without dystonia. However, further studies are necessary.

Phentolamine, an α-adrenergic blocker, is used by intravenous infusion to test the susceptibility of CRPS to sympathetic blockade. It is reported that approximately 30% of patients with sympathetically mediated pain will respond positively to an intravenous infusion test. In these patients, intravenous regional sympathetic blockade may subsequently prove useful. Oral α-blockers have not been found useful because side effects, most importantly hypotension and tachycardia, preclude anything but the smallest doses, which severely limits their utility as analgesics.

Clonidine, an α_2 agonist, has been shown to have significant analgesic properties. It can be administered systemically or neuraxially, and has proven effective for both nociceptive and neuropathic pain. Intravenous regional blockade using 1 mcg per kg clonidine can provide marked pain relief in patients with sympathetically mediated pain. Likewise, transdermal clonidine is believed to be useful, particularly when applied to discreet areas of hyperalgesia. Clonidine has both central and peripheral actions and may be a useful adjunct in the treatment of CRPS. Clonidine is described in more detail in Chapter 10.

3. Regional Anesthesia

A number of regional anesthetic modalities have been used in the treatment of CRPS. The primary indication is as an adjunct to PT in the process of functional restoration. Regional sympatholysis in patients with SMP can be both diagnostic and therapeutic (in conjunction with PT). The regional anesthetic techniques are described in detail in Chapter 12.

(i) Sympathetic Blockade

Temporary sympatholysis of the upper extremity can be accomplished by a stellate ganglion block or a cervical sympathetic block. A lumbar sympathetic block will provide sympathetic blockade in the lower extremities. In addition to providing temporary pain relief, sympathetic blocks can be helpful in determining the extent of the sympathetic component of a patient's pain, thereby predicting potential benefit from pharmacologic therapy, and from spinal cord stimulation (SCS). However, one must keep in mind that some degree of somatic blockade is almost certain to occur in conjunction with these blocks; therefore, the test is not entirely clean. It cannot be overemphasized that the aim of temporary sympatholysis in CRPS is to achieve sufficient pain relief to allow functional restoration during a course of PT. The end point for the combined therapy is either adequate functional restoration, or the point at which the patient is no longer able to increase his or her endurance and workload after sympathetic blockade. A series of blocks may be necessary, in conjunction with the PT sessions.

Sympathetic neurolysis has been advocated in the past but is no longer recommended. Chemical neurolysis lasts only 3 to 6 months, and patients may then suffer a recurrence, or even worsening, of their original pain. There is also a risk of spread of the neurolytic agent to the sensorimotor fibers in close proximity to the targeted nerves (e.g., phrenic nerve, lumbar plexus). In addition, there is a high risk of deafferentation pain, which is worse and harder to treat than the initial pain. More recently, **percutaneous radiofrequency lesioning of the sympathetic trunk** and **endoscopic sympathectomy** have been used in selected patients with clearly demonstrable SMP. Long-term evaluation of these treatments has not yet been completed. However, current experience suggests there may be a similar risk of deafferentation pain.

(ii) Intravenous Regional Blockade

Intravenous regional blockade has been attempted using several different medications, with varying reports of success. A number of the medications previously used for IV regional blockade are no longer available in the United States. If a patient has failed conservative treatment, an IV regional trial may be warranted. However, it is now clearly established that this intervention does not provide long-lasting pain relief. Bretylium and guanethidine can provide up to 3 weeks of relief. Local anesthetic and clonidine often are used in combination. Some practitioners advocate adding ketorolac if the patient is in the acute stage of CRPS when there is a significant inflammatory component. Again, the main purpose of treatment should be pain relief to facilitate PT. Many patients are unable to tolerate the procedure because of severe pain with limb exsanguination and tourniquet placement.

(iii) Epidural Blockade

Lumbar epidural blockade and, less frequently, cervical epidural blockade have been used for extended periods of time to treat cases of CRPS that have been unresponsive to less invasive therapies. Lumbar epidural catheters can be used to provide continuous lumbar plexus blockade for patients who have inadequate pain relief, and have been unable to participate in PT. A low concentration of local anesthetic is used, as high concentrations tend to produce sensory and motor blockade, which hamper functional restoration. Often an opioid or clonidine is used in combination with the local anesthetic to augment pain relief. Temporary epidural catheters have been left in place for up to 6 weeks, allowing successful functional restoration. Obviously, there are risks associated with long-term epidural catheters, and sometimes the external infusion system can interfere with the exercise regime. Implanted epidural infusion systems are more secure and less intrusive, but the risks of the surgical procedure are probably not warranted other than in the most refractory cases.

(iv) Brachial Plexus Blockade

Continuous brachial plexus blockade for patients with CRPS of the upper extremity is sometimes used. This can be accomplished with an axillary, infraclavicular, or supraclavicular catheter. The advantage, as with epidural catheters, is that the prolongation of neural blockade enables patients to make relatively rapid progress in their PT. Under neural blockade, care should be taken to avoid over-extending the passive and active range of motion exercises. As with any catheter treatment, there are risks of dislodgement and infection. A fairly high infusion rate of local anesthetic is needed for successful brachial plexus catheter treatment, which limits the utility of these catheter treatments in outpatients. The treatment is best suited to patients who have been unresponsive to pharmacologic therapy but are likely to have a good and rapid response to PT with adequate sensorimotor blockade.

4. Neuromodulation

(i) Spinal Cord Stimulation

SCS has been shown to be effective in patients with refractory CRPS in several clinical trials. A preliminary report suggests that short-term efficacy of sympathetic blockade may predict a positive response to spinal cord stimulation in patients with CRPS. Stimulation is conducted at the C5 to C7 level for the upper extremities and the T8 to T10 level for the lower extremities. It seems critical to have good overlap between the induced paresthesias and the painful area. Approximately 50% of preselected patients with CRPS will have a positive response to stimulation during the period of a trial. Approximately 70% of these patients will have good-to-excellent long-term benefit. A goal of pain relief is reasonable in view of the refractory nature of the pain in patients selected for this expensive therapy, although if treatment is started early one could hope that functional restoration may be achieved. The recent literature suggests utility for earlier use of SCS in patients with CRPS, although an exact recommendation on timing has yet to be determined. See Chapter 13 for a full description of spinal cord stimulator treatment.

(ii) Peripheral Nerve Stimulation

Peripheral nerve stimulation has been advocated for use in patients with CRPS II, with symptoms entirely or mainly in the distribution of a single major peripheral nerve, who have been unresponsive to other therapeutic modalities. It is not considered an option for patients with CRPS involving an entire limb or further extension to the trunk or other extremities. Peripheral nerve stimulators present a special problem in that they generally cross several mobile joints, and therefore may be dislodged with movement. In select patients, however, early small studies suggest this might be successful treatment for patients with CRPS II who have been unresponsive to other therapies.

5. Psychotherapy

Because of the discrepancy between the subjective complaints of pain made by patients with CRPS and the limited objective evidence of underlying pathology, it may be suggested that psychiatric factors are a major cause of CRPS. Many patients with CRPS become depressed during the course of their illness. There has been a great deal of discussion on whether a premorbid tendency to depression predisposes patients to CRPS, or whether CRPS causes depression or uncovers a preexisting condition, and no consensus has been reached. Early in the illness, only approximately 10% to 15% of patients with CRPS report being depressed; this is similar to the incidence of depression in the general population. Furthermore, when psychological tests are conducted at this stage, the results are similar to those in the general population. As CRPS progresses, anxiety and depression play more of a role. This is confirmed by psychological testing. Clinicians should be aware of the high rate of secondary psychiatric problems in CRPS and refer patients for counseling and medical treatment as needed. A psychiatrist, psychologist, or social worker familiar with CRPS should be involved in caring for patients if at all possible at this juncture. Biofeedback for relaxation and reduction of muscle tension is a useful adjunct to pharmacologic therapy, PT, and psychotherapy.

VI. CONCLUSION

The majority of CRPS cases are best managed with a combination of skilled PT with medication or interventional pain therapy. The aim is always to start treatment early and to optimize function. A simple drug regime, or a simple nerve block (usually sympathetic) or series of blocks, is sufficient in all but the most refractory cases. More complicated procedures, including implanted catheters and stimulators, rarely are needed. With a team approach to the treatment of patients with CRPS, a successful outcome is most likely.

SELECTED READINGS

Baron R, Binder A. Complex regional pain syndromes. In: Pappagallo M, ed. *The neurological basis of pain*. New York: McGraw-Hill, 2005: 359–378.

Becker WJ, Ablett DP, Harris CJ, et al. Long term treatment of intractable reflex sympathetic dystrophy with intrathecal morphine. *Can J Neurol Sci* 1995;22:153–159.

Blumberg H, Janig W. Clinical manifestations of reflex sympathetic dystrophy and sympathetically maintained pain. In: Wall PD, Melzack R, eds. *Textbook of pain*, 3rd ed. Edinburgh, UK: Churchill Livingstone, 1994:685–698.

Bossut DF, Perl ER. Effects of nerve injury on sympathetic excitation of A-delta mechanical nociceptors. *J Neurophysiol* 1995;73:1721–1723.

Bruehl S, Harden RN, Galer B, et al. External validation of IASP diagnostic criteria for complex regional pain syndrome and proposed research diagnostic criteria. *Pain* 1999;81:147–154.

Cepeda MS, Lau J, Carr DB. Defining the therapeutic role of local anesthetic sympathetic blockade in complex regional pain syndrome: a narrative and systematic review. *Clin J Pain* 2002;18:216–233.

Devor M, Wall P, Catalan N. Systemic lidocaine silences ectopic neuroma and DRG discharge without blocking nerve conduction. *Pain* 1992;48:261–268.

Eisenach J, DeKock M, Klimscha W. Alpha 2 adrenergic agonists for regional anesthesia: a clinical review of clonidine (1984–1995). *Anesthesiology* 1996;85:655–674.

Galer BS, Bruehl S, Harden RN. IASP diagnostic criteria for complex regional pain syndrome: a preliminary empirical validation study. *Clin J Pain* 1998;14:48–54.

Harden RN, Bruehl S, Galer BS, et al. Complex regional pain syndrome: are the IASP diagnostic criteria valid and sufficiently comprehensive? *Pain* 1999;83:211–219.

Hord ED, Cohen S, Ahmed S, et al. The predictive value of sympathetic block for the success of spinal cord stimulation. *Neurosurgery* 2003;53(3):626–633.

Hord ED, Oaklander AL. Complex regional pain syndrome: a review of evidence-supported treatment options. *Curr Pain Headache Rep* 2003;7:188–196.

Janig W, Stanton-Hicks M, eds. *Reflex sympathetic dystrophy: a reappraisal*. Seattle, WA: IASP Press, 1996.

Kamibayashi T, Maze M. Clinical uses of alpha 2-adrenergic agonists. *Anesthesiology* 2000;93:1345–1349.

Kingery WS. A critical review of controlled trials for peripheral neuropathic pain and complex regional pain syndromes. *Pain* 1997; 73:123–139.

Kumar K, Toth C, Nath RK, et al. Epidural spinal cord stimulation for treatment of chronic pain—some predictors of success. A 15-year experience. *Surg Neurol* 1998;50:110–120.

Mellick GA, Mellicy LB, Mellick LB. Gabapentin in the management of reflex sympathetic dystrophy. *J Pain Symptom Manage* 1995; 10:265–266.

Merskey H, Bogduk N, eds. Classification of chronic pain. *Description of chronic pain syndromes and definition of pain terms*, 2nd ed. Seattle, WA: IASP Press, 1994.

Mitchell SW. *Injuries of nerves and their consequences*. Philadelphia, PA: JB Lippincott Co, 1872; Reprinted in *Clinical Orthopedics and Related Research* 1982;163:2–7.

Mitchell SW, Morehouse GR, Keen WW, et al. *Gunshot wounds and other injuries of nerves*. Philadelphia, PA: JB Lippincott Co, 1864.

Stanton-Hicks M, Baron R, Boas R, et al. Consensus report. Complex regional pain syndromes: guidelines for therapy. *Clin J Pain* 1998; 14:155–166.

Van Hilten BJ, van de Beek WJ, Hoff JI, et al. Intrathecal baclofen for the treatment of dystonia in patients with reflex sympathetic dystrophy. *N Engl J Med* 2000;343:625–630.

Wheeler DS, Vaux KK, Tam DA. Use of gabapentin in the treatment of childhood reflex sympathetic dystrophy. *Pediatr Neurol* 2000; 22:220–221.

Woolf CJ, Mannion RJ. Neuropathic pain: aetiology, symptoms, mechanisms, and management. *Lancet* 1999;353:1959–1964.

Zollinger PE, Tuinebreijer WE, Kreis RW, et al. Effect of vitamin C on frequency of reflex sympathetic dystrophy in wrist fractures: a randomised trial. *Lancet* 1999;354:2025–2028.

Low Back Pain

James P. Rathmell, Thomas T. Simopoulos,
Zahid H. Bajwa, and Shihab U. Ahmed

Pain is not just a stimulus that is transmitted over specific pathways but rather a complex perception, the nature of which depends not only on the intensity of the stimulus but on the situation in which it is experienced and, most importantly, on the affective or emotional state of the individual. Pain is to somatic stimulation as beauty is to a visual stimulus. It is a very subjective experience.
—*Allan I. Basbaum, "Unlocking the Secrets of Pain: The Science," Medical and Health Annual, Ellen Bernstein, ed., 1998*

I. OVERVIEW

Low back pain (LBP) is one of the most common conditions presenting to both primary care physicians and to pain physicians. It has become a societal problem of unprecedented proportions, accounting for a large proportion of health care costs, as well as lost work days owing to the associated disability. In young adults, the problem often starts with an acute episode, triggered by trivial or substantial injury, which progresses insidiously to chronic pain. In older patients, degenerative changes are the more common cause of chronic back pain. It may be possible to "rescue" younger patients from a prolonged battle with chronic LBP and from reliance on medications by means of active intervention, often with simple conservative measures, early in the course of the pain progression. An evidence-based algorithm for the management of adult LBP from the Institute for Clinical Systems Improvement is published by the National Guideline Clearinghouse. This guideline is a useful resource for physicians treating acute and chronic LBP, and provides the basis for the management approach suggested in this chapter (see Appendix II for useful Websites regarding guidelines for adults with low back pain).

1. Acute Low Back Pain (Less than 6 Weeks' Duration)

Ninety percent of patients with back pain improve within 4 to 6 weeks. During an early presentation, the patient should be encouraged to pursue conservative treatment measures (see Table 1) and to gradually resume normal activities, including return to work, once the pain reaches tolerable proportions. Patients should also be warned that a recurrence of the acute episode is likely and that more than 50% of patients with an acute back pain episode will experience other such episodes. Each acute episode, provided there is resolution between episodes, can be treated independently as a new acute episode.

In rare instances, the sudden onset of back pain has a serious pathologic basis. Serious pathology must be identified or excluded before assuming a more benign cause of pain (see Fig. 1). Initial screening must attempt to identify neurologic deterioration, infection, or tumor progression and to identify patients who require urgent intervention and/or urgent lumbar spine x-rays (see Table 2). The initial screen should also be used to identify patients who need further evaluation (within 2 to 7 weeks), although urgent intervention is not indicated (see Table 3).

2. Subacute Low Back Pain

When the pain does not resolve with conservative measures, comprehensive physical and psychosocial evaluation is indicated (see Table 4). Nerve root compression is identified from history, physical examination, and imaging. If there is neural impingement, surgical assessment is warranted. Strong consideration should be given to performing a single or a series of fluoroscopically guided epidural steroid injections (ESIs) before embarking on

Table 1. Conservative treatment for acute low back pain

- Recommend cold packs or heat
- Prescribe acetaminophen or NSAIDs
- Consider muscle relaxants
- Limit bed rest (only for severe initial symptoms and limited to 2–4 d)
- Modify patient's activity level (maintain nonstressful activities)
- Describe recommended structured exercise program (advice from specialty spine program may be helpful at this stage)
- Provide self-care instructions—educational materials that emphasize absence of serious disease and good prognosis, "hurt does not equal harm," appropriate physical activity is helpful not harmful

NSAIDs, nonsteroidal antiinflammatory drugs.

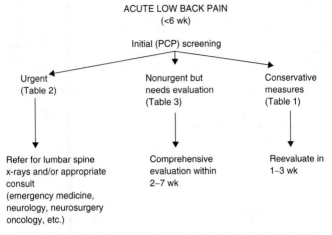

Figure 1. Algorithm for managing acute low back pain of less than 6 weeks duration.

surgery (see Fig. 2). If there is no evidence of nerve impingement (90% of patients), the patient should be encouraged to undergo active rehabilitation (see Table 5). Effective rehabilitation at this stage provides the best hope of stalling the insidious course toward chronic pain. It is reasonable to make maximum use of all treatment options, including opioid medications and interventional procedures, toward the goal of restoration of function and of reduced reliance on medical intervention. The appearance of signs or symptoms of cauda equina syndrome or progressive or severe neurologic deficit calls for urgent surgical referral (see Table 6).

Table 2.   Initial screening of the patient with acute low back pain: identify features requiring urgent evaluation

Urgent evaluation is needed in those patients with:

- Unrelenting nighttime pain or pain at rest
- Fever 100.4°F (38°C) for >48 h
- Pain with distal (below the knee) numbness and/or weakness of leg(s)
- Loss of bowel or bladder control (retention or incontinence)
- Progressive neurologic/neuromotor deficit

Urgent lumbar spine x-rays should be obtained in those patients with:

- Substantial trauma
- Possible cancer
- Osteoporosis
- Chronic steroid use
- Drug or alcohol abuse
- Suspicion of ankylosing spondylitis

Table 3. Initial screening of the patient with acute low back pain: identify features that will require further nonurgent evaluation (within 2–7 wk)

Nonurgent but needs evaluation

- History of injury
- Past history of back symptoms
- Back pain duration >6 wk
- Unexplained weight loss
- History of cancer

3. Chronic Low Back Pain

Many patients with chronic LBP manage without medical intervention, sometimes with the help of medical guidance or benign medical treatment (e.g., over-the-counter pain medication). Only patients with the most intransigent symptoms seek prolonged medical intervention, either from their primary care physicians or

Table 4. Comprehensive physical and psychosocial evaluation

Used in addition to initial screening (Tables 1 and 2) in order to direct the patient to the appropriate specialist.

Medical evaluation

- History and physical examination (physical examination should include palpation for spine tenderness, neuromuscular testing, and straight leg raise[a])
- LBP with radiation below the knee (sciatica) is suggestive of nerve root compression—assess with MRI or lumbar spine CT scan
- LBP without radiation below the knee—assess using AP and lateral plain x-rays of the lumbar spine
- ESR, if inflammatory arthritides or infection are suspected
- Bone scan if bony metastases, inflammatory arthritides, or infection are suspected
- General screening for systemic illness—hematology, chemistry, liver function tests
- EMG/NCV (see Chapter 7)
- Myelography or CT scan enhanced myelography (see Chapter 5)

Psychosocial evaluation
(see also Chapter 15)

- Waddell nonorganic signs
- Nonanatomic pain drawing
- DSM-IV screening checklist for depression
- CAGE alcoholism test (Cut down-Annoyed-Guilty-Eye opener) and CAGE-D

MRI, magnetic resonance imaging; CT, computerized tomography; AP, anterior –posterior; ESR, erythrocyte sedimentation rate; EMG, electromyogram; NCV, nerve conduction velocity; DSM-IV, *Diagnostic and statistical manual of mental disorders*, Fourth Edition.
[a](+) straight leg raise is suggestive of disc herniation; (−) straight leg raise rules out surgically significant disc herniation in 95% of cases.

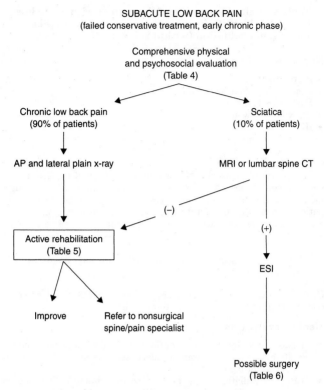

Figure 2. Algorithm for managing subacute low back pain of more than 6 weeks duration that has failed to improve with conservative treatment.

from specialists. When the practitioner takes on a new patient, it will be necessary to repeat the initial screening (see Tables 2 and 3) and the comprehensive physical and psychosocial evaluation (see Table 4) so that any new pathology or psychopathology, if present, can be identified and appropriate specialty care can be sought (see Fig. 3). Chronic intransigent back pain is most appropriately treated with a multidisciplinary approach. Early psychological evaluation and treatment are helpful because motivational, psychological,

Table 5.   Active rehabilitation

- Adopt a multidisciplinary approach
- Assess and manage psychosocial factors
- Begin an exercise program, develop good body mechanics
- Emphasize active self-management
- Encourage gradual resumption of normal activities, as tolerated
- Use medications (including opioids) and interventional procedures to maximize cooperation with active physical rehabilitation
- Refer for vocational counseling (if necessary)

and social issues often dictate how appropriate and meaningful all future biologic interventions will be. An anatomic or other source of pain is sought, and a treatment program is established on this basis. Most often, a logical combination of medications and procedures is used to treat structural sources of pain. Rehabilitation through physical therapy is frequently employed as the next step to restore function. Integration of the various modalities used to treat chronic LBP is essential for optimal results. Ongoing medical, psychological, and rehabilitative intervention is often necessary to treat patients with severe debilitating chronic LBP.

II. EVALUATING THE PATIENT WITH BACK AND NECK PAIN

Important Principles

- Serious causes of neck and back pain (e.g., infection, tumor, and trauma) are rare but must be excluded.
- The etiology of pain in a considerable number of patients with back and neck pain may remain unknown. Nonspecific back or neck pain is a legitimate diagnosis.
- History and physical examination have a limited role in the diagnosis of back and neck pain but are important in ruling out serious pathology.
- It is important to distinguish pain limited to the axis of the spine from radicular pain and radiculopathy (i.e., loss of

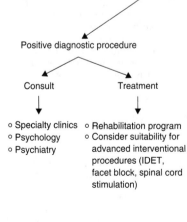

CHRONIC LOW BACK PAIN

New Presentation

Diagnosis

- Repeat comprehensive physical and psychosocial evaluation
- Refer to speciality spine/pain facility for diagnostic procedure (discography, diagnostic facet block, diagnostic nerve blocks)

Positive diagnostic procedure

Negative diagnostic procedure

Consult

Treatment

- Specialty clinics
- Psychology
- Psychiatry

- Rehabilitation program
- Consider suitability for advanced interventional procedures (IDET, facet block, spinal cord stimulation)

- Continue self care (see Table 1)
- Minimize reliance on medications
- Maintain normal activity
- Lifestyle change may be necessary
- Utilize alternative approaches (acupuncture, massage, spiritual healing)
- Utilize behavioral approaches (biofeedback, relaxation)

Figure 3.   Algorithm for managing chronic low back pain.

sensation, weakness, and/or loss of deep tendon reflexes in a dermatomal distribution indicating nerve root dysfunction).

- It is important to reassure patients with acute back and neck pain that most patients recover within weeks, without specific treatment.
- Degenerative disc disease is the single most common cause for axial LBP.
- Cervical facet joints are among the most common sources of axial neck pain.
- Diagnostic local anesthetic blocks can be helpful in establishing an anatomic diagnosis.

1. General Principles

Patients with neck pain or LBP are commonly referred to a pain specialist for evaluation and treatment. In order to guide further diagnostic evaluation and to select proper treatment, several simple characteristics should first be determined by questioning the patient.

- **Duration of symptoms: acute versus chronic pain.** Distinguishing acute back and neck pain (i.e., pain that has been present for days or weeks) from chronic pain (e.g., pain present for more than 6 weeks) will guide therapy. Most episodes of new-onset neck and back pain are self-limited and may require nothing more than symptomatic treatment and reassurance. **Ninety percent of patients with back pain improve within 4 to 6 weeks.** In contrast, patients with chronic axial LBP may present with radicular pain, signaling a new problem that may well require further evaluation. Finally, patients with a chronic, unchanging pattern of axial or radicular LBP, with or without a history of prior surgery, typically do not require further diagnostic evaluation, and attempts at treatment should be targeted toward long-term management.

- **Location of the pain: axial versus radicular pain.** Although many patients will have pain along the axis of the spine (axial pain), as well as pain extending in to one or more extremity (radicular pain), differentiating axial from radicular pain is key to guiding therapy. Radicular pain suggests acute or chronic nerve root involvement. Axial pain suggests pain associated with disc degeneration, facet arthropathy, or other myofascial components of the spine.

Table 6. Indications for surgery

- Fit for surgery
- Cauda equina syndrome
- Progressive or severe neuromotor deficit (e.g., foot drop or functional muscle weakness such as hip flexion weakness or quadriceps weakness)
- Persistent neuromotor deficit after 4–6 wk of conservative treatment (does not include minor sensory changes or reflex changes)
- Chronic sciatica with positive straight leg raising for >4–6 wk

- **Previous diagnostic evaluation.** Understanding any diagnostic evaluation that has already been performed early in the course of obtaining the history and physical examination will help guide questioning and the examination. Attempts should be made to correlate findings on diagnostic imaging or electrodiagnostic testing with the patient's report of pain and the findings during examination. Often, what appear to be important findings on diagnostic tests do not correlate with the pattern of pain reported by the patient. Further evaluation and treatment should always be directed toward the pain reported by the patient and *not* toward the results of diagnostic studies.
- **Previous spine surgery.** "Failed back surgery syndrome" is a term that has worked its way into the medical literature. The term should not be used as if it were a specific diagnosis: every patient with failed back surgery syndrome is unique. To evaluate a patient who has neck pain or LBP following a spinal surgery, it is important to first understand exactly what surgery was performed. The characteristics of the pain preceding and after surgery, as well as the characteristics of the present pain, are the keys to guiding further evaluation and treatment. Following are descriptions of two patients with radicular pain and a history of back surgery. The first is a patient who underwent simple discectomy with complete relief of radicular pain several years earlier and who now presents with acute onset of radicular pain. He likely has a recurrent disc herniation and should be managed accordingly. In contrast, a patient with prior lumbar fusion and long-standing radicular pain likely has a chronic radiculopathy. This form of neuropathic pain should be managed with a very different approach.

2. Medical History

(i) General Medical History

Initial evaluation of any patient with back or neck pain should include a search for signs and symptoms pointing toward a potentially progressive or unstable underlying cause for the pain, including trauma, cancer, or infection (see Fig. 1).

- Screening questions to detect cancer or to determine the status of patients with previous cancer: Any recent history of weight loss; history of prior cancer, including type of cancer, location, and treatment (breast, lung, renal cell, and prostate cancer have a particular proclivity for bone involvement) should be noted. Worsening pain at night, inability to attain relief at rest, and increased pain in the supine position raise suspicions for epidural spinal metastasis.
- Screening questions for infectious causes of spinal pain: Any recent fever, chills, or other symptoms suggestive of an infectious process (e.g., cough, localized erythema or swelling, or antibiotic use); any history of immunosuppression, intravenous drug use, or recent spinal surgery (all are associated with a small but significant incidence of spinal infection) should be determined.

- Screening questions for trauma: Any recent or significant trauma and the diagnostic evaluation that ensued (any patient with a significant mechanism of injury with onset of spinal pain should be evaluated for fracture or ligamentous instability) should be assessed.
- Screening questions for vascular etiologies: Any history of abdominal pain or known abdominal aortic aneurysm or occlusion; history of peripheral vascular disease or claudication should be evaluated.
- Screening questions for progressive or unstable neurologic status: Any worsening numbness or weakness in the extremities; bowel or bladder dysfunction (spinal cord or cauda equina compression may present first with urinary retention followed later by urinary and/or fecal incontinence); numbness extending in to both legs in a saddle distribution (perineal numbness bilaterally extending in to the sacral dermatomes suggests compression of the cauda equina) should be investigated.

Patients with suspected trauma and or progressive or unstable neurologic deficits should be managed urgently, either in collaboration with or by immediate referral to a spine surgeon.

(ii) Pain History

The pain history should document events surrounding the onset of pain. If a motor vehicle injury is the cause of pain, a thorough history including the use of a seat belt, single or multiple car involvement, and whether impact was from the rear or side of the vehicle can be useful in formulating a differential diagnosis. The pain history should also focus on the location of pain, its duration, radiation, character (e.g., deep, superficial, sharp, aching, burning, shooting, pins and needles, etc.), and worsening or relieving factors. When more than one site is involved, each pain complaint should be documented separately. The usefulness of elements in the pain history are as follows:

- **Location.** The usefulness of location is obvious because it often narrows the search to a specific anatomic region. As described earlier, differentiating axial from radicular pain is among the most important features that will guide treatment.
- **Duration.** Acute spinal pain is typically self-limited and requires only conservative management (see Table 1).
- **Character.** The characteristics used by the patient to describe the pain can be very helpful in differentiating somatic pain from neuropathic pain, thereby guiding subsequent therapy. Somatic pain is usually described as aching and well localized. Neuropathic pain is often described as stabbing, shooting, or burning and may be accompanied by symptoms suggesting nerve dysfunction, such as a "pins and needles" sensation in a limited region. The hallmark of neuropathic pain is allodynia, or pain caused by a normally nonpainful stimulus (e.g., light touch to the affected region causes severe pain).

The pain history should also include previous interventions for pain, including medications, nerve blocks, surgery, physical therapy, and behavioral therapy. A review of previous medical records is often quite useful. A brief history of the patient's activities of daily living and limitations secondary to pain is useful for assessing the benefits of future interventions. In all cases, it is important to include a social and family history to assess the psychosocial support needed to cope with the chronic pain condition.

3. Physical Examination

(i) Comprehensive Physical Examination

Physical examination of the patient with neck or back pain is guided by the features gleaned during the initial interview. The physical examination should include vital signs and a description of the patient's general appearance. It is important to apply all of the information obtained in the history to a directed examination using a sound general approach. Although it is impossible to describe what is needed in every case, some examples have been used in subsequent text to highlight how general medical skills and a general physical examination should be directed based on the patient's history.

- A 62-year-old man presents with axial LBP with intermittent pain in both legs, particularly with ambulation. The pain has become progressively worse over the last several months. He has a history of hypertension and emphysema. His blood pressure is 200/120 mm Hg. The history in this case should be directed toward other ravages of atherosclerosis that may need attention, such as unstable angina, syncope, or near syncope, that might point toward coronary artery disease or cerebrovascular disease. On examination, attention should be directed toward the vasculature of the abdomen and lower extremities. Although the symptoms may well be of spinal origin (e.g., lumbar spinal stenosis), they also may be caused by vascular disease (e.g., aortoocclusive disease and an abdominal aortic aneurysm).
- A 50-year-old woman with a history of renal cell carcinoma presents with back pain 6 months after nephrectomy. In this instance, careful questioning and physical examination should be directed toward detecting metastatic cancer. Epidural spinal metastasis with early spinal cord compression often presents first with back pain. The pain often worsens at night, and the patient may describe severe pain shooting to the extremities on movement (Lehrmitte sign). The patient may report a vague feeling of numbness or heaviness in the extremities without describing frank numbness or weakness. On examination, particular attention should be directed toward neurologic examination of the lower extremities. Spinal cord compression may be accompanied by long-track signs (e.g., positive Babinski sign caused by loss of descending inhibitory pathways, and hyperreflexia in the lower extremities). In this case, further evaluation using diagnostic imaging should be done immediately.

(ii) Examination of the Spine

Directed examination of the patient with neck pain or LBP should include inspection, palpation, range of motion, and a detailed neurologic examination. There are several specific tests that can help isolate the specific cause of pain.

- **Inspection.** Examination of the spine begins with taking note of the patient's gait, posture, and any obvious deformity of the spine. Closer examination of the entire length of the spine for scars, rash, or swelling should follow.
- **Palpation.** Light palpation will detect any sensitivity of the skin (allodynia, suggestive of neuropathic pain); firm palpation and/or percussion can then be used to detect any midline tenderness or mass, paraspinous tenderness, or muscle tightness.
- **Range of motion.** Range of motion of the spine should be examined (i.e., flexion, extension, and lateral bending). Sudden increase in axial pain on motion can signal spinal instability (e.g., a dynamic spondylolisthesis). During the range of motion examination, pain with flexion of the spine can be related to disc pathology, whereas pain with extension can indicate facet arthropathy or spinal stenosis; however, pain on range of motion is not specific and may occur with many causes. Lateral flexion of the neck causes a reduction in the size of the neural foramina; patients with neural foraminal compromise caused by a disc herniation or spondylosis will often report radicular pain that is reproduced by lateral flexion.
- **Neurologic examination.** A thorough neurologic examination, including sensation, strength, and deep tendon reflexes, helps rule out associated spinal cord, nerve root, and peripheral nerve pathology. Any practitioner who examines patients with spinal pain should become familiar with the patterns or referred pain, sensation, and loss of deep tendon reflexes associated with each nerve root and peripheral nerve of the extremities.

- **Tests for specific disorders**
    - **Straight leg raise.** Straight leg raise testing is performed with the patient lying flat in a supine position. With the knee held straight in extension, the examiner raises each leg of the patient by lifting the heel. This produces tension on the lumbar nerve roots. A positive straight leg raise occurs when tension on an irritated nerve root causes pain reproduction (the pain must occur in a radicular pattern), and typically is reported with less than 75 degrees of flexion at the hip.
    - **Patrick or FABER (flexion, abduction, external rotation) test.** The knee is flexed and the lateral malleolus of the ankle is placed on the contralateral patella. The knee is then slowly lowered toward the examination table by external rotation of the leg. Pain caused by hip disease (e.g., osteoarthritis of the hip) is produced by this maneuver and is reported as radiating to the groin along the inguinal ligament. During the same maneuver, the examiner presses over the flexed knee while stabilizing the contralateral side of the pelvis over the anterior, superior iliac spine. This maneuver stresses the sacroiliac (SI) joint and any report of pain over the SI joint should raise the suspicion of SI joint etiology.
    - **Gaenslen test.** Gaenslen test, an alternative test for pain arising from the SI joint, is performed by placing the patient

in the supine position along the edge of the examination table. One leg of the patient is placed over the edge of the examination table and lowered toward the floor in hyperextension while the pelvis is held stable. Pain related to the SI joint is reproduced by this maneuver.

4. Diagnostic Testing

- **Plain radiography.** Plain x-ray can be useful in identifying fractures and ligamentous instability. It is important to include flexion and extension films in any case where ligamentous injury or instability is suspected (e.g., when evaluating a patient following spinal fusion, flexion, and extension films can help detect pseudoarthrosis with persistent instability).
- **Computerized tomography.** Computerized tomography (CT) scan uses x-rays to reconstruct axial images of the spine. In recent years, CT scan has become more sophisticated and sagittal, frontal, and even three-dimensional reconstructed images can now be assembled by the most advanced machines. Because CT scan relies on x-ray penetration, it is best for detecting bone abnormalities such as fracture or tumor infiltration that has disrupted bone. CT scan with contrast infusion can delineate vascular abnormalities, including vascular tumors.
- **Magnetic Resonance Imaging.** Magnetic resonance imaging (MRI) is the imaging modality of choice under most circumstances except when fracture is suspected. MRI can detect subtle differences in soft tissue composition, and therefore is the technique that is best used for suspected infection or tumor. Vascular abnormalities including tumor and epidural scarring can be further delineated using contrast enhancement with gadolinium. MRI studies of the spine routinely include detailed sagittal reconstructions, which allow careful examination of the intervertebral foramina for anatomic causes of neural impingement.
- **Provocative discography.** Provocative discography entails inserting a small-caliber needle into the center of an intervertebral disc that is suspected to be the cause of pain. A small volume of radiographic contrast is then placed within the disc and the patient is questioned about reproduction of his or her symptoms. A discogram is said to be concordant when an intradiscal injection at the site of suspected pathology reproduces the patient's typical pain and an injection within an adjacent normal-appearing disc produces no pain. Some practitioners use provocative discography to plan the level of treatment for intradiscal techniques and/or spinal fusion. Discography should only be performed in those patients when further intervention is planned in the event the discogram reveals symptomatic disc degeneration.
- **Electrodiagnostic testing.** Electromyography (EMG) and nerve conduction velocity (NCV) testing are typically performed in parallel to test the physiologic function of nerve conduction, integrity of the neuromuscular junction, and muscle contraction. For the patient with radicular pain, EMG/NCV

can help differentiate acute from chronic radiculopathy, as well as identify patients with peripheral nerve abnormalities.

Further descriptions of history taking, physical examination, and radiologic testing for pain patients can be found in Chapters 4 and 5. Table 7 summarizes the differentiating features of LBP.

III. DISORDERS CAUSING BACK AND NECK PAIN

1. Facet Joint Pain

Pain originating from the facet joints has a similar presentation and may be difficult to distinguish from discogenic pain. Typically, the pain is gradual in onset and is described as a deep, aching pain localized around the midline; standing and sitting intolerance may also be present. Extension and lateral bending of the affected region of the spine are usually painful. Referred pain to the shoulder, buttock, and proximal extremities is also common. Pain is caused by stress of the facet joint capsule secondary to loss of disc or vertebral height and normally accompanies degenerative disc disease. Pain also may be caused by isolated or coexisting osteoarthritis of the facet joints; in those with isolated facet arthropathy, the pain tends to be less severe and is often described as "morning stiffness." In rare instances, facet joint pain may originate from fracture or hemarthrosis following trauma.

Physical examination is usually without focal abnormalities. Many patients will report paraspinal tenderness and pain on extension and lateral bending. Imaging studies may help identify pathology such as loss of disc or vertebral height, spondylolisthesis, or other degenerative changes. Diagnostic local anesthetic block under fluoroscopic guidance is the most accurate way to isolate the facet joint as the source of axial spine pain, but a significant proportion of patients will report temporary relief even when placebo is injected (diagnostic blocks are described in Chapter 12). Radio frequency treatment of the medial branches nerves supplying sensory innervation to the facet joints provides moderately effective long-term therapy for axial spine pain originating from the facet joints.

2. Sacroiliac Joint Pain

Sacroiliac joint dysfunction typically presents with localized pain in the lower back or upper buttock overlying the SI joint. Pain may be referred to the posterior thigh, but pain extending below the knee is unusual. In most cases, the etiology is unclear, and the onset is gradual over months to years. Trauma, infection, and tumor are uncommon causes of SI joint pain. Physical examination may reveal localized tenderness over the joint, and Patrick test (FABER test) and Gaenslen test may reproduce pain in the area of the SI joint (see discussion of physical examination in the preceding text). Degenerative change of the joint on x-ray is uncommon and nonspecific; most patients with SI joint-related pain have normal SI joint appearance on radiography. Resolution of pain following intraarticular injection of local anesthetic under fluoroscopic or CT scan guidance is the best diagnostic tool available to establish the SI joint as the source of pain; as with facet joint pain, definitive diagnosis is hindered by the significant placebo effect of diagnostic injection. Treatment of SI joint pain

Table 7. Differentiating features of low back pain

	Trigger Point	Sitting Intolerance	Sensory or Motor Deficit	Dermatomal Pain Pattern	Pain on Extension	Pain on Flexion	SLR Test	Diagnostic Test
Discogenic Pain	Usually absent	Usually present	Usually absent	Usually absent	May be present	Usually present	Usually absent	Discography
Facet Joint Pain	May be present	May be present	Usually absent	Usually absent	Usually present	Usually absent	Usually absent	Medial branch block
SI Joint Pain	Usually absent	May be present	Usually absent	Usually absent	May be present	May be present	Usually absent	Intraarticular anesthetic block
Spinal Stenosis	Usually absent	Usually absent	May be present	Usually absent	Usually present	Usually absent	May be present	MRI study
Myofascial Pain	Usually present	Usually absent	Usually absent	Usually absent	May be present	May be present	Usually absent	TP injection with anesthetic
Failed Back Surgery Syndrome	May be present	May be present	May be present	May be present	May be present	May be present	May be present	History
Radiculopathy	Usually absent	May be present	Likely to be present	Likely to be present	May be present	May be present	Usually present	EMG

SLR, straight leg raising; TP, trigger point; SI, sacro iliac; MRI, magnetic resonance imaging; EMG, electromyography.

379

remains inadequate and controversial. Currently, periodic intra-articular injection of steroid with local anesthetic is a common therapy for SI joint pain but typically provides only transient relief (see Chapter 12).

3. Spinal Stenosis

Spinal stenosis refers to both central canal narrowing and foraminal narrowing, and is caused by progressive calcification of the spinal elements surrounding the central canal. Hypertrophy and calcification of the facet joints can lead to isolated foraminal stenosis, but when combined with similar changes in the posterior longitudinal ligament and ligamentum flavum, these may produce narrowing of the central spinal canal. Symptoms from central canal narrowing tend to be diffuse compared to foraminal narrowing (where impingement on the exiting nerve root often produces radicular pain in a dermatomal distribution). The clinical presentation of central canal narrowing includes axial spine pain and extremity pain. The degree of axial and extremity pain varies among individuals; pain tends to start over the axis of the spine and gradually involve the extremities. The pain tends to be diffuse (nondermatomal) and is usually characterized as aching or cramping in the extremities with ambulation (neurogenic claudication). The claudication is typically most severe when walking downhill and with other activities that cause extension of the spine (indeed, older patients often describe being most comfortable when walking hunched forward and pushing a grocery cart about—this position significantly increases the dimensions of the foramina). Rest and flexion of the spine usually provide temporary relief. A simple albeit less than perfect way to distinguish neurogenic from vascular claudication is to have patients ride an exercise bike. Patients with neurogenic claudication usually have no pain because they are leaning forward when on the bike, whereas those with vascular claudication will still have ischemic pain when on the bike. Spinal stenosis is more common in older individuals and may be associated with age-related changes of the spine. CT scan or MRI can be useful in delineating the causes and extent of the narrowing.

In mild to moderate cases, periodic epidural steroid injection may reduce claudication symptoms for some time. If there is no improvement from epidural steroid injections, a surgical consultation may be sought to assess the likelihood that decompression surgery may be of benefit. Symptoms stemming from cervical spinal stenosis may involve both upper and lower extremities and an early surgical consultation should be sought.

4. Discogenic Pain

Degenerative disc disease is a leading cause of neck pain and LBP. The patient with neck pain or LBP, originating from the vertebral disc, often presents with deep, aching, axial midline pain. Pain can be referred to the shoulder or scapular regions from cervical discs and the buttocks and posterior thigh from lumber discs but does not extend in to the distal extremities. Patients with discogenic pain are often young and otherwise healthy. Discogenic pain is common in those with jobs that require repetitive motion of the affected spine segment (such as package handlers) or that expose the spine to excessive vibration (such as long-distance truck drivers, helicopter pilots, and jackhammer operators). The onset of symptoms is usually gradual. Pain is experienced with prolonged sitting (sitting intolerance), standing, and bending forward. The referred pain usually remains in the proximal part of the extremity. Results of physical examination are usually nonspecific, with limited range of motion at the affected segment, or pain with movement, particularly on flexion. Straight leg raise is usually normal.

Morphologically, a normal disc has a unilocular, bilocular, spherical or rectangular shape. A degenerated disc loses its water content and may have tears and fissures in the annulus fibrosus. The most common types of annular tears are concentric, radial, and transverse.

MRI and CT scan reveal only nonspecific findings. However, certain MRI findings are highly suggestive of discogenic disease: (a) decreased disc signal intensity on T2-weighted MRI images suggests dehydration; (b) high T2-weighted signal within the annulus has been termed high-intensity zone (HIZ) and is associated with annular tears and a higher incidence of LBP; (c) a "bulging" or "protruding" disc on MRI is more likely associated with disc disruption and pain than a "normal disc"; (d) even a completely normal disc on MRI can be found to be associated with discogenic pain. Decrease in disc height is often seen when internal disc derangement has taken place. For those patients in whom further intervention is warranted [e.g. intradiscal electrothermal therapy (IDET) of surgical fusion], provocative discography is an accepted test to determine whether anatomic abnormality of the discs that are apparent on imaging studies are causing discogenic pain (described in Chapter 12).

Treatment of discogenic pain starts with conservative therapy, including physical therapy (e.g., McKenzie exercises or dynamic lumbar stabilization) and oral nonsteroidal antiinflammatory drugs (NSAIDs). In those patients with prolonged or disabling pain that is confirmed to be of discogenic origin using discography, IDET therapy or surgical referral for spinal fusion may be warranted.

5. Failed Back Surgery Syndrome

A diagnosis of failed back surgery syndrome is given to patients who have chronic pain after spine surgery. The surgery may have been performed only for the purpose of relieving pain or it may have been done for other reasons including stabilization or decompression to relieve neurologic deficit. Although this term is often used indiscriminately, it is important to closely question each patient who presents with pain after surgery to identify those with a new or persistent problem needing further diagnostic evaluation. Pain may vary significantly, and be accompanied by neurologic deficits. In those with chronic pain after previous spine surgery, the first differentiation to be made is to sort those with primarily axial pain from those with predominantly radicular pain. Patients with axial back pain after spinal fusion should first be evaluated by the surgeon to assess the success of the surgical intervention; failure of the fusion to stop mobility in the spinal segment fused (pseudoarthrosis) is a surprisingly common cause for persistent pain after fusion. In those with a distant fusion and worsening axial back pain, the additional wear and tear on the facet joints directly above and below the fused segment may cause significant pain. In contrast, those with persistent radicular pain often have chronic nerve injury and treatment of neuropathic pain will prove most beneficial. Therapy for failed back surgery syndrome should be directed at the suspected etiology as determined by this simple division into axial and radicular pain. For patients with radicular pain, epidural steroid injection via the foraminal or caudal route can be a useful and relatively benign initial intervention. Spinal cord stimulation has proven effective for persistent, neuropathic pain following spinal surgery, particularly radicular pain limited to a single extremity (see Chapter 13).

6. Myofascial Pain

Neck and LBP of myofascial origin is common, especially after trauma and repetitive motion injury. Myofascial pain presents as deep aching and poorly localized discomfort that worsens with activity. Pain is thought to be due to strain or sprain injury to the muscles and ligaments. Patients may complain only of paraspinal muscle discomfort, or the pain may extend to the occipital, scapular, and shoulder areas or buttocks and upper thigh areas. It is important to distinguish somatic referred pain (from disc or facet joint pathology) from pain of muscular origin, but it is quite difficult to make this distinction in most cases. Physical examination may reveal tight, tender muscle bands that produce radiating pain (so-called trigger points). Various physiotherapy techniques (stretching and strengthening exercise, massage, iontophoresis) remain the initial therapy of choice (see Chapter 16). Injection of local anesthetic into the trigger points may be useful, especially if a coordinated physiotherapy program immediately follows the injection. Some physicians add steroid with local anesthetic for trigger point injections; although this is a common practice, the risks and benefits of steroid-containing trigger point injections have not been subjected to scientific scrutiny. Myofascial pain is also described in Chapter 17.

7. Rare Causes of Back Pain

Infection, tumor, aortic aneurysm, sickle cell crisis, retroperitoneal mass, and chronic pancreatitis are among the rare causes of axial spine pain with or without extremity pain. These rare causes of pain highlight the need for a strong general medical background among pain practitioners, the critical need for a thorough medical history and the importance of maintaining a high index of suspicion in those who do not respond to initial treatment attempts.

IV. TREATMENT PRINCIPLES

1. General Principles

Comprehensive and aggressive medical treatment is used to achieve functional restoration, and reduce reliance on long-term medical treatment. Despite these efforts, some cases remain refractory to treatment, and these require a careful multidisciplinary approach. The modalities described here could be utilized as part of an aggressive rehabilitative approach, or used continuously or occasionally as part of a long-term treatment plan. Each modality is described in detail in separate chapters of this book. Here, rationale and principles for their use in LBP are discussed.

2. Medications

Each class of medication has its own set of liabilities, and reliance on medication should be minimized whenever possible.

(i) Nonsteroidal Antiinflammatory Drugs

NSAIDs have been used extensively for the treatment of LBP arising from facet joints, disc herniation, sacroiliac joints, and soft tissues. Nearly all structures in the low back may become acutely inflamed, and ongoing inflammation is appropriately treated with an NSAID. Nevertheless, despite a long history of successful and often benign treatment of back pain with NSAIDs, serious adverse effects may arise, some of which have only come to light recently. The use of standard (nonselective) NSAIDs has been plagued with the side effect of gastrointestinal (GI) toxicity, bleeding, and sometimes death from bleeding. The newer selective *coxibs*, developed expressly to minimize GI toxicity, have now been associated with increased death from myocardial infarction and stroke. These effects are discussed in detail in Chapter 8.

Adverse effects from NSAIDs are much more likely to arise in cases of chronic rather than acute pain management. Manufacturers of standard NSAIDs recommend a maximum course of 10 days, although long-term use of **coxibs** is no longer recommended because of their deleterious cardiovascular effects. NSAIDs do not alter the course of inflammatory disease, but have provided useful pain relief for a large number of patients over many years. New concerns over the safety of both standard NSAIDs and **coxibs** will make the choice between NSAIDs and opioids for long-term treatment of the arthritides even more difficult.

(ii) Opioids

Opioids are a useful adjunct during active rehabilitation (see Table 5). Like all other medications, opioids have major adverse effects; ideally, patients should be weaned from opioid treatment at the end of each period of active rehabilitation. However, certain patients with refractory pain may benefit from long-term opioid therapy. A consensus exists that opioids can relieve pain and improve function in select patients with refractory LBP. In fact, opioid analgesics may be the only medical intervention that brings relief to some patients, and may be safer than NSAID therapy, particularly in older patients. Chronic LBP is frequently a mixture of nociceptive and neuropathic pain and responds better to opioid therapy than does sciatic pain.

The use and liabilities of long-term opioid therapy are fully described in Chapter 30.

(iii) Adjuvant Analgesics

The addition of adjuvant analgesics is indicated if assessment suggests that neuropathic or muscle pain is contributing to a patient's pain. In general, these medications maintain their efficacy over the long term, and therefore, their use has become increasingly popular. The key is to initiate therapy early and to titrate any particular agent to an effective dose while monitoring side effects. Trial and error are often needed in order to determine which medication(s) will be beneficial.

1. **Antidepressants**—Tricyclic antidepressants are particularly helpful in controlling the pain related to inflamed or injured lumbar roots, alleviating muscle-related pain, restoring sleep, and, at higher doses, improving depression.
2. **Antiepileptic drugs**—These are especially useful in controlling the sharp stabbing pain related to nerve root pathology.
3. **α_2 agonists**—Although uncommonly used as monotherapy, these drugs may augment the effects of other medications such as opioids or muscle relaxants.
4. **Skeletal muscle relaxants**—These medications are particularly helpful in alleviating painful muscle spasm, but their effectiveness typically wanes after 10 to 14 days of use.

These drugs are described in more detail in Chapter 10.

3. Physical Therapy

LBP is commonly associated with soft tissue pathology, often with secondary compensatory muscle spasm accompanying the underlying spine pathology, and with particular involvement of the abdominal and paraspinal musculature. Rehabilitation, including strengthening of this musculature through lumbar stabilization has been shown to reduce pain and to improve function. In many instances, muscle pathology is the primary cause of LBP and can be treated in a lumbar stabilization program. Physical therapy is typically short-term and goal directed. Patients are educated on activities to be avoided in order to prevent further injury to the spine. The overall practical goals of physical therapy in the chronic setting are as follows:

- Promote and maintain function
- Prevent further injury
- Alleviate pain and facilitate return of normal function using various modalities [e.g., application of cold or heat, ultrasound, or transcutaneous electrical nerve stimulation (TENS)]

Patients must actively participate in their treatment over the long term to derive benefit in chronic relentless LBP, but most patients can learn a self-care program that can be continued independently. The injection of painful trigger points in taut bands of muscle with either local anesthetic or local anesthetic and corticosteroid may assist physical therapy. Physical treatment modalities are described in more detail in Chapter 16.

4. Psychological Therapies

There are various psychological approaches to altering behavior in patients with chronic pain. In most cases, these modalities are used in combination to treat chronic LBP. These approaches include the following:

- Behavioral therapy
- Cognitive therapy

- Cognitive behavioral therapy
- Biofeedback, relaxation
- Family therapy
- Hypnosis
- Meditation
- Mind–body medicine

These methods involve relaxation training, stress management, positive coping skills, and altering maladaptive thoughts, feelings, and behavior. Assessment and treatment by a psychologist early in the course of LBP may limit the development of passive coping strategies, which are associated with a perception of helplessness and a greater degree of psychological and physical disability. Psychological assessment and treatment are described in more detail in Chapter 15.

Psychiatric illness is prevalent in the chronic LBP population. Depression is most common, followed by anxiety disorder, somatization disorder, and personality disorder. Psychopathology influences the reporting of pain level; in turn, psychopathology may vary in severity depending on the degree of chronic LBP. Because of this complex interaction, psychopathologic conditions require identification and treatment before embarking on interventional therapies. Therapeutic treatment of psychiatric disorder(s) in a patient with chronic LBP does not, however, discount the potential for a true biologic source. More detail can be found in Chapter 36.

5. Interventional Treatments

See Chapters 12 and 13 for a full description of the interventional treatments.

(i) Acute Radicular Pain and Use Of Epidural Steroid Injections

Nerve root inflammation initiated by disc herniation occurs in the epidural space. The nucleus pulposus contains proinflammatory substances such as hydrogen ions, stromelysin, and phospholipase A_2. The deposition of high concentrations of corticosteroid around nerve roots can reduce or eliminate inflammation. Additional potential beneficial effects of corticosteroids include the following:

- Inhibition of phospholipase A_2, which prevents the formation of prostaglandins that are responsible for inflammation and that contribute to central sensitization.
- Reduction of inflammatory edema surrounding the affected dorsal root ganglion and exiting nerve root, with improvement of the microcirculation.
- Inhibition of ectopic discharges originating from an injured nerve root by exerting a membrane stabilizing effect.

ESI is the most commonly used procedure in the management of LBP associated with radicular symptoms, and can be used for both acute and chronic presentations. ESI using a translaminar or transforaminal approach appears to speed resolution of pain in patients with radicular pain due to herniated nucleus pulposus. Recent trials suggest that radiographic guidance and placement of steroids directly on the affected nerve root via a transforaminal approach may preempt or prevent the need for surgical intervention in some of these patients. We routinely use fluoroscopic guidance for ESI because of the improved accuracy of delivering the steroid to the level of pathology.

There are few data to guide the frequency and dosing for ESI. Anecdotally, periodic injections appear to provide ongoing pain reduction in a subset of patients without adverse effects. The steroid preparations commonly used for ESI (e.g., methylprednisolone acetate, betamethasone phosphate/betamethasone acetate suspension, or triamcinolone acetonide) are known to produce suppression of the hypothalamic-pituitary axis for 1 to 3 weeks. Spacing repeated injections at 2 to 3 month intervals therefore seems reasonable to allow for recovery of endogenous corticosteroid production. With 2 to 3 month intervals between injections, the most frequent adverse effect observed is fluid retention in the form of mild pedal edema, but this is uncommon. Serious musculoskeletal complications such as osteopenia, avascular necrosis of the humeral or femoral heads, and muscle wasting are rare.

(ii) Management of Painful Joints in the Low Back

SACROILIAC JOINT INJECTION. The established causes of sacroiliac joint pain include spondyloarthropathies, trauma, infection, and malignancy. Sacroiliac pain is accepted as a valid source of chronic LBP. The specific pathophysiology for the sacroiliac syndrome consisting of pain emanating from the sacroiliac joint radiating to the groin, medial buttocks, and posterior thighs is unknown. Multiple provocative findings from physical examination may suggest that the sacroiliac joint is the source of LBP in a particular patient. Radiographic evaluation is of inconsistent value. Injection of this joint under fluoroscopy can eliminate the pain and support the diagnosis of sacroiliac joint syndrome.

Because of the elusive cause of the sacroiliac syndrome, the treatment of this entity is not clearly established. Initial therapy involves NSAIDs, muscle balancing, pelvic stabilization exercises, and orthoses. Fluoroscopically guided sacroiliac joint injections with local anesthetic and depo-corticosteroid may improve pain and enhance physical rehabilitation in the short term (4 to 8 weeks). Small studies and anecdotal reports describe modalities used to bring about longer-term relief (e.g., radio frequency lesioning of the SI joint), but no therapy has been universally accepted, and there is no long-term outcome data for large patient populations.

LUMBAR FACET JOINT INJECTIONS. Lumbar facet (zygapophysial) joints are an accepted cause of axial LBP with radiation into the buttocks and posterior thighs. Although rheumatoid arthritis and ankylosing spondylitis can affect the lumbar facets, osteoarthritis is by far the most common cause of pain stemming from these joints. The development of painful degenerative facet arthritis is thought to relate to abnormal compressive loads caused by initial intervertebral disc degeneration. The history, physical examination, and radiologic imaging can suggest the possibility of a lumbar facet pain syndrome but are nonspecific; the only means available to establish the diagnosis and begin treatment is with intraarticular injections or blockade of the nerve supply to the joints under fluoroscopic guidance. As with sacroiliac joint syndrome, multiple blocks may be needed to confirm the diagnosis of facet pain.

Many patients derive symptomatic pain relief from periodic intraarticular injections of corticosteroid. If medial branch blockade (the nerve supply to the facet joints) offers similar benefit to intraarticular injections, one can proceed to neuroablation. We typically use medial branch blocks to establish that pain relief can be obtained from targeted neural blockade before proceeding to radio frequency treatment. It is also reasonable to proceed directly with radio frequency treatment in patients who report temporary relief with intraarticular facet injection.

(iii) *Management of Discogenic Low Back Pain*

Degeneration of the intervertebral discs occurs with aging and may lead to internal disc disruption in the form of concentric or radial tears within the annulus fibrosis. Internal disc disruption may lead to painless loss of disc height or significant axial back pain. Pain from internal disc disruption is thought to be caused by chemical and mechanical activation of nociceptors within the torn annulus. Because anatomic abnormalities of the intervertebral discs on diagnostic imaging studies are ubiquitous, even in patients without symptoms, diagnostic discography has been used to identify those abnormal discs that are the cause of pain. The usefulness of discography remains controversial, largely because it is a subjective test that relies on the patient's report of pain during the test to identify problematic discs. The management of discogenic LBP continues to be challenging and controversial, but has traditionally consisted of conservative therapy. Until recently, the only alternative for those with persistent and debilitating pain was surgical fusion. Newer intradiscal procedures, particularly IDET have shown limited effectiveness for treating early discogenic pain in patients with well-preserved disc height. A growing number of minimally invasive alternatives to disc surgery now exist that appear promising. Intradiscal treatments are described in greater detail in Chapter 12. For those with persistent discogenic pain unresponsive to more conservative treatment or for those who have persistent pain following spinal fusion, use of neuromodulation techniques may be useful (see further discussion in the subsequent text).

(iv) *Management of Chronic Radicular Pain*

A subgroup of patients who have acute radicular pain associated with herniated nucleus pulposus will go on to have persistent radicular pain. Indeed, despite surgical decompression, persistent radicular pain is not uncommon. Likewise, a subset of patients who undergo various types of spinal surgery will have persistent or new onset of radicular pain. It is important to separate those patients who have new onset of radicular symptoms after complete resolution of prior symptoms following surgery. This group warrants detailed diagnostic evaluation to rule out recurrent disc herniation and other mechanical causes of radicular pain (e.g., hardware impinging on an exiting nerve root).

Electrodiagnostic testing (EMG/NCV) can be useful in identifying the affected nerve root as well as separating acute from chronic radiculopathies, but all too often EMG/NCV are completely normal even in the face of severe radicular pain. For those with persistent radicular pain and no identifiable mechanical cause, treatment is limited. Treatment should begin with adjuvant analgesics directed at treatment of neuropathic pain (see discussion of adjuvant analgesics in the preceding text). In patients with severe radicular pain that does not respond to more conservative therapy, spinal cord stimulation can provide significant long-term pain relief (see further discussion in the subsequent text).

(v) Use of Neuromodulation in the Treatment of Chronic Low Back and Radicular Pain

These are described in detail in Chapter 13.

SPINAL CORD STIMULATION. Pain that arises from a lumbosacral radiculopathy may no longer be responsive to oral medications, injection methods, lysis of adhesions, radiofrequency lesioning, or further lumbar spine surgery. At this point, a nerve root(s) has likely incurred have significant injury related to spinal pathology. Arachnoiditis or epidural fibrosis that can follow lumbar spine surgery may also be the cause of persistent neuropathic pain. The etiology of persistent pain related to lumbosacral rhizopathy is often multifactorial. Regardless of the cause, spinal cord stimulation can provide significant long-term pain reduction.

The most challenging aspect of pain therapy with spinal cord stimulation is patient selection. The patients chosen for a trial of spinal cord stimulation have referred neuropathic pain into the lower extremities and have exhausted most of the treatment options or cease to be candidates for those treatments. The pain should be characterized as severe and neuropathic, persisting for longer than 6 months. A psychological evaluation is important to address motivational, social, psychological, and support issues that might predispose to a poor outcome. Chemical dependence, secondary gain, unrealistic expectations, personality disorders, ongoing litigation, and depression are common contributors to failure of spinal cord stimulation. The failure of earlier therapies may depend more on these issues than a pure inability to control the biologic cause of the pain.

INTRATHECAL DRUG THERAPY. Implantable intrathecal drug delivery systems are reserved for patients with severe refractory pain. Such therapy has been used to manage both chronic axial LBP and chronic, neuropathic radicular pain, but should be considered only after all other possibilities have been exhausted. The same psychological screening used for spinal cord stimulators applies to implantable pumps. In general, most practitioners would choose spinal cord stimulation over intrathecal therapy in those patients with radicular pain in a single extremity. Both spinal cord stimulation and intrathecal therapy have been used successfully for treating chronic axial LBP, and the advantage of one therapy over the other is unclear. There is no data to guide this choice, but the complexity of intrathecal therapy is greater and mandates periodic return for refill of the pump throughout the entire long-term course of treatment. All patients undergo intrathecal drug trials to assess for side effects and analgesic efficacy.

Successful management of patients with implanted drug delivery systems requires frequent and meticulous evaluation. Polyanalgesic mixtures of intrathecal drugs, often including an opioid, local anesthetic, and α_2-agonist are necessary to control symptoms. Baclofen is added in many cases for refractory spasm and for its analgesic properties, especially for neuropathic pain. Patients are usually seen monthly for refill of the pump reservoir. Tolerance to the analgesic effects of opioids often arises over time, sometimes necessitating dose escalation to neurotoxic doses. Consideration should always be given to weaning the patient from intrathecal opioid therapy when this occurs, even if the therapy is reestablished at lower dose later in the treatment course.

V. CONCLUSION

In most cases of LBP, the anatomic diagnosis remains unclear. LBP and neck pain of unclear etiology is a legitimate diagnosis. Most of the initial painful episodes will resolve without specific treatment, but most patients will also have recurrent pain at some point later in life. Providing symptomatic relief using a short course of acetaminophen, an NSAID, or a short-acting opioid analgesic with or without a skeletal muscle relaxant is common and accepted practice. All patients should be encouraged to remain active, as bed rest simply prolongs the time required for full functional recovery. If no improvement is seen within 3 weeks, physical therapy may be helpful. Physical therapists can assist with return to full ambulation as well as providing instruction in use of proper body mechanics to avoid further injury, and symptomatic relief using modalities such as heat, ultrasound, and iontophoresis. If axial neck pain or LBP lasts for more than 12 weeks, an attempt should be made to establish an anatomic diagnosis; the evaluation, including use of diagnostic imaging, electrodiagnostic testing, or diagnostic nerve blocks is best guided by the pattern of symptoms, as discussed throughout this chapter.

SELECTED READINGS

Abram SE. Treatment of lumbosacral radiculopathy with epidural steroids. *Anesthesiology* 1999;91:1937–1941.

Barnsley L, Lord S, Wallis B, et al. False positive rates of cervical Z-joint blocks. *Clin J Pain* 1993;9:124–130.

Bogduk N. Low back pain. *The clinical anatomy of the lumbar spine and sacrum*, 3rd ed. Edinburgh, UK: Churchill Livingstone, 1999a: 188–189.

Bogduk N. *Acute lumbar radicular pain.* Newcastle, UK: Cambridge Press, 1999b:5.

Bogduk N, Aprill C. On the nature of neck pain, discography and cervical Z-joint pain. *Pain* 1993;54:213–217.

Cohen SP, Mullings R, Abdi S. The pharmacologic treatment of muscle pain. *Anesthesiology* 2004;101:495–526.

Kapural L, Mekail N, Korunda Z, et al. Intradiscal thermal annuloplasty for the treatment of lumbar discogenic pain in patients with multilevel degenerative disc disease. *Anesth Analg* 2004;99:472–476.

Kuslich SD, Ulstrom CL, Michael CJ, et al. The tissue origin of LBP and sciatica: a report of pain response to tissue stimulation during operation on the lumber spine using local anesthesia. *Orthop Clin North Am* 1991;22:181–187.

Maigne JY, Aivaliklis A, Pfefer F. Results of SI joint double block and value of sacroiliac pain provocation tests in 54 patients with LBP. *Spine* 1996;21:1889–1892.

Manchikanti L, Staats PS, Singh V, et al. Evidence-based practice guidelines for interventional techniques in the management of chronic spinal pain. *Pain Phys* 2003;6:3–81.

Schwarzer AC, Aprill CN, Derby R, et al. The false positive rate of uncontrolled diagnostic blocks of the lumber Z-joints. *Pain* 1994;58: 195–200.

Schwarzer AC, Aprill CN, Derby R, et al. The prevalence and clinical features of internal disc disruption in patients with chronic low back pain. *Spine* 1995;20:1878–1883.

Waddell G, McCulloch JA, Kummel E, et al. Nonorganic physical signs in low-back pain. *Spine* 1980;5:117–125.

Warfield CA, Bajwa ZH. *Principles and practice of pain medicine.* New York: McGraw-Hill, 2004.

28

Headache

Fred Michael Cutrer and David F. Black

I have a pain upon my forehead here.
—*William Shakespeare, 1564–1616, Othello, Act 3, Scene 3*

Headache descriptions and treatments can be found in pre-Christian Sumerian and Egyptian writings. Aretaeus of Cappadocia in 2nd-century Turkey writes of people with headaches who "hid from the light and wished for death." Headache is a common affliction; in 1985, a large-scale survey-based study in the United States reported that headaches occur in 78% of women and in 68% of men. It is estimated that 40% of adults in North America have experienced a severe, debilitating headache at least once in their lives.

Despite its long history and great prevalence in the population, the complaint of recurrent headache is still met with widespread indifference and suspicion among many health care providers. As a result, the patient with headaches must often contend with haphazard and sometimes even inappropriate treatment. Such an attitude is unnecessary and can lead to tragic results because headaches not only can be the presenting symptom for a serious, even life-threatening abnormality, but also are liable to show a good response to therapy in most patients.

I. ANATOMY OF HEAD PAIN

More than 50 years ago, epilepsy surgery performed on the brains of conscious patients under local anesthesia indicated that brain tissue itself was relatively insensate to electrical or mechanical stimulation, whereas electrical stimulation of the meninges or meningeal blood vessels produced a severe penetrating headache. The meninges and meningeal vessels are richly supplied with C-fibers (small fibers) and are the key structures involved in the generation of headache. The C-fibers from the meninges converge into the trigeminal nerve and project to the trigeminal nucleus caudalis in the lower medulla where they synapse. From the caudal brainstem, fibers carrying nociceptive signals project to more rostral trigeminal subnuclei and the thalamus (ventral posterior medial, medial, and intralaminar nuclei). Projections from the thalamus ascend to the cerebral cortex, where painful information is localized, and reaches consciousness (see Fig. 1).

II. PATHOPHYSIOLOGY OF HEADACHE

Head pain results from the activation of the pain fibers that innervate intracranial structures regardless of the activating stimulus. In a small number of patients, an identifiable structural or inflammatory source for the headache can be found using neuroimaging or other laboratory investigations. However, most patients encountered in clinical practice have primary headache disorders such as migraine or tension-type headache in which physical examinations and laboratory studies are unrevealing. Research into the pathophysiology of headache has been limited by the subjective nature of the complaints and the paucity of animal models with which to test hypotheses.

1. Genetic Underpinning of Primary Headache Disorders

It is becoming increasingly clear that primary headache disorders such as migraine are strongly influenced by heterogeneous genetic factors. Familial hemiplegic migraine (FHM), an uncommon autosomally dominant subtype, has been shown to occur because of defects within a single gene. In roughly 60% of families studied, the mutation is located on chromosome 19 and codes the α_1 A subunit of a brain-specific P/Q type calcium channel. In another 20% of families, the mutation lies in a gene on chromosome 1 that encodes the α_2 subunit of a Na^+ K^+ pump. Even within a rare subtype such as FHM, the genetic basis is complex, which predicts even greater heterogeneity for the more common forms such as migraine with and without aura. Several genetic linkage sites have been identified for these more common forms.

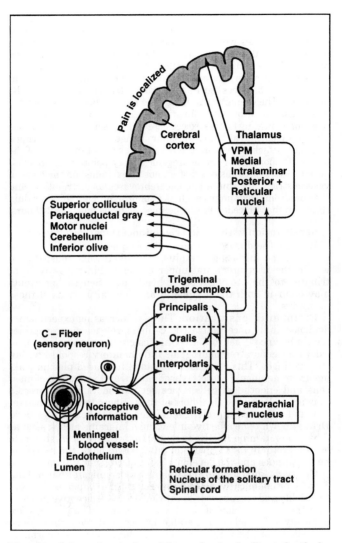

Figure 1.   Schematic overview of the mechanism leading to headache pain perception after activation of trigeminovascular nociceptive neurons.

2. Traditional Theories of Migraine: Vasogenic versus Neurogenic

In the late 1930s, investigators proposed the **vasogenic theory** of migraine, which hypothesized that intracranial vasoconstriction was responsible for the aura of migraine and that the headache resulted from rebound dilation and distention of cranial vessels. This theory was based on the observations that: (a) cranial vessels were important in the generation of headache; (b) extracranial vessels became distended and pulsated during a migraine attack in many patients; and, (c) vasoconstrictive substances such as ergots could abort the headache, whereas vasodilatory substances such as nitrates tended to provoke the headache. The competing **neurogenic theory** held that migraine was caused by a brain dysfunction. According to this hypothesis, when precipitating factors exceed cerebral threshold, a migraine attack occurred, and although vascular changes might occur during a migraine attack, they were the result rather than the cause of the attack. Proponents of the neurogenic theory pointed out that migraine aura symptoms could often not be explained on the basis of vasoconstriction within a single cerebrovascular distribution, and that prodromal symptoms such as euphoria, hunger, thirst or fluid retention that preceded headache in some by as much as 24 hours.

3. Sensitization within the Trigeminocervical Pain System

Because the duration of headache frequently exceeds the duration of the initiating stimulus, it is likely that sensitization within the trigeminal and upper cervical pain pathways contributes to the prolongation of headaches. Sensitizing events may occur in both the peripheral and central portions of these pathways.

Peripheral sensitization: There is increasing experimental evidence that, once activated, C-fibers release neuropeptides (i.e., substance P, neurokinin A, and calcitonin gene–related peptide) that generate a neurogenic inflammatory response within the meninges. This response consists of increased plasma leakage from meningeal vessels, vasodilation, and activation of mast cells and endothelial cells. Once set into motion, this process may act to lower the threshold of the C-fibers to further activation and, as a result, prolong and intensify the headache attack. Drugs known to be effective in ending a migraine attack such as dihydroergotamine (DHE) or sumatriptan have been shown to act at serotonin (5-HT) receptor subtypes to block the release of neuropeptides and the development of neurogenic inflammation.

Central Sensitization: Animal studies indicate that inflammatory or chemical C-activation results in expansion of receptive fields and recruitment of previously nonnociceptive neurons into the transmission of painful information. The changes are clinically reflected as hyperalgesia (lowered pain thresholds) and allodynia (the generation of a painful response by normally nonpainful stimuli). Analogous clinical phenomena are seen in headache disorders. For example, minor head movements, bending, or coughing, which normally do not cause pain, are perceived as painful during or in the hours following a migraine attack. Recent studies by Burstein et al. have demonstrated the stimulation of meningeal nociceptors, causes a lowering of the activation thresholds for convergent previously nonpainful skin stimulation. Subsequent studies of human subjects during migraine attacks have also demonstrated the development of cutaneous allodynia both within the areas innervated by the trigeminal nerve and in extratrigeminal areas.

III. CLINICAL APPROACH TO ACUTE HEADACHE

When faced with a patient in the emergency room (ER) whose primary complaint is that of a severe headache, the first question to ask is whether the headache is symptomatic of a potentially serious underlying abnormality requiring rapid and appropriate treatment. In most cases, the headache will represent a particularly severe episode in a primary headache disorder. However, the distinction between primary and secondary (symptomatic of another cause) headache must be made as rapidly and as accurately as possible. It is crucial to use the history and physical exam to decide whether the patient is at high or low risk, to order diagnostic tests, and to provide therapy accordingly. Laboratory tests and imaging studies ordered without good clinical indication are usually unhelpful and always expensive.

1. Important Questions to Ask

(i) **Is this headache the first of its kind?** If the headache is unlike anything experienced previously, the risk increases. If it is similar (even if of greater intensity) to attacks experienced over many months or years, the likelihood that it is a benign process increases. This question becomes increasingly important for patients older than 40 years because the incidence of the first attack of migraine decreases and the incidence of neoplasm and other intracranial pathology increases after this age.

(ii) **Was this headache of sudden onset?** A persistent headache that begins and reaches its maximal intensity within a few seconds or minutes is more suggestive of an ominous vascular cause.

(iii) **Has there been any alteration in mental status during the course of the headache?** Generally, a family member or friend who has been with the patient must answer this question. Although patients with migraine can appear fatigued, especially after prolonged vomiting or analgesic use, obtundation and confusion are more suggestive of meningitis, encephalitis, or subarachnoid hemorrhage.

(iv) **Has there been recent or coexistent infectious disease?** Infection in other locations (i.e., lungs, paranasal, or mastoid sinuses) may precede meningitis. Fever is not a feature of migraine or a primary headache disorder. Fever also may occur in association with subarachnoid hemorrhage, although this usually happens 3 to 4 days after the actual hemorrhage. Patients who are immunocompromised may exhibit fewer overt signs of infection initially.

(v) **Did the headache begin in the context of vigorous exercise or seemingly trivial head or neck trauma?** Although effort induced migraine or coital migraine certainly exist, the rapid onset of headache with strenuous exercise, especially when minor trauma has occurred, increases the possibility of carotid artery dissection or intracranial hemorrhage.

(vi) **Does the head pain tend to radiate posteriorly?** Pain radiation between the shoulders or lower is not typical of migraine and may indicate meningeal irritation from subarachnoid blood or infection.

(vii) **Other important points not to be overlooked in a careful history:**

   a. Do other family members have similar headaches? Migraine has a strong familial tendency.
   b. What medications does the patient take? Certain medications can cause headache. Anticoagulants and oral antibiotics place the patient in a higher risk group for hemorrhage or partially treated central nervous system (CNS) infection.
   c. Does the patient have any other chronic illness or a history of neurologic abnormality? These may confuse the neurologic examination.
   d. Is the headache consistently in the same location or on the same side? Benign headache disorders tend to change sides and locations at least occasionally.

2. Important Physical Findings

It is crucial to examine each patient carefully, especially when there are atypical elements in the history. A basic neurologic examination should be performed that addresses the following six components.

(i)   **Mental status:** What is the patient's level of consciousness? Is the patient able to maintain normal attention during the examination? Are language and memory normal?
(ii) **Cranial nerves:** Each cranial nerve should be tested separately. Are there asymmetries? Is there papilledema?
(iii) **Motor:** Are motor strength and muscle tone symmetrical and within the normal range? Are there any abnormal involuntary movements?
(iv) **Sensory:** Are there asymmetries of pain, temperature or proprioceptive sensation?
(v)   **Coordination:** Is there dysmetria or gait ataxia?
(vi) **Reflexes:** Is there asymmetry of reflexes in either the upper or lower extremities?

Three findings on examination should be considered as signs of possible serious pathology:

(a) **Nuchal rigidity:** This can be an indicator of either meningitis or subarachnoid hemorrhage.
(b) **Toxicity:** Is there a low-grade fever or persistent tachycardia? Does the patient appear more acutely ill than most patients with migraine?
(c) **Previously unnoticed neurologic abnormality:** Subtle findings such as a slight pupillary asymmetry, a unilateral pronator drift, or extensor plantar response are important and should lead to further investigation.

3. When to Order Laboratory Tests or Imaging Studies

Laboratory tests should be obtained to confirm the presence of abnormalities suspected from the history and physical examination and should be appropriate for the pathology suspected. Laboratory, electroencephalographic, or neuroimaging "fishing trips" are discouraged because they rarely provide useful information, can delay treatment, and can divert attention away from more relevant findings. At present, the computerized tomography (CT) scan is the imaging study most likely to be available in the acute setting. There are three major indications for an urgent CT scan:

- The presence of papilledema
- Any impairment of consciousness or orientation
- The presence of localizing or lateralizing findings on neurologic examination

CT scanning is most useful for identifying recent intracerebral and extracerebral hemorrhages, hydrocephalus and brain abscesses, or other space-occupying lesions.

IV. DIFFERENTIAL DIAGNOSIS OF SECONDARY HEADACHES

Headache can be symptomatic of many underlying abnormalities. The relative frequency of secondary headaches is small when compared to that of primary headache disorders. However, it is vital that these headaches are diagnosed quickly and treated appropriately. The most common etiologies are listed in Table 1.

Table 1. Secondary headache etiologies

Vascular
Subarachnoid hemorrhage
Subdural hematoma
Cerebellar hemorrhage
Arteriovenous malformations
Intracerebral arterial occlusion
Occlusion of cerebral venous sinus (e.g., cavernous sinus thrombosis)
Carotid artery dissection

Infectious
Meningitis
Meningoencephalitis
Brain abscess
Acute sinusitis
Upper respiratory or systemic viral infection
Acquired immunodeficiency syndrome

Neoplastic

Inflammatory
Temporal arteritis
Autoimmune inflammatory process

Hypertensive
Acute pressor response to an exogenous agent
Phaechromocytoma
Malignant hypertension (including hypertensive encephalopathy)
Preeclampsia or eclampsia

Glaucoma
Pigmentary glaucoma
Acute angle closure glaucoma

Substance abuse headache

Benign intracranial hypertension (pseudotumor cerebri)

V. DIFFERENTIAL DIAGNOSIS OF PRIMARY HEADACHES

In clinical practice, most patients investigated because of head pain will ultimately prove to have a primary headache disorder (i.e., recurrent headaches for which no underlying structural, infectious, or other systemic abnormality can be found). Migraine and tension-type headaches are the most commonly diagnosed disorders in this population, but cluster headache and other less common syndromes are also occasionally seen. In order to classify and investigate primary headaches, the International Headache Society (IHS) has developed Classification and Diagnostic Criteria for Headache and Facial Pain. These criteria are invaluable for clinical research and are presented in Table 2 with the caveat that many patients do not fall neatly into a diagnostic category.

Table 2.   Diagnostic criteria for common headache types

Headache Type	Diagnostic Criteria	
Migraine without aura	The patient must have had at least five attacks which fulfill each of the following categories:	(a) Headache attacks lasting 4–72 h (untreated or treated unsuccessfully) (b) Headache has at least two of the following characteristics: • unilateral location • pulsating quality • moderate or severe intensity • aggravation by or causing avoidance of routine physical activity (c) During headache, at least one of the following symptoms is present: • nausea and/or vomiting • photophobia and phonophobia (d) Not attributed to an other disorder
Migraine with aura	In addition to fulfilling the criteria of migraine without aura, the patient must have experienced at least two attacks with three of the four following characteristics:	(a) Aura consisting of at least one of the following, but no motor weakness: • fully reversible visual symptoms including positive and/or negative features • fully reversible sensory symptoms including positive and/or negative features • fully reversible dysphasic speech disturbance (b) At least two of the following: • homonymous visual symptoms and/or unilateral sensory symptoms

Table 2. *Continued*

Headache Type	Diagnostic Criteria
	• at least one aura symptom develops gradually ≥5 min and/or different aura symptoms occur in succession ≥5 min • each symptom lasts ≥5 min and ≤60 min (c) Headache fulfilling criteria for migraine without aura begins during or follows aura within 60 min (d) Not attributed to another disorder
Tension-type headache	The patient must have had at least ten headaches that fulfill each of the following categories:
	(a) Headache lasting from 30 min to 7 d (b) Headaches have at least two of the following pain characteristics: • pressing/tightening (non pulsatile) quality • mild or moderate intensity bilateral location • no aggravation by routine physical activity (c) Both of the following: • no associated nausea or vomiting • either photophobia or phonophobia may be present, but not both (d) Not attributed to another disorder
Cluster headache	The patients must have experienced at least five attacks that fulfill each of the following criteria:
	(a) Severe unilateral orbital or supraorbital and/or temporal pain lasting 15 to 180 min if untreated (b) Headache is accompanied by at least one of the following ipsilaterally: • conjunctival injection and/or lacrimation • nasal congestion and/or rhinorrhea • eyelid edema • forehead and nasal sweating • miosis and/or ptosis • a sense of restlessness or agitation (c) Attacks have a frequency from one every other day to 8/d (d) Not attributed to another disorder

From International Headache Society Classification Subcommittee. International classification of headache disorders, 2nd ed. *Cephalagia* 2004;24(Suppl. 1), with permission.

1. Migraine

It is estimated that approximately 18% of women and 6.5% of men in the United States meet the diagnostic criteria for migraine. In a large epidemiologic study, 52% of the 28 million patients with migraine in the United States were not diagnosed with migraine by their physicians. Patients with migraine frequently have family members who also have recurrent headaches. Migraine falls into two categories: **migraine without aura** (previously called common migraine) and **migraine with aura** (previously called classic migraine). Patients with migraine often report premonitory symptoms, which begin 24 to 48 hours before a headache attack. These symptoms can include hyperactivity, mild euphoria, lethargy, depression, cravings for certain foods, frequent yawning, and other atypical symptoms. Premonitory symptoms should not be confused with the migraine aura, which occurs within 1 hour of the onset of the headache and consists of specific neurologic symptoms. Typical migraine aura symptoms include the following:

- Homonymous visual disturbance, classically a scintillating scotoma
- Unilateral paresthesias and or numbness, often affecting the distal extremities or the perioral region of the face
- Unilateral weakness
- Aphasia or other language disturbance

The aura symptoms in some patients localize to the brainstem. These include visual symptoms in the temporal and nasal fields of both eyes, dysarthria, vertigo, tinnitus, decreased hearing, double vision, ataxia, bilateral paresthesias, bilateral weakness, and decreased level of consciousness.

(i) Basilar-type Migraine

Patients in whom brainstem symptoms predominate are generally given the diagnosis of basilar migraine. One must bear in mind that many of these symptoms are subject to misinterpretation as they can occur with anxiety and hyperventilation. In many patients, basilar attacks are intermingled with typical attacks. Dizziness is frequently reported as a feature of an otherwise typical attack of migraine with aura.

(ii) Migraine with Prolonged Aura (Formerly, Complicated Migraine)

Migraine attacks in which the aura symptoms persist for more than 1 hour, but less than 1 week, and in which neuroimaging studies are normal. Aura symptoms may last longer than 1 week in persistent aura without infarction.

(iii) Hemiplegic Migraine

Hemiplegic migraine attacks are marked by reversible hemiparesis. Previously considered a type of migraine with aura, it is now categorized separately. Hemiplegic migraine may be sporadic or familial and has been associated with mutations on chromosomes 19 and 1 (see preceding text).

2. Tension-type Headache

Tension-type headache is probably the most common primary headache disorder. It has been referred to by many names in the past including muscle contraction headache, essential headache, stress headache, and psychomyogenic headache. The exact pathogenesis of tension-type headache and the importance of muscle contraction to its generation are still poorly understood. Pericranial muscle spasm or tenderness may or may not be present. Tension-type headache occurs in both episodic and chronic forms.

3. Cluster Headache

Cluster headaches are much less common than migraine or tension-type headaches. They afflict men five to six times more often than women, and the age of onset is typically 20 to 40 years. The syndrome derives its name from the fact that attacks occur in series lasting for weeks or months (the so-called cluster periods) separated by remissions, which usually last for months or years. During cluster periods, headache attacks could be provoked by alcohol, histamine, or nitroglycerine. The pain is very severe with a throbbing, at times sharp, quality. During a cluster headache a patient is often agitated and frequently paces, unlike a migraine patient who prefers to avoid movement in a quiet, dark room. In some instances, the clustering pattern of the episodic form can change into the chronic form in which there is no remission.

4. Miscellaneous Benign Headaches

There are several headache syndromes that are not associated with a structural cause but are distinct from migraine, tension-type, or cluster headaches. The following is a brief listing and description of these syndromes.

Paroxysmal hemicrania is a relatively rare syndrome in which attacks occur that are similar to cluster headache. It differs from cluster headache in that attacks occur with greater frequency (>5 per day for more than half the instances) and tend to be very brief (2 to 30 minutes), women are affected more frequently than men, and attacks are very responsive to low dose indomethacin. Attacks may be episodic (with remissions of at least 1 month), or chronic (with attacks occurring for 1 year without remission or with remissions lasting less than 1 month).

Hemicrania continua is a rare headache syndrome in which unilateral orbital or temporal pain is present almost constantly.

Primary stabbing headache, a series of ice-pick-like jabbing pains.

Frequently occurs in migraineurs on the side frequently affected by migraine attacks. Attacks often respond to oral indomethacin (25 mg three times per day).

Primary exertional headache can be precipitated by any form of exercise. These headaches are generally bilateral in location and can last from several minutes up to 24 hours.

Cold stimulus headache can result from either exposure to low ambient temperatures or passage of a cold liquid or solid material over the palate or posterior pharynx (e.g., ice cream headache).

Orgasmic headache can occur in susceptible individuals as a result of masturbation or sexual intercourse.

Primary cough headache may only be diagnosed after a structural lesion has been excluded with neuroimaging.

VI. REFRACTORY HEADACHES

1. Chronic Daily Headache

The IHS classifies headaches that are present for at least 15 days per month during at least 3 months per year as chronic headaches. Patients usually describe these headaches as being tension-type in quality, although more severe attacks similar to migraine may be interspersed. Prophylactic therapy in patients taking daily analgesic or ergotamine containing medications is frequently ineffective. Discontinuation of daily analgesic or ergotamine use often results in improvement.

2. Status Migrainosus

Migraine attacks that persist for longer than 72 hours despite treatment are classified as status migrainosus. Inpatient treatment is necessary (see section entitled Treatment).

VII. RATIONAL APPROACH TO PHARMACOLOGIC TREATMENT OF PRIMARY HEADACHES

Pharmacologic treatment of patients with headache can be divided into two broad categories: acute therapy given during an attack to end it and prophylactic treatment given daily to decrease the frequency and severity of future attacks. The reader is referred to Appendix VII or to the *Physicians' Desk Reference* (PDR) for more detailed descriptions of the drugs used in the management of headache.

1. Treatment of Migraine

(i) Acute Therapy

FOR TREATMENT OF MILD OR MODERATE ATTACKS. **Acetaminophen.** Occasionally, patients will have mild attacks that when found early will respond to over-the-counter analgesics such as acetaminophen (650 to 1,000 mg). Mild to moderate attacks during pregnancy should be treated with acetaminophen in the first instance.

Nonsteroidal antiinflammatory drugs (NSAIDs) including aspirin (900 to 1,000 mg), ibuprofen (1,000 to 1,200 mg), Naproxen (500 to 825 mg), and ketoprofen (100 to 200 mg) can be used to treat mild to moderate attacks.

Midrin is a combination medication containing acetaminophen, isometheptene mucate (a mild vasoconstrictor) and dichloralphenazone (a mild sedative). Two tablets should be taken at the onset of headache followed by one each hour until relief occurs or up to a maximum of five capsules within a 12-hour period. Anecdotally, Midrin appears less likely to generate a rebound headache syndrome than many of the other combination medications, although daily use of any of these treatments is not recommended.

FOR TREATMENT OF SEVERE ATTACKS.   **Butalbital** is a barbiturate combined with caffeine, acetylsalicylic acid, and/or acetaminophen in several medications (including Fiorinal, Fioricet, Phrenilin, and Esgic). The recommended dosage is two tablets every 4 hours, not to exceed six per day. These medications are best suited for treatment of infrequent moderate to severe headaches. If used to treat headaches occurring more than twice per week, patients may develop rebound headaches. Physicians should be careful to avoid prescribing these drugs in escalating doses.

Oral opioid-containing medications have little place in the treatment of chronic recurrent primary headaches and should be avoided until all other treatment alternatives have been considered. Under certain conditions they are the only viable option (e.g., pregnancy, severe vascular disease). Physicians should discuss the risks of rebound headache (medication overuse headache) and dependency before prescribing.

Ketorolac is a potent NSAID that is available in the injectable form. It can be given intramuscularly (IM) or intravenously (IV) for the treatment of severe migraine attacks with early and prominent vomiting. Although ketorolac is expensive, and not clearly superior to cheaper medications, some patients respond well. Because of its potency, the risk of side effects is actually greater than with other NSAIDs, and the manufacturers recommend short-term use only (see Chapter 8).

Ergotamine containing medications are available in oral, sublingual, and suppository formulations in the United States. Ergotamines are the classical antimigraine agents and can be effective if patients tolerate the side effects of nausea and peripheral vasoconstriction. They are typically most effective if given early in the migraine attack. A potential problem is overuse, which can result in a chronic daily headache syndrome and, in extreme cases, the gangrene-like complications of ergotism. When physicians are prescribing the suppository, patients should be instructed to cut the suppository in half or into quarters in order to find the lowest effective dose and thereby to reduce ergotamine induced nausea. Contraindications include coronary artery disease, angina, peripheral vascular disease, Raynaud phenomenon, uncontrolled hypertension, or severely impaired renal or hepatic function.

DHE is a hydrogenated ergot that until recently was the mainstay of nonopioid treatment of acute severe headache attacks. It has less potent peripheral arterial vasoconstrictive effects and can be effective even when given well into the attack. It is associated with less nausea than ergotamine; however, an antiemetic given before treatment is usually required. DHE is available in injectable and intranasal formulations. To give DHE in the acute stage, early in the attack, administer 1 to 2 mg IM or subcutaneously (SQ), repeated up to an additional 3 mg in 24 hours. Well into a severe attack, administer prochlorperazine 5 mg IV, or metoclopramide 10 mg IV, followed in 5 to 10 minutes by DHE 0.75 to 1 mg IV over 2 to 3 minutes. If the attack has not subsided after 30 minutes, give an additional 0.5 mg of DHE as IV.

Sumatriptan (Imitrex) and the "triptans." Sumatriptan is the prototype of the "triptan" class of drugs, which selectively bind to $5\text{-HT}_{1B/D/F}$ receptors. It exerts both direct vasoconstrictor and antineurogenic inflammatory effects on dural vessels. Sumatriptan treatment is also associated with improvement in the nausea, vomiting, photophobia, and phonophobia, which accompany many migraine attacks. It has been shown to be effective when given up to 4 hours after the onset of a headache attack. Sumatriptan is available in injectable (6 mg SQ), oral (25, 50, and 100 mg), and intranasal (20 mg) formulations.

Other 5-HT$_{1B/D/F}$ receptor agonists include **naratriptan (Amerge), zolmitriptan (Zomig), rizatriptan (Maxalt), almotriptan (Axert), frovatriptan (Frova), and eletriptan (Relpax).** The overall efficacy and side effect profiles of these agents do not vary greatly from sumatriptan. However, there are differences in half-life, relative affinity for the h5-HT$_{1D}$ and h5-HT$_{1B}$ receptor subtypes and blood–brain barrier penetration. **Naratriptan** (2.5 mg tablets), **almotriptan** (6.25 and 12.5 mg tablets), and **frovatriptan** (2.5 mg tablets) have been reported to have overall lower incidence of side effects than sumatriptan, but the onset appears to be somewhat slower. Duration may be longer however. The side effect profiles of both **zolmitriptan** (2.5 and 5 mg tablets) and **rizatriptan** (5 and 10 mg tablets and rapidly dispersible wafers) and **eletriptan** (20 and 40 mg tablets) are similar to sumatriptan, but trials suggest that the onset of action may be slightly faster than oral sumatriptan. Triptans have become the *de facto* drugs of choice in the outpatient treatment of moderate to severe migraine attacks in patients without risk factors for coronary disease or prolonged neurologic symptoms.

Neuroleptics.   Neuroleptics including chlorpromazine, prochlorperazine, and metoclopramide have been used as an alternative to meperidine or vasoactive medications in the ER setting for the treatment of severe migraine attacks. The risks of hypotension, sedation, and akathisia limit the use of neuroleptics.

Opioids.   Meperidine is the opioid most frequently chosen by ER physicians for the treatment of severe migraine headache. It is commonly given in combination with an antiemetic. The choice of meperidine, or in fact any other opioid, is questionable for this indication, and there is no evidence in the literature to support this practice. In fact, in one double-blind comparison study, meperidine was found to be inferior to chlorpromazine for aborting a migraine attack. Its main beneficial effect may be that of induction of sleep with resultant resolution of the attack. The use of parenteral opioids should be limited to patients with infrequent attacks, or patients in whom other treatments are contraindicated. The use of meperidine is generally discouraged because of the toxicity of its metabolite normeperidine, and because of the preference of addicts for this particular opioid (see Chapter 9). Suitable alternatives would be morphine or hydromorphone.

(ii) Treatment of Status Migrainosus

If efforts to end a migraine attack in the ER are unsuccessful and the patient requires hospitalization, with intravenous treatment with DHE as the treatment of choice, provided there are no contraindications. The following protocol is recommended:

- Metoclopramide 10 mg IV plus DHE 0.5 mg IV given over 2 to 3 minutes.
- If the headache stops but nausea develops, no DHE is given for 8 hours, then 0.3 or 0.4 mg DHE plus 10 mg metoclopramide is given every 8 hours for 3 days.
- If the head pain persists and no nausea develops, 0.5 mg DHE is repeated in 1 hour; if headache is relieved but nausea develops, DHE 0.75 mg IV every 8 hours for 3 days plus metoclopramide 10 mg; if headache is relieved and no nausea develops, DHE 1.0 mg every 8 hours plus metoclopramide 10 mg for 3 days.
- If the headache stops and no nausea develops, DHE 0.5 mg plus metoclopramide 10 mg IV every 8 hours for 3 days.

The DHE should be given undiluted through an IV heplock. Metoclopramide may be discontinued after six DHE doses.

Diarrhea is a common side effect of the DHE protocol and can be controlled with oral diphenoxylate (Lomotil). Contraindications to IV DHE include Prinzmetal angina, pregnancy, coronary artery disease or uncontrolled hypertension, peripheral vascular disease, severe renal disease, or severe hepatic disease.

When patients are hospitalized and given intravenous DHE, special attention should be given to the amount of analgesic medications they were taking before admission. Status migrainosus is frequently associated with overuse of abortive medications and patients should be watched carefully for evidence of barbiturate or opiate withdrawal. If no prophylactic regimen is in place in a patient with episodes of status migrainosus, then initiation of prophylactic therapy is appropriate.

(iii) Prophylactic Therapy

See Table 3 for the prophylactic medications that are used in migraine.

Abortive drug treatment of headache is largely for symptomatic relief and has no benefit beyond the single attack. In many patients who have infrequent attacks, an effective abortive agent is sufficient. However, the frequent use of abortive agents rapidly becomes a part of the problem. Once a patient has slid into the insidious cycle of analgesic rebound, prophylactic therapy may be futile and the headaches just keep getting worse. If attacks occur more than once or twice per month and are sufficiently severe to prohibit normal activities, or the patient's dread of the attacks is intrusive, then prophylactic therapy should be considered. The regime should be individualized to the patient. Concurrent medical problems may contraindicate certain prophylactic medications, or occasionally the prophylactic medicine can be used to treat migraine as well as a preexistent illness. Prophylactic medications are empiric treatments, and to date, their mechanism of action is unknown. Most of these medications were originally used for other indications and their antimigraine effects were found coincidentally. It is likely that in many cases their effect in migraine is unrelated to the action for which they were originally prescribed. Most prophylactic agents are associated with increased appetite, and patients should be warned about potential weight gain.

Table 3.   Prophylactic medications useful in migraine

Drug	Supplied Doses (mg)	Daily Oral Dose (mg)
β-Blockers		
Propranolol (Inderal)	10, 20, 40, and 80	40–240
Nadolol (Corgard)	20, 40, 80, 120, and 160	20–80
Atenolol (Tenormin)	25, 50, and 100	50–150
Timolol (Blocadren)	5, 10, and 20	20–60
Metoprolol (Lopressor)	50 and 100	50–300
NSAIDs		
Naproxen sodium (Aleve, Anaprox)	220, 275, and 550	480–1,100
Naproxen (Naprosyn)	250 and 500	750–1,000
Ketoprofen (Orudis)	25, 50, and 75	150–300
Aspirin	375	1,000–1,300
Antidepressants		
Amitriptyline (Elavil)	10, 25, 50, 75, 100, and 150	10–120
Calcium channel blockers		
Flunarizine	Not available in the United States	
Verapamil (Calan)	40, 80, and 120	120–480
Anticonvulsants		
Divalproex Sodium (Depakote)	125, 250, and 500	250–1,500
Gabapentin (Neurontin)	100, 300, 400, and 600	600–3,600
Topiramate (Topamax)	15, 25, and 100	50–200
Botulinum toxin type-A (Botox)	Contingent on dilution	25–100 units
Monoamine oxidase inhibitor		
Phenelzine (Nardil)	15	30–60

Prophylactic medications fall into a two-tiered hierarchy. First-line agents are those that are likely to be effective without intolerable side effects. Second-line agents may be effective when the first-line agents have failed, but second-line agents carry with them the risk of more frequent or potentially serious side effects.

FIRST LINE AGENTS. **Adrenoceptor Blockers.** β-blockers shown to be effective migraine prophylactic agents in clinical trials include propranolol, nadolol, atenolol, timolol, and metoprolol. The antimigraine activity of these medications does not depend on CNS penetration, cardioselectivity or 5-HT binding. The only common pharmacologic property that separates the β-blockers effective in migraine prophylaxis from those that are ineffective is the lack of partial sympathomimetic activity. Because of differences in pharmacologic properties among the various agents, failure of one agent is not an indicator of failure of others. Side effects occur in 10% to 15% of patients and include hypotension, fatigue, dizziness, gastrointestinal disturbance (diarrhea, constipation), depression, insomnia, memory disturbance. Contraindications include asthma, congestive heart failure, chronic obstruction pulmonary disease, peripheral vascular disease, cardiac conduction defects, and brittle diabetes.

NSAIDs. Although NSAIDs inhibit platelet function as part of their spectrum of activities (see Chapter 8), it has been difficult to correlate prophylactic efficacy with inhibition of platelet function. NSAIDs that have been shown to exhibit prophylactic effects in controlled clinical trials include aspirin, naproxen/naproxen sodium, tolfenamic acid, ketoprofen, mefenamic acid, and fenoprofen. The NSAIDs are described in detail in Chapter 8.

There have not been any trials comparing different NSAIDs for migraine prophylaxis. The only agent shown to be effective in controlled studies for treatment of menstrually associated migraine is naproxen sodium. This, coupled with its proven efficacy in double blind studies, make it the first choice among the NSAIDs in migraine prophylaxis.

Antidepressants. The only antidepressant with significant evidence of efficacy in migraine prophylaxis is the tricyclic antidepressant, amitriptyline. Amitriptyline inhibits reuptake of both norepinephrine and 5-HT. However, reuptake inhibition does not appear to correlate with efficacy in migraine. Clinical trials also indicate that amitriptyline's antimigraine activity is unrelated to its antidepressant activity. In fact, the doses generally useful in the treatment of migraine are well below those required to treat depression. The tricyclic antidepressants are described in detail in Chapter 11.

Calcium channel blockers. These blockers prevent the transmembrane influx of calcium ions through slow voltage dependent channels. They were first introduced for use in the treatment of migraine on the basis of their presumed blockade of the vasospastic phase in a migraine attack, although vasospasm is now considered an unlikely cause of migraine. Of the available blockers, only verapamil has sufficient evidence of efficacy to warrant its use in migraine.

Anticonvulsants. Anticonvulsants are increasingly recommended for migraine prevention. Valproic acid, an anticonvulsant known to inhibit GABA aminotransferase, reduces headache frequency and severity. It should be reserved for use as a second line agent because of its association with birth abnormalities (neural tube defects) in the offspring of women taking it during the first trimester of pregnancy, and with polycystic ovarian syndrome. Gabapentin, a GABA analog, has recently shown efficacy in migraine prophylaxis, and is generally well tolerated, although it may be associated with dizziness and sedation. Although gabapentin has a very favorable side effect profile, the general experience is that it is less efficacious in the treatment of recurrent headaches than valproic acid. However, until information from head-to-head trials is available, any definitive statement as to relative effectiveness is premature.

Topiramate is a newer anticonvulsant that is increasingly being used to prevent migraine. Topiramate's mechanism of action is largely unknown, but data suggest that it potentiates GABA activity. Dosages of 100 or 200 mg per day have been shown to substantially lower migraine frequency and acute medication requirements. Adverse events include impaired concentration, paresthesias, and weight loss.

The anticonvulsants are fully described in Chapter 10.

SECOND-LINE AGENTS.   **Botulinum toxin type A** is a neurotoxin that has recently been recognized to be useful in migraine prevention. Injections are well tolerated and benefit typically lasts approximately 3 months before another injection set is required. Transient increases in neck discomfort can occur depending on injection sites, but botulinum toxin is not absorbed systemically; therefore, there are no systemic side effects or drug–drug interactions. Cost can be prohibitive and some insurance providers still consider botulinum toxin an experimental medication for headache.

Phenelzine is a monoamine oxidase inhibitor that has been shown to be effective in patients with severe migraine. The potential for the generation of a hypertensive crisis after dietary intake of tyramine-containing foods should limit its use to patients with severe migraine who have been refractory to other treatments and who are committed to strict dietary monitoring.

2. Treatment of Tension-Type Headache

(i) Acute Treatment

Most tension-type headaches are of mild to moderate severity and many patients use nonprescription medications quite effectively. NSAIDs are the mainstay of treatment. Those commonly used are listed in Table 4. These drugs are described in detail in Chapter 8. Acetaminophen in both 650 and 1,000 mg doses has been reported to be superior to placebo in the treatment of headache. Muscle relaxants are sometimes used to treat tension-type headache. Such agents include diazepam, baclofen, dantrolene sodium, and cyclobenzaprine hydrochloride. There are no clinical trials of these medications in the treatment of acute tension-type headaches; therefore, their use is largely empiric. The one exception is tizanidine, which has recently been shown to be effective in chronic tension-type headache. In our experience, doses of 4 to 16 mg may be effective.

Table 4.   NSAIDs commonly used in tension-type headache

Medication	Initial Dose (mg)	Repeat Dose (mg)
Aspirin (325 mg)	650–975	975
Ibuprofen	600–800	600
Ketoprofen	50–75	50
Naproxen	500–750	500
Naproxen sodium	550	275
Ketorolac (oral)	20	10
Indomethacin (sup)	50	—

(ii) Prophylactic Treatment

Tricyclic antidepressants are generally considered first-line agents for prophylaxis. Amitriptyline is the drug of choice. Other medications that are sometimes selected for prophylaxis include NSAIDs, atypical antidepressants, and valproate, although evidence supporting their use in this situation is insufficient.

Amitriptyline has been shown to affect headache improvement in double-blind placebo-controlled studies. Dosage ranges from 10 to 100 mg per day or higher if tolerated. In some patients, its use is somewhat limited by its anticholinergic side effects (i.e., sedation, dry mouth, tachycardia, constipation, or urinary retention). To minimize sedation, the drug can be given in a single dose 1 to 2 hours before bedtime. It should be started at a low dosage (10 mg per day) and should be slowly increased over several weeks (10 mg increments at intervals of 1 to 2 weeks).

3. Treatment of Cluster Headache

(i) Acute Treatment

Oxygen inhalation is a safe and effective treatment of individual attacks of cluster headache in many patients. The patient most likely to respond to oxygen treatment is one with episodic-type cluster headaches who is younger than 50 years.

Oxygen is delivered at a rate of 8 liters per minute for 15 minutes via a loose-fitting face mask. Nasal biprongs are less effective because of greater air entrainment and lower oxygen concentration delivered. Patients who respond to oxygen do so usually within 10 minutes. The mechanism of effect of oxygen is unknown.

Ergotamine has been used since the 1940s to treat cluster headache attacks. The sublingual and inhalational routes appear to be superior to oral tablets. Ergotamines are effective and well tolerated in many patients with cluster headaches. DHE also may be of use in the acute treatment of cluster headaches.

Sumatriptan has been found to be effective in reducing both the pain and conjunctival injection of cluster headache within 15 minutes. It is well tolerated in patients with cluster headache. However, it should be remembered that sumatriptan is contraindicated in patients with coronary artery disease, which is quite common among middle-aged men who account for most patients with cluster headache.

(ii) Prophylactic Treatment

In general, prophylactic treatment of cluster headache is given only during the cluster period. Once a remission is established, in most cases within 3 to 6 weeks, the prophylactic agents is tapered and withdrawn.

Verapamil is frequently used in cluster headache, and in many patients it works well, with few side effects. The recommended dosage is 240 to 480 mg per day.

Ergotamine tartrate is the traditional agent used in the prophylactic treatment of cluster headache. In dosages of 2 to 4 mg per day in either oral or suppository form, ergotamine is an effective, well-tolerated medication for many patients with cluster headache.

Lithium carbonate has been shown in more than 20 open clinical trials to be effective in the treatment of chronic cluster headache. Because of its rather narrow therapeutic window, it is important to monitor serum lithium levels during periods of treatment. The serum level should be obtained 12 hours after the last dose and should not exceed 1.0 mmol per L (therapeutic range is usually from 0.3 to 0.8 mmol per L). It is important to remember that certain medications can interact with lithium to increase is the serum level, these include the NSAIDs and the thiazide diuretics). Average daily doses range from 600 to 900 mg but should be titrated according to serum concentrations.

Steroids are widely used in the treatment of both the episodic and chronic forms of cluster headache although documentation of their effect is largely limited to open trials.

Occipital nerve blocks ipsilateral to the pain of cluster headaches also have been shown to be an effective transitional therapy, providing some patients several weeks of benefit while a prophylactic medication can be initiated.

4. Indomethacin Responsive Headaches

There are several headache syndromes that frequently respond to prophylactic treatment with indomethacin. Indomethacin, a potent NSAID, is not effective in migraine, and has significant gastrointestinal side effects. These syndromes for which indomethacin can be effective include chronic paroxysmal hemicrania, hemicrania continua, benign cough headache, effort, and coital migraine and idiopathic jabbing headaches. It is not known why these headaches respond to indomethacin when others do not. Clinical features that indomethacin-responsive headaches share include a tendency to be provoked by certain movements or activities, relatively brief duration, and severe intensity. To treat these syndromes, an initial dosage of 25 mg twice a day is increased over several days until the attacks cease (sometimes requiring up to 150 to 250 mg per day). After relief is stable for several days, the dosage should be titrated downward to the lowest effective maintenance dosage (usually 25 to 100 mg per day). There is great interindividual variation in the maintenance dosage required.

Indomethacin can have potentially serious gastrointestinal side effects when given over long periods. These include dyspepsia, peptic ulcer, and GI bleeding. Other potential side effects include dizziness, nausea, and purpura.

VIII. NONPHARMACOLOGIC TREATMENT OF HEADACHE

Nonpharmacologic treatments include very old treatments such as application of pressure, heat or cold directly to the head, as well as electrical stimulation, dental treatment, acupuncture, hypnosis, relaxation training, biofeedback, and cognitive therapy. All of these techniques have proponents, but the inherent difficulties in designing and carrying out blind, unbiased studies make it almost impossible to make strong statements regarding their efficacy. At this point, it is impossible to predict whether an individual patient will benefit.

IX. HINTS FOR SUCCESSFUL HEADACHE MANAGEMENT

1. Less Is More

In prescribing prophylactic therapy, start with a small dose and titrate upward using small increments at 1 to 2 week intervals. This will allow you to determine the lowest effective dose.

2. Don't Abandon Ship

If a prophylactic medication does not work at a modest dose, titrate upward slowly and systematically. Listen to the patient, and let side effects be your guide.

3. Pregnancy and Prophylaxis Potentially Precipitate Problems

Women who intend to become pregnant should be withdrawn from prophylactic treatment because the effects of many of these drugs on the fetus (especially in the first trimester) are not known. In many cases, pregnancy induces a remission in migraine attacks.

4. All Headaches Are Not Created Equal

Just because a patient has intermittent severe migraine attacks does not mean that every headache that they have is a migraine requiring aggressive abortive therapy. Many migraineurs have frequent simple tension types headaches intermixed, and the frequent use of ergotamines, analgesics, or barbiturate-containing medications can result in an iatrogenic rebound syndrome.

5. Prophylaxis Is Not a Life Sentence

Once a patient has been headache free for 6 to 12 several months, begin to talk with them about tapering down their medications.

SELECTED READINGS

Burstein R, Cutrer FM, Yarnitsky D. The development of cutaneous allodynia during a migraine attack. *Brain* 2000;123(Pt 8):1703–1709.

Burstein R, Yamamura H, Malick A, et al. Chemical stimulation of the intracranial dura induces enhanced responses to facial stimulation in brain stem trigeminal neurons. *J Neurophysiol* 1998;79(2):964–982.

Edmeads J. Emergency management of headache. *Headache* 1988;28: 675–679.

Forsyth PA, Posner JB. Headaches in patients with brain tumors: a study in 111 patients. *Ann Neurol* 1992;32:289.

Gabai IJ, Spierlings ELH. Prophylactic treatment of cluster headache with verapamil. *Headache* 1989;29:167–168.

Mathew NT, Stubits E, Nigam MP. Transformation of episodic migraine into daily headache. *Headache* 1982;22:66–68.

Medina JL, Diamond S. Cluster headache variant: spectrum of a new headache syndrome. *Arch Neurol* 1981;38:705–709.

Olesen J, Tfelt-Hansen P, Welch KMA, eds. *The headaches.* New York: Raven Press, 1993.

Olesen J, ed. IHS classification and diagnostic criteria for headache disorders, cranial neuralgias and facial pain. *Cephalalgia* 1988; 8(Suppl. 7):9–92.

Quality Standards Subcommittee of the American Academy of Neurology. Practice parameter: the utility of neuroimaging in the evaluation of headache in patients with normal neurologic examinations (summary statement). *Neurology* 1994;44:1353–1354.

Raskin HN. *Headache*. New York: Churchill Livingstone, 1988.

Raskin NH. Treatment of status migrainosus: the American experience. *Headache* 1990;30(Suppl. 2):550–553.

Silberstein SD, Neto W, Schmitt J, et al. MIGR-001 Study Group. Topiramate in migraine prevention: results of a large controlled trial. *Arch Neurol* 2004;61:490–495.

Sjaastad O, Spierings ELH. "Hemicrania continua" another headache completely responsive to indomethacin. *Cephalalgia* 1984;4:65–70.

Taylor H, ed. *The Nuprin report*. New York: Louis Harris and Associates, 1985.

Thomas JE, Rooke ED, Kvale WF. The neurologist's experience with pheochromocytoma. *JAMA* 1966;197:754–758.

Welch KMA. Drug therapy in migraine. *N Engl J Med* 1994; 329(20): 1476–1483.

29

Orofacial Pain

Alexandre F. M. DaSilva
and Martin Andrew Acquadro

Pain diminishes or constrains man's power of activity, in other words,
diminishes or constrains the efforts wherewith he endeavours to persist in his own being; therefore it is contrary to the said endeavour:
thus all the endeavours of a man affected by pain are directed to removing that pain.
—*Benedict de Spinoza, 1632–1677, in Ethics, 1677*

Many medical, dental, and other health specialists are involved
in the management of orofacial pain, often exposing the patient to
a variety of referrals and interventions. Many times orofacial pain
is the result of a complex process. The particular patient's pain
problem is then approached from the bias of one particular specialty, when a multidiscipline or multidimensional approach may
provide a more comprehensive treatment. The multiple specialists involved in the treatment of orofacial pain, the rich synaptic
connections with the limbic and autonomic systems, the social
function of the face, and the highly visible and expressive nature
of the face together make orofacial pain unique.

I. NEUROANATOMY AND NEUROPHYSIOLOGY

Tactile, thermal, and painful stimuli are transduced by specialized end organs or free nerve endings in the skin. At the level of the
brainstem, the trigeminal sensory fibers synapse with second-order
neurons in the trigeminal brainstem nuclear complex, which ascends
through specific pathways. One ascending pathway is the **lemnis-
cal trigeminothalamic pathway**, transmitting tactile, thermal,
and some proprioceptive and noxious information. The other ascending pathway is the **ventral trigeminothalamic pathway**,
subdivided into: (a) the **paleotrigeminothalamic tract**, which

mainly carries the affective-motivational aspects of pain (e.g., unpleasantness) processed subsequently by cortical areas such as the anterior cingulated cortex, insula, and prefrontal cortex; and (b) the **neotrigeminothalamic tract**, which mostly conveys the sensory–discriminative aspects of pain (e.g., location, size) and is processed by the somatosensory cortex and anterior insular cortex.

Clinical features of orofacial pain such as referral patterns, autonomic signs, interference with sleep-wake patterns, and the effect of emotional stimulation can be better understood in the context of the rich area of neural interchange described in the preceding text. Peripherally, many facial structures are innervated by branches of multiple nerves producing pathways for referred pain. For example, the periauricular area receives sensory innervation from cranial nerves V, VII, IX, and X, and from cervical roots C2 and C3, with referral patterns to the neck, eye, and face.

II. PSYCHOLOGICAL ASPECTS

The face and the treatment of facial pain are the most visible examples of the biophysical psychosocial model of pain. The face is a window through which we view the world and, in turn, by which we are viewed. Facial pain is therefore a highly visible form of pain, etched on the most expressive area of the body for all to see. This visibility is emphasized by the term "tic douloureux" given to trigeminal neuralgia. The resulting lack of privacy encountered by people who have facial pain compounds the increased rates of anxiety and depression found in many chronic pain states. In addition, people with facial pain may be perceived as angry, sad, or socially negative because of the effects of pain on their facial expression. Psychological factors present before the onset of pain (primary) and because of the pain (secondary) are important in the patient's perception of pain. Modification of the psychological factors can modulate the pain experience. Treatment of anxiety, depression, and sleep disruption should always be undertaken in conjunction with treatment of the primary pain source.

III. TEMPOROMANDIBULAR JOINT ARTICULAR DISORDERS, TEMPOROMANDIBULAR MUSCLE DISORDERS, AND MYOFASCIAL PAIN DISORDERS

(i) Diagnostic Features

It is useful to distinguish true temporomandibular joint (TMJ) articular disorders, temporomandibular muscle disorders (TMD) (i.e., dysfunction and pain of the muscles of mastication), and myofascial pain disorders originating in muscles other that those involved directly with mastication. When it involves the face, the source of pain may be the head and facial muscles, or muscles of mastication. Because of the neuroanatomy described in the preceding text, muscles of the shoulders and neck can refer pain to the face, sinuses, or head. Just as there are involuntary mechanical and muscle compensation in the lower back, hips, and knees associated with lower back and extremity musculoskeletal pathologies, so there are instigating, contributing, and perpetuating factors of myofascial pain of the head, neck, and orofacial areas from outside these areas (see Table 1).

Table 1. Temporomandibular (TM) disorders

Diagnosis	TM Joint Articular Disorders	TM Muscle Disorders	Myofascial Disorder
Region	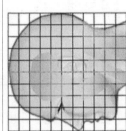		
Diagnostic features	Pain localized in the periauricular area during jaw function (e.g., chewing and talking). Usually, presence of painful click or crepitus during mouth opening. Limited (opening <35 mm), deviated or painful jaw movements.	Tenderness of the masticatory muscles. Dull, aching pain exacerbated by jaw function or palpation.	Diffused dull or aching pain affecting multiple groups of muscles of the head and neck region, as well as other parts of the body.
Diagnostic evaluation	Internal derangement of the TMJ with abnormal function of the disc-condyle complex, or degeneration of the joint surface.	Tenderness during palpation of the masticatory muscles and tendons. Possible limited range of jaw movement and	Presence of trigger or tender points in one or more groups of muscles. Pain can radiate to distant areas with stimulation

415

Table 1. *Continued*

Diagnosis	TM Joint Articular Disorders	TM Muscle Disorders	Myofascial Disorder
	Palpation of the joint is painful. Possible presence of swelling of the joint in acute phases. MRI, CT scan, panoramic radiography, or other imaging study of the TMJ may be necessary to rule out tumors, and advanced degenerative stages.	during passive stretching exam. Can be associated with a parafunctional habit (bruxism-early morning pain).	or not of the trigger points. Rule out presence of lupus erythematosus.
Treatment	Patient education and self-care Medication: NSAIDs, nonopiate analgesics	Patient education and self-care Medication: topical and systemic NSAIDs, nonopiate analgesics, muscle relaxants, antidepressants (usually TCAs over SSRIs), anxiolytics, anticonvulsants, BTX trigger point injections (e.g., corticosteroids, anesthetics), and vapocoolant spray	Patient education and self-care Medication: topical and systemic NSAIDs, nonopiate analgesics, muscle relaxants, antidepressants (usually TCAs over SSRIs), anxiolytics, anticonvulsants, BTX, trigger point injections (e.g., BTX, corticosteroids, anesthetics), and vapocoolant spray
	Physical therapy: exercise program Occlusal splints Oral maxillofacial surgery: arthrocentesis, arthroscopic surgery, open surgery	Physical therapy: TENS, massage, exercise program Occlusal splints Cognitive-behavior: biofeedback, relaxation, coping skills	Physical therapy: TENS, massage, exercise program Occlusal splints Cognitive-behavior: biofeedback, relaxation, coping skills

BTX, botulinum toxin; CT, computerized tomography; MRI, magnetic resonance imaging; NSAIDs, nonsteroidal antiinflammatory drugs; SSRI, selective serotonin reuptake inhibitor; TENS, transcutaneous electrical nerve stimulation; TMJ, temporomandibular joint; TCA, tricyclic antidepressant.

(ii) Clinical Characteristics

TMJ ARTICULAR DISORDERS. True pathologic derangement of the TMJ as the isolated cause for pain is not common. TMJ damage can be the result of direct trauma, wear and tear from chronic pathologic occlusal forces, and overextension of jaw movements. Some other conditions also affect the TMJ, such as congenital and developmental disorders (e.g., hyperplasia and neoplasia), inflammatory disorders (e.g., arthritis), osteoarthritis, and ankylosis. Just as one can find magnetic resonance imaging (MRI) abnormalities of the lumbar spine in patients who are asymptomatic, so can one find evident TMJ pathology in asymptomatic individuals. Many subjects have an "abnormal" TMJ, which "clicks" or has a deviation or displacement during opening and closing of the mandible, but few have accompanying pain. However, if the patient complains of a chronic TMJ dysfunction with pain, he/she deserves assessment by an orofacial pain specialist.

TEMPOROMANDIBULAR MUSCLE DISORDER. TM muscle disorder is characterized by dull aching pain exacerbated by mandibular function, muscle tenderness in one or more masticatory muscles, and often a decreased mandibular range of motion. The pain is commonly described as a dull ache exacerbated by chewing, fluctuating in intensity daily, and associated with remissions lasting months. A range of terms exist, with a variety of classifications and subclassifications. These classifications include myofascial dysfunction, myositis, myalgia, myospasm, and myofibrotic contracture. The absence of clinical features referable to the TMJ and the presence of muscle tenderness distinguish this from primary TMJ articular disorders, although secondary TMJ changes and joint remodeling can occur.

MYOFASCIAL PAIN DYSFUNCTION. Dysfunction of the muscles of the shoulders, neck, head, and face is relatively common in the general population and can aggravate headaches, sinus area pain, and orofacial pain. Fibromyalgia is a type of myofascial dysfunction distinguished as a systemic disease characterized by muscle pain and tenderness in multiple body quadrants. It can be exacerbated by stress, anxiety, and weather changes, and accompanied by a variety of generalized symptoms such as fatigue, morning stiffness, and headache. The patient with fibromyalgia may initially present with facial pain and tenderness in the muscles of mastication; it is important to question patients for systemic features and not focus simply on the local complaint. Other systemic myofascial disorders are polymyalgia, lupus erythematosus, polymyositis, and dermatomyosits. A more common complaint of generalized pain, although usually limited to the upper quadrant of the body, is the direct trauma and whiplash injury to muscles of the neck and shoulders.

(iii) Epidemiology

Myofascial pain disorders occur predominantly in women. Masticatory myalgia and myositis occur in younger women (late teens to 40 years), whereas fibromyalgia most commonly presents in older women (45 to 55 years). The prevalence of TMD ranges from 6% to 12% of the North American population. Patients complaining of TMD pain are likely to be women, with an average age of 40 ($\pm$16) years. Direct trauma to facial muscles producing pain is notable for its greater frequency in men.

(iv) Diagnostic Evaluation, Imaging Studies, and Laboratory Tests

Diagnostic evaluation includes a careful and thorough history and physical examination of the integrity and function of the head and neck structures, with special attention to the TMJ complex (e.g., masticatory muscles, articular structures), and cranial and cervical nerves. Evaluation should include a review for a history of headaches, surgeries, trauma, and psychosocial events and stressors. A review of daily activities along with posture, repetitive movements, habits, and sleep patterns should be included. A history of parafunctional habits (clenching and grinding of teeth), awakening in the morning with sore jaw muscles, clicking or grating noises when opening the mouth, and recent or extensive dental work should be elicited. An examination of the oral cavity for any lesions that may cause a reflex avoidance pattern, pain on extreme opening of the mandible, and abnormal bite should be checked. Teeth sensitivity, painful muscles, and tender points should be examined.

MRI and CT (computerized tomography) scan of the TMJ may be necessary to evaluate possible advanced degenerative pathologies or tumors. However, radiographs frequently report abnormalities of the TMJ disk position in asymptomatic joints that do not need treatment. Therefore, imaging exams of the TMJ, other than panoramic radiography, should only be requested in treatment-resistant chronic pain, unusual pain patterns, and sudden changes in the occlusion. There are no imaging techniques for myofascial pain disorders that are useful in diagnosis or management. Consideration of other rheumatologic or immunologic diagnoses by history and physical examination will dictate additional studies and referral to the appropriate specialist.

(v) Treatment

PHYSICAL THERAPY.   A patient diagnosed with TM disorders may benefit from complete evaluation and treatment by a physical therapist. The treatment program may include stretching, strengthening, and endurance exercises, transcutaneous electrical nerve stimulation (TENS), ultrasound, thermal application, and mobilization (joint and soft tissue). The patient should follow an active exercise program at home with guidance from a physical therapist.

PHARMACOLOGIC THERAPY.   Pharmacologic therapy includes judicious use of nonsteroidal antiinflammatory drugs (NSAIDs), very selective use of tricyclic antidepressants (TCAs), and selective use of anticonvulsants, other analgesics, muscle relaxants, anxiolytics, and, very rarely, opioids. NSAIDs may be used for both their analgesic and antiinflammatory properties. There is marked interpatient variability in response to different agents, necessitating trials of agents until the optimal response is obtained. Because of the ceiling effect of NSAIDs and gastrointestinal and renal toxicity issues, increasing doses, and time of use beyond the recommended maximum is not useful. NSAIDs are of no proven value in the long-term management of TMJ pain, although large doses may provide short-term relief. Patients who are unable to tolerate NSAIDs may use tramadol hydrochloride, a weak and nonaddicting μ-agonist, at a dosage of 50 to 100 mg every 6 hours, as needed. Short-term use of centrally acting muscle relaxants includes cyclobenzapine (Flexeril) and carisoprodol (Soma). These agents decrease excess electromyogram (EMG) activity and muscle spasm. The tertiary amine amitriptyline, having greater anticholinergic effects than the secondary amines desipramine and nortriptyline, in low doses, may improve sleep and may act as indirect analgesics by inhibiting serotonin and norepinephrine reuptake. Benzodiazepines, such as diazepam, decrease muscle spasm, improve sleep, and show anxiolytic activity. A dosage of 0.5 mg once or twice a day is useful in initial therapy. Prolonged use of benzodiazepines should be avoided because of their addiction potential. In patients requiring prolonged treatment of anxiety symptoms, buspirone (Buspar) 5 mg three times daily is effective with little addiction potential, but has no muscle relaxant effects.

TRIGGER POINT INJECTIONS, BOTULINUM TOXIN INJECTIONS, AND PHYSICAL THERAPY.   Pressure on active trigger points (TPs) causes acute pain, and produces spasms when the muscle is used, decreasing the range of motion. Trigger points can be localized by pressure and then inactivated by the topical application of vapocoolant spray (dichlorodifluoromethane), allowing stretching exercises to restore muscle mobility. The injection of local anesthetics in the TP can be performed with subsequent physical therapy. This injection provides prolonged analgesia, allowing the patient a pain-free period to commence physical therapy, with subsequent use of vapocoolants and stretching exercises at home. However, the pain relief may last much longer than the anesthetic effect. Corticosteroids, such as triamcinolone acetonide (Kenalog) can be added to the mixture. Steroid injections should not be repeated any sooner than six weeks, as a *peau d'orange* cosmetic defect may occur.

Botulinum toxin (BTX) injection is proven to be an excellent therapeutic tool for the treatment of myofascial pain. First indicated for involuntary muscle contraction disorders (e.g., blepharospasm and dystonia), BTX seems to disrupt the membrane-fusion and exocytosis of acetylcholine-containing vesicles into the extracellular milieu. The effects are reduction of muscular tone, contractility, and graded chemical denervation in the muscular area injected. Botulinum toxin may also reduce pain, and clinical reports support its use in some chronic pain diseases, including primary headaches (e.g., tension-type headache), inflammatory pain, and even some selected cases of trigeminal, and postsurgical and posttraumatic neuropathic pain. It appears that more injections with lower units per injection over an area of pain are more effective than a single large dose injection. However, randomized control clinical studies are lacking. The beneficial effect of a BTX injection can last for an average of 4 months and may be repeated if indicated. Advantages include no systemic side effects, but the application requires a practitioner skilled in the use of BTX in the head and neck, to avoid unanticipated facial and other head and neck muscular weakness, transient facial deformity, or severe respiratory, masticatory, and swallowing compromise.

PSYCHOLOGICAL THERAPY.   Psychologic intervention including biofeedback, relaxation techniques, and cognitive behavioral therapy addressing aversive behaviors when they exist should be considered.

DENTAL TREATMENT.   Advocates of splint therapy suggest that it temporarily equilibrates bite occlusion, mechanically unloading the TMJ and limiting masticatory muscle activity, thereby decreasing symptoms of TM disorders. Occlusal appliance therapy seems to be beneficial in cases of myofascial pain, even when there are no signs of parafunctional habits (e.g., bruxism). Missing teeth and dental malocclusions have an inconsistent relation to TM disorders. In extreme occlusal discrepancies, oral rehabilitation (e.g., orthodontic and prosthodontic treatments) may improve masticatory function, without guarantee of pain relief.

TEMPOROMANDIBULAR JOINT SURGERY.   Open surgery of the TMJ is associated with high morbidity and a lack of efficacy, unless proper and careful patient selection is utilized by an experienced oral and maxillofacial surgeon. More conservative procedures, such as arthrocenthesis and arthroscopic surgeries, should be considered first.

SUGGESTED TEMPOROMANDIBULAR MUSCLE DISORDER HOME TREATMENT REGIMEN.   Temporary rest of the TMJ is sometimes helpful. Liquid and soft diet is instituted, and gum chewing is stopped. Wide, uncontrolled opening of the jaw is discouraged. Yawning, coughing, laughing, and the eating of large sandwiches are kept to a minimum. A hand or fist placed under the chin during wide mouth opening helps to hold the jaw in place. Heat or ice gel pack therapy can be useful; a heating pad, warm face cloth, or warm water bottle placed to the sides of the jaw and TMJ area will have a soothing and relaxing effect on the muscles. Alternatively, an ice gel pack for 10 to 20 minutes should be tried. Gentle midline opening and closing exercises of the mandible help retrain and relax muscles. Use of a vapocoolant spray also may be helpful in reducing movement-induced pain, so that exercises designed to improve joint mobility can be tolerated. Judicious use of NSAIDs may also help. Consider acetaminophen in patients with NSAID sensitivity, or coxibs in patients with a serious risk for bleeding or other relevant history.

IV. ODONTOGENIC PAIN

(i) Diagnostic Features

Because of the rich innervation of the mouth, pain resulting from tooth or periodontal disease can present with numerous features including local pain, headache, or eye symptoms. Differential diagnosis includes trigeminal neuropathic pain, sinus disease, and primary headaches (e.g., cluster headache and migraine) (see Table 2).

(ii) Epidemiology

Dental disease is common in both male and female adults and children of all ages.

(iii) Diagnostic Evaluation, Imaging Studies, and Laboratory Tests

During the history and clinical examination, odontogenic pain must be adequately assessed. Aggravating and relieving factors,

Table 2. Odontogenic pain

Diagnosis	Pulpitis	Periodontal	Cracked Tooth	Dentinal
Region	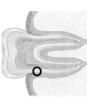			
Diagnostic Features	Spontaneous and/or evoked deep and diffuse pain originating from a compromised dental pulp. The pain can be described as sharp, throbbing or dull.	Localized deep continuous pain originating from a compromised periodontium (e.g., gingiva, periodontal ligament) exacerbated by bite or chewing.	Spontaneous or evoked (bite, chewing) brief sharp pain originating from a tooth with history of trauma, or extensive restorative work (e.g., crown preparation, root canal treatment).	Brief sharp pain evoked by different kinds of stimulus to the dentin (usually hot or cold drinks).
Diagnostic Evaluation	Look for the presence of deep caries, and recent or extensive dental work in the mouth. Pain can be provoked or exacerbated by percussion, thermal,	Percussion of the tooth supported by a compromised periodonto can provoke pain. Look for the presence of inflammation or abscess in the	Presence of tooth fracture, detectable or not by radiographies. Percussion of the tooth should elicit pain. Dental radiographic exams are helpful	Evidence of exposed dentin or cementum because of recession of the periodontium. Possible erosion of dentinal structure. Stimulation of these

421

Table 2. *Continued*

Diagnosis	Pulpitis	Periodontal	Cracked Tooth	Dentinal
	or electric stimulation of the affected tooth. Dental radiographic exams are extremely helpful (periapical).	periodontium (e.g., periodontitis apical abscess). Dental radiographic exams are extremely helpful (bitewings and periapicals).	(periapical exams from different angles).	areas to cold will reproduce the chief painful complaint.
Treatment	Medication: NSAIDs, nonopiate analgesics Dentistry: removal of the carious lesion, restoration of the tooth, endodontic treatment or extraction of the tooth	Medication: NSAIDs, nonopiate analgesics, antibiotics, mouthwashes Dentistry: drainage and debridement of the periodontal pocket, scaling and root planing, periodontal surgery, or extraction of the tooth.	Medication: NSAIDs, nonopiate analgesics Dentistry: depending on the level of the fracture-restoration of the tooth, endodontic treatment, or extraction of the tooth	Medication: mouth washes (fluoride), desensitizing toothpaste Dentistry: application of fluoride or potassium salts, restoration of the tooth, endodontic treatment Patient education and self-care: diet, tooth brushing force and frequency, proper toothpaste

NSAIDs, nonsteroidal antiinflammatory drugs.

duration, and quality of the pain are important key information to differentiate dental pathologies (Table 2). The clinical examination should include probing of the dental surfaces for cavities or fractures, percussion of the teeth in multiple planes for periodontal diseases and fractures, and electric and thermal stimulation for pulpitis. Radiographic examinations contribute greatly to the diagnosis. However, if pathologies of the hard or soft intraoral structures have been ruled out, then one is obliged to consider other uncommon disorders mimicking odontogenic pain.

(iv) Treatment

If dental disease is the obvious source of the pain, then the appropriate referral to a dentist should be made for proper evaluation and treatment. A summary of treatments is provided in Table 2.

V. TRIGEMINAL NEUROPATHIC PAIN DISORDERS

1. Trigeminal Neuralgia

(i) Diagnostic Features

Trigeminal neuralgia is characterized by sudden, stabbing, severe unilateral facial pain in one of the three divisions (most frequently the second) of the trigeminal nerve. Onset is frequently triggered by mechanical stimulation such as touch. Attacks can last from several seconds to minutes. Periods of attacks can last weeks or months, followed by periods of remission of months or years. Limited information is available about the etiology of trigeminal neuralgia other than the possible compression of the trigeminal root by a vessel or tumor. The compression occurs especially at the dorsal area of the cerebellopontine angle (see Table 3).

(ii) Epidemiology

Incidence increases with age, peaking at 75 years, and more commonly presents in women.

(iii) Diagnostic Evaluation, Imaging Studies, and Laboratory Tests

MRI is an important diagnostic test for excluding intracranial masses and multiple sclerosis (MS), particularly in younger patients. MS should be considered in young adults, more common in women than men, with trigeminal neuralgia symptoms. An MRI can show demyelinating lesions of the white matter associated with MS. Symptoms such as diplopia, weakness, and clumsiness are also suggestive of MS.

(iv) Treatment

Carbamazepine has been the first drug of choice in treatment, with an initial beneficial response in more than 75% of patients. More recently, other anticonvulsants with less potential toxicities are used as first-line treatment. Carbamazepine should be started at a dose of 200 mg per day and increased in increments of 200 mg until pain relief or side effects occur. The usual therapeutic dose range is 600 to 1,200 mg per day. Phenytoin is a less effective

Table 3. Trigeminal neuropathic pain disorders

Diagnosis	Trigeminal Neuralgia	Deafferentation Pain	Acute and Postherpetic Neuralgia	Burning Mouth Syndrome
Region				
Diagnostic Features	Brief severe lancinating pain, frequently evoked by mechanical stimulation of a trigger zone (pain-free between attacks). It is usually unilateral and affects more the V2/V3 areas (rarely V1). Possible transitory periods of pain remission that last months or years.	Spontaneous or evoked pain with prolonged after-sensation following tactile stimulation. Trigger zone previously affected by surgery (e.g., tooth extraction) or trauma. Positive and negative pain descriptors such as burning and nagging pain.	Pain associated with herpetic lesions, usually in the V1 dermatome. Spontaneous pain with burning and tingling quality, but may present as dull and aching. Occasional lancinating evoked pain.	Constant burning pain of the mucous membranes of the tongue, mouth, hard or soft palate, or lips. Usually affects women aged >50 y.
Diagnostic Evaluation	MRI for evidence of tumor or vasocompression of the trigeminal tract or root (cerebropontine angle).	History of etiologic factor such as trauma and surgery in the painful area. Order MRI if the	Small cutaneous vesicles (AHN) or scarring (PHN), usually affecting V1 area. Loss of normal	Rule out presence of salivary gland dysfunction (e.g., xerostomia) or tumor,

Table 3. *Continued*

Diagnosis	Trigeminal Neuralgia	Deafferentation Pain	Acute and Postherpetic Neuralgia	Burning Mouth Syndrome
	Rule out MS, especially in young adults.	area is intact to rule out peripheral or central lesions.	skin color and corneal ulceration can occur. Sensory changes in the affected area (e.g., hyperesthesia, dysesthesia).	Sjögrens syndrome, candidiasis, geographic or fissured tongue, and chronic chemical or mechanical irritation. Nutritional deficiencies and menopause can also be an etiologic factor.
Treatment	Medication: anticonvulsants (e.g., carbamazepine, gabapentin); antidepressants (e.g., amitriptyline, nortriptyline, and desipramine); and nonopiate analgesics. The combination of baclofen (antispastic agent) and anticonvulsants can produce good results. Surgery: microvascular decompression of the trigeminal root, ablative surgeries (e.g., rhizotomy, γ knife).	Medication: anticonvulsants (e.g., carbamazepine, gabapentin); antidepressants; nonopiate analgesics; topical agents (e.g., lidocaine 5% patches). The combination of baclofen (antispastic agent) and anticonvulsants can produce good results. Surgery: ablative surgeries (e.g., rhizotomy, γ-knife).	Medication: acyclovir (acute phase) anticonvulsants (e.g., carbamazepine, gabapentin); antidepressants; nonopiate analgesics; topical agents (e.g., lidocaine 5% patches). Surgery: ablative surgeries (e.g., rhizotomy, γ-knife).	Medication: anticonvulsants (e.g., gabapentin); benzodiazepines (e.g., clonazepam); antidepressants; nonopiate analgesics; topical agents (e.g., lidocaine mouthwashes). Cognitive-behavior: biofeedback, relaxation, coping skills.

AHN, acute herpetic neuralgia; BTX, botulinum toxin; MRI, magnetic resonance imaging; MS, multiple sclerosis; PHN, postherpetic neuralgia; V1-ophthalmic/V2-maxillary/V3-mandibular, divisions of the trigeminal nerve.

alternative but can be a useful adjunct to carbamazepine. Baclofen potentiates the action of carbamazepine at the trigeminal nucleus, and can be a useful adjunct. It can be started at a dose of 30 mg per day, increasing to 50 to 60 mg per day. Gabapentin is a safe and well-tolerated adjunct to carbamazepine, titrated to effect from a starting dose of 300 mg at night to a usual range of 900 to 3,000 mg per day. Other agents used less frequently include topiramate, zonisamide, oxcarbazepine, lamotrigine, clonazepam, and sodium valproate. Local anesthetic injections with steroids of V2 or V3 have helped in some cases. Surgical approaches to the treatment of trigeminal neuralgia include microvascular decompression and rhizotomy. Microvascular decompression of the trigeminal nerve at the cerebellopontine angle can provide immediate and long-term pain relief in more than 70% of the patients. Major dysesthesia and pain recurrence seems to be higher after radiofrequency and glycerol trigeminal rhizotomy, as well as alcohol blocks. These procedures are described in more detail in Chapters 12 and 14.

2. Deafferentation Pain

(i) Diagnostic Features

Teeth and dental nerves are commonly amputated. In few cases, these procedures might induce a phenomenon known as phantom tooth pain, which is similar to other phantom pain syndromes, producing pain in previously extracted or endodontically treated teeth. Other facial areas previously harmed by trauma or surgeries (e.g., sinus surgery and Cadwell–Luc procedures) also may induce deafferentation pain. This pain is constant with sharp exacerbations, and is associated with local allodynia (Table 3).

(ii) Epidemiology

Phantom tooth pain rates of 3% closely match rates of 5% for phantom pain following limb amputation. Given the relative frequency of dental procedures when compared to limb amputation, phantom tooth pain is a common cause of facial pain. There is equal distribution between sexes and, although all ages are affected, occurrence in children is rare.

(iii) Diagnostic Evaluation, Imaging Studies, and Laboratory Tests

History and physical examination are important regarding extent of dental work, and other trauma or surgeries in the area. History of prior severe dental pain of the extracted tooth or teeth, as well as prior sinusitis pain, migraine history, and traumatic pain may all suggest possible peripheral or central sensitization. Neuroimaging studies may be ordered to rule out tumors affecting the trigeminal sensory system.

(iv) Treatment

Pain therapies are targeted at both the central and peripheral components of deafferentation pain. The centrally acting drug of choice is gabapentin, starting at a dose of 300 mg at bedtime and increasing to a dose range of 900 to 3,000 mg per day. Some patients may be too sensitive, and therefore will need to start at 100 mg each evening and slowly titrate to higher doses. Clonazepam 1 to 3 mg per day and baclofen 30 to 60 mg per day are useful adjunctive agents. A fixed daily dose of an opioid such as oxycodone has been used successfully but is associated with a risk of dependence, addiction, and possible opioid-induced hyperalgesia. Peripherally acting agents include topically applied drugs and nerve blocks. Ketamine, capsaicin, and clonidine have been applied topically with mixed results. Surgical procedures are mostly ineffective in treatment of phantom tooth pain, and may increase pain severity.

3. Acute and Postherpetic Neuralgia

These are described in more detail in Chapter 25.

(i) Diagnostic Features

Acute herpetic neuralgia (AHN) arises because of herpes zoster infection (shingles) stimulating an acute inflammatory process of the dorsal root ganglion and peripheral nerves. Pain and cutaneous vesicles are located along the distribution of the affected peripheral nerve. Areas commonly affected are thoracic dermatomes (50%), ophthalmic division of the fifth cranial nerve (10% to 20%), and cervical dermatomes (10% to 20%). Shingles is almost always unilateral, and may be recurrent (1% to 8%), usually in the same site. Pain is described as burning, itching, well localized to the dermatome, with lancinating episodes, and is associated with hyperesthesia and hyperalgesia. Intense lancinating pain and paresthesia usually diminish in the second or third week as the skin lesions begin to heal (Table 3).

Pain persisting for longer than 1 month after complete healing of the acute herpes zoster lesions is considered postherpetic neuralgia (PHN). Pain of PHN is diffuse, dull, and aching, with a superficial dysesthetic sensation evoked by clothes or light touch.

(ii) Epidemiology

PHN, increasing resistance to therapy, ophthalmic involvement, and nervous system complications such as stroke, cranial neuropathy, and myelitis are all strongly associated with increasing age and immunocompromise.

(iii) Diagnostic Evaluation, Imaging Studies, and Laboratory Tests

Diagnosis is clinical and is based on the presence or past presence of vesicles. Complications such as stroke should be completely evaluated with CT scan or MRI imaging.

(iv) Treatment

Early effective treatment of acute herpes zoster shortens the acute episode, decreases acute pain, and decreases the incidence of PHN. Antiviral therapy with acyclovir IV 5 mg per kg q8h for 5 days commenced within 72 hours of the shingles eruption is effective, and is particularly useful in immunocompromised patients. Amitriptyline, gabapentin, doxepin, trazodone, fluoxetine, and NSAIDs are useful for pain control of AHN; if pain remains uncontrolled, opioids are then carefully added and tried. Subcutaneous local anesthetic and steroid injections reduce acute and chronic symptoms but should be used with care in immuno-compromised patients.

Tricyclic antidepressants are the mainstay of treatment in PHN. The efficacy of amitriptyline and desipramine has been confirmed in controlled clinical trials, although a secondary amine (desipramine) is preferred with theoretically less cholinergic effects when compared to a tertiary amine (amitriptyline) in the older patients. Anxiolytics and anticonvulsants have been used with less success. Topical agents, such as lidocaine patch 5% and salicylate, prepared as 700 mg aspirin dissolved in 15 to 30 mL of chloroform or diethyl ether, can produce substantial pain relief with minimal systemic absorption. Capsaicin is often poorly tolerated because of cutaneous sensitivity. Opioids should be reserved for patients who are unresponsive to other agents. TENS at or below the involved dermatome level is associated with minimal morbidity and sometimes produces significant benefit. It is underutilized and should always be considered for patients with PHN.

4. Burning Mouth Syndrome

(i) Diagnostic Features

Glossodynia is characterized by burning pain of the mucous membranes of the tongue (most commonly), mouth, hard palate, or lips. The onset of pain is gradual with no precipitating event, and is usually bilateral. Associated symptoms are altered taste and dry mouth. Physical examination of the mouth is normal and excludes causes such as infection and trauma. Although nutritional and menopausal factors, abnormal glucose tolerance, and chronic chemical or mechanical irritation have all been suggested as causes, there is inadequate evidence to pinpoint these factors as the origin of burning mouth syndrome (Table 3).

(ii) Epidemiology

Prevalence rates are 1.5% to 2.5% in the general population. Patients are more likely to be female (3:1) and older than 50 years.

(iii) Diagnostic Evaluation, Imaging Studies, and Laboratory Tests

There are no useful radiographic or laboratory examinations. As always, a careful history and physical examination is required to rule out other treatable causes.

(iv) Treatment

Fifty percent of patients will experience spontaneous resolution within a variable length of time, up to several years after onset. Tricyclic antidepressants such as amitriptyline, nortriptyline, and desipramine titrated in 10 mg increments to a range of 30 to 75 mg, and the serotonin reuptake inhibitor, sertraline may be effective. In a study of 30 patients, clonazepam given at a dose of 0.5 to 1.5 mg per day decreased pain in 70% of patients. A number of drugs including angiotensin-converting enzyme inhibitors and antihypertensives have been associated with burning mouth syndrome that is reversible on drug discontinuation. As pharmacologic therapy is unsuccessful in many patients, psychological support is important.

VI. PARANASAL, PERIOCULAR, PERIAURICULAR, AND HEAD AND NECK CANCER PAIN

1. Paranasal Sinus Area Pain and Headache

(i) Diagnostic Features

Acute sinusitis presents with bilateral or unilateral throbbing or sharp facial pain. In the acute setting, the diagnosis is usually straightforward. Frequently, pain is exacerbated by leaning the head forward (see Table 4).

A sense of pressure is described by 74% of patients. Medial orbital pain with radiation to the temple is a feature of ethmoid sinusitis. Frontal sinusitis features forehead pain and headache; maxillary sinusitis is suggested by pain over the upper teeth, or may be referred to the forehead, or orbit.

Chronic sinus area pain presents more of a diagnostic dilemma. Pain that is perceived as emanating from the sinuses can have other causes, including referred pain from dental, dural, and musculoskeletal areas. The differential diagnosis includes myofascial pain, neurovascular headaches such as migraine, neuralgias, allergies, and dental disease. Other diagnostic features of sinusitis include purulent discharge from the nasal passages or nasopharynx, intermittent fever, smell or taste disorder, tenderness on tapping the maxillary teeth, and tenderness over the maxillary, frontal, or ethmoidal sinuses. A history of recurrent injury in the form of upper respiratory tract infections and allergies may be elicited. A combination of history, anterior endoscopic examination, and CT scan findings is required to accurately diagnose sinusitis, particularly before embarking on surgical treatments (Table 4).

(ii) Epidemiology

There are no distinctive epidemiologic features.

(iii) Imaging Studies and Laboratory Tests

Endoscopic examination is useful in demonstrating inflamed turbinates, sinus ostia edema, and purulent nasopharyngeal discharge. CT imaging reveals opacification of the sinuses and occluded osteomeatal complexes. Additional abnormalities may be demonstrated on imaging, including chronic maxillary atelectasis, mucocele, ossifying fibroma of the maxilla, or fungal involvement. Of note, even the common cold can cause mucosal thickening of the sinuses sufficient to be seen on MRI. Elevations in ESR and C-reactive protein (CRP) are independently predictive of sinusitis but are nonspecific.

(iv) Treatment

Otolaryngologic consultation should be obtained. Endoscopic surgery should be considered when a 6-month trial of medical therapy has failed, or immediately in the case of a significant abnormality on imaging. With careful patient selection, endoscopic sinus surgery can achieve relief of pain in 56% of patients, and substantial improvement in a further 29%. Difficulties arise in patients with chronic sinus area pain that mimics sinusitis but may not be true sinusitis. When imaging repeatedly demonstrates normal sinuses, and there is a lack of any objective evidence for sinusitis, a

Table 4. Paranasal, periocular, periauricular, and head and neck cancer pain

Diagnosis	Paranasal Sinus Pain	Periocular Pain	Periauricular Pain	Head and Neck Cancer
Region				
Diagnostic features	Bilateral or unilateral throbbing or pressure frontal area pain, exacerbated by leaning the head forward or palpation over the sinus.	Pain or tenderness with or without eye movement, deep orbital pain, and referred pain.	Diffuse aching or sudden pain with or without aural discharge (e.g., otitis media).	Wide variety of symptoms. Pain may occur because of tumor growth, nerve compression secondary infection, second myofascial pain, deafferentation, radiotherapy, or chemotherapy.
Diagnostic evaluation	Check history for chronic allergies, frequent URI, sinusitis, history of headaches of various types, or sinus surgery. Referral to ENT specialist for proper endoscopic or CT scan study (e.g.,	Examination of the eyelids, lacrimal apparatus conjunctiva, and, sclera for signs of hemorrhage and inflammation. Direct ophthalmoscopy and referral to ophthalmologist for further exams.	As the area is innervated by multiple cranial and cervical nerves. A complete functional and structural clinical examination must be done (e.g. inspection of the tympanic membrane, TMJ, and	Complete evaluation of multidisciplinary team. CT scan, MRI, endoscopy, biopsy, and surveillance. Treatment coordination by oncologist.

Table 4. Continued

Diagnosis	Paranasal Sinus Pain	Periocular Pain	Periauricular Pain	Head and Neck Cancer
	opacification of the sinus).	Rule out the presence of primary headache (e.g., cluster headache, migraine), temporal arteritis Orbital pseudotumor.	myofascial dysfunction). CT scan and MRI are mastoiditis and cholesteatoma.	
Treatment	Proper ENT evaluation and treatment	Proper ophthalmologic evaluation and treatment	Proper ENT evaluation and treatment	Proper oncologist evaluation and treatment
	Medication: sinusitis— topical decongestants; systemic antibiotics;	Medication: NSAIDs; nonopiate analgesics; corticosteroids; topical or systemic antibiotics, BTX across forehead and glabellar areas in selected cases	Medication: NSAIDs; nonopiate analgesics; systemic antibiotics; topical corticosteroids	Medication: anticonvulsants (e.g., gabapentin); antidepressants (e.g., amitriptyline); opiate or nonopiate analgesics; topical agents (e.g., lidocaine 5% patches), muscle relaxants
	chronic sinus pain— NSAIDs, nonopiate analgesics, topical agents (lidocaine spray), anticonvulsants (e.g., gabapentin); antidepressants (e.g., amitriptyline) Surgery	Surgery	Surgery	Surgery: ablative surgeries

BTX, botulinum toxin; CT, computerized tomography; ENT, ear nose and throat; MRI, magnetic resonance imaging; NSAIDs, nonsteroidal antiinflammatory drugs; TMJ, temporomandibular joint; URI, upper respiratory infection.

431

multidisciplinary, multidimensional approach, including the specialties of neurology, psychiatry, and behavioral medicine, is required. Neuroplasticity, with peripheral and central sensitization, and chronic inflammatory pain should be considered. These patients are unlikely to benefit from surgical intervention.

2. Periocular Pain

(i) Diagnostic Features

Ophthalmic pain results from stimulation of pain fibers relating either directly or indirectly to the orbit. Cranial nerves involved may include the trigeminal, facial, vagus, and glossopharyngeal. The trigeminal sensory complex communicates actively with these cranial nerves, as well as the limbic and autonomic systems, and dips down to the level of C6. As a result, pain may be poorly localized, or be referred from other anatomic structures and areas with shared innervation peripherally and centrally. Pain can be classified as ocular, orbital or referred (Table 4).

OCULAR PAIN.   Corneal irritation or damage is associated with local pain, photophobia, and lacrimation, together with a foreign body sensation. Anterior scleritis presents with severe ocular pain, whereas posterior scleritis is characterized by less well-defined orbital pain; either may be associated with a systemic collagen vascular disease. A triad of red eye, increased intraocular pressure, and a middilated pupil is pathognomonic of acute angle glaucoma. Severe ocular pain is associated with headache; this pain may radiate to the sinuses and teeth and be associated with systemic features such as nausea and vomiting. Atherosclerotic disease of the carotid may present with ocular ischemic pain. Uncorrected refractive error produces pain from excess ciliary body tone, pain that radiates to the head and brow. **Photooculodynia** is an uncommon pain syndrome of unknown etiology in which ocular pain is precipitated by light.

ORBITAL PAIN.   Orbital cellulitis presents acutely with pain exacerbated by palpation and movement. Orbital pseudotumor is an inflammatory process of unknown etiology that presents with pain, chemosis, diplopia, and red eye. Trochleitis is characterized by orbital pain with movement, together with exquisite superonasal point tenderness. Retroocular pain with diminished vision are features of optic neuritis, which may occur alone or as a symptom of a demyelinating disease.

REFERRED PAIN.   The proximity and convergence of afferent pain fibers produce referred pain. Occasionally, pain from the area of the greater occipital nerve presents may radiate to the eye and face (secondary trigeminal neuralgia) because of convergence and communication between the cervical nerves, and the trigeminal sensory complex. Migraine, sinusitis, otitis, mastoiditis, and dental pain can all be referred to the eye. Temporal arteritis presents with visual loss and ipsilateral facial pain, and is diagnosed on temporal artery biopsy.

(ii) Epidemiology

Carotid occlusive disease, glaucoma, and temporal arteritis are more common in the elderly, whereas optic neuritis occurs predominantly in young adults, and MS with optic neuritis in young to middle age adults.

(iii) Diagnostic Evaluation, Imaging Studies, and Laboratory Tests

MRI is indicated in order to detect MS as a cause of optic neuritis. Raeder syndrome requires imaging to rule out a parasellar mass or carotid dissection as causes. Doppler flow studies are useful in detecting carotid stenosis as a cause of orbital ischemia. An erythrocyte sedimentation rate of more than 100 mm per hour, and an increased CRP and fibrinogen levels are strongly associated with temporal arteritis.

(iv) Treatment

If temporal arteritis, optic neuritis, or orbital pseudotumor is suspected, high dose corticosteroids should be started immediately, and the patient should be referred to an ophthalmologist or rheumatologist, depending on the suspected diagnosis. All patients with suspected eye pathology should be examined by an ophthalmologist. Keratitis and orbital cellulitis are treated aggressively with topical and systemic antibiotics, and with surgical drainage of collections and sinusitis as required. Acute angle glaucoma requires urgent ophthalmic referral and topical pupillary constriction, with or without laser iridotomy.

3. Periauricular Pain

(i) Diagnostic Features

Otitis media presents with either dull aching or sudden exquisite pain, with or without aural discharge, an inflamed tympanic membrane, and systemic evidence of infection (malaise and pyrexia). Otitis externa can be exquisitely painful, and is generally an acute process. Mastoiditis and otitis pain may be referred to the eye, pharynx, and neck because of the involvement of cranial nerve VII (supplying branches to both the eye and ear), convergence with the trigeminal sensory complex, and the shared innervations of C2 and C3, and the petrous bone (Gradenigo syndrome). A common cause of otalgia that is frequently overlooked is referred myofascial pain from muscles of the neck and pharynx and from the masticatory muscles (Table 4).

(ii) Epidemiology

Otitis media presents more frequently in childhood and should always be considered in immunocompromised patients. Mastoiditis and infected cholesteatoma are found more frequently in children and young to middle-aged adults.

(iii) Diagnostic Evaluation, Imaging Studies, and Laboratory Tests

Elevated white cell count is supportive but nonspecific evidence for otitis media. CT scan and MRI are invaluable for mastoiditis and cholesteatoma. History and physical examination should direct to an appropriate otolaryngologic referral.

(iv) Treatment

In general, urgent consultation with an otolaryngologist is required. Evidence of petrosal involvement requires broad-spectrum intravenous antibiotics. Pain problems referred to a pain specialist are often from an otolaryngologist who has successfully treated the problem, but the patient still has chronic pain, together with frequent myofascial pain of the neck, head, and orofacial muscles. Treatment is multidimensional and comprehensive, covering possible myofascial, neuropathic, and nociceptive pain

4. Head and Neck Cancer Pain

(i) Diagnostic Features

Head and neck cancer present with a wide variety of symptoms. Frequently, a multidimensional approach is required during diagnosis, treatment, and recovery. Nociceptive and neuropathic pain may occur at any time during the course of disease and treatment, and coordination between surgical, dental, psychiatric, physical therapy, and oncologic consultations are frequently required.

Characteristic effects of the various manifestations of malignant disease and its treatment are discussed in subsequent text. Local tumor growth and invasion result in local tissue destruction, secondary infection, nerve compression with mononeuropathy and plexopathy, secondary myofascial pain from distorted mouth opening and function, diplopia, and ptosis. Surgical resection and reconstruction result in acute postoperative pain, nerve damage and resection, inadequate vascularization of myocutaneous flaps, and sacrifice of the accessory nerve. Chemotherapy with vincristine and cisplatinum results in nerve damage and neuritis. Radiotherapy results in mucositis of the GI tract, osteoradionecrosis, cheilosis (tissue breakdown at the corners of the mouth), loss of salivary glands, secondary infection (fungal and bacterial), and loss of range of motion of the neck, facial, and masticatory muscles (including limited mouth opening and remodeling of the TMJ, with secondary severe myofascial pain and dysfunction). Nutritional deficiencies (secondary to pain, loss of appetite, poor caloric intake, and mismatch between metabolic demands and intake) result in poor fit of dental prostheses (with or without pain), as well as pyridoxine, vitamin B_{12}, and other specific vitamin and mineral deficiencies. Secondary infection results in tissue breakdown and pain. Psychosocial factors contribute to the overall pain response inducing fear, anxiety, lack of self esteem, There are also cosmetic concerns, and fears of tumor recurrence leading to patients' interpretation of symptoms as tumor recurrence rather than the expected secondary complications of therapies (Table 4).

(ii) Epidemiology

Head and neck cancer predominantly occurs in older adults, although lymphoma, adenocarcinoma of the sinuses, and squamous cell carcinoma do occur in younger adults. Smoking and chewing of tobacco; consumption of alcohol; chronic irritation; injury of the intraoral mucosa secondary to habits, damaged dentition, and poorly fitting fixed and removable prostheses; and sun exposure and fair skin are strongly associated with the development of head and neck cancers.

(iii) Diagnostic Evaluation, Imaging Studies, and Laboratory Tests

Radiologic imaging techniques of CT scan and MRI, endoscopy, biopsy, and surveillance are invaluable in the management of head and neck cancer.

(iv) Treatment

Pain from head and neck cancer should be treated on the same principles as those outlined in Chapter 32. With particular reference to head and neck cancer, physical therapy can improve range of motion of the neck, mouth, and TMJ. Myofascial pain of the shoulders, neck and head, and headache, are frequent secondary occurrences, and may also respond to physical therapy. Nutritional consultation may be helpful, as may be dental consultation to aid oral function and cosmetics.

VII. CONCLUSION

Orofacial pain derives from a vast number of complex etiologies, and its successful treatment requires contributions from many different specialties. Orofacial pain is one of the most distressing of all painful syndromes and warrants aggressive and appropriate treatment in a multidisciplinary setting. This chapter outlines some of the etiologies, diagnostic features, and treatments of orofacial pain.

SELECTED READINGS

Acquadro M. Headache and sinusitis. *Curr Opin Otolaryngol Head Neck Surg* 1998;6:2–5.

Barker FG II, Jannetta PJ, Bissonette DJ, et al. The long term outcome of microvascular decompression for trigeminal neuralgia. *N Engl J Med* 1996;334:1077–1083.

Bohr TW. Fibromyalgia syndrome and myofascial pain syndrome: do they exist? *Neurol Clin* 1995;13:365–384.

Borodic GE, Acquadro MA. The use of botulinum toxin for the treatment of chronic facial pain. *J Pain* 2002;3(1):21–27.

Borodic GE, Acquadro M, Johnson EA. Botulinum toxin therapy for pain and inflammatory disorders: mechanisms and therapeutic effects. *Expert Opin Investig Drugs* 2001;10(8):1531–1544.

DaSilva AF, Becerra L, Makris N, et al. Somatotopic activation in the human trigeminal pain pathway. *J Neurosci* 2002;22:8183–8192.

Graff-Radford SB. Facial pain. *Curr Opin Neurol* 2000;13:291–296.

Hu JW, Tsaj CM, Bakke M, et al. Deep craniofacial pain: involvement of the trigeminal subnucleus caudalis and its modulation. In: Jensen TS, Turner JA, Wiesenfeld-Hallin Z, eds. *Proceedings of the Eight World Congress*. Seattle, WA: IASP Press, 1997:497–506.

Huang W, Tothe MJ, Grant-Kels JM. The burning mouth syndrome. *J Am Acad Dermatol* 1996;34:91–98.

Marbach JJ. Orofacial phantom pain: theory and phenomenology. *J Am Dent Assoc* 1996;127:221–229.

Marbach JJ, Lennon MC, Link BG, et al. Losing face: sources of stigma as perceived by chronic facial pain patients. *J Behav Med* 1990; 13:583–604.

Okeson JP. *Orofacial pain, guidelines for assessment, diagnosis, and management/The American Academy of Orofacial Pain*. Chicago, IL: Quintessence Publishing Co, 1996.

Sessle BJ. Acute and chronic craniofacial pain: brainstem mechanisms of nociceptive transmission and neuroplasticity, and their clinical correlates. *Crit Rev Oral Biol Med* 2000;11:57–91.

Truelove E, Sommers E, LeResche L, et al. Clinical diagnostic criteria for TMD. *J Am Dent Assoc* 1992;123:47–54.

Special thanks to Claudio Moreno for constructing the tables.

30

Opioids in Chronic Nonterminal Pain

Jane C. Ballantyne

The Angelic face of Opium is dazzlingly seductive, but if you look upon the other side of it, it will appear altogether a Devil. There is so much poison in this All-healing Medicine, that we ought not to be by any means secure or confident in the frequent and familiar use of it.
—*Thomas Willis, "Medicine in Mans Body," 1621–1673*

I. INTRODUCTION

The earliest evidence of opium use by humans was the discovery of opium poppy seedpods in a 4200 BC burial site in Spain. In fact, throughout the ages, even when medical science was virtually nonexistent, opium was one of the few remedies known to humans, and it maintained a central role in medicine because most diseases were palliated rather than cured. The explosion of medical and scientific knowledge that has occurred over the last hundred years has profoundly altered the role of opioids in our lives. We prolong life, shorten terminal illness, and expect to be pain- and disease-free. Medically, we use opioids to two distinct ends: to treat physical pain and to treat addiction. Regulatory controls, introduced during the 20th century, have given physicians a central role in determining who should and should not receive opioids. We have begun to understand the neurobiologic basis of opioid analgesia, tolerance, dependence, and addiction. We are in a better position now than ever before to understand opioid effects and to use opioids so that they help and do not harm patients. After years of caution brought about by regulatory controls, we use opioids liberally for acute and terminal pain, knowing that we can substantially reduce pain and maintain safety. But the issue of using opioids for chronic nonterminal pain (CNTP) is vastly more complicated and is a key issue in pain management.

II. RATIONALE FOR CHOOSING OPIOID THERAPY

The student reading this book is well aware that there are many ways to control pain, some relying on psychological override, some on physical approaches, some on neural blockade, some on counterstimulation, and others on medication. The choice often depends on culture, background, habit, and fashion rather than on the superiority or the likely success of one medication over another. The link between these indicators of treatment choice and the placebo effect (see Chapter 3) is clear; treatments work better when patients believe in them. Present-day fashion, at least in the Western world, dictates that medications are the most trusted and applicable of the treatment options. Opioids are the only class of pain medication offering powerful analgesia without a ceiling effect, meaning that doses can be increased until pain is overcome. This advantage makes the opioids theoretically attractive options for the management of pain, and the reason that pain advocates believe that all patients with pain have a right to opioid therapy—it being the only therapy that can reliably and effectively relieve pain. But, of course, this is only true in a society or culture that places medications at the top of its hierarchy of effectiveness.

Nobody doubts that opioids are powerful and effective analgesics, and scientific evidence supports this assumption. However, whether analgesic efficacy is maintained with prolonged use is less clear, and other liabilities can also interfere with long-term treatment. There must be sustained and obvious benefit in order to justify continued use. When making the decision to start opioid treatment of CNTP, one can usefully consider two phases—an initial phase, in which opioid treatment is used as part of a multimodal and aggressive rehabilitative approach that aims to restore function and to reduce reliance on medications, followed by a chronic phase, in which opioids are utilized according to strict criteria. The desirable end point of chronic opioid treatment is much debated, but it would seem that some improvement in quality of life must be seen to justify the treatment, whether this is an improvement in function or simply a meaningful reduction in pain.

III. LIABILITIES

1. Loss of Efficacy

Many patients receiving opioid therapy for chronic pain appear to obtain satisfactory and sustained pain relief without dose escalation. This seems counter to our belief that the development of tolerance, a pharmacologic phenomenon, is an inevitable consequence of prolonged opioid use. It is evident, nevertheless, that in many patients, tolerance "levels off," not only in the case of side effects but also in the case of analgesia, and that these patients can derive adequate analgesia at a stable dose.

In other patients, the outcome is less favorable. Satisfactory analgesia is not sustained, and the patients request increasing doses. Tolerance develops to the analgesic and euphoric effects of opioids, as well as to their side effects (except direct bowel effects). Tolerance to opioids can be learned (associative), involving psychological factors and linked to environmental clues; or adaptive (nonassociative), involving down-regulation and/or desensitization of opioid receptors. Mechanisms of pharmacologic tolerance to opioids have not been fully elucidated, but many mechanisms appear to be linked to the N-methyl-D-aspartate (NMDA)-receptor cascade. Alternatively, "apparent" tolerance could arise as a consequence of **opioid-induced hyperalgesia**, a phenomenon that has been largely forgotten for years but one that has been amply described and could sometimes explain resistance to opioid treatment. Recently, the mechanism of **opioid-induced hyperalgesia** has been elucidated, and, interestingly, it is also linked to the NMDA-receptor cascade. This process may represent a form of neurotoxicity, considering that the NMDA-receptor is also implicated in the hyperalgesia associated with neuropathic pain (see Chapter 25). We are now presented with a quandary when a patient presents with escalating pain unresponsive to opioid therapy: Do we, having eliminated the possibility of a change in disease state, assume that the cause is pharmacologic tolerance and will be overcome by dose increase; or would dose increase make matters worse?

2. Unacceptable Side Effects

The side effects of opioids include sedation, respiratory depression, nausea and vomiting, slowing of bowel activity, pruritus, and dysphoria. These side effects are described in more detail in Chapter 9. As mentioned in the preceding text, it is common for tolerance to develop to all these side effects except the bowel effects, which are peripherally mediated and to which tolerance does not develop. Patients starting opioid therapy who experience side effects can be reassured that the side effects will likely subside in time. Patients taking opioids for a long term should always receive bowel prophylaxis to prevent constipation because this is an almost inevitable consequence of chronic opioid therapy. Despite the development of tolerance to side effects, a significant number of patients—one estimate is 50%—will stop taking opioids because of intolerable side effects or because of lack of efficacy.

3. Hormonal Effects

Opioids influence at least two major hormonal systems, the hypothalamic–pituitary–adrenal axis and the hypothalamic–pituitary–gonadal axis. The resultant increase in levels of prolactin and decreases in levels of plasma cortisol, follicular stimulating hormone, luteinizing hormone, testosterone, and estrogen may have deleterious clinical effects including male and female infertility, decreased libido and aggression, menstrual disorders, and galactorrhea. These opioid effects were observed long before they were chemically confirmed in heroin addicts. Later, testosterone depletion was demonstrated in male patients in methadone programs. Testosterone levels can be particularly low in patients receiving intrathecal opioids, to the extent that these patients often feel better and regain energy when they are treated with testosterone. The extent of hormonal changes in patients with

CNTP treated with opioids, and the clinical significance of the change is unknown, but one recent study did find decrements in testosterone and cortisol in these patients. Whether hormonal replacement would improve the well-being of patients with CNTP who are treated with opioids remains uncertain.

4. Immune Effects

Animal and human studies demonstrate the presence of opioid receptors on a wide range of immune cells, and the ability of opioids to alter the development, differentiation, and function of immune cells. Prolonged exposure to opioids appears more likely to suppress immune function than short-term exposure, whereas the abrupt withdrawal of opioids also seems to cause immunosuppression. Few studies have been conducted assessing immune function in patients with CNTP receiving opioids, but the direct evidence that opioids impair immune function does give rise to concern in these patients. Pain itself can produce immunosuppression, so the greatest concern is likely to pertain to patients who receive high doses of opioids and yet do not experience good pain relief.

5. Problematic Opioid Use

Problematic opioid use, comprising addiction, diversion, and other less serious problem behaviors, is an inescapable aspect of opioid treatment of CNTP. To deny these problems is to sweep aside the most challenging aspect of treating long-term pain with opioids, which in turn compromises care, and denies patients appropriate treatment when problematic behavior does arise. Most problematic behaviors are manifestations or harbingers of addiction. Problematic behaviors arise in a substantial proportion of chronic pain patients who are treated with opioids, albeit a minority. Published reports suggest a rate of 3% to 19%.

Typical problematic behaviors for patients with pain who are treated with opioids are listed in Chapter 35, Table 1.

Diversion of opioids from their intended use, usually for profit, occasionally occurs in the pain treatment setting. Sometimes profit seeking is driven by the need of the addict to obtain more drug to satisfy an addiction, but more often it is simply a criminal act. It is not the job of the physician to monitor patients for criminal activity; nevertheless, it would be irresponsible to continue to prescribe opioids to patients who are found to be diverting. A combination of aberrant behavior and a negative drug screen may alert the physician to the possibility that the prescribed drug is being diverted. Occasionally, the whole treatment course is a sham when a patient fabricates pain in order to obtain opioids.

The subject of chronic opioid use, drug abuse, and addiction is covered in detail in Chapter 35. In this chapter, it is important to understand how physical dependence differs from addiction. Although the syndrome of drug addiction is often characterized in part by physical dependence—that is, a state of adaptation manifest as a withdrawal syndrome upon cessation or reversal of the drug—addiction is a syndrome of maladaptive behavior, and maladaptive behavior must be present to diagnose addiction (see Chapter 35, Fig. 2). Physical dependence is likely to develop in almost all patients receiving long-term opioids, but most patients do not become addicted. However, if addiction does arise, physical dependence can be a powerful factor in maintaining the addictive state. Therefore, signs of physical dependence may be manifest in addiction, but the term physical dependence is not synonymous with addiction.

As the medical community grapples with the issues surrounding long-term opioid use, and with its role in treating both pain and addiction, it becomes clearer that the *bona fide* treatment of chronic pain has much in common with the treatment of addiction. Whether addiction arises in only a few patients whose pain was treated with opioids or in most (which may depend on the willingness of treating physicians to diagnose addiction), it is still necessary to provide long-term treatment in a highly structured setting (less restrictive than the methadone clinic, but structured and monitored nonetheless), so that addiction problems can be minimized. How confident can physicians be that during the course of treatment they are treating physical pain and not other life stresses, and how many patients who started self-medicating with illicit opioids did so to relieve similar turmoil or emptiness? What is important is that physicians do not replace poorly controlled pain with poorly controlled pain plus untreated addiction, thereby worsening the lives of their patients. This is why it is necessary to provide long-term opioid therapy only in a structured setting.

IV. STRUCTURED GOAL-ORIENTED APPROACH TO LONG-TERM TREATMENT

The principles of treatment are summarized in Table 1. Ideally, opioids should be used for a short time only, even in the case of CNTP. Early aggressive treatment, using a rehabilitative approach that aims to restore function and reduce reliance on medications, can be utilized when a patient first presents with debilitating pain (see Chapter 19). The structured approach suggested here should be used when the physician and patient decide on a long-term commitment to opioid treatment (see Fig. 1). This approach aims to perform the following functions:

Table 1.   Principles of opioid therapy for CNTP

- First try aggressive rehabilitative approach that may utilize opioids but aims to restore function and reduce reliance on medications
- Consider longer-term treatment a serious undertaking that will require the commitment of both physician and patient
- Ensure that other treatment options have been maximized
- Use goal-directed therapy; set limits and goals and adhere to these
- Consider opioid therapy as an adjunct; sole opioid therapy is rarely successful
- Unless pain is occasional, base regime on long-acting opioids, and avoid breakthrough medication
- Ensure careful and regular follow-up
- Be prepared to wean patient and discontinue if treatment goals are not met
- Maintain good documentation

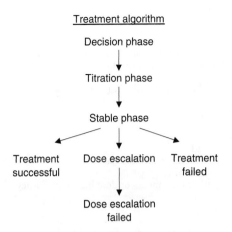

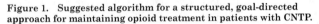

Figure 1. **Suggested algorithm for a structured, goal-directed approach for maintaining opioid treatment in patients with CNTP.**

- Select patients with the best chance of benefiting and the lowest level of risk.
- Continuously monitor patients for achievement of preset goals, and onset of problematic behavior.
- Maintain patients at the lowest effective dose in order to maintain efficacy and minimize liabilities such as toxicity, failed analgesia, hormonal effects, and immune suppression.

1. Decision Phase

The commitment to long-term opioid therapy is a serious one, and should be considered such by both patient and physician. Often, opioid therapy has already been started, but this does not obviate the need for careful review of the implications of long-term treatment once the long-term treatment phase is entered. The pain diagnosis must be clearly established and documented. Both physician and patient must be satisfied that all other treatment options have been explored and do not provide adequate relief. The physician must also be satisfied that the possible risk, particularly the risk of addiction or functional deterioration, does not outweigh the potential benefit of treatment. This is the single most challenging aspect of the decision phase, especially knowing that although we are aware of certain markers of likely risk (see Table 2), the presence of these does not necessarily mean that there will be no benefit from carefully monitored treatment (see Chapter 35, Section V). The physician should carefully describe the complications and risks of long-term opioid therapy and allow the patient to express his or her anxieties. The physician will need to explain the clinic's monitoring policies and the rationale for monitoring. It may be helpful to have an explicit record of the patient's understanding of the liabilities of long-term treatment and the clinic's policies for monitoring, and

Table 2.   Identifying risk of abuse or treatment failure

- History of substance abuse or addiction
- Family history of substance abuse or addiction
- History of depression or anxiety
- Personality disorder
- History of abuse, especially childhood abuse
- Young
- Not working
- On disability
- Litigation pending
- Dysfunctional
- Poor interpersonal relationships
- Difficult personality
- Refusing other treatments or denying their efficacy

this could be in the form of a signed written agreement or consent. As an example, the MGH opioid agreement is included as Appendix IV.

It is helpful, at this stage, to establish and document the goals of treatment. This understanding enables the physician to effectively measure the success of treatment, and to argue for discontinuing the treatment if there is no progress toward meeting the goals. Goals differ: the patient with severe disability may simply want to be able to sit at a table long enough to have a family meal, whereas the patient who was previously a fully functional patient may want to return to work. Whether pain reduction without other improvement is an acceptable goal is debatable, but in view of the complex and broad effects of opioids, it would seem not, especially if pain reduction is accompanied by functional deterioration.

2. Titration Phase

The titration phase aims to find an effective dose as quickly as possible so that the patient can be maintained on a stable dose with known analgesic efficacy. It is usual to start therapy at a low standard dose (see Appendix VII—Drug Appendix), and increase as tolerated to achieve acceptable analgesia. If satisfactory analgesia is not achieved, or if the adverse effects are intolerable, the treatment should be discontinued. In the inpatient setting, the titration phase can be achieved within days, but takes longer in the outpatient setting. It should not, however, take longer than 8 weeks, and it may be necessary to see the patient more often than usual, or to monitor progress by telephone, during the titration phase.

3. Stable Phase

Ideally, the patient should be maintained at a stable dose, and ability to maintain a stable dose is often an indication of successful treatment. For several reasons, including less likelihood of developing addiction, less disruption of normal activity and preference for relying on coping skills rather than focusing on medication, long-acting opioid preparations administered around the clock are usually chosen when treating long-term pain. The issue of long- versus short-acting opioids is discussed more fully in Chapter 35, Section VI, and drug choice are described in Chapter 9. During the stable phase of treatment, it is mandatory (by law in most states) to provide monthly prescriptions, and advisable to conduct regular comprehensive follow-up assessments.

(i) Monthly Refills

In most states of the United States, prescriptions for controlled substances must be provided monthly, and predating of prescriptions is discouraged. It is easier to conduct follow-up evaluations if the patient picks up the prescriptions in person, unless he or she is unable to do so for physical reasons. This is an opportunity for the prescribing physician or an assistant to assess and document the patient's state of health, pain level, and side effects, to treat side effects if necessary, and to arrange for more comprehensive follow-up if there are deviations or other problems.

(ii) Comprehensive Follow-up

Periodically, preferably every 3 months, but at least every year, the patient should undergo comprehensive follow-up. Assessment should be made of pain, the effect of pain on the patient's well-being, the achievement of treatment goals, level of function and quality of life. The use of standard questionnaires such as the SF-36 can help the physician assess function and quality of life and is encouraged (see Chapter 15).

(iii) Toxicology Screening and Identifying Aberrant Behaviors

The patient's presence at monthly clinic visits provides an opportunity to observe aberrant behaviors. Extra visits, requests for interim prescriptions, and frequent telephone calls to the clinic are included in the signs of prescription drug abuse listed in Chapter 35, Table 1. All these should be documented. The physician's regular comprehensive assessments also provide an opportunity to identify problems. Toxicology screening can be a helpful adjunct to monitoring for problematic opioid use, including for addiction and diversion. Some practitioners believe that all patients with CNTP who were treated with opioids should be subjected to random urine screening. In support of this view, in one pain clinic, 43% patients with CNTP who were treated with opioids were judged "problematic," and of these, 49% were identified using toxicology screening, not behavioral parameters. In some practice settings, however, routine or random testing would seem unnecessary. The treating physician must determine the severity of the problem of prescription drug abuse in his or her practice, and institute testing as either an occasional or a routine event. The issue of toxicology screening is covered more fully in Chapter 35, Section VII.

4. Dose Escalation

Sometimes an increase in dose will be needed, but careful consideration should be given before each dose escalation. Tolerance to the analgesic effects of opioids can develop over time, but the more common experience is that tolerance levels out, and most patients can be maintained at stable dose. Therefore, if an increase in dose is needed, it should always alert the physician to the possibility that there are other reasons for the need for increased dose. There may be a change in the patient's pain or underlying disease, which should be sought and treated if necessary. The need for a higher dose may also be a manifestation of psychological need or addiction, which should also be identified and treated if necessary. At high doses, apparent tolerance may be a sign of **opioid-induced hyperalgesia**, which will be made worse by dose escalation. Nevertheless, it is always reasonable to try a controlled dose escalation and see if this improves the pain and overall status of the patient. The aim of each dose escalation is to reach a new, stable dose. For severe pain, it may be helpful to admit the patient to hospital to help with diagnosis and rapid titration.

The use of very high doses of opioids for CNTP is rarely helpful. It is hard to say exactly what dose should be considered a high dose, and the issue of whether there is a clinical ceiling for dose is much debated. The traditional teaching is that opioid dose can be increased in a limitless fashion, and that dose increases are capable of overcoming pain. But clinical experience suggests otherwise, especially with long-term treatment. In the case of acute pain, it seems true that pain can eventually be overcome by high-dose opioid treatment. This also seems true in the early treatment of cancer pain. But now that we see very long survival in patients with cancer, we also see cancer pain that gets out of control, and dose increases that do not seem to help. This observation, together with the basic science observation that there are multiple splice variants of endogenous opioid receptors resulting in much cross-sensitivity between various opioids, was the genesis of the clinical practice of opioid rotation. A switch to a different opioid can provide equal or better analgesia at half or less of the equivalent dose of the first opioid. Opioid rotation is a reasonable way to control dose escalation (opioid rotation is described in more detail in Chapter 32).

Because the highest daily dose of opioid used in existing trials is 180 mg morphine or morphine equivalent, that dose is suggested as the point at which one should begin to consider dose reduction or opioid rotation. That is not to say that some patients do not do well on higher daily doses but rather that clinical experience suggests that most patients do better if the daily dose is maintained below this level. One should also consider that some liabilities, including neurotoxicity, hyperalgesia, hormonal and immune effects, and problematic behavior predominate when high doses are used.

5. Criteria for Success and Failure

In order to decide whether to maintain or terminate opioid treatment, one must establish criteria for success and failure. These criteria tend to be subjective and highly dependent on the treating physician's viewpoint. At MGH, we consider pain relief that improves well-being, progress toward achieving treatment goals, improved function, and improved quality of life as criteria for success. We recommend that at least one of these criteria be achieved to warrant continuing therapy. Our criteria for failure are failure to reach any of the criteria for success, evidence of addiction and repeated noncompliance. If any of these occur, we usually discontinue treatment or refer for appropriate treatment, as in the case of addiction when a psychiatrist and/or addiction specialist should be involved in the patient's care.

6. Discontinuation

If the treatment fails, the patient can be weaned off the medication and the medication can be discontinued. It is important to wean cautiously in order to avoid unpleasant withdrawal, the experience of which can make it hard for the patient to give up the medication a second time. Weaning can usually be accomplished over 10 days, but the exact weaning schedule will depend on dose, drug, and duration of treatment. If there is addiction, discontinuation may not be the appropriate course of action, but addiction therapy will be needed. Many patients, especially those who are not doing well on opioids, report an improvement in well-being, and possibly also in pain, after an opioid wean. If necessary, opioid treatment can be restarted after a period of abstinence. Opioid weaning is not always straightforward, and it may be helpful or even necessary to undergo weaning in a rehabilitation setting.

V. CONCLUSION

The attractions of opioid therapy are plain. Opioids are powerful analgesics, capable of removing most pain at adequate dose, at least in the short term. They will do this instantaneously. In an age when physicians and patients seek sure-fire, rapid solutions to medical problems, opioids seem an obvious answer to the pain problem. But when we try to use long-term opioid treatment, the complexities of the treatment begin to unravel. Opioids are more than just analgesics. Their euphoric effects are therapeutic, but they are intimately involved in the development and maintenance of addiction. Toxicities include neuroendocrine effects, immune effects, and hyperalgesia. Analgesia is not always maintained. There is currently strong commercial pressure to turn to the medicine cabinet to fix all our ills. But pills and opioids are not the only way to effectively control pain; it is not inhumane—in fact, it is good practice—to restrict long-term opioid use to those who cannot obtain relief by other means and to those who are least at risk of deteriorating on opioids.

SELECTED READINGS

American Academy of Pain Medicine and American Pain Society consensus document. The use of opioids for the treatment of chronic pain, 1997.

Ballantyne JC, Mao J. Opioids for chronic pain. *N Engl J Med* 2003; 349:1943–1953.

Katz NP, Sherburne S, Beach M, et al. Behavioral monitoring and urine toxicology testing in patients receiving long-term opioid therapy. *Anesth Analg* 2003;97:1097–1102.

Mao J. Opioid induced abnormal pain sensitivity: implications in clinical opioid therapy. *Pain* 2002;100:213–217.

Model guidelines for the use of controlled substances for the treatment of pain. A policy document of the Federation of State Medical Boards of the United States, Inc., May 1998.

Portenoy RK, Foley KM. Chronic use of opioid analgesics in nonmalignant pain: report of 38 cases. *Pain* 1986;25:171–186.

Pain in Human Immunodeficiency Virus and Acquired Immunodeficiency Syndrome

S. Jane Marshall, Sarah Cox, and Andrew S. C. Rice

I esteem it . . . to be clearly the office of a physician not only to restore health, but also to mitigate the pains and torments of diseases.
—*Francis Bacon, "The Advancement of Learning," 1605, IV ii, in The Works of Francis Bacon, James Spedding, Robert Leslie Ellis, and Douglas Denton Heath, eds. 15 vols, London: Longman and Co, 1860–1864;4:387*

I. INTRODUCTION

Between 40% and 88% of individuals infected with human immunodeficiency virus (HIV) experience pain. This pain may occur as a consequence of the following:

- HIV-induced tissue damage (e.g., myalgia and neuropathy)
- HIV-related infection or malignancy (e.g., herpes virus infections and headache from cerebral lymphoma)
- Immunologic repair as a consequence of HIV treatment (e.g., increased risk of herpes zoster after starting antiretroviral treatment)
- Side effects of HIV treatment (e.g., nucleoside reverse transcriptase inhibitor-induced peripheral neuropathy; indinavir-induced ureteric calculi)
- Causes unrelated to HIV

In general, the principles of pain management in the context of HIV differ little from those of pain management in other scenarios. However, painful peripheral neuropathy is common in HIV and requires particular attention, as does the potential for serious drug interactions with HIV therapy.

II. UPDATE ON HUMAN IMMUNODEFICIENCY VIRUS

HIV, an RNA virus, causes a predominantly cell-mediated immunodeficiency. Humans are susceptible to infection by two types of HIV: HIV-1 and HIV-2. Worldwide, HIV-1 is the most common virus associated with progressive disease, whereas HIV-2 is found predominantly in West Africa, is less infectious, and causes immunodeficiency more slowly than HIV-1.

HIV infection is a pandemic that has exceeded the projections of 10 years ago and now represents one of the ten major causes of death worldwide. The Joint United Nations Programme on HIV/AIDS reports that at the end of 2003, there were approximately 40 million people worldwide living with HIV or acquired immunodeficiency syndrome (AIDS). During the same year, there were three million deaths related to HIV. In developed countries, the prevalence of HIV continues to rise, largely owing to life-prolonging antiretroviral therapy and new infections related to high-risk behavior.

HIV infection generally occurs after transfer of infected bodily fluids. Seroconversion occurs some weeks after acute infection and 75% of individuals recall an associated influenzalike illness.

The clinical consequences of HIV infection largely correlate with the degree of immunosuppression, as reflected in the CD4 T-cell count, which, together with the HIV viral load, is used as a disease marker for monitoring disease activity/progression and the response to therapy. In untreated HIV, the viral load rises and is followed by a falling CD4 count. With effective treatment, the viral load becomes undetectable in the laboratory and the CD4 count may rise, provided immune system damage has not become irreversible. With more advanced immunologic damage, as the CD4 T-cell count falls below 500×10^6 per L, patients experience increased susceptibility to opportunistic infections, diseases of the central nervous system (CNS) and malignancies, some of which are AIDS-defining illnesses, including candidiasis, cytomegalovirus disease, Kaposi sarcoma (KS), lymphoma, and *Pneumocystis carinii* pneumonia. If the CD4 T-cell count falls below 200×10^6 per L, prophylaxis against infection with *P. carinii* pneumonia should be prescribed. At this level of immune dysfunction, patients are also at risk from cerebral toxoplasmosis, progressive multifocal leukoencephalopathy, dementia, and wasting disease. Cytomegalovirus infection causing retinitis and colitis and disseminated nontuberculous mycobacterial infection occur at CD4 T-cell counts less than 50×10^6 per L.

Preventing the immunologic consequences of HIV infection, using complex regimens of antiretroviral drugs [highly active antiretroviral therapy (HAART)], is the most effective way of improving quality of life as well as prognosis. These drugs are administered in combination to reduce the potential for viral mutations that result in the evolution of resistant strains of HIV. The complexity of these treatment regimens dictates that therapeutic decisions must be made by HIV specialists.

Antiretroviral drugs are susceptible to drug interactions and great care should be taken when introducing other drugs to people being treated for HIV. Drug interactions have the potential to compromise the efficacy of antiretroviral drugs, with consequential failure to suppress the viral load and the development of drug resistance (see Table 1).

III. COMMON PAIN SYNDROMES ASSOCIATED WITH HUMAN IMMUNODEFICIENCY VIRUS

1. Painful Peripheral Neuropathies in Human Immunodeficiency Virus

Peripheral neuropathy is commonly associated with HIV and can occur at any stage of HIV disease because of HIV itself, opportunistic infections, or malignancies, or as a consequence of treatment (see Table 2). A proportion of these neuropathies are associated with neuropathic pain, and particularly notable in this regard are AIDS-associated distal sensory neuropathy (AADSN), antiretroviral toxic neuropathy (ATN), and herpes zoster-associated pain.

(i) Acquired Immunodeficiency Virus–associated Distal Sensory Neuropathy (AADSN)

AADSN has an incidence of approximately 35% in subjects with moderate to severe immunosuppression. AADSN has the features of a distal axonal sensorimotor polyneuropathy, predominantly affecting small fibers. Sensory loss, paresthesias, dysesthesias, burning pain, and lancinating pain are frequent features. Large-fiber symptoms such as motor weakness of the intrinsic muscles of the feet can complicate advanced AADSN.

Risk factors for the development of AADSN include increasing age, high viral load (a viral load of >10,000 copies per mL is associated with a 2.3-fold greater risk for the development of AADSN than a viral load of <500 copies per mL), and reduced CD4 count (CD4 <750 $\times$ 10^6 per L increases the risk of AADSN >100-fold, but the association is weaker than with viral load).

The underlying pathologic mechanism of AADSN is unknown, although an hypothesis currently receiving much attention is a HIV glycoprotein 120 (GP120)-induced toxicity of primary sensory neurones, possibly by GP120 acting as a co-ligand for chemokine receptors expressed by dorsal ganglion cells.

(ii) Antiretroviral Toxic Neuropathy

Some of the nucleoside reverse transcriptase inhibitors (NRTIs) used to treat HIV infection have been associated with a distal axonal sensorimotor polyneuropathy, which is possibly a mitochondrial neuropathy. ATN is often clinically indistinguishable from AADSN and the conditions may, of course, overlap. Sometimes, ATN can be deduced from the temporal relation to NRTI use and cessation. Stavudine (d4T), didanosine (ddI), and zalcitabine (ddC) have all been implicated. In individuals receiving ddC, painful peripheral neuropathy has been reported in 15% to 25% of patients. Combining dideoxy-nucleoside analogs has an additive or even synergistic effect on ATN development. Other risk factors include elevated viral load, dose or cumulative dose of NRTI, increased age, preexisting neuropathy, advanced disease, coprescription with other drugs causing neuropathies, for example, thalidomide, isoniazid, or vincristine, or coprescription of hydroxyurea as part of a salvage regime.

Table 1. Examples of drug interactions between antiretroviral drugs and drugs used in pain management

Class of Drug	Example	Comment
Analgesics	Fentanyl	Fentanyl clearance decreased by ritonavir
	Methadone	Methadone withdrawal reported with nevirapine and efavirenz
Antacids		Reduced absorption of delavirdine and protease inhibitors
Antibiotics	Rifampicin	Rifampicin clearance reduced by protease inhibitors
	Metronidazole	Antabuse reaction with alcohol in oral solution of amprenavir and Kaletra
	Isoniazid	Additive toxicity with drugs causing peripheral neuropathy, for example, d4T
Anticonvulsants	Phenytoin	Avoid with all NNRTIs and protease inhibitors, will lead to reduced levels and potentially loss of efficacy of antiretrovirals
	Carbamazepine	As for phenytoin
Antidepressants	Trazadone	Ritonavir inhibits metabolism of these antidepressants leading to increased effects
	Amitriptyline	
Antihistamines	Terfenadine	Avoid with efavirenz as risk of arrhythmias
	Pimozide	Avoid with protease inhibitors because of reduced metabolism of pimozide
Antipsychotics	Haloperidol	Caution with ritonavir as metabolism of antipsychotics is reduced
	Olanzapine	
	Risperidone	
Oral contraceptives		Reduced efficacy with efavirenz, nevirapine, and most protease inhibitors
Sedatives	Diazepam	Caution with ritonavir, which enhanced sedative effect
	Triazolam	Caution with protease inhibitors, enhanced sedative effect
	Alprazolam	
	Midazolam	

NNRTI, nonnucleoside reverse transcriptase inhibitors.
From Davies E. Drugs. In: Gazzard B, ed. *AIDS care handbook*. London, UK: Mediscript, 2002, with permission.

Table 2.   Examples of peripheral neuropathies associated with human immunodeficiency virus

- Early stages (immune dysregulation)
  - Acute inflammatory demyelinating polyradiculopathy
  - Chronic inflammatory demyelinating polyradiculopathy
  - Vasculitic neuropathy
  - Brachial plexopathy
  - Cranial mononeuropathy
  - Multiple mononeuropathies
- Mid and late stages (HIV-1 replication driven)
  - AIDS-associated distal sensory neuropathy (AADSN)
  - Autonomic neuropathy
- Late stages (opportunistic infection and malignancy)
  - CMV polyradiculopathy
  - CMV mononeuritis multiplex
  - Acute herpes zoster/postherpetic neuralgia
  - Syphilitic radiculopathy
  - Tuberculosis polyradiculomyelitis
  - Lymphomatous polyradiculopathy
  - AIDS cachexia neuropathy
- All stages
  - Antiretroviral toxic neuropathy (ATN)
  - Nucleoside reverse transcriptase inhibitors (e.g., ddI, DDC, D4t)
  - Other drugs (e.g., vincristine, ethambutol, thalidomide)
- Other causes, for example,
  - Nutritional (B_{12}, B_6)
  - Alcohol, diabetes, etc.

HIV, human immunodeficiency virus; CMV, cytomegalovirus; AIDS, acquired immunodeficiency syndrome.
From Verma A. Epidemiology and clinical features of HIV-1 associated neuropathies. *J Peripher Nerv Syst* 2001;6:8–13, with permission.

Discontinuing or reducing implicated NRTIs may lead to symptomatic improvement but will reduce therapeutic options for virologic control. Decisions regarding antiretroviral therapy are complex and must be made by a specialist in HIV disease.

After a decision to terminate therapy with a NRTI there can be a "coasting period" of 4 to 8 weeks, when symptoms may even worsen. Signs and symptoms may be more easily reversed with early diagnosis; hence the need to assess those on dideoxy-NRTIs appropriately.

(iii) Pain Management in Peripheral Neuropathy

Because ATN and AADSN present with similar clinical pictures, and no specific disease-altering therapies are currently available, pain management in these conditions will be discussed as a single entity.

Peripheral neuropathies in the context of HIV infection must be appropriately investigated and other neuropathies, both HIV-related and coincidental neuropathies, excluded. This especially applies to other distal axonal sensorimotor polyneuropathies with a similar clinical picture to ATN and AADSN, for example, diabetic neuropathy. A full neurologic assessment and routine blood investigations to exclude other peripheral neuropathies should be undertaken. Because ATN and AADSN predominantly affect small fibers, conventional nerve conduction studies may not reveal any abnormality; however, this investigation may be useful in excluding other etiologies. Quantitative sensory testing (QST) is useful in documenting abnormalities in small fiber function and therefore in the diagnosis and assessment of ATN and AADSN. In our clinic, QST of patients with HIV-related painful peripheral neuropathy reveals the usual pattern as being one of sensory loss to thermal and mechanical stimuli, with little evidence of hypersensory phenomena, such as allodynia and hyperalgesia (i.e., a deafferentation pattern). Epidermal skin fiber density measurement in 4-mm skin punch biopsies is also emerging as a useful tool in the assessment of small fiber neuropathies.

There is currently a paucity of direct evidence from randomized controlled trials supporting analgesic therapies in ATN and AADSN. Therefore, it is reasonable to use the more substantial evidence for other peripheral neuropathic pain conditions to inform analgesic regimen decisions for people with ATN and AADSN. There is sufficient evidence of effectiveness to support the use of gabapentinoids, 5% lidocaine patch, opioids, tramadol, and tricyclic antidepressants as first-line therapies in peripheral neuropathic pain. Opioids should only be prescribed according to published guidelines.

The direct evidence from trials in ATN and AADSN is limited in both quality of study design and size of study populations. The limited evidence base does not support the use of lamotrigine, amitriptyline, mexiletine, acupuncture, capsaicin, peptide T, foot vibration, or cognitive behavioral therapy. There appears to be evidence to support the use of nerve growth factor, but this therapy is not generally available. A limited evidence base would appear to suggest support for the use of gabapentin, topical lidocaine, and acetyl-carnitine, further trials of these therapies are required.

2. Varicella Zoster Virus

Varicella zoster virus (VZV) reactivation is more common in the HIV-infected population, increasing in frequency as CD4 counts fall. Those with a CD4 count less than 200×10^6 per L are most at risk of major neurologic, ophthalmic, and systemic complications of acute shingles.

In a study of VZV-related pain in the context of HIV, no cases were found in early disease but 7% of those with advanced disease were affected. Another study found that acute VZV-related pain in HIV was positively correlated with the number of new skin vesicles, analgesic use, and baseline pain and that postherpetic neuralgia was correlated with baseline pain, pain at 1 month, and duration of lesions. Management of postherpetic neuralgia is as for the non-HIV population, while being aware of potential drug interactions especially with carbamazepine. The substantial evidence for postherpetic neuralgia suggests the following rank order (efficacy—number needed to treat for 50% pain relief) of effective therapies. Oral therapies: tricyclic antidepressants (2.64) > opioids

(2.67) > gabapentin (4.39) > tramadol (4.76) > pregabalin (4.93). Topically administered therapies: aspirin/diethyl ether (1.83) > lidocaine patch (2) > capsaicin (3.26).

3. Headache

Headache has been quoted by one source as the commonest site of pain in HIV infection with 46% of patients affected. The cause varies according to the degree of immunosuppression, but it is of primary importance to identify treatable opportunistic infections or tumors (see Table 3).

Generally, patients with focal brain lesions often complain of headache, whereas in those with diffuse brain lesions headaches are less common and changes in mental state predominate. With opportunistic infections symptoms, including headache, can be mild or absent.

Investigations will depend on the stage of HIV disease, CD4 count, and the presence of clinical signs. Treatment of the underlying cause should accompany symptomatic treatment.

Analgesia follows standard guidelines, always being mindful of potential drug interactions. There have been anecdotal reports of late-stage HIV headache responding to amitriptyline and chronic headaches with CSF pleocytosis responding to a 2-week tapered course of prednisolone (starting at 60 mg). Steroids may also be useful in headaches associated with intracerebral edema.

4. Oral Pain

Causes of oral pain in HIV are listed in Table 4. Several studies have demonstrated the prevalence of most HIV-associated oral lesions to decrease in the era of HAART. These studies, however, still report a prevalence of up to 53%. There is evidence of more oral lesions with a CD4 count less than 200×10^6 per L and higher viral loads (>3000 to >20,000 copies per mL in quoted series). Pain from oral lesions can interfere with nutritional intake and hence contribute to the HIV wasting syndrome. Xerostomia occurs commonly (2% to 10%) in HIV-infected individuals and there is evidence for an increase in HIV salivary gland disease.

Treatment should target the underlying cause when possible. Preventative treatment, for example, good oral hygiene and management of xerostomia, is important. A double-blind, randomized study of thalidomide 200 mg od as therapy for oral apthous ulcers in HIV reported that patients in the thalidomide group showed major improvement in both ulcer healing and discomfort while eating compared to patients taking a placebo. However, nearly 20% of the thalidomide group withdrew because of adverse events. Additional treatments that may be used for pain control include the following:

- Topical granulocyte–macrophage colony-stimulating factor (GM-CSF)
- Coating agents for example, sucralfate, mucilage and polyvinyl–pyrrolidone, and sodium hyaluronate oral gel (Gelclair)
- Topical antiinflammatories, for example, dispersible paracetamol or aspirin used as mouthwash, aspirin in mucilage, or benzydamine hydrochloride mouthwash

Table 3. Headache in human immunodeficiency virus disease

HIV	HIV encephalopathy	Part of the AIDS dementia complex. 14% of those affected have headache.
	HIV aseptic meningitis	Can occur at seroconversion, but more common with progression to the symptomatic stage of HIV disease. Associated with fever, meningism, and cranial nerve palsies. Usually self-limiting. Estimated to occur in 1%–2% of all HIV infections.
	Late-stage HIV headache	Subacute onset of generalized headache; often photophobia but no nuchal rigidity. Usually resolves within 4 weeks.
	Chronic headache with CSF pleocytosis	Resembles tension headaches but with mildly elevated CSF lymphocytes.
Infection	Cytomegalovirus encephalitis	Symptoms include confusion, fits, and ataxia. 30% with headache.
	Cryptococcal meningitis	Can cause hydrocephalus. 88% with headache.
	Cerebral toxoplasmosis	Presents with fever, fits, and focal signs. 55% with headache.
	Other viral infections	Herpes simplex, VZV encephalitis.
	Tuberculous meningitis	More likely in advanced disease. 59% with headache.
	Progressive multifocal leukoencephalopathy	Often presents with focal neurology and personality change without headache, but headache reported in 23%.
	Neurosyphilis	88% complaint of headache.
	Sinusitis	More frequent in the HIV population.
Tumor	CNS lymphoma	Often presents with confusion and focal signs.
	Kaposi sarcoma	Rarely affects the CNS system.
Iatrogenic	Drug induced, e.g., zidovudine (AZT)	Headaches due to AZT may gradually resolve over weeks to months.
Other	Tension headache	An increase in the frequency and intensity of headaches is reported with HIV.
	Migraine	The frequency and intensity may decrease with time after HIV infection, especially in those with HIV encephalopathy or taking antiretrovirals.

HIV, human immunodeficiency virus; CSF, cerebrospinal fluid; VZV, varicella zoster virus; CNS, central nervous system; AZT, azidothymidine.

Table 4.   Causes of oral pain in human immunodeficiency virus disease

Fungal infections	Candidiasis
	Histoplasmosis
	Cryptococcus
Viral infections	Herpes simplex
	Cytomegalovirus
	Herpes zoster
	Hairy leukoplakia
	Human papilloma virus
Bacterial infections	Necrotizing ulcerative gingivitis (NUG) and periodontitis (NUP)
	Mycobacterium
	Treponema pallidum (syphilis)
Malignancies	Kaposi sarcoma
	Lymphoma
	Squamous cell carcinoma
Drug-induced	Zalcitabine, foscarnet
Other	Idiopathic thrombocytopenic purpura
	Apthous ulceration

- Topical local anaesthetic—lidocaine gel 2% qds or viscous lidocaine as a mouthwash
- Topical opioids—Morphine sulfate immediate release liquid as a mouthwash (as an alcohol-free preparation to avoid stinging) or cocaine mouthwash
- Systemic analgesia
- Topical or systemic corticosteroids

5. Esophagitis

Approximately, 30% to 50% of patients with HIV will have esophageal disease at some stage. Esophagitis presents with odynophagia (retrosternal pain on swallowing) and sometimes dysphagia. Patients with HIV have also been reported to have a high incidence of esophageal motility disorders.

Treatment is targeted at the underlying cause. Additional treatments for pain control include coating agents (e.g., sucralfate), topical anaesthetics, drugs to reduce acidity (e.g., proton pump inhibitors), prokinetic drugs to increase the tone of the lower esophageal sphincter and so help prevent reflux (e.g., metoclopramide) and systemic analgesia. For apthous ulceration, corticosteroids or thalidomide 200 mg per day can be helpful. The addition of crushed misoprostol 200 μg suspended in 15 mL of 2% viscous lidocaine has also been reported to help in a small case series.

6. Abdominal Pain

Abdominal pain in AIDS may be related to drug therapy, malignancy, infection, or multifactorial causes. Patients with AIDS are prone to pancreatitis, colic, drug-induced renal colic and lactic acidosis, intraabdominal KS, non-Hodgkin lymphoma (NHL), and cholangitis.

(i) Pancreatitis

The incidence of pancreatitis in HIV infection is 14% to 22%. Antiretroviral therapy is the commonest cause, particularly didanosine. Adding stavudine, hydroxyurea, tenofovir or ribavirin (prescribed for hepatitis C coinfection) to didanosine increases the risk of pancreatitis developing. A recent study failed to show any statistically significant increase in the incidence of hyperlipidaemic pancreatitis in a cohort of patients on protease inhibitors. Other drugs such as intravenous pentamidine and isoniazid also have been implicated. In advanced disease, pancreatitis can be caused by opportunistic infections such as *Pneumocystis carinii*, *Mycobacterium avium* complex, cryptosporidium, and cytomegalovirus.

Treatment, as before, should target the underlying cause and may necessitate a change in the combination of antiretroviral drugs. Analgesic treatment is as for the non-HIV population.

(ii) Intestinal Colic

There are numerous causes of enteritis in HIV disease. These include antiretroviral drugs and infection. The associated diarrhea may be accompanied by diffuse, colicky abdominal pain.

An important differential diagnosis is intussusception. This may be more common than clinically appreciated because of the vague chronic nature of its presentation, and the fact that patients with intussusception frequently develop enteritis. Lead points for the intussusception include lymph nodes involved with mycobacterial infections, KS or lymphoma and adenopathy or small bowel inflammation associated with infectious enteritides. One case study, therefore, suggested that there should be a low threshold for early CT scan in young HIV adults with intestinal colic.

Treatment is of the underlying cause. Cholinergic drugs may exacerbate colic so should be avoided. Hyoscine butylbromide is useful both as an antispasmodic drug for colic and as an antisecretory drug that may help reduce the volume of watery diarrhea. Unfortunately, it is poorly absorbed orally, so parenteral administration either intravenously or by the subcutaneous route is required.

(iii) Ureteric Colic

Indinavir, one of the protease inhibitors, causes renal calculi and hence ureteric colic in as many as 23.6% of recipients. Pure indinavir stones are radiolucent. Treatment involves rehydration, analgesia, and at least temporary cessation of indinavir.

(iv) Lactic Acidosis

Lactic acidosis is an uncommon but serious complication thought to be caused by mitochondrial toxicity due to NRTIs especially stavudine, didanosine, and zalcitabine. A systematic review of patients hospitalized with biochemical evidence of lactic acidosis (median blood lactate 10.5 mmol per L) showed that 45% had abdominal pain. Other gastrointestinal symptoms included nausea, vomiting, diarrhea and, less commonly, abdominal distension. Anorexia and weight loss, weakness, fatigue, dyspnoea, tachypnea and, in 2%, impairment of consciousness were also described. Forty-eight percent of the patients died within 7 days.

This is clearly an important differential in undiagnosed abdominal pain, especially in those on implicated NRTIs. Treatment includes stopping NRTIs and supportive therapy.

(v) Malignancy and Abdominal Pain

KS is a highly vascular tumor associated with human herpes virus 8 (HHV8) infection. KS has been reported to spread to the gastrointestinal tract in up to 50% of those with cutaneous lesions. It can occur anywhere in the gastrointestinal tract, from oropharynx to rectum, and also in the liver, pancreas, and appendix. The nature of pain caused will depend on the site of the lesions. Gastrointestinal KS also can lead to upper or lower gastrointestinal hemorrhage, bowel obstruction or perforation and protein losing enteropathy. The course of KS can be modified by HAART as well as oncologic therapies.

The incidence of NHL is increased almost 100-fold in the HIV population. In HIV extranodal sites, including the gastrointestinal tract or liver are involved in approximately 80% of cases and unusual sites for NHL for example, the anorectum and common bile duct have been reported. Pain and symptoms experienced will depend on the site of disease. Body cavity-based lymphomas, thought to be associated with HHV8, account for approximately 3% of NHL in HIV. If the peritoneal cavity is involved, this can present as a lymphomatous ascites. The addition of HAART to combination chemotherapy improves response rates and survival time.

(vi) Cholangiopathy

AIDS-related cholangitis or cholangiopathy is a form of sclerosing cholangitis most commonly caused by opportunistic infections in individuals with a CD4 count less than 100×10^6 per L. Cryptosporidium, cytomegalovirus (CMV), and microsporidium are the organisms most commonly involved but cases due to *Giardia*, *Mycobacterium avium* complex, *Cyclospora*, and *Isospora* also have been reported.

Abdominal pain occurs in over 90% of cases, usually in the right upper quadrant or mid-epigastric area. This may be associated with fever, nausea, and vomiting. Liver function tests show a cholestatic picture, with marked elevation of alkaline phosphatase, but jaundice is unusual. Cholangiocarcinoma may develop.

Treatment is usually symptomatic, although endoscopic sphincterotomy in cases with papillary stenosis has been shown to relieve pain, but not improve survival. There are isolated case reports of biliary stenting reducing pain and improving liver function tests.

In one series of three patients, CT scan-guided celiac plexus block with bupivacaine and absolute alcohol achieved complete pain relief within 3 days. Antimicrobial treatment is, unfortunately, often ineffective. HAART can modify the course of the illness and improve survival.

7. Anorectal Pain

A study of 180 patients who were HIV positive with anorectal symptoms revealed that the most common symptom was pain (57%), mainly related to anal ulceration. Other causes of anorectal pain included fistulae, abscesses, hemorrhoids, and malignancy

(KS, NHL and squamous cell carcinoma). In addition, 43% had anal condylomata, 10% of which were associated with anal intraepithelial neoplasia (AIN). Surgical treatment of AIN is also a cause of pain in this group.

In addition, anal fissures are more common in the male homosexual population, so are a cause of pain in this subgroup of HIV-seropositive men. Disease specific treatments should be accompanied by stool softeners, topical local anaesthetics, and systemic analgesics.

8. Gynecologic Pain

A study of 67 women hospitalized with HIV reported that gynecologic disease was present in 83%. Herpes simplex virus genital ulceration is a frequent finding in HIV-seropositive women, and other causes include other sexually transmitted infections, cytomegalovirus, and drugs for example, foscarnet. HIV-infected women have a higher incidence of cervical intraepithelial neoplasia (CIN) and invasive cervical cancer. Several reports suggest that HIV positive women are also at an increased risk of developing other human papilloma virus associated lesions including vulval intraepithelial neoplasia (VIN) and possibly invasive vulval cancer.

There are high rates of coinfection of HIV and pelvic inflammatory disease (PID), a cause of acute and chronic pelvic pain. In the United States, HIV seroprevalence among women with PID is reported to range from 6.7% to 27%. Regular gynecologic screening and surveillance is of prime importance in HIV-seropositive women.

9. Musculoskeletal Pain

(i) Musculoskeletal Infections

A recent study of 75 patients with HIV referred to a rheumatology clinic found that septic complications were the most common clinical manifestation. These patients had a mean CD4 count of 250×10^6 per L and mean viral load of approximately 5,000 copies per mL. The diagnoses included septic arthritis, septic bursitis, osteomyelitis, and pyomyositis (which is usually characterized by acute, unilateral thigh pain, swelling, erythema, and induration). Analgesia, following standard guidelines, should accompany antimicrobial therapy and, when necessary, surgical drainage. This study also found a high incidence of bone malignancy.

(ii) Arthritis and Arthropathy

The spondyloarthropathies have been described previously as the most common type of arthritis in the HIV population. HIV-seropositive individuals tend not to have sacroillitis, but have oligoarthritis of the large joints of the lower limbs, enthesopathies of the Achilles, anterior and posterior tibial tendons and plantar fascia, and multidigit dactylitis of the toes. In psoriatic arthritis, these occur in association with various types of psoriatic skin lesions.

An increased prevalence of Reiter syndrome has been reported in the HIV population in some studies. Other studies report a prevalence similar to that for HIV-negative individuals at high risk for gastrointestinal infection or venereal disease. In those with HIV, the syndrome usually begins with urethritis or enteritis followed by skin and joint disease. The cutaneous manifestations, especially keratoderma blenorrhagicum, are more prominent than in HIV-negative individuals but eye disease is less common. Onset may be at the time of the development of immunodeficiency, or may predate this.

Those lacking the skin disease or urethritis of the conditions mentioned in preceding text are categorized as having an undifferentiated spondyloarthropathy.

Nonsteroidal antiinflammatory drugs (NSAIDs) may help mild cases of joint involvement. Intraarticular steroids can be used for symptom control. Otherwise, conventional disease-modifying drugs are used for example, hydroxychloroquine, sulfasalazine, and etretinate. Methotrexate has been associated with the development of pneumocystis carinii pneumonia and KS so its use, if at all, should be reserved for those with a CD4 count greater than 500×10^6 per L.

Nonspecific arthralgias occur in as many as 30% to 40% of those with HIV. These can occur at the time of seroconversion, in association with a mononucleosislike syndrome, or at any time during the course of disease. Any of the limb joints can be affected. The arthralgia can often be controlled with paracetamol or NSAIDs, and is usually short-lived.

Avascular necrosis is also a relatively rare complication in HIV disease. It should be remembered in those presenting with sudden severe pain, especially in the hip or knee.

(iii) Myopathy

Polymyositis is an inflammatory myopathy that may be due to the host response to the HIV virus. It may occur in association with high CD8 levels in early disease. Clinically, it presents with an insidious onset of proximal muscle weakness (especially of the lower limbs), pain, and tenderness. There may be muscle wasting, fever, weight loss, and skin lesions characteristic of dermatomyositis. Serum creatinine kinase levels are elevated and electromyogram shows abnormalities. Polymyositis is treated with corticosteroids. Zidovudine (AZT) also appears to help reduce symptoms.

AZT induced myositis has a similar clinical picture. It has been described starting 3 to 21 months following commencement of the drug. If the myopathy is due to AZT, there should be clinical improvement 1 to 2 weeks following its withdrawal. If this does not occur, muscle biopsy may be required. NSAIDs can help with symptoms.

Opportunistic infections for example, toxoplasmosis also have been associated with myopathy in HIV. Rhabdomyalisis and fibromyalgialike symptoms also can occur.

IV. CONCLUSION

This chapter describes the many and diverse pain syndromes associated with HIV-AIDS. It is clear that pain is a major and frequent complication of this disease, even in the presence of adequate disease-suppressing therapy.

SELECTED READINGS

Cruccu G, Anand N, Attal L, et al. EFNS guidelines on neuropathic pain assessment. *Eur J Neurol* 2004, 11:153–162.

Dworkin RH, Backonja M, Rowbotham MCA, et al. Advances in neuropathic pain: diagnosis, mechanisms, and treatment recommendations. *Arch Neurol* 2003;60:1524–1534.

Frich LM, Borgbjerg FM. Pain and pain treatment in AIDS patients: a longitudinal study. *J Pain Symptom Manage* 2000;19(5):339–347.

Griffin JW, McArthur JC, Polydefkis M. Assessment of cutaneous innervation by skin biopsies. *Curr Opin Neurol* 2001;14(5): 655–659.

Hempenstall K, Nurmikko T, Johnston R, et al. Analgesic therapy in post herpetic neuralgia: a quantitative systematic review *(submitted)*.

Hewitt DJ, McDonald M, Portenoy RK, et al. Pain syndromes and aetiologies in ambulatory AIDS patients. *Pain* 1997;70:117–123.

Jorum E, Arendt-Neilsen L. Sensory testing and clinical neurophysiology. In: Rice ASC, Warfield CA, Justins D, et al., eds. *Clinical pain management*. London, UK: Arnold, 2003;28–38.

Kieburtz K, Simpson D, Yiannoutsos C, et al. A randomized trial of amitriptyline and mexiletine for painful neuropathy in HIV infection. *Neurology* 1998;51:1682–1688.

Marquez J, Restrepo CS, Candia L, et al. Human immunodeficiency virus-associated rheumatic disorders in the HAART era. *J Rheumatol* 2004;31:741–746.

McKeogh M. AIDS. In: Rice ASC, Warfield CA, Justins D, et al., eds. *Clinical pain management*. London, UK: Arnold, 2003;367–394.

Schifitto G, McDermott MP, McArthur JCA, et al. Incidence of and risk factors for HIV-associated distal sensory polyneuropathy. *Neurology* 2002;58(12):1764–1768.

Shembalkar P, Anand P. Peripheral neuropathies. In: Rice ASC, Warfield CA, Justins D, et al., eds. *Clinical pain management*. London, UK: Arnold, 2003;367–381.

Shlay JC, Chaloner K, Mitchell BM, et al. Acupuncture and amitriptyline for pain due to HIV-related peripheral neuropathy. *JAMA* 1998; 280(18): 1590–1595.

Simpson DM, McArthur JC, Olney RA, et al. Lamotrigine for HIV-associated painful sensory neuropathies. *Neurology* 2003;60: 1508–1514.

Singer EJ, Zorilla C, Fahy-Chandon B, et al. Painful symptoms reported by ambulatory HIV-infected men in a longitudinal study. *Pain* 1993;54(1):15–19.

The British Pain Society. Recommendations for the appropriate use of opioids for persistent non-cancer pain. London, UK: The British Pain Society, 2004. Also available at: www.britishpainsociety.org/publications.html.

Verma A. Epidemiology and clinical features of HIV-1 associated neuropathies. *Journal of the Peripheral Nervous System* 2001;6:8–13.

Williams D, Geraci A, Simpson DM. AIDS and AIDS treatment neuropathies. *Curr Pain Headache Rep* 2002;6(2):125–130.

Yusuf TE, Baron TH. AIDS cholangiopathy. *Current Treatment Options in Gastroenterology* 2004;7(2):111–117

Pain Due to Cancer

Pain in Adults with Cancer

Eugenia-Daniela Hord, Jeffrey A. Norton, and
Annabel D. Edwards

We must all die. But that I can save him from days of torture, that is
what I feel as my great and ever new privilege. Pain is a more terri-
ble lord of man than even death.
—*Albert Schweitzer, 1875–1965*

Of all the symptoms that a person experiences during their
course of living with cancer, pain is reported to be the most
feared. At least one-third of patients with cancer have pain at
the time of their diagnosis. Up to two-thirds of patients with advanced cancer rate their pain level as moderate to severe. The
pain of a large portion of all patients with cancer (approximately
90%) can be treated effectively with the multidisciplinary modes
of treatment currently and readily available.

I. DEFINING CANCER PAIN

The term "cancer pain" does not have a specific definition. In
fact, the pain experienced by patients with cancer stems from a
particularly wide variety of causes:

- Tumor invasion or compression of other tissues by the tumor
- Surgical pain/biopsies
- Radiation damage to tissues
- Neuropathies caused by chemotherapy or other treatments
- Ischemia
- Inflammation
- Visceral pain due to blocked or damaged organ structures
- Musculoskeletal pain from decreased mobility and
  arthropathies
- Pathologic fractures

Some pain occurs in direct temporal relationship to an event
such as surgery. Other types of pain start days or months after
an initiating event and get worse with time as with peripheral

neuropathy induced by chemotherapy. It is common for many types of pain to coexist in patients with cancer. In addition, some types of pain are constant, whereas others are incidental to specific movements or intermittent because of physiologic factors. Timing of pain occurrence influences the therapeutic approach used.

The success of pharmacologic pain therapy lies primarily in the proper match between specific pain mechanisms and the pharmacologic effect of the chosen medication(s). The success of nonpharmacologic adjuvant pain therapies, such as relaxation or self-hypnosis, depends on the patient's abilities and beliefs, their practice (or use over time), the modality chosen, and, sometimes, the pain mechanisms.

There is another aspect of pain that is related to the patients' sense of wellness referred to as suffering. Suffering is an emotional state associated with biologic or psychosocial events that threaten the individual's integrity. It can play a major role in a patient's overall quality of life. The experience of pain and suffering are so closely entwined that it makes no sense to treat one without the other. The abolition of physical pain means little when a patient is unable to derive pleasure from life.

II. BARRIERS TO APPROPRIATE CANCER PAIN MANAGEMENT

Unfortunately, it has been demonstrated repeatedly that many barriers still exist to the effective treatment of cancer pain despite the fact that most cancer pain can be treated relatively easily with basic pain management techniques. These barriers are multifactorial and include the following:

- Lack of knowledge about the various mechanisms of cancer pain syndromes
- Lack of knowledge about the variety of medications available
- Failure to properly assess the patient in pain
- Fears of the patient, the patient's family, and health care providers related to addiction and the use of controlled substances
- Fear of complications or side effects of opioid analgesics commonly used in the treatment of cancer pain
- Lack of respect for or knowledge of nonpharmacologic therapies
- Fear that use of opioids may hasten death near the end of life

Patients may, in fact, create major barriers to their own care, which is why a careful assessment of their attitudes and worries is necessary. Patients with cancer have stated in many surveys that they see pain as being inevitable and that they should be able to tolerate it. They worry that physicians will be distracted from treating the cancer if they mention the pain or that they will be considered as complainers. Often, denial is a factor because many patients see worsening pain as a sign of worsening disease and so they do not want to think about it or admit it. Some patients cannot afford the medications prescribed, and, instead of asking whether there is an alternative that is less expensive, simply do not fill their prescriptions. There are also patients who just do not want to take multiple pills.

There are health care system problems as well that can affect pain management efforts. Insurance coverage may make specific forms of therapy unattainable. The availability of medications may be restricted by insurance or pharmacy willingness to carry various products. Instruction about pain and its management is not common in medical school and is barely mentioned in most textbooks. In addition, those practitioners that do provide pain management are often poorly reimbursed for their time.

Some of the systems issues feeding into poor pain management may well be addressed over the next year or two as the new Joint Commission for the Accreditation of Healthcare Organization (JCAHO) regulations relating to pain management are put into place and graded. These regulations will impact all types of health care facilities examined by the JCAHO (see Appendix II for Website address).

III. PAIN ASSESSMENT

Proper assessment of the nature of a patient's pain or pains and the probable cause(s) is essential for effective treatment. Each type of pain needs to be evaluated separately as the mechanisms may be different and require different treatment. Because new pain can develop and old pain can worsen or improve (with disease progression, new health problems, treatment of the disease, etc.), pain should be reassessed regularly.

Pain is a combination of sensory and emotional reactions to intense stimuli. It is inherently a subjective experience. Therefore, a large part of a pain assessment comes from the information the patient provides. The diagnosis of cancer brings with it many emotional responses that may strongly overlay the patient's report. Perhaps this plays a role in providers' tendency to underestimate pain. Understanding how the patient with cancer thinks of himself or herself and of the disease can be important.

1. Pain Descriptions

The two major pieces of information that the patient provides include the level of pain and the description of the pain, that is, what it feels like. Pain level is measured on a scale, most commonly a 0 to 10 scale, in which 0 = no pain and 10 = the worst pain imaginable. Note that 10 does not stand for the worst pain the person has ever had because that person may not have much experience with pain. Scales can be verbal or written, may use colors, numbers, lines, faces and so on, or may rely on behavioral cues. The key is to find a scale that works for the individual patient and to use that scale consistently. The level of pain cannot be compared between patients. The scale can only measure changes (e.g., evaluate the effect of interventions) in the individual patient. In general, we try to get a patient below a 4/10 level of pain but this is purely empirical. Some patients are content with a 4/10 level, whereas others are miserable at this level. The ultimate goal is to achieve a reasonable level of comfort while minimizing side effects; patients and providers need to decide together when this goal has been reached.

Patients' descriptions of pain help identify the mechanisms of pain. When pain is primarily from recent injury (nociceptive), words such as "sharp" and "throbbing" are used, and the patient often can point right to a place that hurts. Pain that derives from damaged nerves may elicit descriptors such as shooting, burning, electrical, painful numbness, or pins and needles. This type of pain tends to be more diffuse or to travel from one place to another. These verbal indicators are not precise but are helpful. Clinical knowledge and experience obviously inform treatment decisions as well.

2. Specific Elements of the History and Physical Examination

All of the usual features of the history and physical examination are relevant (see Chapter 4). The following aspects of the history and physical are of particular importance in patients with cancer.

(i) Review of Medications

This review should include asking about herbal or home remedies, which are very popular and widely advertised to the cancer population. Thus, potentially adverse interactions can be avoided and the treatment plan can be simplified. A careful determination of all pain medications that have been prescribed at one time or another is also warranted. This will ensure that the patient is clear about which medication to take.

(ii) Treatment History

This is a crucial element of the history because it is estimated that approximately 20% of patients with cancer have pain secondary to their treatments. Pain caused by such treatments may confuse the clinical picture for the practitioner and make a patient less willing to continue with the therapeutic plan. Some of these pain problems begin to manifest themselves months and even years after treatment. Examples include the following:

- Pain secondary to radiation includes plexopathy, myelopathy, mucositis, enteritis, proctocolitis, and bone necrosis. Mechanisms include fibrosis, tissue ischemia, necrosis, and inflammation.
- Pain secondary to chemotherapy may be caused by peripheral neuropathy, mucositis, bone necrosis, headaches or herpetic pain. Vincristine, cisplatin, and taxol commonly cause neuropathies. 5-FU, methotrexate, and many other drugs can cause mucositis, which usually starts 1 to 2 weeks into therapy. Intrathecal methotrexate, systemic L-asparaginase and posttransretinoic acid therapy can cause headaches. Mechanisms include inflammation and nerve damage.
- Pain secondary to procedures or surgery includes phantom, stump, postdural puncture headache (PDPH), pleurodesis, bone marrow biopsy, paracentisis, thorocentesis, and nerve injury pain (particularly after nephrectomy, mastectomy, and thoracotomy). Mechanisms are usually nociceptive or neuropathic.

(iii) History of Concomitant Disease

One such disease that frequently afflicts patients with cancer because of their immune-compromised state is shingles. Pain occurs during acute shingles, and can become chronic (postherpetic neuralgia). This is one of the most debilitating and distressing pain states and is extremely difficult to treat. Early and aggressive treatment of the shingles infection and associated acute pain is the best treatment known. Another painful condition associated with immune-compromised states is cryptococcal meningitis, which can cause headaches.

(iv) Pain History

It is important to recognize that some pain syndromes are more likely to occur with specific cancers. For example, bone metastases occur commonly with neoplasms of the lung, bronchus, prostate, breast, rectum, and colon. Frequent sites of disease include the long bones, spine, pelvis, femur, and skull. The pain is usually well-localized somatic pain that is often aggravated by movement (incident pain). The clinician should be aware of the possibility of completed or impending pathologic fracture, as well as the presence of potentially life-threatening hypercalcemia that can accompany widespread bone metastases. Compression of the spinal cord by epidural or spinal metastases is a medical emergency. If treatment of cord compression is initiated when the patient is ambulatory, neurologic function is usually maintained. By contrast, only 50% of patients who have paraparesis before treatment will regain ambulatory function. Patients who are frankly paraplegic rarely if ever regain motor strength. It is important to remember the following:

- Approximately 5% to 10% of patients with cancer develop vertebral body metastases.
- In up to 8% of patients, vertebral metastasis and back pain are the presenting symptoms of cancer.
- Dull, aching, midline back pain presents first in 90% of patients with epidural metastases.
- Symptoms may progress to sharp radicular pains, and neurologic deficits can appear approximately 6 to 7 weeks after initial symptoms.
- Changes in bowel or bladder function as well as sensory changes may herald spinal cord compression.
- Treatment includes immediate high-dose steroids, emergent radiation therapy, and occasionally surgical decompression/ stabilization.

Patients exhibiting classic warning symptoms of impending or actual cord compression should be sent to the emergency room immediately. The characteristics of this and other pain syndromes are summarized in Table 1.

(v) Psychological Assessment

The diagnosis of cancer, regardless of type or prognosis, often brings with it a whole series of automatic assumptions and expectations, mostly negative. It is important to clarify these concerns and to help patients obtain help if necessary (e.g., support groups, counseling, and family discussion).

(vi) Neurologic Examination

A neurologic examination often reveals early or previously missed cancer or cancer treatment effects. Small changes in sensation or strength may be a clue to new or extended tumor

Table 1. Characteristics of pain syndromes in patients with cancer

Area of Involvement	Typical Cancers Involved	Common Pain Description	Potential Pain Issues: Descriptions and Management Considerations
Long bones	Br, C, R, L, B, P	Sharp, achy, throbbing, pressure	Increased pain with use, localized, may fracture, consider plain film, and ± bone scan
Shoulder	L, B, Br		
Pelvis	C, R, P		
Hip	C, R, P		
Cervical vertebrae	Br, MM	Sharp	Can radiate to posterior skull. Can cause sensory/motor loss in upper extremity
Chest wall	Br, L, B	Sharp, throbbing, achy, pressure	Localized, may progress to ribs, intercostal nerves, vertebrae, brachial plexus
Abdomen	C, R, P, Pa, Ov, Ut	Crampy	If retroperitoneal, bending or curling may reduce pain; may radiate to groin, shoulder, back
Abdominal carcinomatosis	P, C, R	Crampy, dull, colicky, ache	May see diarrhea, constipation, ascites, nausea, obstruction
Ribs, intercostal nerves	L, B, Br	Burning, shooting, electric shock	Can increase with deep breath or movement, radiate along nerve root, cause sensory loss
Brachial plexus	Br, L, B	Burning, shooting, electrical	Can radiate down arm, cause numbness, hyperalgesia, allodynia; may progress into epidural space
Lumbar plexus	C, R, P	Burning, shooting, electrical, ache, pressure	Can radiate into anterior or posterior thigh and groin. May cause numbness, edema, weakness, paresthesias
Sacral plexus	P, C, R, Gu, Gyn	Burning, shooting, dull, aching	Mainly felt low back midline; may see bowel and bladder dysfunction, impotence, perianal sensory loss
Spinal cord	Br, L, P, B, K, C, R,MM, ST, Bn, Gl	Aching, dull, bandlike, tight	Pain in back worse when lying down, coughing, weight bearing; can be emergency if indicates impending cord compression

Table 1. *Continued*

Area of Involvement	Typical Cancers Involved	Common Pain Description	Potential Pain Issues: Descriptions and Management Considerations
Postmastectomy pain syndrome	Br	Burning, tight	Can start 1–3 mo after surgery; worse with motion
Postthoracotomy pain syndrome	L, B	Ache, burn, constant, electrical	Can have numbness and scar tenderness; worse with movement; may represent new tumor growth
Painful peripheral neuropathy	(Postchemo) Br, P, L, B, C, R	Tingling, burning	Mild stimuli can be painful; may see loss of reflexes and hand/foot distribution; pain may resolve as neuropathy resolves
Pain associated with steroid use	Br, P, L, B, C, R	Aching, tenderness, throbbing	Mostly transient, in muscles and joints, may be related to taper; may cause aseptic throbbing, necrosis of femur/humerus; worse with motion, may require surgery
Upper extremity radiation fibrosis	Br, L, B	Burning	Can start 6 mo to 20 y after radiation; may feel numbness, tingling, and neurologic deficits; pain may also mean tumor recurrence
Lower extremity radiation fibrosis	C, R, P	Burning, pulling	Can start 1–30 y after radiation; may feel numbness, tingling, and neurologic deficits; bone necrosis may occur
Radiation myelopathy		Aching	Can start 5–30 mo after radiation treatment; not reversible; must rule out impending cord compression

Bn, bone; Br, Breast; B, bronchus; C, colon; Gyn, gynecologic; Gu, genitourinary; GI, gastrointestinal; K, kidney; L, lung; MM, multiple myeloma; Ov, ovarian; P, prostate; R, rectal; ST, soft tissue; Ut, uterus.
From McCaffery M, Pasero C. *Pain: clinical manual*, 2nd ed. St. Louis, MO: Mosby, 1999:532–540, with permission.

involvement. One survey demonstrated that more than 60% of the patients with cancer sent to a pain management center had previously undetected lesions that were picked up in the assessment process at the pain treatment center.

3. Helpful Diagnostic Studies

(i) Radiologic

Many types of imaging are helpful in filling out the details in the evaluation of the cancer pain patient. It is often helpful to acquire and evaluate these studies early in the course of treatment. First, it provides a basis on which to compare disease progression or regression. Second, it provides essential information to the various specialists who become involved in the patient's care. Examples include the following:

- **Conventional radiology or plain films**: excellent for diagnosis of fracture or other bone abnormalities. Some soft tissue (ST) tumors and visceral pathology can be seen on plain films.
- **Computerized tomography (CT) scan**: excellent for bone abnormalities such as metastatic lesions.
- **Magnetic resonance imaging (MRI)**: excellent for soft tissue abnormalities. It is very useful for analysis of spinal pathology and bone metastatic disease.
- **Bone scan**: use of radioactive compound to detect areas of increased bone growth or turnover. Extremely useful for detection of bone metastases.
- **Positron emission tomography (PET) scan**: can identify areas of cancer metastases; distinguish between scar tissue and tumor, and help determine disease response to chemo and radiation therapy.

(ii) Neurophysiological
(See Chapter 7.)

- **Electromyography**: examines muscle activity, an abnormality of which may demonstrate nerve pathology.
- **Nerve conduction studies**: useful for the detection of neuropathy or other disease of the nervous system. Can help, for example, to clarify if tumor is involved in the plexus.

Quantitative sensory testing: includes a variety of noninvasive studies that explore the functioning of sensory nerve pathways. These results often can expose abnormal functioning in specific components of the pain pathway thus helping to clarify possible mechanisms of pain.

IV. CANCER PAIN TREATMENT

1. Primary Treatment of Malignancy

Primary treatment of malignancies with surgical resection, radiation therapy, or systemic chemotherapy is often an effective way to treat related pain. Nevertheless, adding analgesic medications or other methods of pain relief to the patient's primary therapy helps improve the patient's experience with cancer treatment and can be tapered if or when adjuncts are no longer needed. Pain treatment also helps patients to remain "compliant" with often difficult treatment protocols. Early intervention helps prevent long-term pain problems such as postherpetic neuralgia and phantom limb pain.

2. Pharmacotherapy

In an effort to raise awareness of the treatment of cancer pain, as well as functional pain management treatment protocols, the World Health Organization (WHO) developed a stepwise treatment algorithm, which was widely disseminated around the world (Fig. 1). This "WHO analgesic ladder" is composed of three basic steps, which can be outlined as follows: Step 1: Start with nonopioid analgesics for mild pain; Step 2: Begin using opioids such as hydrocodone or codeine for mild to moderate pain, with or without nonopioid analgesics; and Step 3: Use the more potent opioids such as morphine or hydromorphone (Dilaudid) for moderate to severe pain, with or without nonopioid analgesics. Other adjuvant medications (see subsequent text) can be added at any step of the ladder. This logical guide to cancer pain treatment has proved extremely helpful throughout the world. It has provided a simple algorithm to direct cancer pain therapy using widely available and inexpensive medications. However, in the United States and other advanced countries there is now debate about whether the stepladder should be modified. For example, it has been suggested that the concept of "mild" opioids in the

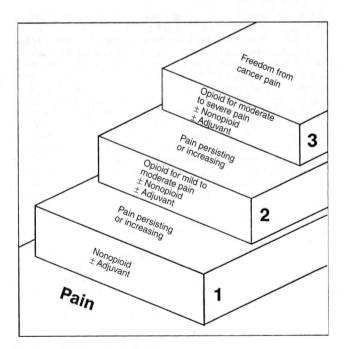

Figure 1. WHO analgesic ladder.

second step should be abandoned because these are really "strong" opioids in formulations that have dose limitations because of the addition of acetaminophen or aspirin. It would seem preferable to give opioids and nonopioids separately, especially because there are now more potent and safer nonopioid analgesics available. Also, because the safety and tolerability of long-acting opioids is well established, should the use of "mild" opioids in the second step be abandoned in favor of long-acting opioids? The ladder step concept also has been extended by some to include two possible higher-level step interventions. Step 4 would be the use of devices as epidural catheters, implanted opioid pumps, and spinal cord stimulators. An additional Step 5 might include cryotherapy, radio frequency lesioning and neurosurgical treatment techniques.

Some practitioners worry that the ladder concept may be misconstrued such that all patients are treated with the same protocol despite differences in their pain level and mechanisms of pain. For example, some patients may present with severe pain and need to be treated at a higher step of the ladder rather than at step one. Obviously, the WHO analgesic ladder is meant to act as a guide, not a predestined treatment plan.

The various classes of medications commonly used to treat cancer pain and related symptoms are summarized in Table 2 and discussed in subsequent text.

(i) Nonopioid Analgesics

This group comprises the nonsteroidal antiinflammatory agents (NSAIDs), acetaminophen, and tramadol. (Tramadol is difficult to classify because it does have μ-opioid receptor activity, but this is not its sole analgesic activity, and the drug does not behave like the standard opioids.) Unlike the opioids, these medications do not cause physiologic dependence, but they all have ceiling effects (in contrast to the opioids). They are often used for their synergism with opioids. When used together, the two agents are effective at lower doses, and as a result the potential toxicity of each agent may be reduced. NSAIDs and acetaminophen are widely prescribed and often provide real benefit. However, because it is common for liver or kidney function to be impaired in patients with cancer, caution must be used when prescribing these medications (see Chapter 8). This caution extends to the use of combination therapies such as Percocet, Percodan, Vicodin, Narco, and Vicoprofen, which contain NSAIDs or acetaminophen. Accidental overdoses of acetaminophen have been associated with the use of these combination therapies because of lack of awareness of their constituents. As widely used as these medications are, they can cause harm.

There are two classes of NSAIDs in the market at this time, the nonselective COX inhibitors (e.g., aspirin, ibuprofen, naproxen sodium) and the COX-2 selective inhibitors or **coxibs** (e.g., celecoxib). The nonselective group causes a higher incidence of side effects related to gastric distress and platelet dysfunction. The coxibs cause fewer gastrointestinal (GI) adverse effects, but are not free of them. These newer agents have only been available in United States in the past few years, and they are still being assessed in patients with cancer. Recently they have been associated with adverse thrombotic effects such as myocardial

Table 2. Drugs commonly used in the management of cancer pain

Chemical Class	Drug	Recommended Adult Dose
Long-acting opioids	Oxycodone (Oxycontin/Oxycodone ER)	Starting dose 10 mg PO bid, with upward titration as needed
	Morphine sulfate (MS Contin/Oramorph)	Starting dose 15 mg PO bid with upward titration as needed
	Transdermal fentanyl	Starting dose 25 mg/h, changed q72h
	Methadone	Starting dose 2.5–5 mg PO q8–12h
Short-acting opioids	Oxycodone	5–10 mg every 3–4 h/m
	Morphine	10–30 mg every 3–4 h/m
	Hydromorphone (Dilaudid)	1–3 mg every 4 h/m
	Hydrocodone	5–10 mg every 4 h/m
Laxatives	Senna	1–2 tablets up to bid
	Lactulose	15–30 mL up to tid PM
	Oral naloxone	0.2–4 mg PO q4h up to four doses or bowel movement
Psychostimulants	Dextroamphetamine	5–10 mg every morning, occasionally repeated at 2 PM
	Methylphenidate	10 mg titrated up to maximum of 40 mg before midday
Nonsteroidal antiinflammatory drugs		
Standard	Ibuprofen	400–800 mg every 8 h
	Naproxen	250–500 mg every 8–12 h
	Ketorolac	15 mg IV/IM every 6 h
	Choline magnesium salicylate	500–750 mg every 8–12 h
Coxibs	Celecoxib	100–200 mg once or bid
Adjuvant medications		
Tricyclic antidepressants	Amtriptyline, nortriptyline	10–50 mg nightly
	Doxepin, desipramine	10–50 mg every h
Anticonvulsants	Gabapentin	300–3,600 mg/d in three divided doses
Other analgesics	Tramadol	50–100 mg up to every 6 h as needed
	Acetaminophen	325–1,000 mg every 4–6 h, not to exceed 4,000 mg in 1 day

infarction and stroke, so their use is under intense scrutiny at present. Their risks are still uncertain, and it remains unclear whether they should replace traditional low side-effect therapies such as choline magnesium salicylate (Trilisate).

Ketorolac is the only NSAID that can be given parenterally for analgesia in the United States . This medication is rarely used in a chronic pain, but it is useful for the short-term management of acute pain and is as efficacious as morphine for mild to moderate pain. It should only be used for 3 to 5 days. Gastric distress and bleeding are the major potential problems with its use.

Acetaminophen is a useful analgesic and antipyretic, but should be avoided in patients with impaired liver function because it is potentially hepatotoxic.

Tramadol is useful for mild to moderate pain, especially for patients who do not wish to take opioids. It is occasionally useful for severe pain in combination with other nonopioid analgesics or adjuncts in patients who cannot tolerate opioids. It is known to lower seizure thresholds so must be used with caution in patients with seizure disorders or brain pathology. Tramadol competes for protein binding sites and may potentiate the effects of coumadin. It should also be avoided in combination with tricyclics, selective serotonin reuptake inhibitors and dextromethorphan.

(ii) Opioids

Opioids are the mainstay of cancer pain treatment and their use can markedly improve the quality of life of patients with cancer with pain. Fears of addiction are unwarranted in patients with cancer. They and their families should be reassured so that fear of addiction does not prevent appropriate opioid use. Another related fear is that opioids will hasten death in patients with terminal cancer. In fact, the contrary appears to be true, and it has been demonstrated that terminally ill patients can have their lives prolonged and the quality of their final days improved by opioid analgesia. Caregivers should not hesitate to use appropriate doses of opioids at the end of life guided by the patient's level of pain and distress.

CHOICE OF OPIOID. The WHO has designated morphine the standard for the treatment of cancer-related pain. This is based on its efficacy, its ready availability throughout the world, widespread familiarity with its use, and its low cost. There are many opioids to choose from, both naturally occurring and synthetic, and each has its advantages and disadvantages in the clinical care of patients with cancer pain. Factors affecting the choice of an opioid agent may include drug potency, half-life, toxicity, and available routes of administration.

SHORT-ACTING VERSUS LONG-ACTING. Another consideration in drug choice relates to the pattern and timing of the patient's pain. For example, if the patient feels their pain primarily related to specific infrequent activities, then use of the intermittent short-acting opioid preparations is preferred. Examples of short-acting opioids include MSIR, oxycodone, hydromorphone, and transmucosal fentanyl. If, by contrast, a patient's pain is constant throughout the day or night, then long-acting opioid preparations would be emphasized, reserving short-acting opioid medications for intermittent exacerbations of the pain (often referred to as breakthrough pain). Examples of long-acting opioids include MS Contin, Kadian, Avinza, OxyContin, Duragesic, and methadone. See Chapter 9 for a full description of these drugs.

NOTE: Methadone is an excellent analgesic, very inexpensive, has additional benefits in the dorsal horn, and is completely legal to use for pain, provided that you write the words "For Pain" on the prescription. It does, however, tend to accumulate (because of its affinity for protein binding sites and its slow rate of metabolism), and may require a downward dose adjustment 5 to 10 days after initiating its use, or after a dose increase.

The concept of "breakthrough" pain is important to understand. It is defined as a transitory exacerbation of pain superimposed on a background of otherwise stable pain treated with analgesic. Reported by 50% to 66% of patients with cancer, it can be due to movement (i.e., bone metastases), general activity, time of day, other physiologic changes, or possibly disease progression. Whenever possible, moments in which breakthrough pain are likely to occur should be anticipated and the analgesic administered 30 to 45 minutes ahead of time (i.e., before taking a shower each morning or changing a dressing).

For many reasons, different patients respond uniquely to specific opiates. The ability of a patient to metabolize specific opioids also can vary; for example, oxycodone, a prodrug of oxymorphone, cannot be metabolized into its active form by 10% of the Caucasian population.

ROUTE OF ADMINISTRATION. Oral administration of opioids is always preferred and usually easily accomplished early in the treatment of cancer-related pain. However, as disease progresses or enters the terminal phase, it may become necessary to use other routes of administration. Patients with face and neck pathology may not be able to swallow and those with gastrointestinal tract pathology may not be able to reliably absorb oral preparations.

The Duragesic (fentanyl) patch provides a 2- to 3-day sustained release opioid therapy, which can be useful for patients with stable pain who have trouble using oral medications or who are active and find regular oral dosing inconvenient. There may be less constipation when using Duragesic because the oral route is avoided. As with any long-acting preparation, one needs to provide breakthrough medication as well.

There also may be problems with Duragesic as a treatment choice in patients with cancer. First, dose changes (up or down) may take up to 18 hours to be fully realized because of the absorption characteristics of both the patch and the subcutaneous depot. Some patients are sensitive to the adhesives in the patch and develop skin irritations. Some patients with cancer become cachectic, thus losing their subcutaneous body fat, which may alter the absorption rate of the fentanyl. Starting a patient on the lowest Duragesic patch, 25 μg per hour, is warranted when the patient is tolerating a consistent daily opioid dose equivalent to no less than 50 mg of morphine.

Parenteral opioids can be delivered intramuscularly (IM), intravenously (IV), or subcutaneously (SQ). We rarely use the IM route because it is irritating and painful. Subcutaneous infusions of opiates are satisfactory if the IV route is not available, although serum levels are not as stable and depend on local perfusion and absorption. The use of the SQ route limits the volume of medication that can be delivered (volumes more than 10 mL per hour tend to cause local irritation and poor absorption) thereby limiting drug choice (e.g., methadone cannot be concentrated to more than 10 mg per mL; hydromorphone and morphine are available in highly concentrated forms). Many patients with cancer have some form of intravenous access in place, which can be utilized for pain medications.

Patients who are alert and wish to have control over their own analgesia often benefit from using a patient-controlled analgesia (PCA) device. PCA machines provide flexibility and can be used for continuous infusion, intermittent injection, or as a combination of the two. They can be carried around with the patient in a fanny pack, a small backpack, or in a pocket. The most commonly used opioids for PCA are morphine and hydromorphone. Other opioids such as fentanyl, methadone, and, rarely, meperidine can also be used.

More invasive opioid delivery systems include epidural and intrathecal catheters. These treatments often benefit patients with cancer who require relatively large doses of systemic opioid, especially when side effects are intolerable, because neuroaxial doses are much smaller. Approximately one-tenth of the IV dose needed for pain control is needed for epidural delivery and 1/100th for intrathecal delivery. The addition of a local anesthetic agent such as bupivacaine can provide supplementary analgesia and reduce the overall amount of opioid needed. Catheters can be used in many formats such as: (a) with an external or subcutaneous injection port for intermittent injections, (b) with an external infusion pump giving a continuous infusion, (c) as patient-controlled epidural analgesia (PCEA), or (d) with a totally implanted delivery system. Unfortunately, catheter placement is contraindicated in patients with infection or coagulopathy. Some chemotherapy agents, such as the antiangiogenesis drugs, would need to be held for up to 3 to 4 weeks to allow for catheter implantation or removal. There should always be a backup pain treatment plan for home because most catheter problems, if they arise, cannot be fixed by phone consultation and require a trip to the hospital often causing a delay before treatment can be reinstated.

SIDE EFFECTS.   The opioids have a number of well-recognized and often troublesome side effects including respiratory depression, nausea, slowing of bowel movements, sedation, euphoria, mental status changes, dysphoria, and pruritis. By incrementally increasing opioid doses as pain levels increase, most side effects can be avoided, including respiratory depression, which is rarely a problem. However, there are two side effects that remain a potentially significant issue for patients with cancer despite how dosing changes are made, namely, constipation and sedation. Constipation can usually be avoided by placing all patients with cancer treated with opioids on a bowel regime consisting of stimulating laxatives [e.g., senna (Senokot), 2 tablets, twice daily] and a stool softener such as docusate. Note that bulk-forming laxatives do not reverse opioid induced constipation and may actually make matters worse if the patient is not well hydrated.

Narcan can be given orally to reduce the opioid's effect on the gastrointestinal mucosa; however, dosing should be kept in the range of 1.6 to 2.0 mg per dose (usually given every 6 hours until effective) to avoid the potential of reversing systemic analgesia.

However effective opioids are in controlling cancer pain, some patients are reluctant to use these drugs because they would rather have pain than feel drowsy and confused. For these patients, feeling alert and interactive (especially with family members) is so important that they will reject pain medication. To counteract sedation, the addition of a stimulant (e.g., dextroamphetamine, methylphenidate or modafinil) may be tried. These drugs do not compromise analgesia. Alternatively or additionally, nonopioid and adjunctive pain treatments can be added and maximized. Doing so may lead to lower opioid dosing.

TOLERANCE. Some degree of tolerance to opioids is common in patients with cancer primarily because these drugs are often used over long periods of time. When tolerance occurs, dose escalations are necessary to achieve the same level of comfort. High opioid dosages may be needed to meet the analgesic requirement and result in opioid toxicity, the symptoms of which can include confusion, sedation, and myoclonus. If tolerance occurs, or even preemptively, a number of strategies might be used in addition to dose escalation that might improve analgesia while reducing side effects:

- **Opioid rotation**: Switching from one opioid to another may be helpful because of partial cross-tolerance between opioids. Switching to methadone may be the best choice because of methadone's additional N-methyl-D-aspartate (NMDA) receptor antagonism. It is often possible to reduce the equianalgesic dose of the new opioid by 1/2 to 1/4, or, in the case of methadone, even to one tenth or less.
- **Resting period off opioids**: In the case of mild to moderate cancer pain, it is sometimes possible to discontinue opioid medication altogether for a while substituting nonopioid analgesics and/or adjuvants. A 1- to 2-week rest from the use of opioids may allow the opioid receptors to "reset" to their baseline level of functioning, thereby reducing or eliminating tolerance.
- **Addition of an NMDA antagonist**: Tolerance is known to be dependent on NMDA receptor activity. Some clinical studies have shown that the coadministration of an NMDA antagonist can reduce opioid tolerance. The NMDA antagonist most often used for this purpose is **dextromethorphan**, which is available as an over-the-counter medication. Ketamine compounded as an oral or nasal spray medication can be tried. Memantine is now also available in the United States.

OPIOID INDUCED HYPERALGESIA. There has been evidence in the literature for many years now that people and animals can become hyperalgesic (an increased response to a stimulus that is normally painful) when given opioids. This state can be mistaken for tolerance. The area of hyperalgesia extends beyond the known area of injury, perhaps even to the whole body. Elements of allodynia may also be present. This state requires opioid rotation, not dose escalation. NMDA antagonists would also be appropriate to use.

(iii) Adjuvant Analgesics

Although the nonopioid analgesics and the opioids described in the preceding text are used primarily for their analgesic effects, there are also drugs that have useful secondary analgesic effects. These are referred to as the adjuvant analgesics, and they come from such drug classes as antidepressants, anticonvulsants, antispasmodics, local anesthetics, and corticosteroids. A full description of these drugs can be found in Chapters 10 and 11. These drugs may be very useful in patients with cancer pain, particularly those used to treat neuropathic pain (e.g., gabapentin), pain associated with depression or insomnia (e.g., tricyclics), or to shrink tumor mass and reduce inflammation (steroids).

NOTE: Patients with cancer are often on complex treatment protocols requiring that they take a number of medications. When at all possible, the treatment regimen should be kept simple or be simplified. When choosing medications, we try to pick those that may give more than one benefit at a time. An example would be the use of nortriptyline, a tricyclic antidepressant. It has been shown to be beneficial in the treatment of neuropathic pain, and it has the secondary benefit of augmenting sleep. In the upper dosing range, it can also treat depression.

(iv) Bisphosphonates and Calcitonin

Severe bone pain frequently accompanies bone metastases. Although this pain responds somewhat to opioids and NSAIDs, it is often more useful to think in terms of treating the causative pathology. As typically seen with metastatic prostate and breast cancers, bone pain caused by osteoclast-induced bone resorption may be responsive to agents that inhibit the osteoclasts themselves, such as the bisphosphonates (e.g., pamidronate, zoledronic acid) and calcitonin. These agents are also used to treat hypercalcemia of malignancy. Although these agents appear to be beneficial in many patients, others show no response. Study findings are mixed and additional studies are warranted to define criteria that may predict clinical efficacy.

3. Interventional Techniques

Somatic nerves usually mediate cancer pain; however, certain forms of chronic cancer pain may be maintained by the sympathetic nervous system. This kind of pain is called sympathetically maintained pain (SMP). In addition, research has shown that peripheral and central sensitization are involved in most types of clinical pain syndromes. Both somatic and sympathetic nerves can be "blocked."

It is important when referring to nerve blockade to note whether it is an anesthetic (reversible) or neurolytic/neurodestructive (longer-lasting to permanent) block. (For a full description of diagnostic and therapeutic procedures used in pain management, see Chapters 12 and 13.) Perhaps the most effective block used in patients with cancer is the celiac plexus block used for the treatment of pain associated with pancreatic cancer and other intraabdominal malignancies. This procedure is usually done in two stages. After needle placement, a local anesthetic is injected. If the pain is significantly abated, a lytic agent such as alcohol or phenol is then injected. The local anesthetic wears off after a few hours. The lytic part of the block may not become effective for a couple of days. This block has a pain-relieving efficacy rate of greater than 80% and can be repeated if necessary. Most patients with pancreatic pain get several months of pain relief from this procedure.

Long-term intrathecal administration of opioids and local anesthetics is now commonly used in patients with cancer. It can be delivered either through a tunneled epidural catheter or implanted pump.

4. Neurosurgical Techniques

With the advent of the use of implantable devices to deliver neuroaxial analgesics, neurosurgical procedures for the management of pain are rarely used. These procedures are indicated in a few select patients and can cause neurologic dysfunction. Examples of these procedures include:

- **Peripheral neurectomy**: rarely used if at all
- **Anterolateral cordotomy**: usually for contralateral somatic pain below the C5 dermatomal level
- **Commisurotomy**: when pain is bilateral
- **Dorsal rhizotomy**: rarely used
- **Hypophysectomy**: best used for widespread hormonally mediated metastatic cancer (i.e., breast or prostate)
- **Cingulotomy**: for refractory cancer pain

These procedures are discussed in detail in Chapter 14.

5. Radiation Therapy

When pain is localized, external beam radiation can be extremely helpful for pain palliation. Radioisotopes can be implanted into some tumor beds as well. If pain is more diffuse as when because of multiple bone metastases, systemic infusion of radionuclides, such as samarium, can afford significant pain relief (see Chapter 20).

V. CONCLUSION

Cancer pain is almost always multifactorial and variable, making ongoing assessment critical to good care. Careful and regular assessment also helps to ensure the best quality of life for patients with cancer. From the initial diagnosis of disease to the final stages of life, currently available pain management techniques can relieve pain in most patients with cancer. It is often helpful to refer patients to a multidisciplinary pain treatment center when they present with a complex pain picture, preferably before the pain and associated symptoms are out of control.

SELECTED READINGS

Ahmedzai S. New approaches to pain control in patients with cancer. *Eur J Cancer* 1997;33(Suppl. 6):S8–S13.

American Medical Association. CME Library Module 10: overview and assessment of cancer pain. Available at: http://www.ama-cmeonline.com/pain_mgmt/module10/index.htm. Accessed 2005.

Cutson T. Management of cancer pain. *Prim Care* 1998;25:407–420.

Du Pen SL, Kharasch ED, Williams A, et al. Chronic epidural bupivacaine-opioid infusion in intractable cancer pain. *Pain* 1992;49: 293–300.

Falkmer U, Jarhult J, Wersall P, et al. A systematic overview of radiation therapy effects is skeletal metastases. *Acta Oncol* 2003;42 (5-6):620–633.

Fitzgibbon D, Galer BS. The efficacy of opioids in cancer pain syndromes. *Pain* 1994;58:429–431.

Grond S, Radbruch L, Meuser T, et al. Assessment and treatment of neuropathic cancer pain following WHO guidelines. *Pain* 1999;79: 15–20.

Levy M. Pharmacologic treatment of cancer pain. *N Engl J Med* 1996; 335:1124–1130.

Mantyh PW, Clohisy DR, Koltzenburg M, et al. Molecular mechanisms of cancer pain. *Nat Rev Cancer* 2002;2(3):201–209.

Mao J. Opioid-induced abnormal pain sensitivity: implications in clinical opioid therapy. *Pain* 2002;100:213–217.

Mercadante S. Opioid rotation for cancer pain. *Cancer* 1999;86: 1856–1866.

Patt RB. *Cancer pain.* Philadelphia, PA: JB Lippincott Co, 1993.

Payne R. Mechanisms and management of bone pain. *Cancer* 1997; 80(Suppl. 8):1608–1613.

Portenoy RK, Hagen NA. Breakthrough pain: definition, prevalence and characteristics. *Pain* 1990;41(3):273–281.

Portenoy RK, Payne D, Jacobsen P. Breakthrough pain: characteristics and impact in patients with cancer pain. *Pain* 1999;81(1-2): 129–134.

Simonnet G, Rivat C. Opioid-induced hyperalgesia: abnormal or normal pain? *Neuroreport* 2003;14(1):1–7.

World Health Organization Expert Committee. *Cancer pain relief and palliative care.* Geneva, Switzerland: World Health Organization, 1990.

Control of Pain in Children with Chronic and Terminal Disease

Alyssa A. LeBel

Infants do not cry without some legitimate cause.
—— *Omnibonus Fenarius*

Pain is the overwhelming concern in children with terminal disease. These patients have complex presentations of acute and chronic somatic, visceral, and neuropathic pain associated with severe illnesses: cancer, acquired immune deficiency syndrome (AIDS), cystic fibrosis, congenital heart disease, neuromuscular disease, and neurodegenerative disorders. Treatment-related and procedure-related pain is prominent and includes problems such as mucositis, pleurisy, pathologic fracture, phantom limb pain, chemotherapy-associated neuropathy, prolonged postdural puncture headache, abdominal pain from intractable vomiting, and radiation dermatitis. The child's sensory experience is accompanied by emotional and behavioral responses modified by parental fears and beliefs, social context, and past experiences, as well.

I. PRESENTATION OF CHRONIC PAIN AND PAIN FROM TERMINAL ILLNESS IN CHILDREN

1. Children with Cancer

A prospective study assessing the prevalence and etiology of pain in children and young adults with cancer treated by the pediatric branch of the National Cancer Institute over a 6-month period demonstrated that pain was present in 54% of hospitalized patients and 25% of outpatients. The individual frequencies of the various causes of pain differed markedly from those reported in a similar adult series. Tumor-related pain accounted for 34% of the pain experienced by hospitalized children and only

18% of the pain experienced by outpatients. Treatment-related pain was commonly reported in children who were both inpatients and outpatients. Even in patients with active malignancy, tumor-associated pain accounted for only 46% of the pain experienced, and therapy-related pain accounted for 39%; pain of both etiologies was reported by 14% of patients.

Several obvious differences between adult and pediatric malignancies contribute to these reported differences. First, the spectrum of malignancies seen in children is different from that in adults. The most common malignancies seen in children (acute lymphoblastic leukemia, primary brain tumors, rhabdomyosarcoma, neuroblastoma, and other soft tissue and bone sarcomas) are rarely seen in adults, whereas carcinoma, the most common adult malignancy, rarely occurs in children. Second, most pediatric malignancies become widely metastatic and are rapidly fatal once they become refractory to standard therapy. An adult, by contrast, may survive for many years with advanced disease. Third, most pediatric cancers are initially managed with aggressive multimodal treatment regimens that combine surgery, radiation therapy, and chemotherapy. These treatments are highly effective in inducing tumor remission but also result in considerable morbidity. Fourth, when conventional therapy is no longer effective, many children continue to receive anticancer treatment (often investigational treatment) until shortly before their death. This approach is designed to test new treatment strategies and to offer an approach that reasonably addresses parental concerns; however, it inevitably leads to an increase in treatment-related morbidity and pain for children.

2. Children with Other Chronic and Terminal Illnesses

In other chronic and terminal illnesses in children, such as AIDS, cystic fibrosis, and congenital heart disease, pediatric patients may have the more "adult" experience of prolonged disability with superimposed acute exacerbations and intervention-related distress.

II. DEVELOPMENTAL ISSUES AND THE PAIN SYSTEM

1. Maturity of the Nervous System

Until recently, many clinicians assumed that "neurologic immaturity" prevents very young children from experiencing pain. Current research disputes this contention. Pain transmission pathways develop during fetal life. Nerve tracts in the spinal cord and brainstem begin to myelinate around the gestational age of 22 weeks and are completely myelinated by 28 to 30 months after birth. More specifically, myelination is complete up to the thalamus by 30 weeks' gestation, and the thalamocortical pain connections to the cortex are myelinated by 37 weeks' gestation. Therefore, pathways that conduct noxious information from nociceptor to cortex are present in the newborn infant. Cortical descending inhibition develops postterm.

Most neurotransmitters and neuromodulators are present in the fetus. Calcitonin gene-related peptide (CGRP) and substance P are present at 8 to 10 weeks' gestation, whereas others such as enkephalin and vasoactive intestinal peptide (VIP) appear 2 to 4 weeks later. Catecholamines are present in late gestation, and, in the human fetus, serotonin has been found at 6 weeks postnatally. Neurotransmitters that enhance the perception of pain are produced earlier in the fetus than are endogenous opioids.

It appears, therefore, that pain processing in the mature fetus and newborn is adequately developed so that the infant may exhibit behavioral and physiologic responses to noxious stimuli and may even have enhanced nociception. The misconception that neonates and infants do not feel pain combined with a fear of using opioids in very young children resulted in gross undertreatment of pain in this population. Recent research has emphasized the importance of providing adequate pain control in newborns and young infants. It is now clear that the undertreatment of pain can have major short-term physiologic effects. The long-term consequences of untreated pain in the developing organism are not yet defined, but some studies suggest that early pain responses influence later pain behaviors.

2. Cognitive Development

Piagetian theory is often used to describe the developmental levels of understanding pain in school-age children; these levels are listed in Table 1. Speculations about younger children have been extrapolated from that framework. However, recent findings have shown that younger children have a more sophisticated understanding of pain than was previously reported. Children of 18 months of age can express and localize pain. Although younger children may recover more rapidly from surgery and report less pain after surgery, they typically have more pain from needle procedures that older children. Young children's limited cognitive development may preclude an understanding of the context of the needle pain, the realization that the pain will be over quickly, and the use of effective cognitive coping strategies.

Coping strategies are influenced by cognitive development. Children as young as 18 months indicate, through structured play sessions, the awareness of ways to eliminate their pain, generally by seeking hugs and kisses and asking for medicine. Children who

Table 1. Development sequence of children's understanding of pain

Age	Expression of Pain
6–18 mo	Fear of painful situations; use of simple words associated with pain; development of localization of pain
18–24 mo	"Hurt" used to describe pain
24–36 mo	Describes pain and external cause of pain
36–60 mo	Defines intensity of pain; use of descriptive adjectives and emotional terms
5–7 y	Clear differentiation of levels of pain intensity
7–10 y	Explanation of why pain hurts
>11 y	Explanation of the value of pain

From McGrath PJ, Craig KD. Developmental and psychological factors of children's pain. *Pediatr Clin North Am* 1989;36:823–836, with permission.

are 3 to 4 years of age spontaneously use distraction and also report that play makes them feel better. Although they may use this technique spontaneously, children cannot deliberately distract themselves or use self-initiated cognitive strategies to decrease pain before the age of approximately 5 years. Cognitive and behavioral strategies, such as relaxation, are generally beyond their capabilities.

Communicating pain is also influenced by cognitive development (see section entitled General Principles in subsequent text).

III. ASSESSMENT OF PAIN

1. General Principles

The assessment of pain in children should be systematic, and requires reevaluation throughout the course of the illness. Because infants cannot communicate verbally, behavioral and physiologic responses can be used to assess pain in the very young, including facial expression, tachycardia, and stress-related hormones. However, these signs may not be specific to pain. The child's cognitive development and ability to understand pain influence the choice of suitable measurement tools.

In children, pain measurement must consider the following:

- The child's report of pain is the best indicator of pain.
- Pain that appears unexplained by known causes may indicate disease progression or other factors, and should be investigated.
- The denial of pain when there is evidence of tissue damage should be investigated.
- Neonates and infants feel pain.
- Developmental factors should be considered before selecting the appropriate measures of pain intensity (this is more difficult in children younger than $2\frac{1}{2}$ years).

Measurement tools are summarized in Table 2.

2. Self-report

Children as young as 18 months can indicate their pain and give a location, but it is not possible to obtain a self-report of intensity of pain before approximately 3 years of age. Children who are 3 years old can give a gross indication, such as "no pain," "a little pain," and "a lot of pain." Similarly, many children at this age can use concrete measures such as "poker chips" representing "pieces of hurt" to convey the intensity of their pain. The use of more abstract self-report instruments, such as the "smiling faces scale" (see Chapter 6, Fig. 1), are generally not valid for use in children younger than 5 years.

Simple self-report measures are recommended for children older than 6 years. Among the most useful scales for measuring intensity of pain are visual analog scales, either vertical or horizontal, and simple numeric scales. For example, "If 0 means no hurt or pain and 10 means the biggest pain you ever have, what is your pain now?" The use of adjectival categorical scales such as "mild," "moderate," "severe," and "excruciating" are not recommended for children younger than 13 years.

Table 2. Behavioral, observational, and self-report scales

CRIES
Score 0–2 assigned by observer for each parameter: **C**rying; oxygen **R**equirement; **I**ncreased vital signs; facial **E**xpression; and **S**leep

FLACC
Score 0–10 total for changes in **F**ace, **L**egs, **A**ctivity, **C**rying, and **C**onsolability; scale is validated from 2 mo to 7 y

CHEOPS (Children's Hospital of Eastern Ontario Pain Scale)
Score ≥4 signifies pain. Assesses cry, facial expression, verbalization,torso movement, child touch of affected site, and leg position

Wong-Baker Faces
Score 0, "no hurt," to 5, "worst hurt you can imagine," using six cartoon faces showing increasing amounts of distress; for children >3 y

Bieri-modified
Score 0–10, using six cartoon faces progressing from a neutral state to tears/crying face; also for children >3 y

Visual analog scale
Score 0–10, using a 10-cm line marked as no pain at one end and worst pain at opposite end; after the child marks the line, it is measured from the 0 end to the mark

From Zempsky WT, Schecter NL. What's new in the management of pain in children. *Pediatr Rev* 2003;24:337–347, with permission.

3. Pain Behavior and Physiologic Variables

Behavioral observations should not be used in lieu of selfreport. However, behavioral observations are invaluable when self-report is not available. For example, in children younger than 2 years or in children without verbal ability because of disability or disease. In the presence of noxious stimuli, behavioral pain indicators may arouse suspicion and prompt investigations even in the absence of a verbal report of pain. Behavioral indicators of pain are listed in Table 3.

Neonates and infants feel pain, and neonates are no less sensitive to noxious stimulation than are older children and adults. Therefore, assessment of pain, although more complex than in older children, should be considered essential in the care of neonates and infants. In infants, reliance on facial expression, crying, posture, and physiologic variables such as heart rate, respiratory rate, blood pressure, and palmar sweating are important as potential indicators of pain, and scoring systems, such as the CRIES scale described by Krechel and Bildner (1995) are useful. There currently are no physiologic measures that reliably indicate pain, and pain treatment should never be withheld solely because of a lack of physiologic evidence.

IV. PAIN MANAGEMENT

The administration of analgesics to children with cancer and terminal illness follows the general principles of the World Health

Table 3.   Behavioral indicators of pain

Crying
Fussing, irritability
Withdrawal from social interaction
Sleep disturbance
Grimacing
Guarding
Not easily consoled
Reduction in eating
Reduction in play
Reduction in attention span

From McGrath PJ. An assessment of children's pain: a review of behavioral, physiological, and direct scaling techniques. *Pain* 1987;31:147–176, with permission.

Organization (WHO) analgesic ladder, a stepwise approach to prescribing analgesics depending on the intensity of pain (see Chapter 32).

1. Pharmacologic Treatment

Table 4 lists the pediatric dosages for common pain medications.

(i) Acetaminophen and the Nonsteroidal Antiinflammatory Drugs

Acetaminophen has been shown to be safe even for newborns in whom the immature hepatic metabolism system is protective, with decreased production of toxic metabolites. In children who are unable to take acetaminophen by mouth, the rectal route is an option. However, in the child with cancer, bacterial seeding is a concern.

Aspirin, salicylates, such as choline magnesium trisalicylate, and several nonsteriodal antiinflammatory drugs (NSAIDs), including ibuprofen (Motrin) and naproxen (Naprosyn), are used, particularly for children with pain of inflammatory origin. Early experience with the use of the coxibs is promising, but the risk versus benefit of these drugs in children is yet to be determined. The use of all the NSAIDs should be limited in children with thrombocytopenia, coagulopathy, or gastritis.

(ii) Opioids

Although there has been a history of avoidance of opioids in the treatment of newborns and infants, our current understanding dictates that there are few contraindications to opioid treatment in the very young. As in adults, opioid analgesics are the drugs of choice for moderate to severe acute and cancer pain. For children with chronic nonterminal pain (CNTP), the same constraints in opioid prescribing that apply to adults are relevant to children (see Chapter 30).

Physiologic factors such as the immaturity of the nervous system, liver and, kidneys force us to alter the method of providing opioid analgesia, but do not preclude the use of these important and effective analgesics. For infants aged 3 to 6 months, clearance

Table 4.   Analgesic medications in children

Drug	Dose	Route	Frequency
Acetaminophen	10–15 mg/kg	PO (PR)	q4h
Amitriptyline	0.2–3 mg/kg	PO	Every night
Aspirin	10–15 mg/kg	PO	q4h
0.1% Bupivacaine	2–7 mL/h	Epidural	Continuous
Choline magnesium salicylate	10–15 mg/kg	PO	q4h
Codeine	0.5–1 mg/kg	PO	q4h
Fentanyl	0.5–2 µg/kg	IV	q1–2h
2 µg Fentanyl/0.1% bupivacaine mix	2–7 mL/h	Epidural	Continuous
Gabapentin	5–45 mg/kg/d	PO	Three divided doses
Ibuprofen	4–10 mg/kg	PO	q6–8h
Morphine	0.01–0.05 mg/kg/h	IV, SQ	Continuous
	0.08–0.1 mg/kg	IV	q2h
	0.1–0.15 mg/kg	IV, IM	q3–4h
	0.2–0.4 mg/kg	PO	q4h
Morphine sustained release	0.3–0.6 mg/kg	PO, PR	q12h
Meperidine	0.8–1.3 mg/kg	IV	q2h
	0.8–1 mg/kg	IV, SQ	q3–4h
Methadone	0.1 mg/kg	IV, PO	q4h × 2, then q6–12h
Naproxen	5–7 mg/kg	PO	q8–12h
Naloxone	0.5–1 µg/kg	IV	q10–15 min

PO, orally; PR, rectally; IV, intravenously; IM, intramuscularly; SQ, subcutaneously; q, every.
From Berde CB, Ablin A, Glazer J, et al. Report of the Subcommittee on Disease Related Pain in Childhood Cancer. *Pediatrics* 1990;86:818–825, with permission.

and analgesic effects of morphine, fentanyl, sufentanyl, and methadone resemble those for young adults. Six-month-old infants show no more respiratory depression from fentanyl than do adults. It is the general clinical impression that all opioids, including morphine, have a wide margin of safety and excellent efficacy for most children older than 6 months of age with cancer pain and resistant chronic pain. Premature and full-term infants show reductions in clearance of most opioids. Pharmacologic guidelines for opioid use in the newborn and infant are described in Chapter 22. For nonintubated infants younger than 3 to 6 months, opioids must be used with caution and only with close observation. The dose should be approximately one third to one fourth of that used for older children. In contrast to respiratory effects, the cardiovascular depressant effects of opioids in newborns are mild and may actually be beneficial in some situations.

For children with cancer, the oral route is most effective. However, the use of this route may be limited by nausea, mucositis, and difficulty with swallowing pills or elixirs. The principles of opioid therapy for treating cancer pain (Chapter 32) apply equally to adults and children. Long-acting preparations are used as the basis of chronic opioid therapy, reserving short-acting opioids for breakthrough pain. However, in small children (<20 kg), the use of long-acting preparations is limited by the lack of availability of low dose preparations. Tramadol (Ultram), a weak opioid agonist (chiefly at the μ receptor) with additional norepinephrine and serotonin reuptake inhibition, is an option for oral analgesia with fewer side effects than pure opioid agonists. However, the concomitant use of standard opioids, or use in patients dependant on opioids, should be avoided because of unpredictable interactions.

When parenteral administration is required, the intravenous or subcutaneous route can be used. Intramuscular injections should not be used because they are painful and frightening, and children may accept pain rather than asking for a "shot." In cases of severe pain in a patient whose dosage requirement is unknown, 0.05 to 0.1 mg per kg of morphine can be given and reassessed every 15 minutes, with additional increments of 0.05 mg per kg administered until relief is obtained. Intermittent bolus injections of morphine can then be provided round the clock. Continuous infusions of morphine may begin at a starting dose of 0.01 to 0.05 mg/kg/hour for children older than 6 months. Occasionally, an alternative opioid may be indicated, in which case equianalgesic dosages can be substituted for morphine (see Appendix VII). Patient-controlled analgesia (PCA) is effective for children and adolescents aged 5 years and older (see Chapter 22). However, some children and adolescents may not have the cognitive, emotional, or physical resources to use PCA.

The pharmacologic approach to the management of side effects is similar to that in adults. However, children may have difficulty communicating subjective symptoms that reflect difficulties with pruritus, nausea, and dysphoria. Therefore, if an infant or child becomes restless or irritable with increased opioid dose, treatment of side effects is suggested empirically, as is a change to an alternative opioid. For acute respiratory depression, as dictated by professional judgment, children may receive naloxone titrated to the desired effect. The initial dose of naloxone in a child is 0.5 to 1.0 μg per kg.

(iii) Adjuvant Medications

Adjuvant medications such as tricyclic antidepressants and stimulants are beneficial as a coanalgesics in children with cancer pain, with doses extrapolated from the adult dosage by weight (see Chapter 32 and Appendix VII). In general, the starting dose is low, approximately 0.2 mg per kg of amitriptyline (Elavil) with an increase to approximately, 1 to 3 mg/kg/day. A baseline electrocardiogram (ECG) may be useful in patients who have received other cardiotoxic medications. Neuropathic pain may respond to anticonvulsant/sodium channel blocking agents such as gabapentin (Neurontin), up to 45 mg/kg/day, titrating from qhs (5 mg per kg) to tid, and mexiletine, 2 to 3 mg per kg, bid or tid. The starting dose for stimulants, such as dexamphetamine and methylphenidate, is 0.05 mg per kg. Corticosteroids are helpful owing to their antiinflammatory, antiemetic, and mood-altering effects.

(iv) Topical Preparations

Infants and children also may receive viscous lidocaine for mucosal analgesia. A single mucous dose of lidocaine should not exceed 4 mg per kg; a repeated oral administration of up to 2 mg per kg is generally safe. Infants and young children should receive dilute lidocaine sprays, such as 1% in neonates and 2% in children versus the 4% to 10% used in adults. The use of transdermal 5% lidocaine patch (lidoderm), applied to dermal areas of localized peripheral neuropathic pain, one to three patches per 12 hours, is currently being studied in children. Eutectic mixture of lidocaine and prilocaine (EMLA) use is now considered safe in neonates and preterm infants. Sucrose solutions, which may activate the descending analgesic system, are effective until approximately 4 to 6 months of age.

2. Regional Anesthesia and Analgesia

Regional blockade techniques have been developed for children of all ages, including newborns, and are generally performed with sedation or light general anesthesia because of patients' fear of needles. Regional, caudal epidural, and lumbar epidural blockade provide excellent analgesia with wide margins of safety. Hemodynamic and respiratory effects of epidural or subarachnoid blockade in infants are mild. The distribution and clearance of bupivacaine and lidocaine following regional blockade in children older than 6 months resemble those in adults. Bupivacaine clearance is mildly delayed in newborns. Epidural and subarachnoid infusions of opioid and local anesthetics have been effectively used in infants and children who have refractory cancer pain, deafferentation pain, and complex regional pain syndrome, type I (CRPS I). It is important to administer local anesthetic slowly in children, with constant assessment for clinical signs of intravascular effect.

3. Other Techniques

Children are excellent subjects for hypnosis, relaxation, and biofeedback training, all of which are especially useful for recurrent pain such as headache and for brief painful medical procedures. Some of these techniques are described in Chapter 22. Children older than 7 years generally benefit from such programs, but some behavioral treatment strategies have applied to children as young as 3 to 4 years.

V. CONCLUSION

Thankfully, chronic pain and serious illness are rare in the pediatric population of the developed world. Pain management in developing countries is advancing, generally through the efforts of WHO and International Red Cross. Whenever pain and illness occur, their effects are devastating, not only to the children but also to their families and caregivers. Pain treatment in this population is challenging for many reasons, including caregivers' insecurity about pediatric dosing, difficulties in assessing pain, and resistance to opioid use because of misguided fears. It is, however, critically important to give the benefit of adequate analgesia to these vulnerable patients, although this may require the involvement of experts in developing safe and effective treatment regimes.

SELECTED READINGS

Anand KJS, Hickey PR. Pain and its effects in the human neonate and fetus. *N Engl J Med* 1987;317:1321–1329.

Berde CB. The treatment of pain in children. In: Bond MR, Charldon JE, Woolf CJ, eds. *Proceedings of the Seventh World Congress on Pain.* New York: Elsevier Science, 1991;435–440.

Berde CB, Ablin A, Glazer J, et al. Report of the Subcommittee on Disease Related Pain in Childhood Cancer. *Pediatrics* 1990;86:818–825.

Beyer JE, Wells N. Assessment of cancer pain in children. In: Patt RB, ed. *Cancer pain.* Philadelphia, PA: JB Lippincott Co, 1993.

Burrows FA, Berde CB. Optimal pain relief in infants and children. *Br Med J* 1993;307:815–816.

Eliott K, Foley KM. Neurologic pain syndromes in patients with cancer. *Neurol Clin* 1989;7:333–360.

Ferrell BR, Rhiner M, Shapiro B, et al. The experience of pediatric cancer pain. Part 1: impact of pain on the family. *J Pediatr Nurs* 1994;9:368–379.

Krechel SW, Bildner J. CRIES: a new neonatal postoperative pain measurement score. Initial testing of validity and reliability. *Paediatr Anaesth* 1995;5:53–61.

Leahy S, Hockenberry-Eaton M, Sigler-Price K. Clinical management of pain in children with cancer: selected approaches and innovative strategies. *Cancer Pract* 1994;2:37–45.

McGrath PJ, Beyer J, Cleeland C, et al. Report of the Subcommittee on Assessment and Methodologic Issues in the Management of Pain in Childhood Cancer. *Pediatrics* 1990;36:814–817.

McGrath PJ, Craig KD. Developmental and psychological factors in children's pain. *Ped Clin North Am* 1989;36:823–836.

Yaster M, Krane EJ, Kaplan RF, et al. *Pediatric pain management and sedation handbook.* St. Louis, MO: Mosby–Year Book, 1997.

Zeltzer LK, Altman A, Cohen D, et al. Report of the Subcommittee on the Management of Pain Associated with Procedures in Children with Cancer. *Pediatrics* 1990;86:826–831.

Zempsky WT, Schecter NL. What's new in the management of pain in children. *Pediatr Rev* 2003;24:337–347.

Palliative Medicine

Constance M. Dahlin, Andrew Tyler Putnam, and J. Andrew Billings

You are outside life, you are above life, you are afflicted with ills the ordinary person does not know, you transcend the normal level, and that is what people hold against you, you poison their quietude, you corrode their stability. You feel repeated and fugitive pain, insoluble pain, pain outside thought, pain which is neither the body, nor the mind, but which partakes of both. And I share your ills, I am asking: who should dare to restrict the means that bring us relief.
—Antonin Artaud, 1895–1948

I. WHAT IS PALLIATIVE CARE?

Palliative care is comprehensive interdisciplinary care that focuses on the quality of life of patients with a life-limiting advanced disease or terminal disease and for their families. Care is "comprehensive" because it aims to prevent and relieve all the sources of suffering, including not only pain and other disagreeable physical symptoms but also emotional, sociocultural, and spiritual distress. A core palliative care team typically consists of a physician, nurse, social worker, and chaplain who meet regularly to provide coordinated, interdisciplinary care and to promote a patient-derived concept of quality of life. Teams may also include a bereavement counselor, volunteer coordinator, volunteers, nutritionist, physical therapist, and so on. The goals of care grow out of an exploration of the well-informed patient's definition of living well until death comes and the management options provided by specially trained professionals—an individualized and changing view of a "good death." Palliative medicine is the branch of medicine encompassing the knowledge, attitudes, and skills of the clinician that are a requisite for a practicing clinician on such a palliative care team.

Palliative care should not be confused with the dismissal or abandonment conveyed when physicians say to a dying person, erroneously and perhaps cruelly, "Nothing more can be done." It is not "comfort measures only," but it is rather an aggressive, active, idealistic team approach to making the best of limited time. Palliative care is based on the hospice philosophy of care but is not subject to regulations in the United States that limit hospice care to persons with a prognosis of 6 months or less who have decided to forego all "aggressive," expensive, and life-prolonging interventions. Indeed, palliative care is not an alternative to conventional care; it coexists comfortably with curative or life-prolonging measures. Therefore, it has a role in the earliest phases of management of a life-limiting or terminal condition, while also aggressively pursuing comfort, support, and quality of life through all appropriate means in the final phases of life.

II. WHAT IS A GOOD DEATH?

Although all medical decisions should reflect patient values, preferences, beliefs, and goals, nowhere in medicine are individualized notions of good care—and of a good death—more important to be recognized than in palliative medicine. Patients' desire for comfort, to avoid hospitalization and medical procedures, and to be at home or in homelike settings with their family present may be more of a priority than such common medical goals as prolonging life, curing an illness, or correcting a metabolic disorder. Weighing benefits and burdens often leads to a decision to discontinue a variety of "aggressive" interventions—diagnostic or therapeutic maneuvers, many of which require institutional care and that would seem appropriate at most times of life but not when one is dying. Simple measures (e.g., sublingual or buccal medication for a patient unable to swallow rather than an intravenous line) are often favored because they are easier to carry out at home and do not entail regular nursing attention or much discomfort or expense.

Areas typically addressed in a palliative care plan of care include the following:

Pain and Symptom Control: Patients who are dying often experience a myriad of disagreeable physical symptoms that interfere with their ability to function and enjoy their remaining life. These symptoms may include pain, as well as nausea, vomiting, anorexia, dyspnea, weakness, fatigue, and bowel and bladder problems. The fear of unrelieved pain and suffering can be enormously disturbing and can make the patients wish that they were already dead. Although studies of what patients and family members want most when they are terminally ill tend to identify primarily nonphysical matters, excellent pain and symptom control are essential substrates that allow for good psychosocial and spiritual coping and a good death. Attention to all physical symptoms and meticulous treatment of even minor distress can contribute greatly to the patient's overall well-being. Current palliative care textbooks describe treatments that can alleviate most of these common symptoms.

Sense of Control: Control of different aspects of life can be important to many patients. Indeed, loss of control from health-related issues can be overwhelming for some patients. As a terminal illness progresses, there is increased loss of control. People may feel diminished when they sense they are being treated merely as patients, subject to the orders of doctors and nurses and requiring family for assistance with everyday tasks.

An individualized care plan reflecting sensitivity to concerns about control helps patients feel more themselves rather than passive victims. For example, using a patient-controlled analgesia (PCA) device rather than relying on nurses or family to bring medications may bolster a patient's sense of active involvement in the care process and result in better pain and symptom management.

Patient-centered Decision Making: By current bioethical standards, competent adults can choose what medical treatment to accept. They have the right to refuse any proposed life-sustaining treatment. More important, in order to create a plan of care that includes personal values and goals, patients have the right to be helped to understand all reasonable diagnostic and treatment options and the likely consequences of carrying out such procedures.

Patients need professional collaboration in making good choices—shared decision making. If the patient is incapable of making decisions or prefers to delegate them, then a designated proxy or, by default, the closest family member needs to consider carefully what the patient would want. For a patient who is incompetent, a process called "substituted judgment" is requested, asking the proxy to determine what the patient would choose if he or she were able to make a decision. The proxy might be asked questions such as the following: Has the patient ever said anything about similar diagnostic or treatment options in the past? Would the patient want to live this way? How did the patient react about other people's decisions in such situations or their deaths? Answers to these sorts of questions provide clues to how substituted judgment can be carried out. An important aspect of substituted judgment is that it does not require the proxy or family to decide what they think is right or what they want; it simply asks them about the patient's values so that the health care team can base their decisions on them. Only when no such information about patient preferences is available is the proxy or family asked to help make a decision on behalf of the patient, based on what they think is right. Finally, in situations in which no proxy is available, decisions in the best interest of the patient are left to the medical team, generally assisted by a patient representative, an ethics consultant, or, occasionally, a court-appointed guardian.

Avoid Inappropriate Prolongation of Dying When Quality of Life is Diminished: Patients and families fear painful, depersonalized, costly, prolonged dying. Many fear a medical system that uses technology to keep a patient alive but does not know when to stop such measures. Patients and families should be reassured that their wish to avoid prolonging the dying process will be honored. At the same time, they should never feel abandoned or that the intensity of support and attention to their comfort will be lessened because they have rejected any treatment options.

Great importance may be placed on protecting the patient from a "bad death." Would it make more sense to let the patient die from a potentially reversible infection or metabolic disorder rather than to rescue him briefly from death but leave him to face great pain and suffering? Is an effective treatment, perhaps involving prolonged hospitalization or invasive procedures, less desirable than a less definitive, simple, easily handled approach that can be carried out in the home? Neither excessive reliance on medical technology nor crude and inflexible dismissal of the most elaborate technical approaches is appropriate.

Identify Meaning and Purpose in Life and Redefine Hope for the Remaining Time: Facing death paradoxically involves seeking meaning and purpose in life. Patients who recognize their terminal condition regularly ask spiritual questions: Why me? Did I live a good life? What happens after I die? Will I be remembered? Exploring these questions, perhaps in the context of religious beliefs, is part of making sense of mortality and of facing death. The answers to these questions are also the basis for hope for the future—not necessarily hope of living forever, but hope of living longer, of making the best of whatever time is left, of taking some pride in one's life, of experiencing a sense of completion, or of feeling one has made an enduring contribution. Patients often hope to fulfill key duties or wishes in their remaining time; for example, putting one's affairs in order, or surviving long enough to see a new grandchild or to attend a family wedding may be attainable goals. Reconciliation with loved ones may be important. Patients can be helped by questions about "unfinished business": If you died tonight, what would be left undone? What do you still hope to accomplish?

Assistance in Preparation for Death: Dying patients may want assistance with practical issues such as completing a health care proxy, executing a durable power of attorney, writing a will, or making funeral arrangements. Often patients are hesitant to ask about their future or to share their worries about the dying process, although they regularly harbor deep fears (e.g., of a crescendo of intractable pain or of suffocation). Although clinicians cannot foresee the future, they can reassure patients about providing comfort and nonabandonment, and they often can reassure patients about unnecessary fears (e.g., "You really do not need to worry about suffocation with this kind of cancer"). Ask patients what is on their mind: What are your concerns now? Have you had thoughts about what the future holds? Are you thinking about death? What are your worst fears?

Psychosocial and Spiritual Care of the Family: Because the patient's medical condition usually is our primary focus, professional caregivers may overlook the suffering of family and friends. Although the patient is dying, those close to the patient may experience anticipating grieving, each struggling with his or her own imminent loss. They also benefit from the caring and support offered by palliative care professionals. Could a chaplain or priest be helpful at the bedside? Would a social worker facilitate the family in more effective coping with their grief? How are they managing the financial burden of terminal illness (which proves devastating to about a third of families) or the need for assisting the patient at home? Unhappy memories of a relative's difficult death or the perception that one did not fulfill an expected role can cause suffering that complicates grief long after the patient dies. Family support should extend through the period of intense bereavement, typically the first year, and specialized resources may be required for selected survivors.

III. ALTERNATIVES TO AN ACUTE CARE HOSPITAL

Patients and their families commonly wish to be at home for most, or all, of the course of a terminal illness. In the United States, hospice programs specialize in appropriate end-of-life care in the home. Such programs have been shown to provide improved outcomes at lower cost for dying persons in the final months of life. Unfortunately, government-mandated admission requirements, including a likely prognosis of 6 months or less and a rejection of costly, "aggressive" life-sustaining measures, have hindered appropriate referral of patients to hospice. Most patients use such services only in the last few weeks of life. Palliative care programs—features of care that are well established throughout the United Kingdom, Australia, and Canada and that are currently developing in many academic centers in the United States—are more flexible in serving patients and families earlier in the course of the illness and are willing to entertain all forms of diagnostic and therapeutic interventions that might benefit the patient.

Home Care: At home, the patient often finds comfort, privacy, security, and a sense of control. The close involvement of family and friends and the convenience of being at home are also appreciated. Most patients express the wish to be cared for and often even to die at home. Home hospice generally provides medications, durable medical equipment, occasional nursing visits, home health aide visits, and 24-hour on-call assistance, while offering support from volunteers, chaplains, social workers, and bereavement coordinators. For most of the day, families are usually the direct caregivers in the home. When properly arranged, home hospice can be a rewarding experience and a powerful source of satisfaction for the family, leaving them with the feeling that they did everything they could for their loved one.

Institutional Care: When the patient's medical condition and comfort require more attention or skilled care than is available at home from the "formal" services of trained health service providers and from the "informal" assistance of family and friends, institutional care is required. Inpatient hospices and palliative care units, typically located in acute care hospitals, chronic care hospitals, or nursing homes, provide such an option. These units ideally provide a homelike atmosphere and ready access to family, friends, and pets, but also consistent professional assistance. By unburdening the family of difficult patient care responsibilities that are often physically and psychologically exhausting, these units allow the family to support a loved one in a more comfortable, appropriate manner.

Discharge Planning: The process of discharge planning from an acute care facility is a process, not a single event. Patients and their families, assisted by various health professionals, need to be educated about providing care and the common problems and crises they might encounter. Discussion includes availability of 24-hour assistance when problems arise and planning for where the death is likely to occur. The requirements for professional help and durable medical equipment need to be assessed. Complex medication regimens from the hospital can often be simplified, and drugs not essential for comfort may be eliminated. Families can then have a better sense of their care-giving capabilities and can consider realistic options and appropriate settings.

IV. PAIN MANAGEMENT AT THE END OF LIFE

Pain is frequently a problem at the end of life. Important principles in pain management in this situation include the following:

Opioids are the Mainstay of Cancer Pain Treatment: Many terminally ill patients with pain can be successfully managed with opioids alone, without resorting to other analgesics or interventional treatments. Opioids can also play an important role in managing dyspnea and anxiety, both common terminal symptoms. Some patients benefit from adjunctive therapies such as nonsteroidal antiinflammatory drugs (NSAIDs), neuropathic pain medications, and various psychotropic medications. A small number with unremitting, poorly controlled pain may benefit from an interventional procedure. The celiac plexus block is relatively simple to perform and helpful for patients with intraabdominal malignancies, particularly pancreatic cancer. Simplicity is the key in terminally patients; many of them are cared for at home by nonprofessionals who are easily overwhelmed by complex treatments. Treatment choices are described in Chapter 32.

The Oral Route is Preferred: The oral route for pain relief generally allows the greatest freedom and comfort for the patient and greatest ease for home management. Long-acting forms are convenient. In general, avoid the following: (a) painful intramuscular injections; (b) intravenous injections or infusions that require skilled personnel, regular monitoring, and continuous access [although the availability of relatively long-lasting peripherally inserted central catheter (PICC) lines has made PCA pumps more practical at home]; and (c) epidural or intrathecal pumps that often intimidate families and home health nurses, may fail at home, and are unacceptable at some post–acute care facilities.

When Patients Cannot Swallow, Simple Alternatives May be Used: If a patient loses the ability to swallow pills and liquids, concentrated opioid elixirs can be taken sublingually or buccally. Analgesia from sublingual/buccal administration of morphine or oxycodone is roughly equivalent to that from the same dosage of oral medication, since medications are absorbed via the GI tract.

Transdermal administration of medications is commonly used for pain control at the end of life when patients cannot swallow reliably, or earlier in the course of an illness when the oral route is not feasible. The fentanyl patch may provide basal pain control, whereas the sublingual or rectal route is reserved for additional (prn) medication. The smallest patch (25 μg per hour) is roughly equivalent to 90 mg of oral morphine over 24 hours, and clinicians should beware of starting the patch when the patient's opioid requirements are significantly lower than this daily dosage. Transdermal preparations of other medications, including opioids, are popular in some hospices although little evidence supports their efficacy, and they may be costly.

The **rectal** route may also be useful. A few opioids are commercially available as suppositories, but a pharmacist can often prepare suppositories of a desired medication and dosage—typically placed in KY jelly or in a gel cap to assist in breakdown and absorption. Analgesic levels from rectal administration are generally comparable to that achieved with the same dosage given orally. Limited experience with long-acting opioid formulations suggests that they can be used by the rectal route.

Subcutaneous infusion should be considered in place of intravenous or intramuscular medication for patients being managed at home, in a subacute care facility, or when intravenous access is problematic. Both intermittent and continuous infusions can be used, generally delivered through an intravenous infusion needle or a specially designed needle placed in the subcutaneous tissue. Such needles are easily inserted, and accidental removal poses no hazard of bleeding. Absorption appears roughly equivalent to that achieved with an intravenous infusion, if somewhat delayed, and with limits on the rate of infusion. Considerable experience has now accumulated on combining opioids with other agents in subcutaneous infusions, although the mixing of drugs may prevent titration of individual agents. Subcutaneous administration of fluids (hypodermoclysis) also can be considered.

Addressing Tolerance: Many terminal patients take opioids for long periods of time. Tolerance and the need for high dosages may lead to inconvenient regimens with many pills or patches. Toxicity, including sedation or other side effects, particularly myoclonus, is not infrequent. Opioid rotation—switching from one drug to another—may allow for use of lower doses, and may produce better pain control, either from improved analgesia or reduced toxicity. Methadone is often chosen when a component of neuropathic pain is suspected. The opioid equivalency found in equianalgesic tables is not appropriate once a patient has developed opioid tolerance because there is incomplete cross-tolerance between the opioids. A dose half of the equivalent dose is normally used when a different opioid is started (1/10th to 1/20th in the case of methadone), with slow upward titration to achieve the desired effect if necessary. The principle of opioid rotation and alternative ways to control tolerance are described in Chapter 32.

Appropriate Use of Opioid Infusions: Continuous intravenous opioid infusions are regularly used in inpatient settings to ensure good analgesia, relieve breathlessness, and/or provide sedation in the last few days of life. Common indications include (a) inability to take oral medication (due to vomiting and dysphagia) or uncertain oral or transdermal absorption, and (b) need for fine tuning or rapid titration of analgesics, including for breakthrough or incident pain or dyspnea, and even agitation. For patients with severe distress, analgesic effects may need to be monitored every 5 to 15 minutes.

When prescribing continuous opioid infusion for a patient who is dying, write orders for a generous dose range so that the patient's fluctuating symptoms can be quickly relieved. In addition to the constant infusion, there should be orders for boluses "as necessary" (e.g., morphine sulfate 1 to 8 mg q15 min) to be used whenever the patient complains of pain or dyspnea or appears agitated or distressed. Providing relief immediately with a bolus injection is preferable to waiting for the effects of an increase in infusion rate (typically requiring five half-lives to reach a new equilibrium). Boluses can be administered by a PCA pump or by injection—clinicians should be mindful that very ill patients might not have the capacity to operate a PCA system.

Addressing Inappropriate Fears about Hastening Death: All health professionals are concerned about causing a patient's death. Unfortunately, some clinicians avoid opioids or prescribe them at ineffective dosages to avoid any hint of hastening death. In reality, opioids prescribed and titrated appropriately for physical distress will rarely produce life-threatening toxicity, except perhaps constipation. Dosages required to alleviate severe pain or dyspnea generally are not associated with serious sedation.

In unusual situations, clinicians are faced with a difficult choice in prescribing the right dose of an opioid. Higher opioid dosages that produce good symptom control may cause serious sedation (generally when nonsedating analgesics and added psychostimulants have been ineffective) whereas lower opioid dosages allow for greater alertness but do not control symptoms well. Patient goals and values should play an important role in deciding on appropriate therapy.

In situations in which sedation or, more rarely, respiratory depression, is a desirable goal and may conceivably hasten death, clinicians should be familiar with the **principle or rule of double effect,** which makes a distinction between intended effects and foreseeable but unintended effects. This principle is widely accepted by bioethicists and medical–legal experts and instructs that when comfort is the primary goal of medical management, a treatment for achieving comfort is justifiable even if that treatment has the potential for causing serious, predictable, but unintended, side effects. The principle of double effect justifies the use of opioids, or the upward titration of opioids, even if the doses necessary for the patient to be comfortable cause unintended, but foreseeable harm to the patient. The importance of keeping a patient comfortable at the end of life is arguably the most important responsibility of the clinician and justifies the risks of medications necessary for that comfort.

In very unusual circumstances, physical or emotional suffering near the end of life is so severe and refractory to usual medications that **sedation for intractable distress in the patient who is dying** (also called **palliative sedation** and often labeled with the misleading term, **terminal sedation**) is necessary. In these situations, continuous infusions of benzodiazepines (e.g., midazolam), barbiturates (e.g., pentobarbital), or anesthetics (e.g., propofol) may be used alone or added to opioid regimens. Opioid dosages should generally be continued to assure adequate pain relief.

V. NONPAIN SYMPTOM CONTROL

To convey the complexity and richness of nonpain symptom control, we have noted a few of the major interventions that are regularly employed by palliative medicine practitioners in Table 1. Details of evaluation and treatment are included in some of the texts referenced below. In all cases, consideration of the underlying etiology, diagnostic testing, and potential specific treatments is appropriate, but purely symptomatic approaches make sense for many patients nearing death.

Table 1. Nonpain symptom control

Agitation: Haloperidol can help organize the patient's thoughts and reduce agitation, and generally produces less somnolence than other antipsychotics. Chlorpromazine is favored when sedation is desirable. Newer ("atypical") neuroleptics are expensive but have occasional advantages.

Anorexia: Common treatments include megestrol and low dosages of glucocorticosteroids. Gastroparesis is a common complication of cancer, and can be treated with metoclopramide. Dronabinol is occasionally useful. Patients and families often require intensive counseling that improved nutrition, including TPN, will neither improve well-being nor prolong life, and thus the patient should eat for pleasure.

Anxiety: Benzodiazepines are usually the anxiolytics of choice, but they can lead to confusion, paradoxical agitation, and excess somnolence, especially in the elderly. In more severe or unresponsive anxiety, haloperidol or chlorpromazine is indicated or an "atypical" neuroleptic.

Ascites: Diuretic treatment can be useful early, but monitoring of hydration and mineral balance may be burdensome. Paracentesis provides symptomatic relief, but ascites usually recurs quickly. The procedure should be performed as infrequently as tolerated because repeated paracentesis can deplete serum proteins, thus aggravating the ascites, and also may lead to infection. Indwelling peritoneal catheters are useful for selected patients requiring regular paracentesis.

Asthenia: Treat the underlying cause if possible (metabolic disturbances, anemia, etc.). Patients may be counseled on reducing unnecessary exertion and saving strength for key activities. Otherwise, corticosteroids and psychostimulants may provide some short-term relief.

Cachexia: Treatments focus on anorexia, if present, as described in the preceding text, but no treatments for progressive wasting from cancer have proven to increase length of life.

Constipation: Laxatives, such as senna and magnesium salts, are the mainstay of treatment especially for a patient on opioids. For difficult opioid-induced constipation, oral naloxone is helpful.

Cough: Remove airborne irritants. Nebulized saline may be effective as a mucolytic agent. Opioids are the mainstays of treatment, and anticholinergic agents may assist in reducing respiratory secretions, including the "death rattle."

Dehydration: This common late-stage consequence of cancer is generally not uncomfortable as long as good mouth care is maintained. Hydrating a patient often causes more distress in the form of excessive edema and increased GI or respiratory secretions.

Table 1. *Continued*

Depression: This syndrome is common in the course of a terminal illness, but it is often dismissed inappropriately as a normal response to dying. Conventional SSRIs and tricyclic antidepressants are often effective but require considerable time to achieve therapeutic benefit. For most people who are dying, a psychostimulant, such as methylphenidate or dextroamphetamine, can alleviate depression within a few days.

Diarrhea: Loperamide or diphenoxylate are the most common symptomatic treatments for patients not receiving opioids.

Dyspepsia: Antacids, H_2-receptor antagonists, proton pump inhibitors, and gastrokinetic agents are the most common treatments. The choice depends on the likely cause and the severity of the discomfort.

Dysphagia: Appropriate treatments for candidiasis or mucositis may be helpful. In patients with head and neck cancers, alternative feeding routes are often appropriate. In some patients, dietary manipulation may be sufficient, especially near the end of life. Having a terminally ill patient eat nothing by mouth should only be ordered after all the alternatives are considered.

Dyspnea: This unpleasant subjective feeling of difficulty breathing, not to be confused with tachypnea, is often associated with anxiety and advanced cachexia, as well as a host of systemic and cardiopulmonary problems. Pleural fluids may be drained, often followed by paracentesis. An open window or a cool breeze from a fan may help. Opioids are the treatment of choice, usually in low or moderate dosages; treat dyspne-like pain. Benzodiazepines help the symptom by treating the anxiety. Corticosteroids can act as bronchodilators or can alleviate dyspnea due to cancer in the lungs. Studies of nebulized morphine have not indicated convincing benefit. When massive hemoptysis or other catastrophic events lead to severe breathlessness or a sense of suffocation, vigorous use of opioids and benzodiazepines are recommended to ensure prompt, deep sedation.

Fatigue: Fatigue is a very common occurrence in end stage disease, particularly in patients with cancer. Causes are multifactorial depending on diagnosis. Fatigue profoundly affects a patient's quality of life. Treatment focuses on reversible causes such as anemia, hypothyroidism, or depression. Other strategies include exercise, energy conservation techniques, and attention to rest/sleep patterns.

Hepatic failure/encephalopathy: In a patient who is dying, dietary protein restriction and oral lactulose are the mainstays of treatment. Oral neomycin also may be helpful, and can replace some lactulose when diarrhea from this laxative is troubling.

Hiccups: Common bar remedies, such as quickly swallowing a tablespoon of sugar, are worth trying, as is pharyngeal stimulation. Gastric irritation is a common cause, and may respond to antacid regimens. Protracted, unresponsive hiccups can often be relieved with chlorpromazine. Many other agents have been reported as useful, including baclofen and nifedipine.

Insomnia: When this symptom cannot be attributed to physical discomfort, anxiety, depression, drug side effects, or one of the many other etiologies of a sleep disorder, patients should be counseled on good sleep hygiene and offered a short-acting benzodiazepine. Difficulty remaining asleep may respond to trazodone or other antidepressants.

Malignant small bowel obstruction: Most patients will not require nasogastric suction and intravenous fluids. Time often leads to resolution, and, meanwhile, oral liquids, perhaps supplemented with small amounts of parenteral fluids, may be given to maintain minimal hydration. Regardless, prescribe opioids for pain, antispasmodics for cramps, and antiemetics for nausea and vomiting. For symptomatic treatment, octreotide reduces the amount of gastrointestinal secretions. A venting gastrostomy may be considered for patient comfort.

Nausea and vomiting: Consider the common etiologies of the nausea and treat with an appropriate medication. Frequent causes are gastric stasis (use metoclopramide), intestinal irritation (use various classes of antacids), CTZ stimulation by medications or accumulating metabolites (treat with D-2 inhibitors [phenothiazines, haloperidol] or 5-HT3 receptor antagonists), vestibular or CTZ stimulation communicated to the emesis center (use H-1 antihistamines or antimuscarinic agents), psychological causes (modified by benzodiazepines), or cerebral edema (reduced by corticosteroids and mannitol).

Pressure ulcers: The best treatments are preventive: relieve pressure, avoid friction, and keep the skin dry and clean. Active treatment should be appropriate to the stage of the ulcer. When terminal patients are not bothered by decubiti, difficult and often painful treatment may be foregone.

Pruritus: When the cause cannot be reversed or specific treatments are not available (e.g., cholestyramine for cholestasis), corticosteroids, or antihistamines (H-1 and possibly H-2 blockers) often provide relief.

Putrid wounds: Powdered metronidazole sprinkled over the wound will often control the growth of the anaerobes causing the smell.

Somnolence: Methylphenidate or amphetamines can reduce medication-induced sedation or somnolence due to other causes.

Stomatitis: Preventative treatment is the mainstay. Keep the mouth clean and moist. Topical anesthetics for pain and appropriate treatments for candidiasis or other infections are important.

Xerostomia: Vaseline on the lips and artificial saliva to the mouth provide effective symptom control.

TPN, total parenteral nutrition; CTZ, chemoreceptor trigger zone; SSRI, selective serotonin reuptake inhibitors.

501

VI. COMMUNICATION WITH PATIENTS AND FAMILIES

Taking care of a patient with a terminal disease can be stressful for clinicians. We naturally feel distress when someone is suffering greatly from an incurable disease. Patients whom we particularly like or who are similar to ourselves or to our loved ones can make the clinician particularly uncomfortable, reminding us of our mortality and that of persons close to us. Some clinicians believe that they or the medical system have failed patients who are dying, and so they feel ashamed or guilty. Others believe that because we cannot cure the illness, there is "nothing more to do." Consequently, clinicians will often avoid spending time with patients who are dying or will not talk with them about emotionally charged matters. Yet, many terminally ill persons wish to share their concerns about dying, and find few people who will really listen. They turn to their health care providers for help with their fears and concerns and for safe passage through an unfamiliar journey.

Talking with a patient who is dying is similar to talking with any patient. Confusional states are very common, particularly near the end of life, so the patient's mental status should be assessed carefully. Communication primarily requires basic listening skills, rather than knowing what to say.

Introduction: Patients meet many clinicians in the hospital. They cannot always read nametags or remember names. Clinicians should introduce themselves and explain their role in the patient's care.

Sit down for a discussion of any length: Studies show that patients feel the seated clinician has given them more attention and been present for a longer time. Try to sit at roughly the same eye level as the patient.

Body language: Body language conveys interest in what is being said. In general, lean toward the speaker, make good eye contact, and nod to show you are listening and to encourage elaboration.

Physical contact: Physical contact can be positive if the clinician and patient feel comfortable with it. A light touch on the arm or shoulder for emphasis or to comfort the patient or family member can help form an important connection.

Avoid jargon: The clinician is responsible for ensuring that the patient understands the substance of the conversation.Use words and expressions that the patient knows. Medical terminology, including our many three-letter acronyms, should be used cautiously. Explain complicated matters in clear, simple language.

Open-ended questions: Open-ended questions allow patients to tell their stories and to feel that they are being heard. More directed, closed questions are useful for clarification after the patient has laid out a broad response to open-ended questions. Clinicians tend to cut off the patient early and concentrate on topics they consider important, thus often missing what the patient wants to convey.

Avoid interruptions and tolerate silence: Asking another question before the previous one is answered can give the impression that the questioner is not interested in the answer. Let the patient tell his or her story at his or her own pace. Avoid the normal tendency to fill up silences with your own words or new questions. Tolerating silence can be especially difficult for busy clinicians who generally prefer quick, fact-oriented history taking. But silence encourages the patient to lead a conversation, and can also convey tolerance of difficult feelings.

Listen for and respond to the affect: Patients quickly learn from their medical interviewers whether feelings are supposed to be part of an interview. History taking should not be just about "the facts." Make comments that acknowledge affect ("So, that really upset you" or "I can see how troubling that must have been") and encourage its expression ("How did that make you feel?").

Facilitate conversation and support the patient: Statements of encouragement ("Yes, good, go on" or "Say more") or nonverbal encouragement through head nodding also helps patients feel they have been heard and encourages them to deepen the conversation.

Encourage the patient to talk with clinicians, family, and friends: Many dying persons will not talk unless encouraged, feeling that others do not wish to listen. Families will often have a hard time talking about death and may need gentle encouragement. Giving permission to both family and patient to discuss the dying process and coaching them on or modeling this discussion can be among the most important intervention a clinician makes.

VII. THREE ESSENTIAL QUESTIONS FOR PATIENTS FACING A TERMINAL ILLNESS

1. *If you become temporarily or even permanently unable to make decisions for yourself—perhaps from an accident or stroke or because of medications—whom would you like to make decisions on your behalf?*

   - Does this person know you want him or her to take responsibility? Does he or she accept the role? Have you created a formal health care proxy document?
   - Have you discussed the preferences you would have if various situations arose and decisions would need to be made about using cardiopulmonary resuscitation or artificial ventilation or similar life-sustaining procedures? I strongly advise you to review advanced care planning documents with your proxy and family, and to consider writing out a living will or similar document.

2. *How much information about your illness would you like to have?*

   - Do you want the frank truth or prefer to be shielded from distressing information?
   - Would you like to be told everything first or would you prefer that we talk with a family member or someone else of your choosing who would decide what to share with you?

3. *Strong pain medicines can sometimes make people sleepy or confused. In general, we can control pain without causing serious mental clouding. However, in some circumstances, pain treatment can interfere with alertness. Given the choice, would you rather have some pain and a clear mind, or would you rather have no pain even if that required enough medicine to make you sleepy or confused?*

Table 2.   Guidelines for breaking bad news to patients

1. Choose an appropriate setting: quiet, privacy, comfort, lack of interruptions.
2. Consider involving family or other health professionals, but beware that the family's information needs may differ dramatically from those of the patient.
3. Ask yourself what the patient absolutely needs to know now. Very little new, distressing information can be absorbed in a single meeting. What would be better shared over time as the patient becomes capable of or in interested absorbing more information?
4. Begin by asking what the patient and family already know. Consider reviewing the facts as they have developed up to the present.
5. Ask what they wish to know, including who should be hearing it.
6. Fire a warning shot: "I'm afraid I have some bad news."
7. Keep it very simple and clear. Often a few sentences are quite adequate. Avoid jargon.
8. Encourage questioning. Let the patient's understanding, concerns, and questions guide further discussion.
9. Listen carefully. What sense are they making of the news?
10. Maintain honesty. Avoid both false reassurance and excessive bluntness.
11. Repeat key points.
12. Support the patient and family. Reassure them of your continuing attention to their well-being.
13. To minimize helplessness, try to explain the next steps or offer a realistic plan for making the best of things in this changed situation.
14. Arrange for prompt follow-up that addresses information sharing and support.

See Table 2 for guidelines for breaking the bad news about the terminal illness to patients.

VIII. FAMILY MEETINGS

Family meetings, either with or without the patient, provide an important means for sharing key information, assessing family coping, and providing family support. The communication strategies described in the preceding text are also important when talking with families. The following guidelines apply to situations in which the patient is unable to participate, typically because of cognitive impairment.

Begin a meeting with appropriate introductions by making sure that everyone knows everyone else present and their roles. State the general purpose of the meeting such as "to help determine how Mr. Smith would wish to be taken care of now." Next, find out what the family knows by asking them their understanding of the patient's current medical condition and how they think he is doing. Some of the health professionals may then give their own views on how the patient is doing. Inviting other care providers who have had close contact with the patient can be invaluable in both describing the patient's condition and facilitating expression of family concerns. Clear up any important misconceptions. Ask the family to express their concerns. Listen for questions that have not been fully expressed, and speak about worries that are not being said out loud.

If the patient is cognitively impaired and unable to participate in decisions, seek "substituted judgment," as described earlier. Later, interpret the patient's values and goals in terms of a reasonable management plan. If the family has just received bad news, try not to ask that any important decisions be made immediately. If urgent decisions are necessary, make that explicit. At the end of the meeting, quickly review the discussion. Also, make a plan on how to be in contact again. A family spokesperson is helpful for disseminating information in larger families. Document the discussion and make sure that all involved clinicians are aware of the outcome of the meeting.

IX. EUTHANASIA AND PHYSICIAN-ASSISTED SUICIDE

"Doctor, I do not want to live anymore. Can you help me?" Physicians usually dread hearing those words, and often manage to cut off patients from expressing these common sentiments near the end of life. Society and physicians are divided as to whether a physician may, in certain circumstances, be the agent of a patient's death. Regardless of how one feels about helping a patient take his own life, clinicians should foster discussions about hastening death and even ask patients directly if they are entertaining such thoughts.

Once the topic is broached, further inquiry is productive. What are the factors that make life intolerable? What sort of relief for physical and emotional suffering might make life bearable or even worthwhile? Is the patient troubled by current treatable pain or symptoms or perhaps frightened by the possibility of future, accelerating symptoms? Can we treat a depression or a delirium? Is dependency on others intolerable? Are there worries about burdening the family with physical or emotional demands of personal care or its financial implications? Sit with the patient and try to explore the fear and sadness that led to this call for help. How can we maximize the quality of the life that is left to the patient? What does the patient value that may lead to a wish to live? In many instances, psychiatric consultation will be helpful.

Once the clinician explores and responds to these issues, few patients persistently request for death to be hastened. Data from Oregon and the Netherlands where physician-assisted suicide has been legalized suggests that difficulty tolerating dependency and lack of control are the major reasons that patients seek to hasten death. Where assisted suicide is legal, a very small number (around 0.1%) of patients who are dying request and are offered assisted suicide, and about half of them actually go on to suicide.

X. CONCLUSION

In the context of caring for terminally ill patients, pain physicians are called on to offer expert advice about pain management, possibly, but rarely to give advice on interventional therapy. The guidance of the palliative care team is indispensable in terms of formulating reasonable treatment plans that fit patients' needs as well as those of families and other caregivers, often within the constraints of caring for patients at home with or without the aid of hospice.

SELECTED READINGS

Abrahm JL. *A physician's guide to pain and symptom management in cancer patients.* Baltimore, MD: The Johns Hopkins University Press, 2000.

Barnard D. The promise of intimacy and the fear of our own undoing. *J Palliat Care* 1995;11:22–26.

Berger A, Portenoy RK, Weissman DE, eds. *Principles and practice of palliative care and supportive oncology,* 2nd ed. Philadelphia, PA: Lippincott Williams & Wilkins, 2002.

Block SD. For the ACP-ASIM End-of-Life Care Consensus Panel. Assessing and managing depression in the terminally ill patient. *Ann Intern Med* 2000;132:209–218.

Block SD, Billings JA. Patient requests to hasten death: evaluation and management in terminal care. *Arch Intern Med* 1994;154: 2039–2047.

Cassell ES. The nature of suffering and the goals of medicine. *N Engl J Med* 1982;306:639–645.

Cassem EH. The person confronting death. In: Nicholi AM Jr, ed. *The new Harvard guide to psychiatry.* Cambridge, MA: Belknap Harvard University Press, 1998:728–758.

Doyle D, Hanks GWC, Cherny NI, et al. *Oxford textbook of palliative medicine,* 3rd ed. New York: Oxford University Press, 2004.

Ferrell BR, Coyle N. *Textbook of palliative nursing.* New York: Oxford University Press, 2001.

National Consensus Project for Quality Palliative Care. *Clinical practice guidelines for quality palliative care.* Available at: http://www.nationalconsensusproject.org. Accessed 2004.

Waller A, Caroline NL. *Handbook of palliative care in cancer.* Boston, MA: Butterworth-Heinemann, 2000.

Wanzer SH, Federman DD, Adelstein SJ, et al. The physician's responsibility toward hopelessly ill patients: a second look. *N Engl J Med* 1989;320:844–849.

Woodruff R. *Palliative medicine: symptomatic and supportive care for patients with advanced cancer and AIDS,* 3rd ed. Melbourne, FL: Oxford University Press, 1999.

VIII

Special Situations

Long-term Opioid Therapy, Drug Abuse, and Addiction

Barth L. Wilsey and Scott Fishman

He jests at scars that never felt a wound.
—William Shakespeare, Romeo and Juliet, Act 2, Scene 2

The utilization of opioids for chronic nonterminal pain (CNTP) remains controversial in the midst of growing awareness of the public health crisis of undertreated pain. Much of the controversy surrounding the prescribing of these medications is related to addiction and diversion. A national survey on drug use showed that the number of new nonmedical users of prescription pain relievers increased from 600,000 in 1990 to more than 2 million in 2001. This survey also showed that the prevalence of opioid abuse is now similar to that of cocaine and only second to that of marijuana (see Fig. 1). In March 2004, the Bush administration disclosed an ambitious plan, The President's National Drug Control Strategy, to curb the growing menace of prescription drug abuse (i.e., analgesics, tranquilizers, stimulants, and sedatives), which it stated, "now touches and harms more than 6 million Americans." As part of its new policy, the administration has radically increased the funding for the control of prescription drug diversion (from $20 million to $138 million). A portion of the new funding will be directed toward reducing the illegal distribution of opioids, which are among the most commonly prescribed medications in the United States. The issue of how pain medications such as Oxycontin and Vicodin are being diverted has been regularly highlighted in the media. Although prescription drug abuse is a very serious problem, restraining legitimate prescription of opioid medications is unlikely to benefit the war on drugs but carries the likely risk of limiting necessary treatments for the individuals in need of the same.

Pain specialists and regulatory agencies are now actively debating how widely and readily pain medicines should be made available and whether these medicines should be prescribed only by specialists. At the same time, the Justice Department and Drug

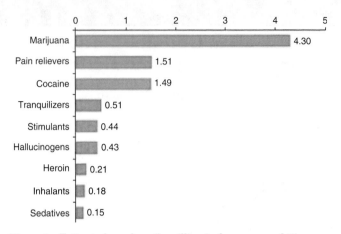

Figure 1. Estimated numbers (in millions) of persons aged 12 or older with past year illicit drug dependence or abuse, by drug. [From the 2002 National Survey on Drug Use and Health (NSDUH) report on the nonmedical use of prescription pain relievers. Available at: http://oas.samhsa.gov/2k4/pain/pain.html. Accessed 2005.]

Enforcement Administration (DEA) of the United States have become more aggressive in prosecuting doctors and pharmacists who they believe are inappropriately prescribing and dispensing prescription opioids. In recent years, a dozen or so health practitioners have been charged for their prescribing practices and several have been incarcerated. But patient advocates fear that the government has strayed from its mandate to recognize chronic pain, and they believe that such activities have had a "chilling effect" on appropriate prescribing practices. A middle ground must be found because it is imperative that patients with pain disorders are provided pain relief with opioid medications while drug diversion is curtailed.

Beyond regulatory scrutiny, treating pain has its own intrinsic difficulties stemming from the subjective nature of pain and the lack of conclusive objective markers. For instance, a history of substance abuse and the manifestation of prescription drug abuse are the two areas that require special attention because they pose special dilemmas for even the most experienced physician. This chapter explores the rational use of opioids for pain in relation to addiction and the monitoring of adherence to a treatment regimen. We hope to assist the clinician in developing an approach to opioid use that allows for vigilance for potentially adverse effects while suspending judgment and maintaining compassion in the service of effective analgesic intervention.

I. OPIOID USE IN THE ATMOSPHERE OF REGULATORY OVERSIGHT

Each state in the United States has its own regulations governing the prescription of controlled substances, and physicians prescribing these drugs should be familiar with the regulations in their state. The California triplicate prescription law was established in 1939 for controlled substances and was the longest continuously running multiple copy prescription program in the United States. This program was replaced by tamper-resistant prescription pads in July 1, 2004, after it became apparent that the old law posed an unnecessary barrier to effective pain management. The rationale for multiple copy or serialized prescriptions was to provide a means of tracking these medications and thereby reducing their illicit use. Unfortunately, this law did not lead to a reduction in illicit drug trafficking. One possible reason for its ineffectiveness in reducing drug trafficking is that most drug abusers [i.e., those meeting the *Diagnostic and Statistical Manual of Mental Disorders,* Fourth Edition (DSM-IV) criteria for the diagnosis of abuse of Schedule II drugs] probably obtain the drugs from sources other than their physician (by their own report). Although regulatory scrutiny seeks to prevent drug misuse associated with addiction, it also risks causing problems by its secondary disincentive for adequate pain management. Probably the most difficult question is what degree and type of regulation actually controls addiction and illicit drug use and what merely stands in the way of adequate pain treatment.

Concerns over forgery, theft, excessive dosages, regulatory investigation, and addiction are cited as reasons why pharmacists are asked to uphold the "letter of the law" and are often reluctant to fill prescriptions for strong opioids. Prohibiting preferred drug regimens, restricting allotment to a 30-day maximum supply, and allowing only a 3-day emergency supply limits access to medications. It is not surprising that regulations and their ramifications have discouraged the prescribing of Schedule II drugs. Proposed electronic data transfer (EDT) of pharmacy information to centralized processing points is likely to be enacted in the near future, which will make it easier to identify unscrupulous physicians or patients with multiple prescribers. At the time of writing this chapter, the United States Congress was considering a national prescription monitoring program, and individual state governments were also considering modifying their approaches to drug abuse by adopting the revised Uniform Controlled Substances Act and/or by establishing state pain initiatives. Taken together, these programs may some day alleviate the need for regulations requiring restriction of pain prescriptions to a specific number of dosage units and/or using multiple copy prescriptions for controlled substances.

To avoid misinterpretation by regulatory agencies, physicians contemplating long-term opioid therapy for patients with chronic pain may be well advised to follow clear and consistent procedures to limit diversion of medications and drug abuse. At the very least, it is essential to perform a thorough initial history and physical examination, maintain a written treatment plan, and consult with knowledgeable colleagues, as needed. Minimum assessment should include a substance abuse, family, and psychiatric history. This is important because a history of substance abuse or a lifestyle where drug use is accepted or pervasive might indicate the need for additional measures before and after initiating opioid therapy. On the physical examination, one should note the patient's affect and mood, evidence of loss of interest in personal grooming, needle marks, and/or any signs of intoxication or withdrawal. If any of these signs are detected, one should proceed with a laboratory evaluation. This examination should include determination of γ-glutamyl transpeptidase (GGT) level for evidence of hepatocellular damage; red cell volume [mean cell volume (MCV)] for evaluation of megaloblastic anemia associated with alcoholism; in the case of positive signs of intravenous drug use, hepatitis B and C antigen titers; and a human immunodeficiency virus (HIV-1) ribonucleic acid level. Because opioids never cure the underlying disorder that causes pain, consultation with a specialist in the area of the patient's pain problem may be necessary when initiating opioid therapy. Although all these steps go a long way toward minimizing the risk of regulatory action for the patient and the clinician, the practitioner must also maintain the skills required for recognizing and responding to possible prescription drug abuse.

II. PRESCRIPTION DRUG ABUSE

Careful assessment for possible prescription drug abuse is essential to limit a physician's liability with regard to regulatory scrutiny. Many practitioners rely on their impression of the patient's "drug-seeking behavior" for a rationale to refuse prescribing opioids. But there is controversy about the meaning of "drug-seeking behavior" because the term is often used pejoratively and signs of these behaviors can easily be based upon false impressions and may lead to false conclusions. One of the more common reasons for such labeling is that patients often self-escalate their opioid prescription and run out of medications early. They then call in for an early refill, disrupting the doctor's practice with multiple phone calls or showing up at the office without an appointment. If such incidences are related to what has become known as pseudoaddiction, this occurs when a weak opioid (e.g., hydrocodone, codeine, and oxycodone) is given for a pain condition with an unrecognized need for a stronger medication. The solution involves rotating the patient from a weak opioid to a more potent opioid (e.g., slow-release morphine, slow-release oxycodone, transcutaneous fentanyl, and methadone). In other instances, the patient displays overt signs of drug-abuse with self-escalation of opioids that does not improve after opioid rotation. This scenario is complicated from the standpoint of clinical decision making because the patient may be taking medication for comorbid psychological conditions or may have developed opioid tolerance. Instances of abuse in patients who self-medicate with illicit substances are more clearly evident when urine toxicology reveals drugs of abuse. Alternatively, urine toxicology screening may demonstrate that the patients may not be taking their prescribed medications, suggesting the possibility of drug diversion. Interpretation of repeated prescription loss, multiple prescribers, or requests for early refills may range from simple manifestations of inadequate analgesia to signs of true abuse or diversion. Pseudoaddiction, a phenomenon first described in the patients with cancer, occurs when patients who are undertreated for their pain manifest a "drug-seeking behavior." Unlike addiction, this behavior resolves once the pain is under

Table 1.   Signs of prescription drug abuse

Self-escalation of dosage
Repeated prescription loss with "classic" excuses:
  "The pills fell into the toilet bowl."
  "I left the prescription in the changing room."
  "The airline lost my luggage."
  "The dog ate it."
  "The vial was stolen from my medicine cabinet."
  "The pills were ruined in the laundry."
Multiple prescribers
Frequent telephone calls to the office
Multiple drug intolerances described as "allergies"
Focusing mainly on opioid issues during visits
Visiting office without an appointment

adequate control. Table 1 lists various aberrant behaviors that a patient may manifest in association with opioid use and abuse. Different responses are in order for these behaviors.

Unfortunately, the psychiatric literature on addiction and pain has been, and still remains, a source of confusion about addiction in the patient with chronic pain. To diagnose addictive disease, the DSM-IV diagnostic criteria for substance dependence requires evidence of certain drug-seeking behaviors whereby "important social, occupational, or recreational activities are given up or reduced because of substance use." But classic evidence of compulsive opioid use may be missing in patients with pain because opioid medication is being prescribed and is therefore readily available. In addition, patients with pain usually do not have to compromise their lifestyle or run the risk of endangering their lives by visiting seedy parts of town to obtain the prescribed opioid. Likewise, an illicit lifestyle (i.e., involvement in criminal activity and drug diversion) is generally not seen in patients with chronic pain. The form of addiction seen in the patient with pain is different from the type seen in the street addict. The subtle signs of prescription drug abuse (see Table 1) are deciphered from multiple observations and encounters.

If there is evidence of emotional distress accompanying prescription drug abuse, visits to a mental health provider should be encouraged to evaluate psychosocial issues. In cases of comorbid addiction and chronic pain requiring opioid therapy, it may be prudent to coordinate care with both a pain and an addiction specialist.

III. DISTINGUISHING BETWEEN PHYSICAL DEPENDENCE, TOLERANCE, AND ADDICTION

Recently, it has become possible to decipher the chemical "trigger zones" in which individual drugs of abuse initiate their habit-forming actions. Addiction and physical dependence are believed to be subserved by distinct anatomic areas within the central nervous system. Drugs belonging to different categories, such as heroin, cocaine, nicotine, alcohol, phencyclidine, and cannabis, activate a common reward circuitry in the brain. The area of the brain in a rat that is responsible for opioid reward, the ventral tegmental dopaminergic area (mesolimbic pathway), is anatomically distant from the locus ceruleus, a noradrenergic area in the periventricular gray matter thought to have a major role in maintaining physical dependence. Several lines of evidence support the involvement of noradrenergic neurons in the development of withdrawal phenomena. Norepinephrine levels change in the brain following opioid dependence. Furthermore, administration of an α_2 agonist, such as clonidine, or a β-antagonist, such as propranolol, reduces the severity of opioid withdrawal. The disparate anatomic and biochemical basis of addiction and withdrawal of the different drugs complement their differentiation in the clinical setting.

Despite the substantial differences between addiction and the pharmacologic states of physical dependence and tolerance, these concepts and labels are frequently misunderstood and are used inappropriately. Physical dependence is characterized as a physiologic state in which abrupt cessation of a drug results in a strong counterreaction called **withdrawal**. Such reactions are common to many drugs such as alcohol, benzodiazepines, and caffeine. Physical dependence also occurs with drugs that have almost no abuse potential, such as clonidine. Opioid withdrawal can result from abrupt cessation or administration of an opioid antagonist. The withdrawal syndrome for opioids is often characterized as a "flulike" condition with runny nose, chills, yawning, sweating, aching muscles, abdominal cramps, nausea, and diarrhea. The syndrome is self-limited, usually lasting 3 to 7 days. To avoid the syndrome, medications can be tapered by 10% to 15% every 48 to 72 hours. Usually, a 2- to 3-week period is necessary for completion of the tapering process. Occasionally, it is also necessary to add clonidine, 0.2 to 0.4 mg per day, to ward off particularly bothersome symptoms of withdrawal in select patients.

The Liaison Committee on Pain and Addiction, a collaborative effort of the American Academy of Pain Medicine, the American Pain Society, and the American Society of Addiction Medicine, defines tolerance as a form of neuroadaptation to the effects of chronically administered opioids (or other medications). Tolerance occurs when exposure to the opioid results in a higher dose requirement to sustain the same level of effect. Although this is a common feature of chronic opioid therapy in animal models, in clinical circumstances, it is not commonly a barrier to effective opioid analgesia. Dose escalation can alternatively indicate other problems such as disease progression or potentially reduced pain tolerance as a result of opioid-induced hyperalgesia. Opioid-induced hyperalgesia has been conceptualized as a coexisting antagonist process to opioid-induced analgesia and has been proposed to be an alternative explanation for the development of analgesic tolerance to opioids.

Fortunately, tolerance to most of the nonanalgesic effects of opioids (e.g., sedation, cognitive impairment, and decreased motor reflexes) appears to occur more reliably (opioid bowel effects are an exception and a stimulating laxative protocol is often provided on a long-term basis to prevent constipation).

I. ADDICTION

Addiction is a primary, chronic, neurobiologic disease, with genetic, psychosocial, and environmental factors influencing its development and manifestations. It is characterized by behaviors that include one or more of the following: impaired control over drug use, compulsive use, continued use despite harm, and craving.

II. PHYSICAL DEPENDENCE

Physical dependence is a state of adaptation that is manifested by a drug class specific withdrawal syndrome that can be produced by abrupt cessation, rapid dose reduction, decreasing blood level of the drug, and/or administration of an antagonist.

III. TOLERANCE

Tolerance is a state of adaptation in which exposure to a drug induces changes that result in a diminution of one or more of the drug's effects over time.

Figure 2.   Definitions related to the use of opioids for the treatment of pain. (From Savage S, Covington EC, Ehit HA, et al. Definitions related to the use of opioids for the treatment of pain. A consensus document from the American Academy of Pain Medicine, the American Pain Society, and the American Society of Addiction Medicine, 2001, with permission.)

Addiction in the context of pain treatment with opioids was defined by this same Liaison Committee on Pain and Addiction as being characterized by a persistent pattern of dysfunctional opioid use (see Fig. 2). This pattern could involve adverse consequences, loss of control over the use of opioids, and/or preoccupation with obtaining opioids despite the presence of adequate analgesia. Addiction implies a psychiatric or behavioral state in which the subject pursues a self-indulgent drug effect despite its damaging impact. Although the term **addiction** may include the signs and symptoms of physical dependence, in addition to tolerance, physical dependence and/or tolerance are not synonymous with addiction. In the patient with chronic pain who takes opioids over the long-term, physical dependence and tolerance can be anticipated; however, the maladaptive behavioral changes associated with addiction do not necessarily follow.

The occurrence of dysfunction appears to be a crucial component of addiction, particularly when it involves the treatment of pain. The difference between the dysfunction that marks addiction and the improved function that marks effective pain management must necessarily be recognized. Therefore, addiction and effective pain treatment have diametrically opposite endpoints and are distinguishable. In the chronic state, functional improvement is usually the guiding outcome for opioid therapy, allowing us to clarify situations where there are subjective reports of effective pain relief in the face of dysfunction. Unless there are mitigating factors in such cases, their outcome would not be considered successful.

Addiction to opioid analgesics is estimated to occur in 3% to 19% of patients with chronic pain. The exact number of patients is difficult to calculate because of unclear terminology and ongoing changes in the nomenclature. Doctor shopping, multiple prescribers, prescription loss, visiting without a prescription, frequent telephone calls to the clinic, multiple drug intolerances or "allergies," and frequent dose escalations are the common manifestations of addiction in patients with pain. However, there is rarely a single behavior or event that confirms the diagnosis of addiction. Making this diagnosis requires careful consideration of diverse information, and firm conclusions cannot always be supported. The diagnosis of addiction can range from crystal clear to murky and elusive. Often, the decision to alter or discontinue opioid therapy is based on partial suspicion of dysfunction and addiction but may be more securely based on the collateral finding of insufficient gains in function from the therapeutic trial of opioids.

IV. DIFFERENTIATING ADDICTION FROM EFFICACY IN OPIOID THERAPY

Restoration of function should be one of the primary treatment goals for the patient with chronic pain. Unlike the patient whose level of function is impaired by substance use, the level of function of the patient with chronic pain may improve with adequate, judicious use of medications, including opioids. Analgesic trials for chronic pain should use function as an objective outcome while lack of functional gain or malfunction should indicate treatment failure. As in the case of treatment failure in any therapeutic trial, the possibility of toxicity being responsible for the failure must be considered. An increase in function means that the patient's activities of daily living increase or improve in quality as a result of therapy. Specific improvements in increasing the participation of the patients in recreation and in the time spent shopping, socializing with friends and relatives, performing yardwork, and doing household chores should be sought. Return to work is another outcome that might be sought in specific cases (see Table 2). Improvements in functionality should be made part of the patient's treatment plan and reviewed on each visit after initiating therapy with opioids. Often, it is necessary to gather collateral information from family members or others. Using improvement as the main outcome goal in opioid prescribing allows one to deemphasize pain and to provide a behaviorally oriented program to induce desirable outcomes. On the other hand, when a patient is not becoming more functional, one should forego sanctioned dosage escalations and eventually taper the dosages of these medications.

Table 2.   Desirable functional outcomes

Participating in recreation
Shopping
Socializing with friends and relatives
Performing yardwork
Doing household chores
Return to work

V. HISTORY OF SUBSTANCE ABUSE

Until relatively recently, a history of substance abuse has been considered to be a contraindication to opioid therapy for CNTP. A retrospective review sheds light on this issue by reviewing the records of 20 patients with a history of substance abuse who were treated with long-term opioid therapy for CNTP. Almost one-half of the group showed signs of prescription drug abuse. Individuals who showed signs of drug abuse (Table 1) were more likely to have a prior history of opioid abuse or a recent history of polysubstance abuse, whereas patients with either isolated alcohol abuse or a remote history of polysubstance abuse were more likely to manage their medications appropriately. Therefore, isolated alcohol abuse and distant polysubstance abuse do not appear to be absolute contraindications to opioid therapy for CNTP.

There is controversy over whether recent substance abuse should be a contraindication to opioid treatment of CNTP. The key question is whether the likelihood of abuse recurrence is unacceptably high, and existing studies and reports have such mixed results that there is no clarity on the issue. If such care is to be embarked upon, far greater than normal resources will have to be in place to help either prevent addiction or detect addiction if it should recur. Such resources may be well beyond those available to the average clinician. However, if there are ample resources in place, a reasonable approach is to prescribe, but with a higher than normal threshold, for starting opioid therapy after making attempts to find other options. Thereafter, the clinician must remain especially vigilant in follow-up, watch carefully for signs of dysfunction or deterioration, and invite, if not require, the participation of an addiction specialist or psychiatrist. A carefully structured program of treatment may be preferable to less structured options.

VI. LONG-ACTING VERSUS SHORT-ACTING OPIOIDS

Stimulation of reward centers in the brain is both important to addiction and relevant to the variable responses that are seen to different opioid drugs and preparations. Stimulation of reward centers is usually associated with euphoria, although this may not be the case in late stages of opioid addiction. This euphoria correlates with drugs and drug delivery systems that produce a rapid rise of circulating drug levels. The rate of onset of drug action is thought to influence the abuse potential of benzodiazepines and abusable intravenous substances, including parenteral opioids. Therefore, it has been an unproven belief of many who treat pain with chronic opioids that drugs that accrue blood levels slowly have less potential for abuse than those that are rapidly active.

Whether long-acting opioids offer less risk of stimulating addiction than short-acting opioids has not been well studied. Nonetheless, the higher risk for the short-acting opioids is suggested by the preponderance of short-acting medications diverted for nonmedical use (see Fig. 3). The predilection for abuse of rapidly active opioids is further supported by the conversion of the long-acting oxycontin back to its rapidly active and short-acting state by crushing the pills and administering them by an alternate route (intravenous injection or nasal inhalation). It is logical that short-acting opioids, with their fast onset and high

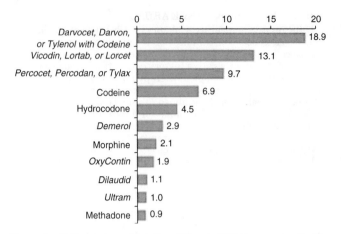

Figure 3.   Estimated numbers (in millions) of lifetime nonmedical use of selected pain relievers, among persons aged 12 or older. [From the 2002 National Survey on Drug Use and Health (NSDUH) report on the nonmedical use of prescription pain relievers. Available at: http://oas.samhsa.gov/2k4/pain/pain.htm. Accessed 2005.]

serum peak levels, are better suited than long-acting opioids for inducing psychoactive nonanalgesic effects. Theoretically at least, the euphoric effect of short-acting preparations (e.g., oxycodone, hydrocodone, and codeine) might then foster compulsive use. The use of long-acting opioids (e.g., sustained-release preparations of morphine and transdermal fentanyl) has been championed because of their gradual onset with reduced chance that a euphoric effect may be produced. Therefore, to reduce the incidence of prescription opioid abuse, it can be extrapolated by this line of reasoning that sustained-release opioids will be better than short-acting opioids for CNTP. But physicians generally prefer prescribing short-acting opioids. Presumably, the smaller amount of medicine in the short-acting opioids or compounding with dose-limiting coanalgesics such as acetaminophen or anti-inflammatories may appear safer and may be less likely to induce addiction. Although an appealing rationale, this rationale is not without counterargument. As stated in the preceding text, the rate of onset of drug action is known to influence the abuse potential of benzodiazepines and intravenous substances of abuse. In the case of prescription opioids, the strategy of reducing abuse potential with longer-acting delivery systems is embodied in transdermal delivery systems and in controlled-release oral formulations. The reduction in abuse potential is presumably derived from decreased rate of onset or fluctuation of effects. However, these slow delivery systems can be bypassed by crushing or extracting the opioids from the slow-release matrix, as is now well documented for OxyContin. The dose in each tablet is intended for 12-hour use, not for immediate effect, and is usually reserved for patients who are already opioid tolerant. Manufacturers are countering this misuse by developing opioid preparations that include an opioid antagonist that will induce withdrawal if the original matrix is disturbed and the opioid is injected. Clinical trials are being conducted to ensure that the addition of a small amount of opioid antagonist does not affect analgesia when the medication is taken as directed.

For ongoing intractable pain, short-acting opioids require frequent administration and undermine attempts to improve functionality by maintaining and reinforcing attention to pain and analgesic dosing. Long-acting opioids are intended to maintain steady opioid serum levels (and a steady level of analgesia) with fewer doses. The need for fewer analgesic interventions helps reduce the focus on pain.

Although long-acting opioids may be preferable for CNTP in general, there are exceptions. For patients who are opioid naive or for those with major pulmonary disease or sleep apnea, short-acting opioids may be the most appropriate agents, at least initially. In addition, because opioid-induced disorientation and confusion is common in patients with underlying cognitive deficits, persons suspected of having increased risk of opioid-induced toxicity are best started, and possibly maintained, on short-acting preparations. Patients who reject long-acting opioids and find acceptable level of analgesia only with frequent daily dosing of short-acting opioids may be expressing a conditioned preference and are not necessarily problematic or addicted. However, this conditioned preference should raise suspicions of abuse and should prompt close observation and methods of adherence monitoring discussed in the subsequent text.

VII. MONITORING ADHERENCE TO AN OPIOID REGIMEN

A wide variety of prescription opioids are available on the street. The mark-up from pharmacy cost can be considerable, with the price per pill ranging from $0.25 to $80. Given the high value placed on diverted drugs, one should always maintain a degree of suspicion for diversion, particularly if there is evidence of prescription drug abuse. If suspected, closer control of opioid prescribing is indicated and clearly defined parameters must be maintained. These parameters may include use of random urine samples to determine whether patients are taking the prescribed drug or, alternatively, to establish whether they are taking illicit substances. Recurrent excuses for lost or stolen prescriptions are likely to increase one's index of suspicion and may suggest drug diversion, particularly if random testing of the urine reveals lack of evidence of medication intake. Requests for specific drugs of high abuse potential or request for "name brand" only (e.g., Dilaudid, Percocet, Vicodin, and OxyContin) may also indicate a problem, although occasionally the preference may be a conditioned response to a particular drug or due to a placebo effect (see Chapter 3). A high level of suspicion should be balanced by efforts to avoid erroneous assumptions. Valuable information may be gathered from family members, friends, or pharmacists, and if appropriate, early refill requests due to lost prescriptions or unexpected travel may be validated by documentation such as police reports of theft or airline tickets, respectively.

Conventional methods of measuring compliance such as tablet counts, diaries, and patient interviews usually overestimate adherence to prescription regimens. But these techniques may still be valuable as a means of emphasizing the attention to detail that goes into prescribing controlled substances. Because of the possibility of deception, laboratory testing plays a large role in the assessment of compliance in the patient suspected of prescription drug abuse. Although opioid levels can be detected in multiple body compartments (i.e., serum, urine, hair, and saliva), urine screening is the most commonly used method for routine drug surveillance. The advantages of testing urine include the relative ease of sampling, simpler testing method, lower cost, and longer duration of a positive result compared to that in serum. Unfortunately, routine urine assays provide only qualitative results (i.e., the presence or absence of a representative from a specific drug class, e.g., opioid and benzodiazepine). This is simply a screening method, which needs to be followed by a second confirmatory test. The preliminary test result must be validated when the consequences of a false-positive result are crucial, such as in the case of ongoing litigation. The second confirmatory test is aimed at providing the identity of the drug (e.g., morphine, hydromorphone, and codeine) rather than simply identifying that a class of substances is present [screening methods for opioids include urine immunoassays and thin layer chromatography (TLC)]. Technically more complex confirmatory tests include high-pressure liquid chromatography (HPLC) and gas chromatography–mass spectrometry (GC–MS).

Results from urine analysis of opioids must be interpreted by taking into consideration each laboratory's specific procedures because toxicology laboratories have different handling practices for screening and confirmatory tests. It is imperative to know about local laboratory policies (to determine whether the laboratory automatically proceeds with the confirmatory test or whether this must be determined by the physician ordering the test). In addition, it needs to be recognized that a negative screen can only rule out opioids that are detectable by that particular assay. For example, some assays detect oxycodone and oxymorphone only at very high concentrations. Consequently, patients taking normal dosages of oxycodone may test negative by urine opioid screening and might therefore be suspected of diversion of medication. Other opioids (including buprenorphine, butorphanol, and pentazocine) are not detected by common opioid assays. Urine screening may also produce false-positive results, for example, recent ingestion of poppy seeds can return a positive screen for morphine.

Following ingestion, opioids may be detected in urine for approximately 10 days. However, this detection period is only an estimate that depends upon many factors. For example, dehydration and impaired renal function may slow drug clearance, thereby prolonging the duration of a positive urine result. Consumption of large amounts of fluid can accelerate clearance, a tactic sometimes employed by individuals wishing to foil drug screen detection.

VIII. SCREENING FOR RISK

Since an early attempt by Chabal et al. (1997) to identify aberrant behaviors suggestive of substance abuse disorder in patients on a chronic opioid regimen, several investigators have attempted to develop measurement tools that could be used to help predict and identify problematic opioid use. To be widely applicable, the tool would need to be relatively simple and practicable, and its predictive ability would need to be tested and validated. A great deal of progress has been made toward developing such an instrument, and the process of validating the prototypes is also underway. A validated behavioral screening tool could improve physicians' ability to identify potential and actual problems, although it may be incapable of capturing all problematic usage, as illustrated by one recent study that found approximately 25% of seemingly uncomplicated patients with abnormal urine toxicology findings. The area of risk assessment in therapeutic use of potentially abusable drugs is actively developing, and the interested reader is referred to the bibliography for more in-depth information.

IX. OPIOID CONTRACTS/AGREEMENTS

Contracts or agreements are often employed in the chronic administration of opioids and are intended to improve adherence to a treatment regimen. The term **"agreement"** has become preferred over "contract" because of its less litigious connotation. However, any bilaterally agreed upon plan will meet criteria as a contract and is probably enforceable against clinicians who break their own terms irrespective of what they call the document ("contract," "agreement," consent, etc.) or even regardless of whether the agreement is written or verbal. Although no contract or agreement is perfect, an example is provided in Figure 4. In addition to enhancement of adherence or compliance, contracts can provide education and informed consent. The "opioid contract" often includes clear descriptions of what constitutes medication use and abuse, terms for random drug screening, consequences of contract violations, and measures for opioid discontinuation should this become required.

The efficacy of opioid contracting is not known. Studies reviewing use of contracts for patients in methadone programs suggest a benefit. Mandatory structured contingency contracting system involving weekly urine toxicology screens has been scrutinized in this population. When the participants continued using illicit drugs, the initial contingency was to lower their methadone dose. Tapering (detoxification) and discharge followed subsequent violations. Illicit opioid use decreased substantially for subjects utilizing such stringent contracts.

Anecdotal reports in the pain population have described the implementation of similar formal treatment agreements. Key features included acknowledgment that previous treatment strategies had failed, listing of side effects and the risks of opioid therapy (including the potential for addiction), and the contingencies of treatment including the importance of pain relief coupled with enhanced function through the active participation in other therapies. A survey comparing opioid contracts from major academic centers disclosed substantial consistency among many contracts across the country. The major impetus of contracting was to improve care through distribution of information, facilitating a mutually agreed-upon course, and enhancing compliance with medications. Therefore, although there is limited scientific

MGH PAIN MANAGEMENT CENTER
CONTROLLED MEDICATION AGREEMENT

I _____agree to participate in a program of pain management with the physicians of the MGH Pain Center. I may be provided with controlled medications such as opioids, for the treatment of _____ pain only while actively participating in the program, if I adhere to the following regulations:

1. **Risks:** I understand that some risks associated with long-tem controlled medications are dependence, addiction, tolerance, constipation, sleep changes, potential for increased pain, risk to unborn children, changes in appetite, coordination, sexual desire and sexual performance. Stopping such medications suddenly can cause withdrawal. Combination with other drugs (including alcohol and nicotine) can lead to breathing and other problems. I will notify my Pain Physician if I experience any of these conditions.

2. **Treatment Plan:** I agree to adhere to the treatment plan the physician discussed with me regarding controlled medication including; type of drug, method of drug delivery, frequency, and dosage.

3. **Prescription Source:** I will receive controlled substances for the treatment of pain only from the PAIN MANAGEMENT CENTER. Should a new or worsening condition be diagnosed and controlled medicaton is provided by a physician outside the Pain Center, I will notify the Pain Center of this as soon as possible.

4. **Pharmacy:** I will use only one pharmacy _____ # _____for controlled medication prescriptions. If I need to change my pharmacy, I will notify the Pain Center.

5. **Safety of Medications:** I understand that I am solely responsible for the safe keeping of my medication. In the event that it is lost, stolen, destroyed or used other that than prescribed, the Pain Center **will not** replace the prescription until the due date of my next refill. To aid with the signs and symptoms that I may experience due to withdrawal, a prescription of clonidine may be called in to my local Pharmacy. I will be required to provide a police report on or before my next scheduled appointment.

6. **Discontinued Therapy:** Controlled medication may be discontinued if they fails to achieve set goals. I agree to participate in a drug detoxification program if prescribed. Discharge from the Pain Center will occur if I obtain multiple controlled medication from multiple practitioners, fill prescription at multiple pharmacies, sell or give away or otherwise divert the medication from its intended use, or alter prescriptions. Patients that miss three (3) consecutive appointments (cancellation or no show) will be discharged to the care of their Primary Care Physician.

7. **Testing:** I understand that my urine and/or blood my be tested at any time for levels of the substances in my system. I may be requested to bring in my medication for the physician to inspect.

8. **Appointments:** If I am on stable doses of controlled medication, I still need to schedule and keep appointments with my Pain physician to assure that I do not run out of my medications.

9. **Consent:** I give my consent for the physician and staff to speak with my pharmacist and other physicians to exchange pertinent information regarding my medical condition.

10. **Primary Care Physician (PCP):** I understand that I must have an active PCP while being treated by the MGH Pain Center. If I change PCP's I must notify the Pain Center and provide the name, address and phone number of my current PCP. I understand that the Pain Center physician will communicate with my PCP to provide updates of my treatment plan and that I will be returned to the care of my PCP at the discretion of the MGH Pain Center physicians.

I have been provided with a copy of this agreement and understand that I may discuss any questions or concerns about the contents with my physician at any time.

Signature of patient: _____   Date:_____

Signature of physician: _____

Review date: _____

Review date: _____

Figure 4. The Massachusetts General Hospital Pain Management Center controlled medication agreement.

evidence to support success with contracts in the pain population, the practice seems to be widespread.

A model for tracking prescription drug abuse with a log for monitoring contract violations has been championed. Known as "three strikes and you're out," the patients are given a maximum of three minor infractions (e.g., early refills, multiple prescribers, and self-escalation of dosage) before the medications are tapered and the patients are discharged from care. Other prescribers are more stringent and will taper the medications and discharge a patient after one or two instances of prescription drug abuse. Certainly, unlawful activities such as forging prescriptions, selling drugs, and/or resumption of alcohol or illicit drug intake are considered grounds for such a lower threshold for tapering and discharge. A recent study reported on an opioid contract that engaged the patient, pain care clinician, and the primary care physician (PCP), and was termed the Trilateral Opioid Contract. The results indicate that such a patient agreement can facilitate improvement in long-term collaborative care between pain specialist and continuity care providers.

X. OPIOID RESPONSIVENESS

There is disagreement in the literature about the overall beneficial effects of opioids on the treatment of patients with chronic pain. There have been many open label trials in which opioids have been shown to be effective. Several clinical trials have been performed demonstrating the efficacy of opioids in chronic pain. However, there are also reports of improvement in pain level when patients are detoxified from opioids. In the latter studies, neither psychological profiles nor a history of substance abuse differentiated the groups that improved after opioid withdrawal. Most patients were said to have experienced an improved sense of well-being with abstinence. These conflicting outcomes are explicable by assuming that there is a spectrum of patients with chronic pain. Patients who are successfully treated with opioids often experience analgesia without noticeable side effects or functional deterioration. The studies in which patients improved after withdrawal of opioids may have had a selected population referred to them for that purpose—patients who abused their medications, prompting their physicians to refer them for detoxification. It is possible that these patients became dysfunctional while receiving opioids and only improved after withdrawing from these medications. This possibility supports the practice of using function as a primary determinant of long-term treatment of CNTP with opioids to gauge analgesic efficacy and addictive side effects simultaneously.

XI. CONCLUSION

It is ironic that the current atmosphere of increased concern about legal scrutiny over aggressive opioid prescribing is occurring at the same time when physicians are increasingly criticized for focusing more on quantity rather than quality of life, particularly when it comes to undertreated pain. Regulations and social stigma around opioid prescribing continue to send mixed messages to clinicians who are being increasingly held to their obligation to treat pain. Fortunately, there are many tools and strategies that can help with the risk management responsibilities that each prescriber must accept if he or she is to offer rational and safe opioid therapies. At the heart of rational chronic opioid therapy is the recognition that function is a critically important outcome measure and that lack of functional improvement (or dysfunction) is a sign of treatment failure and possible addiction.

SELECTED READINGS

Adams LL, Gatchel RJ, Robinson RC, et al. Development of a self-report screening instrument for assessing potential opioid medication misuse in chronic pain patients. *J Pain Symptom Manage* 2004;27:440–459.

Butler SF, Budman SH, Fernandez K, et al. Validation of a screener and opioid assessment measure for patients with chronic pain. *Pain* 2004;112:65–75.

Cami J, Farre M. Drug addiction. *N Engl J Med* 2003;349:975–986.

Chabal C, Erjavec MK, Jacobson L, et al. Prescription opiate abuse in chronic pain patients: clinical criteria, incidence, and predictors. *Clin J Pain* 1997;13:150–155.

Clark JD. Chronic pain prevalence and analgesic prescribing in a general medical population. *J Pain Symptom Manage* 2002;23(2): 131–137.

Compton P, Darakjian J, Miotto K. Screening for addiction in patients with chronic pain and "problematic" substance use: evaluation of a pilot assessment tool. *J Pain Symptom Manage* 1998;16:355–363.

Dunbar S, Katz N. Chronic opioid therapy for nonmalignant pain in patients with a history of substance abuse: report of 20 cases. *J Pain Symptom Manage* 1996;11(3):163–171.

Fishman SM, Bandman TB, Edwards A, et al. The opioid contract in the management of chronic pain. *J Pain Symptom Manage* 1999; 18:27–37.

Fishman SM, Mahajan G, Jung SW, et al. Bridging the pain clinic and the primary care physician through the opioid contract. *J Pain Symptom Manage* 2002;24(3):254–262.

Fishman SM, Papazian JS, Gonzales S, et al. Regulating opioid prescribing through balanced prescription monitoring programs. *Pain Med* 2004;5(2):255–257.

Fishman SM, Yang J, Reisfield G, et al. Compliance monitoring and drug surveillance with chronic opioid therapy. *J Pain Symptom Manage* 2000;20(4):293–307.

Joranson DE, Ryan KM, Gilson AM, et al. Trends in medical use and abuse of opioid analgesics. *JAMA* 2000;283:1710–1714.

Passik SD, Kirsh KL, Whitcomb L, et al. A new tool to assess and document pain outcomes in chronic pain patients receiving opioid therapy. *Clin Ther* 2004;26:552–561.

Portenoy R. Opioid therapy for chronic nonmalignant pain: a review of the critical issues. *J Pain Symptom Manage* 1996;11(4):203–217.

Savage SR, Joranson DE, Covington EC, et al. Definitions related to the medical use of opioids: evolution towards universal agreement. *J Pain Symptom Manage* 2003;26(1):655–667.

Wilsey B, Fishman S. Issues of addiction in opioid therapy. *Progress in Anesthesiology* 2000;14(5):71–83.

Pain and Affective Disorders

Daniel M. Rockers and Scott Fishman

Happiness is not being pained in body or troubled in mind.
—Thomas Jefferson, 1743–1826

Most patients in chronic pain have comorbid psychiatric conditions, ranging from mild (e.g., anxiety, adjustment, and dysthymic disorders) to severe (e.g., delusional and psychotic disorders). The chronology of these conditions often makes it difficult to determine whether the pain caused the psychiatric condition or the psychiatric condition caused the pain, or whether the condition and the pain occurred simultaneously. Depression and anxiety are known to enhance perceptions of pain and may be a predominating component of some pain syndromes. Some psychiatric conditions may even manifest as pain or painlike symptoms. For example, it has been suggested that complex regional pain syndrome (CRPS) is a conversion-like disorder (Ochoa and Verdugo, 1995). Many psychiatric conditions are caused by or are accompanied by neurochemical abnormalities. These abnormalities may help determine what type of pain medication is prescribed and may have a significant affect on the pain condition. For example, serotonin is considered an important factor in pain as well as mood states. The extensive overlap of drugs used to treat pain with those prescribed for psychiatric disorders suggests that common mechanisms may be at work in the two conditions. Because of this, comprehensive pain management requires an understanding of basic principles of psychiatric diagnoses and how they might affect or be affected by pain.

I. MOOD DISORDERS

Mood disorders are often split into two general categories: unipolar and bipolar disorders. Unipolar disorders include major depression and dysthymia (a less severe variant of depression); bipolar disorders include bipolar I (combination of manic and depressive episodes), bipolar II (combination of depressive and hypomanic episodes), and cyclothymia (a less severe variant of bipolar disorder).

(i) Description

Depression is the psychologic issue most frequently associated with chronic pain. Major depression is found in 8% to 50% of patients with chronic pain, and dysthymia may be seen in more than 75% of patients with chronic pain. At particular risk for major depression are women—those of lower socioeconomic status, those separated or divorced, those with a family history of depression, those with negative stressful events, those not having a confidant, and those living in urban areas.

For a clinical diagnosis of depression, the following are required: (a) at least 2 weeks of either depressed mood or the loss of interest or pleasure in nearly all activities, and (b) any four of the following additional symptoms: changes in appetite or weight, sleep difficulties, changes in psychomotor activity, decreased energy, feelings of worthlessness or guilt, difficulty in thinking, recurrent thoughts of death, or suicidality. In addition, these symptoms must substantially impair an individual's social, occupational or other functioning.

It is important to distinguish between clinical depression and naturally occurring mood states such as bereavement or normal sadness. The use of rapid assessment instruments such as the Beck Depression Inventory or the Hamilton Rating Scale for Depression (HAM-D) augments and documents interview impressions but does not replace them. Collateral information can be used as well; patients themselves may be poor historians or may not recognize when these feelings began to emerge—some of the symptoms include an inability to think, concentrate, or make decisions—and these feelings may impair their ability to recall. Depression may manifest in a number of various symptom constellations; for example, children may experience depression more in terms of somatic complaints, social withdrawal, or irritability.

(ii) Concerns

Suicide risk is greatest for those depressed patients with psychotic functioning, a history of past suicide attempts, a family history of suicides, or concurrent substance abuse. The astute practitioner is aware of when a depressed patient exhibits a loss of impulse control or when cognitive faculties are compromised to the point of poor judgment. When patients are judged to present a significant risk of suicide, standard precautions should be taken, such as having them sign a written contract promising not to harm themselves, determining appropriate social support, and helping elucidate reasons to continue living. For patients who cannot be left alone, family or friends' assistance should be secured or hospitalization should be considered. When treating those in imminent danger of harming themselves or others, one should remain mindful that most state laws mandate that any treating clinician, including a pain specialist, must take action to ensure safety, as well as formal psychiatric evaluation.

(iii) Course and Treatment

Symptoms of depression may develop over days or weeks; there may be a prodromal phase characterized by slight anxiety or mild depressive symptoms. The duration of this stage is variable. An untreated depression typically lasts 6 months or longer, regardless of age of onset. Although most patients experience remission, a significant minority (20% to 30%) continue to have symptoms over a period of 1 to 2 years. In addition, two out of three will experience a recurrence.

There are many contemporary models of depression, including **cognitive, learned helplessness, reinforcement, biogenic amine, neurophysiologic,** and **final common pathway**. Cognitive or psychologic models suggest cognitive and behavioral treatments, whereas biologic models tend to suggest pharmacologic treatments. Beck's cognitive triad characterization of depression is that the self is seen in a negative light, the current situation is viewed negatively, and the future is viewed negatively. These cognitions are very common in a chronic tormenting condition such as pain. According to Seligman's learned helplessness model, the depressed person views his or her responses to the environment as ineffective—they will not bring relief.

Many patients with chronic pain experience depressive hopelessness about their pain condition, and it is easy to experience negative thoughts or feelings of helplessness when faced with ceaseless pain. The pain seems to (and frequently does) control life. The experience is one of a tormenting, unremitting taskmaster. Psychosocial treatment of unipolar depression consists of behavioral therapy, cognitive-behavioral therapy, or interpersonal therapy. These treatments are discussed in Chapter 15 and can result in significant reduction in depressive symptoms and can maintain their effect after treatment is terminated. The goal in these treatments is for the patients to (a) accept the chronicity of their pain condition, (b) restructure negative beliefs, and (c) experience a sense of self-efficacy in life. Acceptance is crucial, and without it, forward progress out of the depressive state is unlikely.

Pharmacologic treatment of depression is typically accomplished through antidepressant drugs such as tricyclic antidepressants (TCAs); selective serotonin reuptake inhibitors (SSRIs), which have recently gained in favor because of their safety and reported efficacy; and a third class called **atypical antidepressants**. Antidepressants are discussed in detail in Chapter 11. TCAs have documented analgesic effects, which are independent of the antidepressant effects. To date, the SSRIs have not consistently demonstrated such effects.

2. Dysthymia

When an individual experiences less severe depressive symptoms that persist for a long time (2 years), they may be diagnosed as having dysthymia. Many of the symptoms are the same as for depression, but individuals typically experience fewer vegetative symptoms (e.g., sleep difficulties, weight change, psychomotor agitation, or psychomotor retardation). Dysthymia is a risk factor for major depression—75% of those diagnosed with dysthymia go on to develop major depression within 5 years. Women are two to three times more likely to develop dysthymia than men. Lifetime prevalence is approximately 6%.

3. Bipolar Disorder

(i) Diagnosis

Bipolar disorder is characterized by cyclic mood fluctuations between mania and depression. These fluctuations may be predominately manic, with depressive episodes (bipolar I) or depressive episodes may predominate, with hypomanic episodes also occurring (bipolar II). Risk factors for bipolar I include higher socioeconomic status, being separated or divorced, and having a family history of depression. The first episode in men is likely to be manic, whereas the first episode in women is likely to be depressive.

A manic episode is a discrete period in which a number of somatic and cognitive responses are accelerated. Patients in a manic phase experience an elevated, expansive, or irritable mood. They may have an expanded or grandiose sense of themselves or have flights of ideas or racing thoughts. Vegetative or behavioral symptoms include a decreased need for sleep, talkativeness, increase in goal-directed activity, and excessive involvement in pleasurable activities such as unrestrained buying sprees or sexual indiscretions. The patients' judgment is often impaired. At its extreme, the mania escalates into psychotic behavior. A depressive episode meets the criteria for major depression, as described in the preceding text. The same caveats for depression diagnosis apply to bipolar disorders, and collateral information is a very important aspect because patients may be poor historians when manic or depressed.

(ii) Concerns

Suicide attempts are made by 25% of patients with bipolar disorder and 10% to 15% of patients commit suicide—this is a genuine and important concern. There may be abuse or violent behavior when an individual is in a manic episode, as well. Safety may be a paramount concern in fulminant cases. Many drugs common to pain management can induce mania, such as corticosteroids or antidepressants, and must be used with caution.

(iii) Course and Treatment

Mean age of onset for a manic phase is 20 years, although some cases begin at a younger age and some begin as late as 50 years. Sleep deprivation or abrupt changes in sleep–wake cycles can initiate manic or depressive episodes. The course of these episodes is chronic; 90% of those with one manic episode go on to have future episodes. The frequency and intensity of episodes tend to decrease as an individual ages. It is important to recognize that manic episodes and depressive episodes can "color" perceptions of pain, so the nature of a patient's pain may change when the bipolar condition is treated.

A leading conceptualization of bipolar disorder is that it is a disorder of biologic regulation that is activated or maintained by stressful or negative life events. Therefore, treatment should be both pharmacologic and psychosocial. Because the disorder is viewed chiefly as a dysregulation of biology, the primary treatment prescribed is pharmacologic. Lithium is the classic agent for treating bipolar disorder, although recently many other agents such as anticonvulsants have gained popularity. Pharmacologic treatments should be maximized using medications that target both the pain and bipolar condition if possible. For example, membrane stabilizers used for neuropathic pain are often mood stabilizers as well (see Chapter 11).

Psychosocial treatments include psychoeducation, individual psychotherapy, and family therapy. Psychosocial treatments are especially important because bipolar disorder can have devastating effects on an individual's life as well as on his or her family. For example, it is not unusual for an individual to acquire thousands of dollars of debt during a manic phase. Individual psychotherapy helps patients to understand their condition better, decrease relapses, and adhere to pharmacologic therapies.

Patients in chronic pain with comorbid bipolar disorder need appropriate education about both bipolar disorder and chronic pain. The challenge is to maintain the course through speeding highs and dark, immobilizing lows. This challenge includes maintenance of medication for both disorders and the clear overarching knowledge that the current phase will eventually change.

II. ANXIETY DISORDERS

In the spectrum of comorbid pain and affective disorders, anxiety ranks high. For some patients, the anxiety is a response manifestation of the pain, and for others it is a separate entity that can amplify and distort pain and pain perception. There are many disorders with the common characteristic of anxiety. The scope of this section includes panic disorders, posttraumatic stress disorder (PTSD), and generalized anxiety disorder (GAD).

1. Generalized Anxiety Disorder

(i) Description

GAD is considered the "basic" anxiety disorder. It is characterized by excessive anxiety and worry for at least 6 months, often about routine things. The extent of worry and anxiety is out of proportion to the likelihood of the negative consequences occurring, and the individual has great difficulty controlling the worry. Diagnosis requires at least three of the following symptoms: restlessness, a tendency to become easily fatigued, difficulty concentrating, irritability, muscle tension, and sleep disturbance.

Current models of GAD advocate that there exists a biologic and psychologic vulnerability. This vulnerability, combined with the feeling that situations are outside one's control, leads to neurobiologic changes and excessive self-evaluation. This further fuels the feelings of external control and the cycle intensifies.

Lifetime prevalence estimates are around 5%. Some cultures tend to display anxiety in more cognitive symptoms, whereas others have more somatic symptoms. It is uncommon for GAD to begin after the age of 20 years. The course of GAD is chronic but tends to worsen during stress.

(ii) Treatment

Regarding psychologic treatment, studies have shown that active treatments are superior to nondirective treatments. The most common successful therapies involve some variant of relaxation therapy combined with cognitive therapy. The task is to bring the stress under the individual's control, which is often done through cognitive restructuring and through exposure using graded practice. Several studies have shown cognitive-behavioral therapy superior to benzodiazepine treatment.

Although GAD is typically perceived by clinicians as a "worry" or otherwise as a cognitive disorder, many of the symptom manifestations are somatic. As noted in the preceding text, there may be associated muscle tension, trembling, twitching, muscle aches, soreness, nausea, diarrhea, sweating, headaches, or irritable bowel symptoms. It is possible for an individual to present in the pain clinic with undiagnosed GAD.

2. Panic Disorders

(i) Description

Panic attacks are periods of intense fear or discomfort that rapidly develop and reach a peak within 10 minutes. They are commonly characterized by a number of discrete cognitive or somatic symptoms, taken from the following list: palpitations, sweating, trembling or shaking, shortness of breath or sensations of smothering, feeling of choking, chest pain, nausea, dizziness, derealization (the surrounding environment seems unreal), depersonalization (the individual feels unreal, but the environment seems real), fear of losing control or "going crazy," fear of dying, parasthesias (numbness or tingling), chills, or sweats.

Panic disorder with its variants (with agoraphobia, without agoraphobia, etc.) comprises the actual diagnoses that involve panic attacks. Keep in mind that to meet criteria for panic disorder, these symptoms should not be attributable to the use of substances such as stimulants or caffeine. There must be at least one panic attack for diagnosis (at least four of the symptoms mentioned in preceding text, manifesting and peaking within 10 minutes) followed by at least 1 month of persistent concern of having another attack. Patients with this diagnosis usually have other intermittent feelings of anxiety and may have a sense of being demoralized. This is because (a) the attacks are often crippling, (b) the attacks may appear to arise of their own accord, and (c) the individual begins to feel little self-efficacy and is unable to get things done.

(ii) Course and Treatment

Panic disorder usually begins in an individual's teens and early twenties. There may be prodromal symptoms of mild anxiety, or the attack may simply erupt without warning. There is often no way for a patient to predict when the next attack will occur, and this unpredictability leads to anticipatory anxiety. A current leading model of anxiety disorders suggests that certain individuals have a biologic predisposition to such conditions, and when placed in a stressful situation involving loss of control, anxiety and panic occur. Lifetime prevalence figures indicate that panic disorder with or without agoraphobia occurs in about 3.5% of the population.

Fifty percent to 65% of individuals with panic disorder also have a diagnosis of major depression. Some individuals may be self-treating their anticipatory anxiety, panic, or depression with substances such as alcohol or drugs; thereby developing a comorbid substance abuse disorder. From the physician's point of view, be careful not to unwittingly treat panic symptoms with analgesics.

Treatment involves educating the patient about the nature of anxiety and panic, coping skills, and *in vivo* (systematic desensitization or flooding) exposure. Patients are often taught relaxation and diaphragmatic breathing techniques to help combat physiologic symptoms. The course of the disorder fluctuates, and some symptoms may persist even after treatment. The main goals are to decrease subjective anxiety while improving objective function and the ability to travel.

It is not uncommon to see diagnosable panic disorder in the patient with pain. Chronic pain with panic disorder often includes a component of apparent uncontrollability Many patients begin to experience panic or extreme anxiety about impending and unending pain. They fear pain as an entity in itself and often experience pain as a tormenting entity with its own volition. Patients with pain should also understand that stimulants may exacerbate both pain and anxiety and so should be utilized with caution.

3. Posttraumatic Stress Disorder

(i) Description

When subjected to extreme traumatic stressors, individuals may develop a characteristic disorder that involves ongoing residual anxiety, a state known as PTSD. Diagnostic criteria require that the traumatic stressor be extreme, and that the individual's response involve intense fear, helplessness, or horror. Examples of extreme traumas include involvement in hostage situations, terrorist attacks, torture, war combat, physical or sexual abuse, or automobile-related injuries. The residual anxiety manifests in re-experiencing events related to the stressor, avoidance of reminders of events, and persistent increased autonomic system arousal. The hyperarousal may show up in sleep disturbance, irritability, hypervigilance, or an exaggerated startle response. Management of the disorder is accomplished by avoiding thoughts of, or feelings about, the event. The disorder may also show up as amnesia for a part of the event. Diagnosed individuals may also have a restricted range of affect and feel detached from others.

Associated with PTSD is an increase in somatic complaints such as pain, or increased autonomic arousal. In pain clinics, it is not unusual to encounter patients who are war veterans or assault or abuse victims. Lifetime prevalence of PTSD is estimated at 8% of the adult population. About half of those diagnosed with PTSD experience complete recovery in 3 months.

(ii) Treatment

The accepted and empirically supported treatment approach for PTSD includes exposure therapy and anxiety management techniques. Exposure therapy usually consists of imaginal as well as exposure type treatments (*in vivo*—systematic desensitization or flooding), and anxiety management techniques include relaxation, breathing retraining, trauma education, guided self-dialog, cognitive restructuring, and anger management. Pharmacologic therapies may involve treatments with antidepressants as well as other psychiatric drugs.

III. CONCLUSION

Because there is an affective component to all pain, patients with chronic pain commonly present with comorbid affective disorders. In addition, a chronic stressor such as pain taxes the affective regions of the psyche, which can manifest as an affective disorder. Conversely, an affective disorder can present as a pain disorder. Regardless of primacy, attempts to identify and treat affective disorders should occur simultaneously with identification and treatment of somatic pain disorders.

SELECTED READINGS

American Psychiatric Association. *Diagnostic and statistical manual of mental disorders*, Text Revision, 4th ed. Washington, DC: American Psychiatric Association, 2000.

Maxmen JS, Ward NG. *Essential psychopathology and its treatment*, 2nd ed. New York: WW Norton & Co, 1995.

Nathan PE, Gorman JM. *A guide to treatments that work*. New York: Oxford University Press, 1998.

Ochoa JL, Verdugo RJ. Reflex sympathetic dystrophy: a common clinical avenue for somatoform expression. *Neurol Clin* 1995;13:351–363.

Emergencies in the Pain Clinic

Asteghik Hacobian and Milan P. Stojanovic

Though an arrow is always approaching its target, it never quite gets there, and Saint Sebastian died of fright.
—*Tom Stoppard*

The use of fluoroscopic guidance and contrast injection markedly decreases the complication rate of pain procedures. However, complications do occur and can have disastrous consequences if the clinic is not prepared to deal with these emergencies. This chapter reviews some of the emergency problems encountered in the pain clinic. Every pain management clinic specializing in interventional pain management procedures should be equipped with emergency equipment including an airway cart, oxygen tanks, resuscitation equipment, and emergency medication, and all providers in the pain clinic should be familiar with their use and their location. There should always be personnel trained in resuscitation present in the clinic when there are patients in the clinic undergoing or recovering from procedures. Finally, a safety officer should be identified, and a regular check of the emergency equipment should be carried out and documented by him or her.

I. PROCEDURE-RELATED EMERGENCIES

1. Vasovagal Syncope

Syncope is one of the most common reactions that occur in a pain clinic. Patients commonly fear needles and procedures. The best prevention is reassurance. If there is any suspicion that the patient may be very anxious, insertion of an intravenous line with the consent of the patient is recommended. Sometimes, an anxiolytic agent before the procedure is helpful, although anxiolytic agents may provide pain relief and may diminish the diagnostic value of blocks. Unfortunately, vasovagal syncope can occur even during minor procedures.

Vasovagal syncope is always associated with brachycardia. During any kind of procedure, standard monitors, including noninvasive blood pressure cuff and pulse oximeter, and, in most cases, a three-lead electrocardiograph (ECG), should be used and patient baseline values should be documented.

To avoid possible patient injury from a fall due to loss of consciousness, avoid performing procedures with the patient in the standing or sitting position.

(i) Symptoms and Signs

Presyncopal symptoms and signs include nausea, epigastric distress, perspiration, light headedness, confusion, tachycardia, and pupillary dilatation. Syncopal signs include loss of consciousness, generalized muscle weakness, loss of postural tone, pallor or cyanosis, and brief tonic–clonic seizure-like activity. Hypotension can also occur.

(ii) Treatment

In the event of any complaint from the patient, including feeling faint, nauseated, or sweating, do the following:

- Place the patient in the Trendelenburg position.
- Administer oxygen, evaluate and protect the airway, and support ventilation, depending on the severity of the case.
- Monitor oxygenation, ventilation, and vital signs.
- Establish intravenous access (if not present), administer atropine 0.4 to 1 mg IV for a heart rate of less than 45 beats per minute or for a rapidly decreasing heart rate.
- Apply standard monitors and evaluate ECG tracing for other possible causes of bradycardia (e.g., junctional rhythm).
- Continue to monitor and keep patient supine.
- Make sure that all the vital signs are stable and that the patient is stable before being discharged home.

2. Systemic Local Anesthetic Toxicity

Systemic local anesthetic toxicity can manifest as minor symptoms such as tinnitus, a metallic taste in the mouth, numbness of the lips, light headedness, or visual disturbance, and may progress to loss of consciousness, seizure activity, and decrease in myocardial contractility. Obviously, the toxicity depends on the dose of local anesthetic being absorbed into the systemic circulation. Toxicity may result from an accidental intraarterial injection, an overlarge bolus, a high infusion rate, or frequent boluses. Toxicity can present with central nervous system (CNS) manifestations or cardiovascular or both. The cardiotoxic effects of local anesthetic result in a depression of myocardial contractility and can also produce refractory arrhythmias. The CNS symptoms can progress to loss of consciousness, generalized seizure activity, or even coma.

(i) Treatment

- Airway should be protected.
- Oxygen should be administered by mask or bag as soon as the first sign of toxicity develops; in mild cases, this may be the only treatment needed.

- Airway, breathing, and circulation should be assessed, and standard monitoring should be applied.
- If seizure activity interferes with ventilation or if prolonged, give midazolam 1 to 2 mg IV or diazepam 5 to 10 mg IV.
- If the patient's airway is compromised, give thiopental 50 to 200 mg and intubate the trachea; succinylcholine 1.5 mg per kg IV may be given to facilitate intubation; it should be kept in mind that muscle relaxation abolishes muscle activity but the neuronal seizure activity continues.

(ii) Treatment of Cardiovascular Toxicity

- Airway, breathing, and circulation should be supported according to the acute cardiac life-support (ACLS) protocol; oxygen should be administered and emergency assistance should be called.
- Ventricular tachycardia should subside over time secondary to drug distribution; adequate circulatory support, including lidocaine 100 mg IV, should be provided in the meanwhile.
- Bupivacaine-induced ventricular arrhythmia may be more responsive to bretylium 5 to 10 mg per kg IV every 15 to 20 minutes to a maximum of 30 mg per kg followed by lidocaine; prolonged cardiopulmonary resuscitation (CPR) or cardiopulmonary bypass may be required until the cardiotoxic effects subside.

3. Complications of Epidural and Intrathecal Procedures

(i) Epidural Hematoma

Epidural hematomas are extremely rare if coagulation parameters are normal. However, in a patient with rapid onset of neurologic deficit and severe back pain, the diagnosis of epidural hematoma should be entertained. Sometimes the only symptom is severe pain in the back. The treatment includes immediate magnetic resonance imaging (MRI), steroids, surgical consultation immediately for decompression, and laminectomy for evacuation of the hematoma.

(ii) Epidural Abscess

Epidural abscess is a rare complication, but it should be considered a possibility in a patient with severe back pain, local back tenderness, fever, and leukocytosis with or without neurologic deficit after an epidural or intrathecal injection or catheter placement. An immediate MRI, preferably with gadolinium, emergency surgical consultation for possible decompression laminectomy, and intravenous antibiotics will be needed.

(iii) High Spinal Anesthetics

With fluoroscopy and contrast dye, the incidence of complications in high spinal anesthetics is rare. However, it may still occur as a result of an unintentional subarachnoid injection of local anesthetic during an epidural block, celiac plexus block, lumbar sympathetic block, stellate ganglion block, or occipital nerve block.

SYMPTOMS AND SIGNS.   Symptoms and signs may include nausea; vomiting; hypotension; bradycardia; dyspnea; high sensory level, which can progress to apnea; and unresponsiveness.

TREATMENT
- Establish adequate airway, administer oxygen, and assess sensory and motor level.
- Support ventilation if muscles of respiration are affected; endotracheal intubation may be necessary if the airway cannot be protected.
- Support blood pressure and heart rate until the local anesthetic wears off.

(iv) Accidental Overdose via Neuraxial Pump

Intrathecal or epidural pumps implanted on the anterior abdominal wall are a common mode of continuous delivery of opioids into the intrathecal or epidural space. Some of these pumps have two ports, the catheter access port and the drug reservoir port. In case of accidental overdose of morphine, the most common opioid used for intrathecal pump delivery, the patient may experience respiratory depression with or without CNS depression.

In the event of possible morphine overdose do the following:

- Establish airway access, breathing, and circulation.
- Intubate, if necessary.
- Give naloxone 0.04 to 2 mg IV.
- Withdraw 30 to 40 mL of cerebrospinal fluid (CSF) through the catheter access port to decrease the concentration of morphine in the CSF.
- Stop the pump infusion.
- Monitor the patient's vital signs.
- Repeat the dose of naloxone every 2 to 3 minutes. Because the half-life of naloxone is considerably shorter than that of intrathecal/epidural morphine, repeated administration or continuous infusion may be necessary.

In severe cases, intrathecal naloxone may be indicated.

4. Hypotension

Immediate systemic causes of hypotension include vasovagal syncope, allergic reaction, myocardial ischemia, adrenal insufficiency, pulmonary embolism, and others. Patients with a preexisting condition such as hypothyroidism, cardiac dysrhythmias, left ventricular dysfunction, and sepsis are predisposed to hypotension. Iatrogenic causes include the following:

- Intrathecal or subdural injection of local anesthetic
- High neuraxial block
- Celiac plexus block (neurolytic or with local anesthetic) without adequate preblock hydration
- Lumbar sympathetic block
- Tension pneumothorax
- Rapid release of tourniquet during Bier block, causing release of drugs such as labetalol, guanethidine, and bretylium
- Intravenous phentolamine

Symptoms and signs include pallor, light headedness, vomiting, tachycardia, tachypnea, pupillary dilation, confusion, and decreased muscle tone.

Treatment

- Give supplemental oxygen.
- Immediately establish intravenous access, if not already established.
- Give intravenous fluid, boluses of lactated Ringer solution in case of no contraindication.
- Monitor the patient's vital signs, ECG tracing, oxygen saturation, and verbal communication.
- Put the patient in Trendelenburg position or elevate lower extremities.
- Administer vagal pressures if necessary, ephedrine 10 mg every 5 to 10 minutes or phenylephrine 50 to 100 μg IV bolus or start phenylephrine infusion at 100 μg per minute and maintain at 40 to 60 μg per minute.
- Transfer patients with cardiac involvement to an inpatient cardiac unit, if required.

5. Hypertension

Hypertension could be due to acute pain or an exacerbation of chronic pain. Anxiety, preexisting disease, and essential hypertension are other common causes. Rebound hypertension after a sudden discontinuation of α-blockers (e.g., clonidine) or beta blockers (e.g., propranolol) can cause hypertension, and both types of drugs are occasionally used for treating pain. Drug interactions can cause hypertension, for example, monoamine oxidase inhibitor (MAOI) interactions with meperidine, tricyclic antidepressants (TCAs), and ephedrine. Accidental vascular injection of vasopressors (e.g., epinephrine in local anesthetic solutions) or absorption of vasopressors from topical solutions (e.g., cocaine) also can induce hypertension. Other causes include hypoxia and hypercarbia.

Treatment

- Provide supplemental oxygen.
- Ensure adequate ventilation.
- Treat underlying cause.
- Cancel planned procedures when diastolic blood pressure is greater than 110 mm Hg.
- Treat with nifedipine 10 mg sublingual or labetolol 2.5 to 5 mg IV every 5 to 10 minutes.
- Depending on the severity, the patient may need to be transferred to an inpatient facility or be followed up with primary care physician.

6. Pneumothorax

Pneumothorax may occur as a complication of intercostal nerve block, stellate ganglion block, celiac plexus block, intrascalene nerve block, supraclavicular nerve block, and also trigger point injections in the chest and anterior abdominal wall. The incidence of pneumothorax with intercostal nerve blocks is rare in experienced hands. Pneumothorax has been reported with transforaminal selective thoracic epidural blocks. However, in experienced hands, the incidence is rare.

(i) Symptoms and Signs

A small pneumothorax usually causes no symptoms, although chest pain and dyspnea may occur. Depending on the severity of the pneumothorax, signs on physical examination include tachypnea, asymmetrical expansion of the chest on the affected side, deviation of the trachea away from the pneumothorax, hyperresonance to percussion, and diminished breath sounds on the affected side. Despite these specific diagnostic features, pneumothorax is difficult to diagnose with a stethoscope, and a chest x-ray (taken in the upright position and the end of maximal expiration) is often needed to confirm the diagnosis. Tension pneumothorax manifests as decreased breath sounds, wheezing, hypotension, and circulatory collapse.

(ii) Treatment

- If the situation is life-threatening and cardiovascular collapse is imminent, a large bore 14-G catheter should be inserted in midclavicular line in the second intercostal space just above the ribs. To prevent air from entering the intrapleural space, a syringe should be placed over the catheter before insertion. This should be followed by insertion of a chest tube with placement on waterseal and suction.
- Airway breathing and circulation should be supported and standard monitoring applied. Oxygen should be administered.
- A small pneumothorax occupying less than 25% hemithorax in asymptomatic individuals can be treated on an outpatient basis without removing the area. Serial chest x-rays to exclude nonexpansion should be obtained. The pneumothorax should spontaneously resolve in 7 to 10 days.

II. MEDICATION-RELATED EMERGENCIES

1. Anaphylaxis

(i) Symptoms and Signs

Anaphylaxis presents with cardiovascular manifestations including hypotension; tachycardia and dysrhythmias; pulmonary manifestations including bronchospasm, dyspnea, pulmonary edema, laryngeal edema, hypoxemia and cough; and dermatologic manifestations including urticaria, facial edema, and pruritus. In its mildest form, urticaria may be the only symptom; in its worst form, complete cardiovascular collapse occurs, usually with severe bronchospasm.

(ii) Treatment

- Stop the administration of the drug.
- Administer oxygen.
- Assess the airway and ventilation.
- Intubate the patient if necessary.

- Epinephrine is the absolute treatment of choice; give 50 to 100 μg IV, or for persistent bronchospasm, 0.5 μg per minute IV, then titrate against the patient's response.
- Administer IV fluids.
- H_1 blocker (diphenhydramine hydrochloride 50 to 100 mg IV), H_2 blocker (cimetidine 50 to 300 mg IV).
- Steroids, hydrocortisone 500 mg per kg IV, or dexamethasone 1 to 5 mg per kg IV.

(iii) In the Event of Circulatory Collapse
- Provide endotracheal intubation.
- Administer epinephrine 1 to 5 mg IV, or via endotracheal tube if no IV access, titrate to response.
- For cardiac arrest, follow ACLS protocol.

2. Opioid Overdose

(i) Symptoms and Signs
Miosis, sedation, hypoventilation, apnea, and coma.

(ii) Treatment
First establish an airway, support ventilation, and give supplemental oxygen.

Give naloxone 0.04 to 0.4 mg IV. If the patient has been on chronic opioid therapy, it is wise to administer no more than 0.04 mg every 2 minutes, which will help avoid inducing a withdrawal syndrome. Because naloxone has a half-life of 1 hour, monitoring and repeated injections might be needed. Close monitoring and a naloxone infusion (0.5 to 1.2 mg per hour) might be required, depending on the half-life and mode of administration of the opioid being reversed. Because vomiting is associated with naloxone administration, it is safer to keep the patient in the lateral decubitus position to prevent aspiration (endotracheal intubation should also be considered).

When treating a patient on chronic opioid therapy, where opioid overdose is causing sedation but not significant hypoventilation, observation for a few hours is the best therapeutic approach.

3. Opioid Withdrawal
Opioid withdrawal rarely causes life-threatening symptoms. The exception is the patient on chronic opioids who receives naloxone.

(i) Symptoms and Signs
- Hypertension, nausea, and vomiting.
- Aspiration pneumonia might be a complication.
- Fever, chills, runny nose, yawning, sweating, irritability, diarrhea, abdominal cramping, and muscle aches.

(ii) Treatment
Resumption of opioid treatment, in general, is the best way to stop the withdrawal syndrome. Generally, 25% to 40% of the previous dose will abort most of the symptoms. In severe cases, clonidine 0.2 to 0.4 mg per day can be added. For symptomatic treatment of nausea, use prochlorperazine, metoclopramide, or

droperidol. For treatment of muscle aches and for abdominal cramping, use nonsteroidal antiinflammatory drugs (NSAIDs) (see Chapter 8 and Appendix VII). It may be helpful to admit the patient to an addiction service unit and taper off the drug, with the patient in a monitored setting.

For a full description of opioid tolerance and withdrawal, see Chapters 9 and 35.

4. Steroid Overdose and Adrenal Insufficiency

When used inappropriately and excessively in a cyclical weekly fashion, epidural tiamcinolone (150 to 300 mg) has been shown to suppress adrenal production of cortisol and the pituitary synthesis of endogenous corticotropin.

(i) Symptoms and Signs

Adrenal insufficiency presents as weakness, fatigue, hypotension, weight loss, and anorexia. In its ultimate form, adrenal crisis—nausea, vomiting, and abdominal pain—may become persistent. Lethargy may deepen to somnolence. Hypovolemic shock may be precipitated with a poor hemodynamic performance, although such poor hemodynamic performance is usually not evident when exogenous hormone is available, because mineralocorticoid activity of the adrenal medulla is still maintained.

(ii) Treatment

It is recommended practice to supplement patients who have undergone treatment with repeat epidural steroid injections within the last month with stress-dose steroids before major surgery, or if other stressors develop (e.g., infection, hypoglycemia in diabetes).

This recommendation is not universally agreed, and some authorities do not give supplementary steroids unless their patients have been on high-dose systemic steroids. Should acute adrenal insufficiency occur, immediate treatment is necessary. First-line therapy is fluid and electrolyte resuscitation and steroid replacement.

III. CONCLUSION

Many of the unwanted sequelae of pain procedures are life-threatening and require immediate and expert intervention. It is important to be prepared for these events in terms of personnel training, equipment, equipment maintenance, and protocol development. Thankfully, bad events are rare, but vigilance and preparedness are necessary to avoid adverse outcomes from these events.

SELECTED READINGS

Barash PG, Cullen BF, Stoelting RK. *Clinical anesthesia*, 4th ed. Philadelphia, PA: Lippincott Williams & Wilkins, 2000.

Cousins M, Bridenbaugh P. *Neural blockade in clinical anesthesia and management of pain*, 3rd ed. Philadelphia, PA: Lippincott Williams & Wilkins, 1998.

Goldman L, Ausiello D. *Cecil textbook of medicine*, 22nd ed. Philadelphia, PA: WB Saunders, 2003.

Kasper D, Braunwald E, Fauci A, et al. *Harrison's principles of internal medicine*, 16th ed. New York, NY: McGraw-Hill, 2004.

Dermatomes and Nerve Distribution

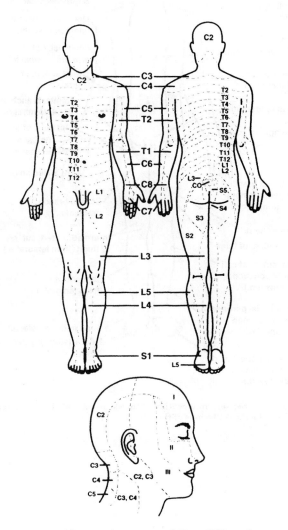

Figure 1.   Sensory dermatomes. I, II, and III are the three divisions of the trigeminal nerve (cranial nerve V).

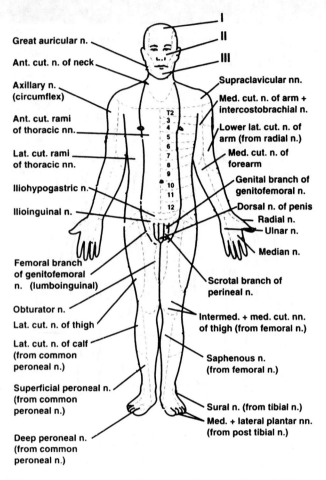

Figure 2. Sensory innervation of the skin—partial view. I, II, and III are the three divsions of the trigeminal nerve (cranial nerve V).

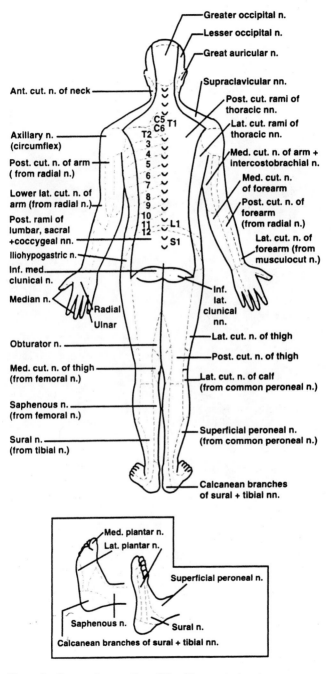

Figure 3.   Sensory innervation of the skin—posterior view.

Useful Addresses and Websites

AMERICAN ACADEMY OF CRANIOFACIAL PAIN

Organization that focuses on the diagnosis and treatment of TMJ.
Executive Director: Cordelia Mason
516 West Pipeline Road
Hurst, TX 76053
Phone: 800-322-8651 or 817-282-1501
Fax: 817-282-8012
E-mail: central@aacfp.org
www.aacfp.org

AMERICAN ACADEMY OF OROFACIAL PAIN

Organization of health care professionals dedicated to alleviating pain and suffering through the promotion of excellence in education, research, and patient care in the field of orofacial pain and associated disorders.
19 Mantua Road
Mt. Royal, NJ 08061
Phone: 856-423-3629
Fax: 856-423-3420
E-mail: aaopco@talley.com
www.aaop.org

AMERICAN ACADEMY OF PAIN MANAGEMENT

Information and Referral, National Pain Data Bank; provides credentialing, accreditation of facilities, networking opportunities, continuing education, and quality publications; holds annual clinical meeting.
Executive Director: Kathryn Padgett, PhD
13947 Mono Way #A
Sonora, CA 95370
Phone: 209-533-9744
Fax: 209-533-9750
E-mail: aapm@aapainmanage.org
www.aapainmanage.org

AMERICAN ACADEMY OF PAIN MEDICINE

A medical specialty society representing physicians practicing in the field of pain medicine.
4700 West Lake Avenue
Glenview, IL 60025-1485
Phone: 847-375-4731
Fax: 877-734-8750
E-mail: aapm@amctec.com
www.painmed.org

AMERICAN ALLIANCE OF CANCER PAIN INITIATIVES

A national network of state-based pain initiatives dedicated to promoting cancer pain relief.
1300 University Avenue, Room 4720
Madison, WI 53706

Phone: 608-265-4013
Fax: 608-265-4014
E-mail: mebennet@wisc.edu
www.aacpi.org

AMERICAN CHRONIC PAIN ASSOCIATION

Support and informational system for people with chronic pain; several hundred ACPA support group chapters meet worldwide; written materials available.
P.O. Box 850
Rocklin, CA 95677
Phone: 1-800-533-3231
Fax: 916-632-3208
E-mail: acpa@pacbell.net
www.theacpa.org

AMERICAN COLLEGE OF OSTEOPATHIC SCLEROTHERAPEUTIC PAIN MANAGEMENT

Organization that provides training and education for physicians interested in practicing prolotherapy/sclerotherapy.
President: John L. Sessions, DO
303 S. Ingram Court
Middletown, DE 19709
Phone: 800-471-6114 or 302-376-8080
Fax: 302-376-8081
E-mail: admin@ACOPMS.com
www.acopms.com

AMERICAN COUNCIL FOR HEADACHE EDUCATION

Nonprofit patient–health professional partnership dedicated to advancing the treatment and management of headache; educational resources, 50 support groups nationwide.
19 Mantua Road
Mount Royal, NJ 08061
Phone: 856-423-0258
Fax: 856-423-0082
E-mail: achehq@talley.com
www.achenet.org

AMERICAN HEADACHE SOCIETY

Professional society of health care providers dedicated to the study and treatment of headache and facial pain.
19 Mantua Road
Mount Royal, NJ 08061
Phone: 856-423-0043
Fax: 856-423-0082
E-mail: ahshq@talley.com
www.ahsnet.org

AMERICAN PAIN FOUNDATION

Information, resource, and patient advocacy organization serving people with pain.
Will Rowe, Executive Director
201 N. Charles Street, Suite 710
Baltimore, MD 21201

Phone: 888-615-PAIN (7246)
www.painfoundation.org

AMERICAN PAIN SOCIETY

Multidisciplinary organization of basic and clinical scientists, practicing clinicians, policy analysts, and others to advance pain related research, education, treatment, and professional practice.
4700 West Lake Avenue
Glenville, IL 60025-1485
Phone: 847-375-4715
Fax: 877-734-8758
E-mail: info@ampainsoc.org
www.ampainsoc.org

AMERICAN SOCIETY OF ADDICTION MEDICINE

The nation's medical specialty society dedicated to educating physicians and improving the treatment of individuals suffering from alcoholism and other addictions.
President: Elizabeth F. Howell, MD, FASAM
4601 North Park Avenue, Arcade Suite 101
Chevy Chase, MD 20815
Phone: 301-656-3920
Fax: 301-656-3815
www.asam.org

THE AMERICAN SOCIETY OF INTERVENTIONAL PAIN PHYSICIANS

To promote the development and practice of safe, high quality, cost-effective interventional pain management techniques for the diagnosis and treatment of pain and related disorders.
81 Lakeview Drive
Paducah, KY 42001
Phone: 270-554-9412
Fax: 270-554-5394
E-mail: asipp@asipp.org
www.asipp.org

AMERICAN SOCIETY OF LAW, MEDICINE, AND ETHICS

Educational information at the nexus of law, medicine, and ethics, access to research projects on pain under-treatment.
Executive Director: Benjamin Moulton, JD, MPH
765 Commonwealth Avenue, Suite 1634
Boston, MA 02215
Phone: 617-262-4990
Fax: 617-437-7596
E-mail: info@aslme.org
www.aslme.org

AMERICAN SOCIETY FOR PAIN MANAGEMENT NURSING

Organization of professional nurses dedicated to promoting and providing optimal care to individuals with pain through education, standards, advocacy, and research.
7794 Grow Drive
Pensacola, FL 32514
Phone: 888-342-7766 or 850-473-0233

Fax: 850-484-8762
E-mail: aspmn@puetzamc.com
www.aspmn.org

AMERICAN SOCIETY OF REGIONAL ANESTHESIA AND PAIN MEDICINE

Provides schedules of upcoming meetings, information about fellowships in pain management.

(For the consensus statement on Neuraxial Anesthesia and Anticoagulation, go to www.asra.com, click on "consensus conferences" tab, on the right-hand side click "Second Consensus Conference on Neuraxial Anesthesia and Anticoagulation, April 25–28, 2002.")

President: Richard W. Rosenquist, MD
520 N. Northwest Highway
Park Ridge, IL 60068
Phone: 847-825-7246
Fax: 804-282-0090
E-mail: g.hoormann@asahq.org
www.asra.com

ARTHRITIS FOUNDATION

National nonprofit organization that supports more than 100 types of arthritis and related conditions through advocacy, programs, services, and research.

President and CEO: John H. Klippel, MD
P.O. Box 7669
Atlanta, GA 30357
Phone: 800-568-4045 or 404-872-7100
www.arthritis.org

CANCER CARE

Offers free professional help to people with all cancers through counseling, education, information and referral, and direct financial assistance.

275 7th Avenue
New York, NY 10001
Phone: 800-813-4673
www.cancercare.org

CANCER PAIN EDUCATION RESOURCE (CAPER)

A resource for use by various educators regarding cancer pain (A 28-member interdisciplinary team designed CAPER World Wide Website.)

www.caper.tufts.edu

CANDLELIGHTERS CHILDHOOD CANCER FOUNDATION

Provides information, support, and advocacy for families of children with cancer, survivors of childhood cancer, and the professionals who care for them.

Executive Director: Ruth Hoffman
National Office
P.O. Box 498
Kensington, MD 20895

Phone: 800-366-2223 or 301-962-3520
Fax: 301-962-3521
E-mail: staff@candlelighters.org
www.candlelighters.org

CFIDS ASSOCIATION OF AMERICA

Charitable organization dedicated to conquering chronic fatigue and immune dysfunction syndrome (CFIDS) through advocacy, information, and research.
P.O. Box 220398
Charlotte, NC 28222-0398
Info Line: 800-442-3437
Resource Line: 704-365-2343
Fax: 704-365-9755
E-mail: info@cfids.org
www.cfids.org

CITY OF HOPE BECKMAN RESEARCH INSTITUTE

Pain/Palliative Care resource center.
1500 E. Duarte Road
Duarte, CA 91010
Phone: 626-359-8111 x63829
www.cityofhope.org/prc

COMMISSION ON ACCREDITATION OF REHABILITATION FACILITIES (CARF)

Accredits comprehensive inpatient and outpatient pain management programs. (A list of accredited pain programs can be obtained by contacting CARF.)
4891 East Grant Road
Tucson, AZ 85712
Phone: 520-325-1044 or 888-281-6531
Fax: 520-318-1129
E-mail: webmaster@carf.org
www.carf.org

COMMUNITY OF INTEREST (COIN) IN PAIN MANAGEMENT & PALLIATIVE CARE CME COURSES

Free CME Web-based courses in pain management and palliative care.
CEO: Marlene Von-Friedrichs-Fitzwater, PhD, APR
Health Communications Research Institute
3550 Watt Avenue, Suite 140
Sacramento, CA 95821
Fax: 916-979-7046
www.cme-webcredits.org/COIN.html

GUIDELINES FOR ADULT LOW BACK PAIN

Guidelines for adult low back pain from the Institute for Clinical Systems Improvement.
www.icsi.org/knowledge/detail.asp?catID=29& itemID=149
Or at National Guidelines Clearinghouse:
www.guideline.gov/summary/summary.aspx?
doc_id=5883&nbr=3869&string=sciatica>

INTERNATIONAL ASSOCIATION FOR THE STUDY OF PAIN (IASP)

International, multidisciplinary, nonprofit professional association dedicated to furthering research on pain and improving the care of patients in pain.

(For the IASP Classification of Chronic Pain, go to www.painbooks.org/class.html to purchase Classification of Chronic Pain: Descriptions of Chronic Pain Syndromes and Definitions of Pain Terms, 2nd Ed. *Editors: Harold Merskey and Nikolai Bogduk; IASP Press, 1994.)*

[Members may print the book for free by signing in to the Members section of the IASP web site. Click on "Book: 'Classification of Chronic Pain – 2nd Edition' (1994)."]

IASP Secretariat
909 NE 43rd Street, Suite 306
Seattle, WA 98105-6020
Phone: 206-547-6409
Fax: 206-547-1703
E-mail: iaspdesk@iasp-pain.org
www.iasp-pain.org

INTERSTITIAL CYSTITIS ASSOCIATION

Offers information and support to IC patients and their families, educates the medical community about IC, and promotes research to find effective treatments

President: Vicki Ratner, MD
1100 North Washington Street, Suite 340
Rockville, MD 20850
Phone: 301-610-5300 or 800/help.ica
Fax: 301-610-5308
E-mail: icamail@ichelp.org
www.ichelp.org

JOINT COMMISSION ON ACCREDITATION OF HEALTH CARE ORGANIZATIONS

An independent, not-for-profit organization that is considered the nation's predominant standards setting and accrediting body in health care.

One Renaissance Boulevard
Oakbrook Terrace, IL 60181
Phone: 630-792-5000
Fax: 630-792-5005
www.JCAHO.org

NATIONAL ASSOCIATION OF STATE CONTROLLED SUBSTANCES AUTHORITIES

Provides a mechanism for state and federal agencies, and regulated industries, to increase effectiveness of efforts to prevent and control drug abuse, yet provide mechanisms to make controlled substances available to persons who have a true medical need.

Executive Director: Katherine Keough
72 Brook Street
Quincy, MA 02170
Phone: 617-472-0520
Fax: 617-472-0521

E-mail: kathykeough@nascsa.org
www.nascsa.org

NATIONAL CHRONIC PAIN OUTREACH ASSOCIATION

National support group list; does physician referrals.
P.O. Box 274
Millboro, VA 24460
Phone: 540-862-9437
Fax: 540-862-9485
www.chronicpain.org

NATIONAL FOUNDATION FOR THE TREATMENT OF PAIN

Not-for-profit organization dedicated to providing support for patients who are suffering from intractable pain, and their families and friends; resources for medical professionals and attorneys.
P.O. Box 70045
Houston, TX 77270
Phone: 713-862-9332
Fax: 713-862-9346
www.paincare.org

NATIONAL HEADACHE FOUNDATION

Resources for headache sufferers and health care professionals.
820 N. Orleans, Suite 217
Chicago, IL 60610
Phone: 888-NHF-5552
E-mail: info@headaches.org
www.headaches.org

NATIONAL MULTIPLE SCLEROSIS SOCIETY

Has written material; support groups and physician referrals through local chapters.
733 3rd Avenue
New York, NY 10017-3288
Phone: 800-344-4867
www.nmss.org

NATIONAL NETWORK OF LIBRARIES OF MEDICINE

Program coordinated by the National Library of Medicine to provide access to biomedical information for health professionals and the public.
8600 Rockville Pike
Bldg. 38, Room B1-E03
Bethesda, MD 20894
Phone: 301-496-4777
Fax: 301-480-1467
www.nnlm.nlm.nih.gov

NATIONAL VULVODYNIA ASSOCIATION

Organization created to improve the lives of individuals affected by vulvodynia.
P. O. Box 4491
Silver Springs, MD 20914-4491
Phone: 301-299-0775

Fax: 301-299-3999
www.nva.org

NEUROPATHY ASSOCIATION

Organization committed to raising awareness of neuropathy, established by people with neuropathy and their families or friends to help those who suffer from disorders that affect the peripheral nerves.

60 E. 42nd Street, Suite 942
New York, NY 10165
Phone: 212-692-0662
E-mail: info@neuropathy.org
www.neuropathy.org

ONCOLINK

The first multimedia oncology information resource placed on the Internet; contains information about specific types of cancer, updates on cancer treatments, and news about research.

Abramson Cancer Center of the University of Pennsylvania
3400 Spruce Street – 2 Donner
Philadelphia, PA 19104-4283
Fax: 215-349-5445
www.oncolink.com

PAIN.COM

A world of information on pain; program of the Dannemiller Memorial Education Foundation.

www.pain.com

PAIN MANAGEMENT ROUNDS

Newsletter on pain related topics; a publication of the MGH Pain Center.

www.painmanagementrounds.org

PAIN ONLINE JOURNAL

The Journal of the International Association for the Study of Pain, publishing original research on the nature, mechanisms, and treatment of pain.

www.sciencedirect.com/pain

PEDIATRIC PAIN: SCIENCE HELPING CHILDREN

Pediatric pain research lab located in the IWK Health Centre and the Psychology Department of Dalhousie University in Halifax, Nova Scotia, Canada; research, resources, and information on pediatric pain management, self-help for children in pain and their parents, Pediatric Pain Letter, downloadable copy of the Faces Pain Scale in several languages.

www.is.dal.ca/~pedpain/pedpain.html

PROMOTING EXCELLENCE IN END OF LIFE CARE

A national program of the Robert Wood Johnson Foundation dedicated to long-term changes in health care institutions to substantially improve care for dying people and their families.

The University of Montana Practical Ethics Center
1000 East Beckwith Avenue
Missoula, Montana 59812

Phone: 406-243-6601
Fax: 406-243-6633
E-mail: excel@mso.umt.edu
www.promotingexcellence.org

REFLEX SYMPATHETIC DYSTROPHY SYNDROME ASSOCIATION

Has written material; about 100 support groups nationwide; will send a list of physicians in patient's area.
P.O. Box 502
Milford, CT 06460
Phone: 203-877-3790 or 877-662-7737
Fax: 203-882-8362
E-mail: info@rsds.org
www.rsds.org

SICKLE CELL DISEASE ASSOCIATION OF AMERICA, INC.

Has written materials, support links, message board.
16 S. Calvert Street, Suite 600
Baltimore, MD 21202
Phone: 800-421-8453 or 410-528-1555
Fax: 410-528-1495
E-mail: scdaa@sicklecelldisease.org
www.sicklecelldisease.org

SOCIETY FOR NEUROSCIENCE

World's largest organization of basic scientists and physicians devoted to the study of the brain, spinal cord, and peripheral nervous system.
11 Dupont Circle, NW, Suite 500
Washington, DC 20036
Phone: 202-462-6688
Fax: 202-462-9740
E-mail: info@sfn.org
www.sfn.org

STOPPAIN.ORG

Information on pain and palliative care put together by the department of Pain and Palliative Care at Beth Israel Medical Center in New York.
Department of Pain and Palliative Care
Beth Israel Medical Center
First Avenue at 16th Street
New York, NY 10003
Phone: 877-620-9999 or 212-844-8930
Fax: 212-844-1503
E-mail: stoppain@chpnet.org

TMJ ASSOCIATION

Has written material, strives to develop standards for safe, effective research-based diagnostics, treatments, and prevention of TMJ diseases.
P.O. Box 26770
Milwaukee, WI 53226-0770
Phone: 414-259-3223

Fax: 414-259-8112
E-mail: info@tmj.org
www.tmj.org/index.asp

TRIGEMINAL NEURALGIA ASSOCIATION

Has written materials for patients and professionals, support groups nationwide.
2801 SW Archer Road
Gainesville, FL 32608
Phone: 352-376-9955 or 800-923-3608
Fax: 352-376-8688
E-mail: tnanational@tna-support.org
www.tna-support.org

THE VULVAR PAIN FOUNDATION

Information, research seminars, personal support, and resource network.
P.O. Drawer 177
Graham, NC 27253
Phone 336-226-0704
Fax: 336-226-8518
www.vulvarpainfoundation.org

VZV RESEARCH FOUNDATION

Written material on zoster/shingles pain and post-herpetic neuralgia.
24 East 64 Street
New York, NY 10021
Phone: 212-371-7280
Fax: 212-838-0380
E-mail: Vzv@vzvFoundation.org
www.Vzvfoundation.org

Standards of Treatment: The American Pain Society's Quality Assurance Standards for Relief of Acute and Cancer Pain

In most patients with acute pain and chronic cancer pain, comfort can be achieved with the attentive use of analgesic medications. Historically, though, the outcomes of analgesic treatment have often not been satisfactory, largely because clinical care units have not had systems in place to ensure that the occurrence of pain is recognized and that when pain persists, there is rapid feedback to modify treatment. These suggested standards are offered as one approach to developing such a system. Individual facilities may wish to modify these standards to suit their particular needs.

The guidelines are intended for hospitals and chronic care facilities in which only conventional analgesic methods are used (e.g., intermittent parenteral or oral analgesics) and for those using the most modern technology for pain management. In either case, a dedicated pain management team would enhance the quality of pain control if its personnel acquire special training in pain relief. Newer, more aggressive methods of pain control, such as patient-controlled analgesia, epidural opiate administration, and regional anesthetic techniques, may provide better pain relief than intermittent parenteral analgesics in many patients, but these carry their own risks. If institutions choose to use these methods, they must be delivered by an organized team with frequent follow-up and titration and with adequate briefing of the primary caregivers. Such teams should be organized under one of the recognized medical departments of the facility. Specific standards for such methods, monitored by that department, might well augment the general guidelines articulated here.

I. RECOGNIZE AND TREAT PAIN PROMPTLY

Chart and Display Pain and Relief (Process)

A measure of pain intensity and a measure of pain relief are recorded on the bedside vital sign chart or a similar record that facilitates regular review by members of the health care team and is incorporated in the patient's permanent record.

1. The intensity of pain or discomfort is assessed and documented on admission, after any known pain-producing procedure, with each new report of pain, and at regular intervals that depend on the severity of pain. Each clinical unit will select a simple, valid measure of intensity. For children, age-appropriate pain intensity measures will be used.
2. The degree of pain relief is determined after each pain management intervention, once sufficient time has elapsed for

the treatment to reach peak effect (e.g., 1 hour for parenteral analgesics and 2 hours for oral analgesics). Each clinical unit will select a simple, valid measure of intensity.

Define Pain and Relief Levels to Trigger Review (Process)

Each clinical unit will identify values for pain intensity rating and pain relief rating that will elicit a review of the current pain therapy, documentation of the proposed modifications in treatment, and subsequent review of its efficacy. This process of treatment review and follow-up should include participation by physicians and nurses involved in the patient's care. As the general quality of treatment improves, the clinical unit will upgrade this standard to encourage a continuous process of improvement.

Survey Patient Satisfaction (Outcome)

At regular intervals to be defined by the clinical unit and the quality assurance committee, each clinical unit will assess a randomly selected sample of patients who have had surgery in the past 72 hours, have another acute pain condition, or have a diagnosis of cancer. Patients will be asked whether they have had pain during the current admission. Those patients who have experienced pain will then be asked about the following:

1. Current intensity of their pain
2. Intensity of the worst pain they have experienced in the last 24 hours (or other interval selected by the clinical unit)
3. Degree of relief obtained from pain management interventions
4. Satisfaction with the staff's responsiveness to their reports of pain
5. Satisfaction with relief provided.

II. MAKE INFORMATION ABOUT ANALGESICS READILY AVAILABLE (PROCESS)

Information about analgesics and other methods of pain management, including charts of relative potencies of analgesics, is made available on the unit in a way that facilitates writing and interpreting orders. Nurses and physicians can demonstrate the use of this material. Appropriate training to treat their patients' pain is available to health professionals and is included in continuing education activities.

III. PROMISE PATIENTS ATTENTIVE ANALGESIC CARE (PROCESS)

Patients are informed on admission, orally and in writing, that effective pain relief is an important part of treatment, that their communication of unrelieved pain is essential, and that health professionals will respond quickly to their reports of pain.

IV. DEFINE EXPLICIT POLICIES FOR USE OF ADVANCED ANALGESIC TECHNOLOGIES (PROCESS)

Advanced pain control techniques, including intraspinal opioids, systemic or intraspinal patient-controlled anesthesia or continuous opioid infusion, local anesthetic infusion, and inhalational analgesia, are governed by policy and standard procedures that define the acceptable level of monitoring of patients and define appropriate roles and limits of practice for all groups of health care providers involved. Such policy includes definitions of physician accountability, nurse responsibility to the patient and the physician, and the role of pharmacy.

V. MONITOR ADHERENCE TO STANDARDS (PROCESS)

1. An interdisciplinary committee, including representation from physicians, nurses, and other appropriate disciplines (e.g., pharmacy), monitors compliance with the standards mentioned in preceding text, considers issues relevant to improving pain treatment, and makes recommendations to improve outcomes and their monitoring. Where a comprehensive pain management team exists, its activities are monitored through the parent department's quality assurance body. In a nursing home or very small hospital where an interdisciplinary pain management committee is not feasible, one or several individuals may fulfill this role.
2. At least the chairperson of the committee has experience working with issues related to effective pain management.
3. The committee meets at least every 3 months to review the process and outcomes related to pain management.
4. The committee interacts with clinical units to establish procedures for improving pain management where necessary and reviews the results of these changes within 3 months of their implementation.
5. The committee provides regular reports to administration and to the medical, nursing, and pharmacy staffs.

Massachusetts General Hospital Pain Center Guidelines on Prescribing Controlled Substances for Patients with Nonmalignant Chronic Disease

1. Controlled substance prescriptions are not sent by mail.
2. Prescriptions are not written as "brand name medically necessary" or "no substitution" unless it is absolutely necessary.
3. The Pain Center does not act as a primary care facility. Therefore, patients must be under the care of a primary care physician, and all decisions regarding pain management are shared with that physician.
4. When chronic opioid therapy is initiated, the primary referring physician must agree with this decision and must agree to continue to care for the patient. All decisions regarding continuance of opioid therapy are agreed to by the Pain Center and the primary care physician.
5. Discovery that the patient has obtained concurrent prescriptions for controlled substances from multiple physicians usually results in termination of the Pain Center's relationship with the patient.
6. A second instance of lost or early depletion of a prescription is considered a possible sign of misuse, and treatment is either restructured or discontinued.
7. Prescription refills are provided only by appointment.
8. Appropriate adjunctive services are arranged during opioid treatment as well as during an opioid wean.
9. Massachusetts state regulations require that prescriptions for opioids be written on a monthly basis. Patients must pick up their prescriptions in person unless there are extenuating circumstances.

Drug Enforcement Administration Prescription Guidelines[1]

The Drug Enforcement Administration has issued guidelines for prescribers of controlled substances (i.e., Schedules II–V). These guidelines have been endorsed by the American Medical Association.[2] The Massachusetts Board of Registration in Medicine endorses these general guidelines.

1. Controlled substances have legitimate clinical usefulness and the prescriber should not hesitate to consider prescribing them when they are indicated for the comfort and well-being of patients.
2. Prescribing controlled substances for legitimate medical uses requires special caution because of their potential for abuse and dependence.
3. Good judgment should be exercised in administering and prescribing controlled substances so that diversion to illicit uses is avoided and the development of drug dependence is minimized or prevented.
4. Physicians should guard against contributing to drug abuse through injudicious prescription writing practices or by acquiescing to unwarranted demands of some patients.
5. Each prescriber should examine his or her individual prescribing practices to ensure that all prescriptions for controlled substances are written with caution.
6. Physicians should make a specific effort to ensure that patients are not obtaining multiple prescription orders from different prescribers.

[1]Massachusetts Board of Registration in Medicine. To access, go to www.massmedboard.org/regs/ and scroll to Policy (Guideline), Prescribing Practices Policy and Guidelines (August 1, 1989). Note: Policy was amended on 12/12/01.
[2]American Medical Association, *Prescribing Controlled Drugs Source Book*, 1986.

U.S. Food and Drug Administration State Drug Schedules

There are five established schedules of controlled substances, to be known as Schedules I, II, III, IV, and V. Such schedules currently consist of the substances listed as follows:

Table 1.   Schedules for controlled substances prescribed for patients in pain

Schedule I

The drug or other substance has a high potential for abuse.

The drug or other substance has no currently accepted medical use in treatment in the United States.

There is a lack of accepted safety for use of the drug or other substance under medical supervision.

None

Schedule II

The drug or other substance has a high potential for abuse.

The drug or other substance has a currently accepted medical use in treatment in the United States or a currently accepted medical use with severe restrictions.

Abuse of the drug or other substances may lead to severe psychological or physical dependence.

Opioids: morphine, codeine, fentanyl, hydromorphone, meperidine, levorphanol, oxycodone.

Stimulants: amphetamine, methylphenidate.

Marihuana: dronabinol.

Schedule III

The drug or other substance has a potential for abuse less than the drugs or other substances in Schedules I and II.

The drug or other substance has a currently accepted medical use in treatment in the United States.

Abuse of the drug or other substance may lead to moderate or low physical dependence or high psychological dependence.

Opioids: nalorphine; mixtures of limited specified quantities of codeine, dihydrocodeine, hydrocodone, morphine, or opioid with noncontrolled medicinal ingredients.

Schedule IV

The drug or other substance has a low potential for abuse relative to the drugs or other substances in Schedule III.

The drug or other substance has a currently accepted medical use in treatment in the United States.

Abuse of the drug or other substance may lead to limited physical dependence or psychological dependence relative to the drugs or other substances in Schedule III.

continued

Table 1.   *Continued*

Opioids: pentazocine.
Benzodiazepines: Diazepam, clonazepam, flurazepam, midazolam, triazolam.

Schedule V

The drug or other substance has a low potential for abuse relative to the drugs or other substances in Schedule IV.

The drug or other substance has a currently accepted medical use in treatment in the United States.

Abuse of the drug or other substance may lead to limited physical dependence or psychological dependence relative to the drugs or other substances in Schedule IV.

Opioids: cough suppressant preparations.

Appendix VII

Drugs Commonly Used in Pain Practice

Delbert R. Black, Gary Jay Brenner,
Salahadin Abdi, and Jatinder Gill

NOTE: This table provides a ready reference to the drugs frequently used in pain practice. The information provided is not comprehensive and the reader is encouraged to refer to the Physicians' Desk Reference *(PDR) or to other sources for a complete description of these drugs.*

Acetaminophen (Tylenol)

Description:	Analgesic, antipyretic
Indications:	Used to relieve mild to moderate pain and has minimal antiinflammatory effects
Dosage:	325 to 1,000 mg PO every 4 to 6 hours, not to exceed 4,000 mg per day
Side Effects:	Overdoses of acetaminophen can cause severe, even fatal, hepatic dysfunction. Allergies to this drug can also occur
Precautions:	Use with caution in presence of alcoholism or liver disease. Daily use of alcohol, especially when combined with phenobarbital, may enhance acetaminophen's hepatotoxicity. It may produce a slight increase in prothrombin time in patients receiving oral anticoagulants, but the clinical significance of this effect is not clear.

Acetylsalicylic acid (see NSAIDs)
Actiq (see Opioids)
Almotriptan (see Triptans)
Amerge (see Triptans)
Amitriptyline (see TCAs)
Amoxapine (see TCAs)
Anafranil (see TCAs)
Anaprox (see NSAIDs)
Ansaid (see NSAIDs)
Asendin (see TCAs)
Aspirin (see NSAIDs)
Atarax (see Hydroxyzine)
Ativan (see Lorazepam)
Axert (see Triptans)

Books@Ovid
Copyright © 2002 by Department of Anesthesia and Critical Care,
Massachusetts General Hospital
Published by Lippincott Williams & Wilkins
Jane C. Ballantyne
The Massachusetts General Hospital Handbook of Pain Management

Baclofen (see Lioresal)
Benadryl (see Diphenhydramine)
Benylin (see Dextromethorphan)

Butalbital-caffeine-acetaminophen/aspirin (Fioricet/Fiorinal)

Description:	Barbiturate, caffeine, and analgesic mixture
Indications:	Tension (or muscle contraction) headache and conditions in which a simultaneous sedative and analgesic action is required, such as mixed migraine headache, postdural puncture headache, and menstrual and postpartum tension and pain
Dosage:	Two tablets or capsules at once, followed, if necessary, by one tablet or capsule every 3 to 4 hours; up to six capsules or tablets daily
Side Effects:	Bloating; dizziness, or lightheadedness; drowsiness; nausea, vomiting, or stomach pain
Precautions:	Use with caution in patients with history of alcohol abuse, heart disease, mental depression, kidney and liver disease, diabetes mellitus, porphyria.

Butazolidin (see NSAIDs)

Capsaicin (Zostrix, topical)

Description:	Topical analgesic, antipruritic, antineuralgic
Indications:	Arthritis, shingles, diabetic neuropathy
Dosage:	Apply to affected areas (rub well) three to four times a day
Side Effects:	Warm, burning feeling, stinging, redness
Precautions:	Avoid contact with eyes or on other sensitive areas of the body.

Carbamazepine (Tegretol)

Description:	Anticonvulsant, antineuralgic
Indications:	Neuropathic pain medication, especially useful for trigeminal neuralgia
Dosage:	Usually initiated at 100 mg PO bid with escalation by 100 mg every 12 hours as tolerated. Effective dose for pain may range from 200 mg to 1,200 mg per day
Side Effects:	Dizziness, drowsiness, blurred vision, pruritus and rash, hematologic and hepatic complications
Precautions:	Obtain baseline hematologic function test and subsequently monitor on the basis of clinical indication. Perform liver function tests before initiating therapy and periodically thereafter. Use with caution in patients with history of bone marrow depression and liver dysfunction.

Celebrex (see Celecoxib)

Celecoxib (Celebrex)

Description:	NSAID, selective COX-2 inhibitor
Indications:	Pain with peripheral inflammatory component
Dosage:	100 mg PO bid to 200 mg PO bid
Side Effects:	Lower incidence of GI complications than with traditional NSAIDs. Usual doses do not appear

to affect platelet aggregation. Renal toxicity similar to traditional NSAIDs.

Precautions: Sulfonamide allergy. Use with caution in patients with history of GI bleeding, ischemic heart disease, fluid retention, or renal impairment. Continued use may increase risk of myocardial infarction or stroke.

Chlorpromazine (Thorazine)

Description: Phenothiazine, dopamine antagonist, antipsychotic, antiemetic, sedative

Indications: Psychoses, hiccups, anxiety, and nausea and vomiting

Dosage: 10 to 50 mg PO/IM bid or qid

Side Effects: Constipation, drowsiness, vision changes or dry mouth, extrapyramidal symptoms, occasional tardive dyskinesia

Precautions: Use with caution in presence of extreme hypertension or hypotension, liver or heart disease, alcohol or drug dependencies, history of neuroleptic syndrome.

Choline magnesium trisalicylate (see NSAIDs)
Clinoril (see NSAIDs)
Clomipramine (see TCAs)

Clonazepam (Klonopin)

Description: Benzodiazepine, sedative-hypnotic, anxiolytic, amnestic, anticonvulsant, skeletal muscle relaxant

Indications: Patients with chronic neuropathic pain who exhibit sleep disturbances, anxiety and restlessness, skeletal muscle spasm

Dosage: Start at 0.5 mg PO at bedtime. May be given as a tid dose for patients with daytime anxiety/panic attack, usually not exceeding 3 to 4 mg per day with largest dose given at bedtime

Side Effects: Sedation, drowsiness, increased salivation, constipation

Precautions: Avoid alcohol; use with caution in patients with hepatic impairment and in case of positive results of liver function tests; periodic blood counts should be taken.

Clonidine (Catapres)

Description: Centrally acting α2-agonist, antihypertensive, suppresses manifestations of opioid withdrawal syndrome, adjunct analgesic

Indications: Neuropathic pain with sympathetic dependency; opioid withdrawal

Dosage: Clonidine has been used orally, topically, and neuraxially for pain; start at 0.1 mg PO bid or tid and gradually escalate by 0.1 to 0.2 mg per day every few days until side effects, or maximum dose of 2.4 mg per day; use 0.2 to 0.4 mg per day for opioid withdrawal

Transdermal: 0.1 to 0.3 mg once every 7 days

Epidural: 2 to 10 μg per kg (about 150 to 800 μg for a normal adult) bolus, and 10 to 40 μg per hour continuous infusion

Spinal: 10 to 30-μg bolus

Side Effects: Bradycardia, hypotension, sedation, xerostomia, constipation, urinary retention, impotence, pruritus, and insomnia

Precautions: Patients should be warned about the risk of rebound hypertension with abrupt discontinuation. Use with caution in patients with coronary artery disease, cerebrovascular disease, Raynaud disease, and depression.

Codeine (see Opioids)
Compazine (see Prochlorperazine)

Cyclobenzaprine (Flexeril)

Description: Skeletal muscle relaxant; structurally and pharmacologically related to TCAs

Indications: Myofascial pain in conjunction with physical therapy, usually short-term effect

Dosage: Usually 10 mg PO tid with gradual increase to maximum of 60 mg per day

Side Effects: Drowsiness, dry mouth, fatigue, tiredness, blurred vision, constipation, flatulence

Precautions: Follow the guidelines for tricyclic antidepressants.

Demerol (see Opioids)
Desipramine (see TCAs)

Dexamphetamine (Dexedrine)

Description: Central stimulant; central nervous system (CNS) and respiratory stimulant with weak sympathetic activity

Indications: Excessive sedation due to opioids, especially in patients with cancer

Dosage: 5 to 10 mg PO is administered in the morning after a 2.5 mg test dose; maximum daily dose is 20 mg per day

Side Effects: Nervousness, insomnia, anorexia, angina, tachycardia, thrombocytopenia, leukopenia

Precautions: Tolerance and psychological dependence may occur. Use with caution in seizure disorder, psychiatric symptoms. Contraindicated in presence of uncontrolled hypertension, significant coronary artery disease and in patients exhibiting anxiety, agitation.

Dexedrine (see Dexamphetamine)

Dextromethorphan (Benylin)

Description: Antitussive, weak analgesic with some N-methyl-D-aspartate (NMDA) receptor antagonism

Indications: Combined with opioids to decrease the development of tolerance; second-line medication for neuropathic pain

Dosage: 30 mg PO every 6 to 8 hours; dosage can be titrated as high (typically up to 90 mg PO tid) as tolerated

Side Effects: Dizziness, drowsiness, nausea, and vomiting

Precautions: Asthma, chronic bronchitis, emphysema, diabetes, liver disease

Diazepam (Valium)

Description: Benzodiazepine, sedative hypnotic, anxiolytic, amnestic, anticonvulsant, skeletal muscle relaxant

Indications: Patients with chronic neuropathic pain exhibiting sleep disturbances, anxiety and restlessness, skeletal muscle spasm

Dosage: Start at 5 mg PO at bedtime; may be given as a tid dose for patients with daytime anxiety/panic attack, usually not exceeding 3 to 4 mg per day, with largest dose given at bedtime

Side Effects: Sedation, drowsiness, increased salivation, constipation

Precautions: Not recommended for use in depressive neurosis or in psychotic reactions; avoid alcohol; be careful when given to elderly or seriously ill patients with limited pulmonary function, to those with hepatic or renal disease, to debilitated patients, or to those with organic brain syndrome.

Dibenzyline (see Phenoxybenzamine)
Diclofenac sodium (see NSAIDs)
Diflunisal (see NSAIDs)

Dihydroergotamine (DHE 45, Ergomar, Ergostat)

Description: Antihypotensive, vascular headache suppressant, ergot alkaloid

Indications: Severe throbbing headaches, such as migraine and cluster headaches

Dosage: For the abortion of migraine with aura (also called classic migraine) or migraine without aura (also called common migraine); intranasal dose of dihydroergotamine mesylate is 0.5 mg (one spray) administered in each nostril (1 mg total) initially, followed by 1 mg [one spray (0.5 mg) in each nostril] 15 minutes later for a total dose of 2 mg; for rapid response, dihydroergotamine mesylate may be administered IV (total IV dose should not exceed 2 mg; and total weekly IM or IV dosage should not exceed 6 mg); for the prevention or abortion of vascular headaches, the usual adult

IM dose of dihydroergotamine mesylate is 1 to 2 mg initially, followed by 1 mg at 1-hour intervals until the attack has abated or until a total of 3 mg has been given in 24 hours

Side Effects: Dizziness, drowsiness, stomach upset (nausea and vomiting), anxiety, tremor

Precautions: Liver, kidney, or vascular disease; hypertension, poor circulation; arterial vasospasm when given with heparin; ischemic heart disease (e.g., angina pectoris, Prinzmetal angina, myocardial infarction, and documented silent myocardial ischemia); and peripheral vascular disease, coronary artery disease, uncontrolled hypertension.

Dilaudid (see Opioids)

Diphenhydramine (Benadryl)

Description: Antihistamine, antiemetic, sedative–hypnotic

Indications: Nausea, vomiting, and itching

Dosage: For PO, use 25 to 50 mg every 4 to 6 hours; for IV/IM, use 10 to 50 mg every 4 to 6 hours (not to exceed 400 mg per day)

Side Effects: Antihistaminic effect, such as, drowsiness, sedation, dry mouth, vertigo, urinary retention

Precautions: Use with caution in patients with GI obstruction, seizure, increased intraocular pressure.

Disalcid (see NSAIDs)
Dolobid (see NSAIDs)
Dolophine (see Opioids)
Doxepin (see TCAs)

Droperidol (Inapsine)

Description: Butyrophenone, dopamine antagonist, antipsychotic, antiemetic

Indications: Nausea/vomiting and anxiety

Dosage: 0.625 to 1.25 mg IV every 4 to 6 hours; higher doses for anxiolysis

Side Effects: Shares toxic potential of phenothiazines: dysphoria, hypotension, sedation, and respiratory depression, especially in combination with opioids

Precautions: Black-box warning from U.S. Food and Drug Administration secondary to possible prolongation of QT interval; continuous electrocardiogram monitoring must be used; contraindicated in patients with Parkinson disease and with a history of neuroleptic syndrome.

Effexor XR (see Venlafaxine)
Elavil (see TCAs)
Eletriptan (see Triptans)
Etodolac (see NSAIDs)
Feldene (see NSAIDs)

Fenoprofen (see NSAIDs)
Fioricet (see Butalbital)
Flexeril (see Cyclobenzaprine)

Fluoxetine (Prozac)
Description:	Selective serotonin reuptake inhibitor (SSRI), first-line antidepressant
Indications:	Depression, panic disorder, obsessive-compulsive disorder
Dosage:	10 to 80 mg per day PO
Side Effects:	Rare but include headaches, stimulation or sedation, fine tremor, tinnitus, rare extrapyramidal symptoms, palpitations, nausea and vomiting, bloating, and diarrhea
Precautions:	Known sensitivity, interactions with monoamine oxidase inhibitors (MAOIs).

Flurbiprofen (see NSAIDs)
Frova (see Triptans)
Frovatriptan (see Triptans)

Gabapentin (Neurontin)
Description:	Anticonvulsant, adjunct antineuralgic
Indications:	Commonly used neuropathic pain medication marketed as anticonvulsant
Dosage:	Start at 300 mg PO qhs or lower (100 mg) in elderly patients; gradual escalation in dose every 3 to 5 days to the range of 1,200 mg tid as tolerated; maximum dose varies depending on efficacy and patient's tolerance of side effects; beneficial effects expected in 1 to 3 weeks of therapy
Side Effects:	Usually well tolerated, with self-limiting mild to moderate side effects; somnolence, dizziness or fatigue, ataxia (CNS), mild dyspepsia (GI), and diplopia and amblyopia
Precautions:	Do not discontinue abruptly; reduce dose in renal dysfunction.

Gabitril (see Tiagabine)
Haldol (see Haloperidol)

Haloperidol (Haldol)
Description:	Butyrophenone, antipsychotic, antiemetic
Indications:	Nervous, mental, and emotional conditions (e.g., agitation, confusion); Tourette syndrome
Dosage:	0.5 to 5 mg PO bid or tid
Side Effects:	Drowsiness, dizziness, or blurred vision, stomach upset, loss of appetite, headache, drooling, dry mouth, sweating, sleep disturbances, or restlessness
Precautions:	Difficulty in urinating, Parkinson disease, glaucoma, lung disease, heart or blood vessel disease, seizure disorder, or disease of the thyroid, kidney, liver, or prostate gland.

Hydromorphone (see Opioids)
Hydrocodone (see Opioids)

Hydroxyzine (Atarax, Vistaril)
Description: Antihistamine, antiemetic, sedative-hypnotic
Indications: Itching, emesis, anxiety
Dosage: For PO and IM use, 25 to 100 mg q6h; adjust
                  dose to patient response
Side Effect: Drowsiness, dry mouth, dizziness, discomfort
                  at site of injection
Precautions: Epilepsy, prostatic hypertrophy, glaucoma, he-
                  patic disease.

Ibuprofen (see NSAIDs)
Imipramine (see TCAs)
Imitrex (see Triptans)
Inapsine (see Droperidol)
Indocin (see NSAIDs)
Indomethacin (see NSAIDs)
Kenalog (see Triamcinolone)
Keppra (see Levetiracetam)
Ketoprofen (see NSAIDs)

Ketorolac (Toradol)
Description: Potent, injectable NSAID
Indications: Acute postoperative pain, acute inflammatory
                  pain, available for intravenous, intramuscular
                  and oral use; recommended for short-term use
                  only; superior adjunct drug for patients with
                  inadequately controlled postoperative pain
Dosage: 15 to 30 mg IV or IM every 6 hours; 10 mg PO
                  q6h; it is used preferably as a fixed regimen;
                  lower dose for elderly, low-weight patients and
                  for renal impairment; total usage not to exceed
                  5 days
Side Effects: Dizziness, nausea, vomiting, pain/redness at
                  the injection site may occur; enhanced risk of
                  bleeding, adverse GI effects, renal function im-
                  pairment and some concerns about bone re-
                  modeling in acute fractures and bone fusion
                  procedures
Precautions: Use with caution in presence of hematologic,
                  GI, and renal dysfunction. Use minimum ef-
                  fective doses and adjust for low weight, age,
                  and renal impairment.

Klonopin (see Clonazepam)

Lactulose
Description: Laxative
Indication: Constipation
Dosage: 10 to 40 g per day or two divided doses
Side Effects: Skin rash, abdominal cramping, potassium loss
Precautions: Use with caution in presence of kidney disease,
                  heart disease, high blood pressure, intestinal
                  blockage (ileostomy/colostomy), inflamed bowel.

Lamictal (see Lamotrigine)

Lamotrigine (Lamictal)

Description:	Anticonvulsant, antineuralgic
Indications:	Neuropathic pain; beneficial effects may be slow to occur, as dose escalations are gradual
Dosage:	Initial dose is 25 mg PO qd for 2 weeks; increase to 50 mg PO qd for 2 weeks; then, may increase by 50 mg per day each week to a maximum dose of 200 mg PO bid
Side Effects:	Somnolence, dizziness, ataxia, visual changes, nausea and vomiting, maculopapular rash (rare Stevens-Johnson syndrome); rapid dose escalation increases risk of rash
Precautions:	Discontinue if rash develops. Dose adjustment required with concomitant anticonvulsant medications. Reduce dose in renal or hepatic dysfunction. Do not discontinue abruptly.

Levetiracetam (Keppra)

Description:	Anticonvulsant, antineuralgic
Indications:	Antiepileptic drug potentially useful for treatment of neuropathic pain
Dosage:	Start at 500 mg PO bid; may increase by 1,000 mg per day q2wk to a maximum of 1500 mg PO bid; it is unlikely that dose escalation to this level will be necessary
Side Effects:	Somnolence, weakness, infection, dizziness; generally well tolerated
Precautions:	Do not discontinue abruptly. Reduce dose in renal dysfunction.

Levo-Dromoran (see Opioids)
Levorphanol (see Opioids)

Lidocaine (Xylocaine) patch, ointment, oral gel, infusion, eutectic mixture

Description:	Local anesthetic, antiarrhythmic
Indications:	Itching and pain of various disorders [postherpetic neuralgia (PHN), peripheral diabetic neuropathy (PDN), burns]; irritation and inflammation in the mouth and throat; as an infusion, this is a diagnostic test for neuropathic pain
Dosage:	As a diagnostic test for neuropathic pain, prepare an IV infusion of 1 to 5 mg per kg in 20 to 100 mL of normal saline and infuse for 20 to 60 minutes; for postherpetic neuropathy (PHN), Lidoderm patch 12 hours on and 12 hours off; for painful diabetic neuropathy (PDN), apply lidocaine cream/ointment to affected areas one to four times a day
Side Effects:	Stinging, burning, redness, tenderness, swelling, or rash
Precautions:	Heart disease, serious illness, infections, or allergies.

Lioresal (Baclofen)
Description:	Antispastic analgesic
Indications:	Myofascial pain in conjunction with physical therapy, spasticity; may also be used for the treatment of facial pain (trigeminal neuralgia)
Dosage:	Usually started at 5 mg PO tid; dose escalations of 15 mg every 3 days, as tolerated, to a maximum of 40 to 80 mg per day; intrathecal administration is often beneficial for cases of severe spasticity
Side Effects:	Drowsiness, fatigue, nausea, vertigo, hypotonia, muscle weakness, mental depression, and headache may occur
Precautions:	Seizure disorder, peptic ulcer disease, and psychotic disorders.

Lodine (see NSAIDs)

Lorazepam (Ativan)
Description:	Benzodiazepine, sedative hypnotic, anxiolytic, amnestic, anticonvulsant, skeletal muscle relaxant
Indications:	Patients with chronic neuropathic pain exhibiting sleep disturbances, anxiety and restlessness, skeletal muscle spasm
Dosage:	Initial adult daily oral dosage is 2 mg in divided doses of 0.5 mg, 0.5 mg, and 1 mg, or of 1 mg and 1 mg; the daily dosage should be carefully increased or decreased by 0.5 mg depending on tolerance and response
Side Effects:	Drowsiness, dizziness, weakness, fatigue and lethargy, disorientation, ataxia, anterograde amnesia, nausea, change in appetite, change in weight, depression, blurred vision and diplopia, psychomotor agitation, sleep disturbance, vomiting, sexual disturbance, headache, skin rashes, and GI, ear, nose, and throat, musculoskeletal, and respiratory disturbances
Precautions:	Not recommended for use in depressive neurosis or in psychotic reactions; avoid alcohol; use with caution in elderly or seriously ill patients with limited pulmonary function; hepatic or renal disease, and in debilitated patients and in those with organic brain syndrome.

Lorcet (see Opioids)
Lortab (see Opioids)
Maxalt (see Triptans)
Meclofenamate (see NSAIDs)
Meclomen (see NSAIDs)
Meloxicam (see NSAIDs)
Meperidine (see Opioids)

Metaxalone (Skelaxin)
Description:	Muscle relaxant, centrally acting
Indications:	Muscle spasm

Dosage: Usually given tid-qid, with maximum dose of 800 mg qid in adults; start with lower dose and titrate upward

Side Effects: Dizziness, drowsiness, paradoxical stimulation, abdominal pain, nausea/vomiting, headache, nervousness; serious reactions (uncommon) include hemolytic anemia, leucopenia, hepatotoxicity

Precautions: Use with caution in patients with impaired liver or renal function. Contraindicated in patients with history of drug-induced, hemolytic, or other anemias.

Methadone (see Opioids)

Methylphenidate (Ritalin)

Description: Central stimulant; CNS and respiratory stimulant with weak sympathetic activity, similar to amphetamines

Indications: For excessive sedation due to opioids, especially in patients with cancer

Dosage: Start at 5 to 10 mg PO in the morning; avoid late evening or night dose; maximum dose 40 mg per day

Side Effects: Nervousness, insomnia, anorexia, angina, tachycardia, thrombocytopenia, leukopenia

Precautions: Periodic blood counts (use clinical judgment), tolerance and psychological dependence may occur. Use with caution in seizure disorder, psychiatric symptoms. Contraindicated in presence of uncontrolled hypertension, significant coronary artery disease, and in patient exhibiting anxiety, agitation.

Methylprednisolone (Medrol, Solu-Medrol, Depo-Medrol)

Description: Corticosteroid, antiinflammatory

Indications: Swelling, arthritis, skin diseases (psoriasis, hives), asthma, chronic obstructive pulmonary disease, pain

Dosage: Epidural: 20 to 80 mg

Side Effects: Dizziness, nausea, indigestion, increased appetite, weight gain, weakness, or sleep disturbances

Precautions: Extreme hypertension or hypotension, liver or heart disease, Reye syndrome, alcohol or drug dependencies, neurologic disease.

Metoclopramide (Reglan)

Description: Dopamine antagonist, antiemetic, peristaltic stimulant

Indications: Nausea and emesis

Dosage: Oral, IM, IV, 10 mg up to qid

Side Effects: Restlessness, drowsiness, anxiety, headache, extrapyramidal symptoms

Precautions: Contraindicated in obstructive GI pathology, neuroleptic syndrome. Use with caution in presence of seizure disorder and depression.

Mexiletine (Mexitil)

Description:	Sodium channel blocker, antiarrhythmic, antineuralgia adjunct
Indication:	Adjunct medication for neuropathic pain
Dosage:	Starting dose is 150 mg PO qhs, gradually titrated as tolerated up to 900 mg per day in three divided doses
Side Effects:	Nausea, vomiting, heartburn, dizziness, tremor, changes in vision, nervousness, confusion, headache, fatigue, depression, rapid heartbeat, general weakness
Precautions:	Use with caution in patients with cardiac disease, especially congestive cardiac failure, hypotension, liver disease; a history of seizures or allergies, especially allergies to amide-type anesthetics (e.g., lidocaine, tocainide).

Mexitil (see Mexiletine)
Mobic (see NSAIDs)

Modafinil (Provigil)

Description:	Wakefulness promoting agent
Indications:	Excessive sleepiness associated with narcolepsy, obstructive sleep apnea/hypopnea syndrome, and shift-work sleep disorder; useful for excessive sedation due to opioids, especially in patients with cancer
Dosage:	Start at 100 mg PO every morning; may increase up to 400 mg PO QAM as necessary for desired effect and as allowed by side effects; usual dosage is 200 mg PO once daily
Side Effects:	Generally well tolerated. Headache, nausea, anxiety, dizziness, insomnia, chest pain, nervousness
Precautions:	Ischemic heart disease, mitral-valve prolapse, hypertension, psychotic mental illness. May elevate blood levels of concurrent diazepam, propranolol, phenytoin, TCAs, and SSRIs. Reduce dose in renal or hepatic insufficiency. Reduce dose in elderly patients.

Morphine (see Opioids)
Motrin (see NSAIDs)
MS Contin (see Opioids)
Nalfon (see NSAIDs)
Naratriptan (see Triptans)

Naloxone (Narcan)

Description:	μ-Opioid receptor antagonist
Indication:	Reversal of opioid effects
Dosage:	0.02 to 0.04 mg IV every 2 to 3 minutes, titrated to effect; avoid high doses to prevent complete reversal of opiate effects; use higher doses 0.4 to 2 mg every 2 to 3 minutes to a maximum of 10 mg in emergency situations

only; infusions may be required to prevent renarcotization; used orally 1.2 to 2.4 mg every 4 to 6 hours until the first bowel movement or to a maximum of 5 mg for reversing opioid-induced constipation

Side Effects: Acute cardiovascular and CNS excitability caused by rapid reversal of opioid effects, acute withdrawal symptoms

Precautions: Use low doses and titrate to effect. Use with caution in the presence of opioid dependence.

Naproxen (see NSAIDs)
Naproxen sodium (see NSAIDs)
Narcan (see Naloxone)
Neurontin (see Gabapentin)
Norco (see Opioids)
Norpramin (see TCAs)
Nortriptyline (see TCAs)

NSAIDs (nonsteroidal antiinflammatory drugs)

Description: Nonsteroidal antiinflammatory agents, prostaglandin inhibition secondary to cyclooxygenase (COX) inhibition; Celecoxib is a "coxib," a subclass of selective COX-2 inhibitors

Indications: First-line medications in mild to moderate pain, especially of musculoskeletal origin; valuable adjuncts in severe pain by attacking the peripheral inflammatory cascade; opioid sparing; CNS effects not clearly elucidated but under investigation

Dosage: See Table 1

Side Effects: Prostaglandin inhibition leading to decreased platelet adhesion, gastric mucosal damage with or without GI bleeding, and renal function impairment; coxibs are associated with less GI damage and bleeding

Precautions: Use with caution in elderly patients and in the presence of peptic ulcer disease, ischemic heart disease (especially coxibs), coagulopathy, and renal impairment. Continued use of coxibs is associated with increased risk of myocardial infarction and stroke. Use lowest effective doses.

Ondansetron (Zofran)

Description: 5HT-3 receptor antagonist, antiemetic
Indications: Nausea and emesis
Dosage: Oral or IV (4 mg IV every 6 hours), higher doses used for patients undergoing chemotherapy and/or radiation treatment
Side Effects: Headache, blurring vision, diarrhea, unspecified chest pain, pruritus, fever
Precautions: Rapid intravenous injections may increase the risk for headache.

Table 1.   Commonly used oral NSAIDs

Generic Name	Trade Name	Adult Oral Dosage
Acetaminophen	Tylenol	650–975 mg q4–6h
Acetylsalicylic acid	Aspirin	650–975 mg q4–6h
Celecoxib	Celebrex	100–200 mg bid
Choline magnesium trisalicylate	Trilisate	500–750 mg q8–12h
Diclofenal sodium	Voltaren	25–75 mg q8–12h
Diflunisal	Dolobid	250–500 mg q8–12h
Etodolac	Lodine	200–400 mg q6–8h
Fenoprofen calcium	Nalfon	200 mg q4–6h
Flurbiprofen	Ansaid	100 mg q8–12h
Ibuprofen	Motrin	400–800 mg q6–8h
Indomethacin	Indocin	25–50 mg q8–12h
Ketoprofen	Orudis	25–75 mg q6–8h
Ketorolac	Toradol	10–50 mg q6–8h
Meclofenamate sodium	Meclomen	50 mg q4–6h
Meloxicam	Mobic	7.5–15 mg qd
Naproxen	Naprosyn	250–500 mg q8–12h
Naproxen sodium	Anaprox	250–550 mg q6–8h
Phenylbutazone	Butazolidin	100 mg q6–8h
Piroxicam	Feldene	10–20 mg qd
Salsalate	Disalcid	500 mg q4 h
Sulindac	Clinoril	150–200 mg q12h
Tolmetin	Tolectin	200–600 mg q8h

Opioids

Description: Ligands at endogenous opioid receptors; opium constituents (e.g., morphine, codeine, and thebaine) or their derivatives (e.g., hydromorphone, buprenorphine, and oxycodone) or synthetic (e.g., levorphanol, methadone, meperidine, and fentanyl)

Indications: Potent analgesics for severe pain including postoperative pain and cancer pain; controversial, but gaining acceptability in chronic nonterminal pain

Dosage: See Table 2

Routes: PO, IM, SC, transdermal, IV, nasal, sublingual, epidural, intrathecal; start at lowest dose and gradually titrate to effect; dose depends on effect versus side effects; add adjuncts for opioid-sparing effects; tolerance to analgesic effects and to side effects is common; rotate opioid if excessive tolerance develops; new opioid can be started at half to one fourth of the calculated equivalent dose of the new opioid because of incomplete cross-tolerance; approximate conversion ratio for intrathecal:epidural:IV:PO is 1:10:100:300; use

Table 2. Standard doses of commonly used opioids

Generic Name	Trade Name	Equianalgesic Doses		Typical First Dose	
		Oral	Parenteral	Oral	Parenteral
Codeine		200 mg	120 mg	30 mg q3–4 h	10 mg q3–4 h
Fentanyl patch	Duragesic	N/A	N/A	N/A	25 μg/h patch q72h[a]
Fentanyl oralet	Actiq	N/A	N/A	N/A	200 μg[b]
Hydrocodone	Vicodin[c], Lorcet[c], Lortab[c], Norco[c]	N/A	N/A	10 mg q3–4h	N/A
Hydromorphone	Dilaudid	7.5 mg	1.5 mg	2–4 mg q3–4h	1.5 mg q 3–4h
Levorphanol	Levo-Dromoran	4 mg	2 mg	4 mg q6–8h	2 mg q6–8h
Meperidine	Demerol	300 mg	100 mg	100 mg q3h	100 mg q3h
Methadone[d]	Dolophine	2–4 mg	10 mg (acute) 2–4 mg (chronic)	5 mg q8–12h	5 mg q8–12h
Morphine		30 mg	10 mg	15 mg q3–4h	10 mg q3–4h
Morphine SR	MS Contin	N/A	N/A	15 mg q8–12h	N/A
Oxycodone	Percocet[c], Percodan[c]	N/A	N/A	5 mg q3–4h	N/A
Oxycodone CR	OxyContin	N/A	N/A	10 mg q8–12h	N/A

[a]Lowest available dose. Risk of overdose in opioid-naïve patients. 25 μg per hour patch = 50 to 75 mg oral morphine per 24-hour period. Conversions should be made conservatively (consult product literature) and titrated slowly.

[b]Lowest available dose. Contraindicated in opioid-naïve patients, especially children. Not for use in children whose weight is <10 kg; 200 μg oralet = 2 mg IV morphine; 800 μg oralet = 10 mg IV morphine.

[c]Combination formulations, with either acetaminophen or aspirin.

[d]The equianalgesic conversion dose for methadone decreases significantly with increasing dose of previous opioid. Caution guided by experience is mandatory.

long-acting opioids for background analgesia and short-acting opioids for breakthrough or incidental pain; avoid rapid or frequent dose escalations in chronic nonterminal pain

Side Effects: Respiratory depression, sedation, euphoria, dysphoria, weakness, agitation, seizure, nausea, vomiting, constipation, biliary spasm, urinary retention, sweating, flushing, bradycardia, tolerance, physical dependence, and addiction

Precautions: Use with caution in elderly patients, opioid naïve patients, respiratory disease, infants, hepatic or renal disease, patients with history of drug abuse, and patients performing tasks requiring high mental alertness.

Orudis (see NSAIDs)

Oxcarbazepine (Trileptal)
Description: Anticonvulsant, antineuralgic
Indications: Neuropathic pain
Dosage: Start at 150 mg PO bid; may increase by 150 mg every 3 to 5 days to maximum dose of 600 mg PO bid
Side Effects: Hyponatremia, dizziness, somnolence, diplopia, fatigue, gastrointestinal symptoms, ataxia, vision changes; generally well tolerated
Precautions: Do not discontinue abruptly. Reduce dose in renal dysfunction. Reduce dose in geriatric patients. Periodically measure, serum sodium levels.

Oxycodone (see Opioids)
OxyContin (see Opioids)
Pamelor (see TCAs)
Percocet (see Opioids)
Percodan (see Opioids)

Perphenazine
Description: Phenothiazine, dopamine antagonist, antipsychotic, antiemetic, sedative
Indications: Psychoses, anxiety, nausea, and vomiting
Dosage: PO or IM 4 mg two to four times daily
Side Effects: Constipation, sedation, vision changes or dry mouth, extrapyramidal symptoms, occasional tardive dyskinesia
Precautions: Extreme hypertension or hypotension, liver or heart disease, alcohol or drug dependencies, history of neuroleptic syndrome. Avoid in children.

Phenergan (see Promethazine)
Phenoxybenzamine (Dibenzyline)
Description: α-adrenergic blocker
Indications: Sympathetically mediated/maintained pain

Dosage:	Start at 10 mg PO tid and increase by 10 mg every 2 days, titrating to effect and as tolerated; maximum dose (as an antihypertensive agent) 90 to 120 mg per day
Side Effects:	Orthostatic hypotension, reflex tachycardia, meiosis, lethargy, nausea, vomiting, nasal congestion, and headaches
Precautions:	Use with extreme caution in the elderly and in presence of cardiovascular disease.

Phentolamine (Regitine)

Description:	α-adrenergic antagonist
Indications:	Diagnostic IV injection in suspected sympathetically mediated/maintained pain
Dosage:	Infuse 35 to 70 mg in 250 mL normal saline over 20 minutes
Side Effects:	Hypotension, dizziness, reflex tachycardia, syncope
Precautions:	Monitor heart rate and blood pressure; patent IV access; preload with 500 mL normal saline or lactated Ringer solution before infusion; propranolol pretreatment (2 mg) for preventing reflex tachycardia recommended; have resuscitation equipment available.

Phenylbutazone (see NSAIDs)

Phenytoin (Dilantin)

Description:	First-generation sodium channel blocking anticonvulsant, adjunct antineuralgic
Indications:	Seizures, epilepsy, and neuropathic pain
Dosage:	PO 100 mg tid
Side Effects:	Constipation, dizziness and drowsiness, blurred vision, unsteadiness, nausea, mood changes or confusion, slurred speech, rash, insomnia, or headache
Precautions:	Porphyria, liver disease, myocardial insufficiency, cardiac arrhythmias, hypotension. Measure therapeutic levels.

Piroxicam (see NSAIDs)

Prednisolone

Description:	Corticosteroid, anti-inflammatory
Indications:	Suppression of inflammatory and allergic disorders including asthma, chronic obstructive pulmonary disease, rheumatic disease, pain due to inflammation
Dosage:	Usual starting dosage is 10 to 30 mg PO per day
Side Effects:	Dizziness, nausea, indigestion, increased appetite, weight gain, weakness, or sleep disturbances
Precautions:	Extreme hypertension or hypotension, liver or heart disease, Reye syndrome, alcohol or drug dependencies, neurologic disease.

Prilocaine (see Lidocaine—eutectic mixture)

Prochlorperazine (Compazine)

Description:	Antiemetic
Indications:	Nausea and vomiting
Dosage:	Oral 5 to 10 mg tid–qid, usually not exceeding 40 mg; rectal, 25 mg twice daily; IM, 5 to 10 mg every 3 to 4 hours, not to exceed 40 mg per day; IV, 2.5 to 10 mg every 3 to 4 hours, not to exceed 40 mg per day
Side Effects:	Extra pyramidal syndrome, neuroleptic malignant syndrome, drowsiness, postural hypotension, leukopenia, anorexia, dyspepsia, hyperpyrexia
Precautions:	Use with caution in elderly patients and patients with seizure disorder, glaucoma, and prostate hypertrophy.

Promethazine (Phenergan)

Description:	Phenothiazine, dopamine antagonist, antipsychotic, antiemetic, sedative, antihistamine
Indications:	Nausea and vomiting
Dosage:	Can be used PO, IV, or IM for antiemesis, 12.5 to 25 mg every 4 hours, not to exceed 100 mg per day
Side Effects:	Shares the side effects of antihistamines, anticholinergic effects (dry mouth, blurring vision), phenothiazines (extrapyramidal symptoms), leukopenia, obstructive jaundice
Precautions:	Use with caution with cardiovascular or hepatic disease, and in the presence of other CNS depressants.

Protriptyline (see TCAs)
Provigil (see Modafinil)
Prozac (see Fluoxetine)
Regitine (see Phentolamine)
Reglan (see Metoclopramide)
Relpax (see Triptans)
Ritalin (see Methylphenidate)
Rizatriptan (see Triptans)

Salsalate (see NSAIDs)

Senna (Senokot)

Description:	Laxative
Indication:	Constipation
Dosage:	One to two tablets PO once or twice per day
Side Effects:	Diarrhea, nausea, vomiting, rectal irritation, stomach cramps, or bloating
Precautions:	Kidney disease, heart disease, high blood pressure, edema, or allergies, especially to tartrazine.

Sertraline (Zoloft)

Description: Selective serotonin reuptake inhibitor (SSRI), first-line antidepressant

Indications: Depression, panic disorder, obsessive-compulsive disorder

Dosage: PO 50 to 200 mg per day

Side Effects: These are rare but include headaches, stimulation or sedation, fine tremor, tinnitus, rare extrapyramidal symptoms, palpitations, nausea and vomiting, bloating, and diarrhea

Precautions: Known sensitivity, interactions with MAOIs.

Sinequan (see TCAs)
Skelaxin (see Metaxalone)
Sodium valproate (see Valproic acid)
Sulindac (see NSAIDs)
Sumatriptan (see Triptans)

TCAs (tricyclic antidepressants)

Description: Norepinephrine and serotonin reuptake inhibitors

Indications: Depression, neuropathic pain, evening dose may improve overnight sleep

Dosage: Usually given once daily at bedtime; start at 25 mg (10 mg for elderly patients) and gradually escalate dose in small increments every 3 to 5 days as tolerated to a maximum of 75 to 150 mg at bedtime (see Table 3 for range of doses); beneficial effects may be noticed in 1 to 3 weeks

Side Effects: Dry mouth, blurred vision, urinary retention, constipation, reflux (anticholinergic), weakness, lethargy, fatigue, paradoxical excitement, exacerbation of psychiatric symptoms (CNS), postural hypotension, cardiac arrhythmias

Table 3. Commonly used tricyclic antidepressants (TCAs)

Generic Name	Trade Name	Adult 24-Hour Dosage Range (mg)
Amitriptyline[a]	Elavil	10–300
Amoxapine	Asendin	50–400
Clomipramine[a]	Anafranil	25–300
Desipramine[a]	Norpramin	10–300
Doxepin	Sinequan	10–300
Imipramine[a]	Tofranil	10–300
Nortriptyline[a]	Pamelor	10–200
Protriptyline	Vivactil	10–60

[a]Commonly used for neuropathic pain.

Precautions: Benign prostatic hypertrophy, urinary retention, closed-angle glaucoma, severe respiratory
disease, seizure disorder, cardiac dysrhythmias,
other cardiac disease.

Tegretol (see Carbamazepine)
Thorazine (see Chlorpromazine)

Tiagabine (Gabitril)
Description: Anticonvulsant, antineuralgic, selective GABA
reuptake inhibitor
Indications: Neuropathic pain
Dosage: Start at 4 mg PO qd; after 1 week, may increase to 4 mg PO bid; maximum antiepileptic
dose is 56 mg per day; however, 4 to 8 mg per
day is recommended effective dose for pain
management, which minimizes side effects
Side Effects: Somnolence, dizziness, nervousness, fatigue,
gastrointestinal symptoms, tremor, cognitive
impairment; generally well tolerated
Precautions: Do not discontinue abruptly. Reduce dose in hepatic dysfunction. Pharmacokinetics unchanged
with renal insufficiency.

Tizanidine (Zanaflex)
Description: Antispasmodic
Indications: Myofascial pain (muscle spasms)
Dosage: Start with 2 to 4 mg PO qhs, then gradually in-
crease to maximum of 36 mg per day in divided
doses
Side Effects: Nausea, drowsiness, dizziness, constipation,
unusual weakness, or dry mouth
Precautions: Caution in patients with hypotension, hepatic,
cardiac, renal, or eye diseases.

Tofranil (see TCAs)
Tolectin (see NSAIDs)
Tolmetin (see NSAIDs)
Topamax (see Topiramate)

Topiramate (Topamax)
Description: Anticonvulsant, adjunct antineuralgic
Indications: Second-line medication for neuropathic pain.
May act by inhibiting voltage-dependent sodi-
um channels, enhancing activity of inhibitory
neurotransmitter α-aminobutyric acid (GABA)
and antagonism of NMDA receptor
Dosage: Usually start at 50 mg qhs and gradually increase by 25 mg every week up to a maximum
of 200 mg bid as tolerated; gradual improvement may be noticed over weeks, as doses are
titrated gradually
Side Effects: Weakness, tiredness, drowsiness, dizziness, tingling sensations, loss of appetite and weight,

unsteadiness, slowing or shakiness, speech problems, mental/mood changes, stomach/abdominal pain, or vision problems may occur

Precautions: Use with caution in patients with renal or hepatic disease.

Toradol (see Ketorolac)

Tramadol (Ultram)
Description: Analgesic, weak μ-agonist with additional inhibition of norepinephrine and serotonin reuptake
Indications: Mild to moderate pain, adjunct in severe pain; useful in patients who cannot tolerate opioids.
Dosage: PO 50 to 100 mg every 4 to 6 hours as needed; start at low dose to minimize side effects (not to exceed 400 mg per day).
Side Effects: Dizziness, vertigo, headache, constipation, nausea and vomiting, dyspepsia, pruritus, and sedation
Precautions: At high doses, seizures may occur, especially if used in combination with TCAs. Respiratory depression, constipation, and dependence are extremely rare. Prolonged international normalized ratio (INR) in presence of warfarin; reduce dose in renal impairment and the elderly.

Triamcinolone (Aristocort, Kenalog)
Description: Corticosteroid, antiinflammatory
Indications: Inflammation, swelling, and pain
Dosage: For epidural or nerve root injection, 10 to 80 mg as a single dose
Side Effects: Increased or decreased appetite, insomnia, indigestion, nervousness
Precautions: Extreme hypertension or hypotension, liver or heart disease, Reye syndrome, alcohol or drug dependencies, neurologic disease.

Tricyclic antidepressants (see TCAs)
Trileptal (see Oxcarbazepine)
Trilisate (see NSAIDs)

Triptans
Description: Selective 5HT-1 agonists
Indication: Migraine headache attacks
Dosage: See Table 4; do not use to treat more than three to four headaches in 30-day period
Side Effects: Tingling sensations, feelings of warmth or heaviness, dizziness, flushing, drowsiness
Precautions: Ischemic heart disease, high blood pressure, cerebrovascular disease, elderly patients, kidney disease, liver disease.

Tylenol (see Acetaminophen)
Ultram (see Tramadol)
Valium (see Diazepam)

Table 4. Commonly used triptans

Generic Name	Trade Name	Adult Dose	Adult Maximum 24-hour Dose
Almotriptan	Axert	6.25 to 12.5 mg PO (may repeat >2 h)	25 mg
Eletriptan	Relpax	20 to 40 mg PO (may repeat >2 h)	80 mg
Frovatriptan	Frova	2.5 mg PO (may repeat >2 h)	7.5 mg
Naratriptan	Amerge	2.5 mg PO (may repeat >4 h)	5 mg
Rizatriptan	Maxalt	5 to 10 mg PO (may repeat >2 h)	30 mg
	Maxalt-MLT	5 to 10 mg PO Orally disintegrating tablets (may repeat >2 h)	30 mg (MLT)
Sumatriptan	Imitrex	25 to 100 mg PO (may repeat >2h)	200 mg PO
		6 mg SQ (may repeat >1h)	12 mg SQ
		5 to 20 mg intranasal (may repeat >2 h)	40 mg intranasal
Zolmitriptan	Zomig	1.25 to 5 mg PO (may repeat >2 h)	10 mg PO
		5 mg intranasal (may repeat >2 h)	10 mg intranasal
	Zomig-ZMT	2.5 mg PO Orally disintegrating tablets (may repeat >2 h)	10 mg PO (ZMT)

Valproic acid (Depakene)

Description: Anticonvulsant, adjunct antineuralgic

Indications: Seizure disorders, migraine headache prophylaxis, manic phase of bipolar disorder, neuropathic pain

Dosage: 15 mg/kg/day in two or three divided doses, increasing every week up to maximum dose of 60 mg/kg/day

Side Effects: Stomach pain, loss of appetite, change in menstrual periods, diarrhea, mild hair loss, unsteadiness, dizziness, drowsiness, rash, or headache

Precautions: Liver disease, bleeding disorder.

Venlafaxine (Effexor XR)

Description:	Antidepressant, potent inhibitor of serotonin and norepinephrine reuptake and weak inhibitor of dopamine reuptake
Indications:	Antidepressant medication useful for migraine prophylaxis and potentially useful as adjuvant neuropathic pain medication
Dosage:	Start at 37.5 mg PO qd for 4 to 7 days; may slowly titrate up to 150 mg PO qd
Side Effects:	Sustained hypertension, insomnia, nervousness, gastrointestinal intolerance, anorexia, activation of mania, vivid dreams, acute angle-closure glaucoma, sexual dysfunction, sweating, cholesterol elevation
Precautions:	Use with caution in patients with history of seizures. Discontinue if seizures develop. Reduce dose in renal or hepatic dysfunction. Consider measurement of cholesterol with long-term treatment.

Vistaril (see Hydroxyzine)
Vicodin (see Opioids)
Vivactil (see TCAs)
Voltaren (see NSAIDs)
Zanaflex (see Tizanidine)
Zofran (see Ondansetron)
Zoloft (see Sertraline)
Zolmitriptan (see Triptans)
Zomig (see Triptans)
Zonegran (see Zonisamide)

Zonisamide (Zonegran)

Description:	Anticonvulsant, antineuralgic
Indications:	Neuropathic pain
Dosage:	Start at 100 mg PO qd; may increase by 100 mg every 2 weeks to maximum dose of 400 mg PO qd
Side Effects:	Renal stones, renal insufficiency, anorexia, somnolence, dizziness, headache, nausea, irritability
Precautions:	Sulfonamide allergy. Discontinue use if rash develops. Do not use in patients with renal failure. Do not discontinue abruptly.

Subject Index